Phytochemicals Beneficial to Human Health

Phytochemicals Beneficial to Human Health

Editors

José Antonio Morales-González
Nancy Vargas Mendoza

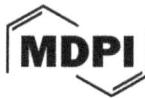

Basel • Beijing • Wuhan • Barcelona • Belgrade • Novi Sad • Cluj • Manchester

Editors

José Antonio
Morales-González
Escuela Superior de Medicina
Instituto Politécnico Nacional
Ciudad de México
Mexico

Nancy Vargas Mendoza
Escuela Superior de Medicina
Instituto Politécnico Nacional
Ciudad de México
Mexico

Editorial Office
MDPI
St. Alban-Anlage 66
4052 Basel, Switzerland

This is a reprint of articles from the Special Issue published online in the open access journal *Plants* (ISSN 2223-7747) (available at: www.mdpi.com/journal/plants/special_issues/phytochemicals_beneficial).

For citation purposes, cite each article independently as indicated on the article page online and as indicated below:

Lastname, A.A.; Lastname, B.B. Article Title. *Journal Name* **Year**, *Volume Number*, Page Range.

ISBN 978-3-7258-1320-9 (Hbk)
ISBN 978-3-7258-1319-3 (PDF)
doi.org/10.3390/books978-3-7258-1319-3

© 2024 by the authors. Articles in this book are Open Access and distributed under the Creative Commons Attribution (CC BY) license. The book as a whole is distributed by MDPI under the terms and conditions of the Creative Commons Attribution-NonCommercial-NoDerivs (CC BY-NC-ND) license.

Contents

About the Editors . . . . **vii**

Preface . . . . **ix**

Nancy Vargas-Mendoza, Eduardo Madrigal-Santillán, Isela Álvarez-González, Eduardo Madrigal-Bujaidar, Liliana Anguiano-Robledo and José Leopoldo Aguilar-Faisal et al.
Phytochemicals in Skeletal Muscle Health: Effects of Curcumin (from *Curcuma longa* Linn) and Sulforaphane (from *Brassicaceae*) on Muscle Function, Recovery and Therapy of Muscle Atrophy
Reprinted from: *Plants* **2022**, *11*, 2517, doi:10.3390/plants11192517 . . . . **1**

César Esquivel-Chirino, Mario Augusto Bolaños-Carrillo, Daniela Carmona-Ruiz, Ambar Lopéz-Macay, Fernando Hernández-Sánchez and Delina Montés-Sánchez et al.
The Protective Role of Cranberries and Blueberries in Oral Cancer
Reprinted from: *Plants* **2023**, *12*, 2330, doi:10.3390/plants12122330 . . . . **25**

Maria Vrânceanu, Simona-Codruța Hegheș, Anamaria Cozma-Petruț, Roxana Banc, Carmina Mariana Stroia and Viorica Raischi et al.
Plant-Derived Nutraceuticals Involved in Body Weight Control by Modulating Gene Expression
Reprinted from: *Plants* **2023**, *12*, 2273, doi:10.3390/plants12122273 . . . . **48**

Eduardo Osel Olvera-Roldán, José Melesio Cristóbal-Luna, Yuliana García-Martínez, María Angélica Mojica-Villegas, Ricardo Pérez-Pastén-Borja and Gabriela Gutiérrez-Salmeán et al.
Effects of *Spirulina maxima* on a Model of Sexual Dysfunction in Streptozotocin-Induced Diabetic Male Rats
Reprinted from: *Plants* **2023**, *12*, 722, doi:10.3390/plants12040722 . . . . **74**

Eduardo Madrigal-Santillán, Jacqueline Portillo-Reyes, Eduardo Madrigal-Bujaidar, Manuel Sánchez-Gutiérrez, Jeannett A. Izquierdo-Vega and Julieta Izquierdo-Vega et al.
Opuntia spp. in Human Health: A Comprehensive Summary on Its Pharmacological, Therapeutic and Preventive Properties. Part 2
Reprinted from: *Plants* **2022**, *11*, 2333, doi:10.3390/plants11182333 . . . . **87**

Germán Chamorro-Cevallos, María Angélica Mojica-Villegas, Yuliana García-Martínez, Salud Pérez-Gutiérrez, Eduardo Madrigal-Santillán and Nancy Vargas-Mendoza et al.
A Complete Review of Mexican Plants with Teratogenic Effects
Reprinted from: *Plants* **2022**, *11*, 1675, doi:10.3390/plants11131675 . . . . **125**

Erika Anayetzi Chávez-Bustos, Angel Morales-González, Liliana Anguiano-Robledo, Eduardo Osiris Madrigal-Santillán, Cármen Valadez-Vega and Olivia Lugo-Magaña et al.
Bauhinia forficata Link, Antioxidant, Genoprotective, and Hypoglycemic Activity in a Murine Model
Reprinted from: *Plants* **2022**, *11*, 3052, doi:10.3390/plants11223052 . . . . **152**

Maria Vrânceanu, Damiano Galimberti, Roxana Banc, Ovidiu Dragoș, Anamaria Cozma-Petruț and Simona-Codruța Hegheș et al.
The Anticancer Potential of Plant-Derived Nutraceuticals via the Modulation of Gene Expression
Reprinted from: *Plants* **2022**, *11*, 2524, doi:10.3390/plants11192524 . . . . **167**

Tassanee Ongtanasup, Nuntika Prommee, Onkamon Jampa, Thanchanok Limcharoen, Smith Wanmasae and Veeranoot Nissapatorn et al.
The Cholesterol-Modulating Effect of the New Herbal Medicinal Recipe from Yellow Vine (*Coscinium fenestratum* (Goetgh.)), Ginger (*Zingiber officinale* Roscoe.), and Safflower (*Carthamus tinctorius* L.) on Suppressing PCSK9 Expression to Upregulate LDLR Expression in HepG2 Cells
Reprinted from: *Plants* **2022**, *11*, 1835, doi:10.3390/plants11141835 . . . . **200**

Idowu J. Adeosun, Itumeleng T. Baloyi and Sekelwa Cosa
Anti-Biofilm and Associated Anti-Virulence Activities of Selected Phytochemical Compounds against *Klebsiella pneumoniae*
Reprinted from: *Plants* **2022**, *11*, 1429, doi:10.3390/plants11111429 . . . . **230**

About the Editors

José Antonio Morales-González

José Antonio Morales-González graduated as a surgeon physician from FES-Iztacala, National, Autonomous University of Mexico (UNAM). He engaged in Doctoral studies in Biological Sciences at the UNAM. Dr. Morales-Gonzalez has received diverse recognition: he was awarded the Gustavo Baz Prada Medal and the Alfonso Caso Medal for academic merit by the UNAM and was distinguished by the National System of Researchers (SNI) as National Researcher Level 2 (2017–2025). Additionally, he has served as the director for 16 undergraduate and 100 postgraduate theses. He is the author of 103 internationally published articles, with more than 5000 citations. He is also the editor and coordinator of 28 specialized books and is the author of 43 chapters in specialized books. Dr. Morales-Gonzalez is a full-time tenured professor and researcher at the Escuela Superior de Medicina, IPN.

Nancy Vargas Mendoza

Nancy Vargas Mendoza has a degree in Nutrition and a Master of Science from the Autonomous University of the State of Hidalgo, as well as a Ph.D. in Medicine Research from the National Polytechnic Institute. As a consultant on sports nutrition topics, she has taught classes at undergraduate and graduate levels. She is the author of more than 30 academic products (articles, books, and book chapters). She is an expert in the field of sports nutrition.

Preface

Plant materials and derivatives have been widely studied worldwide for the countless benefits they bring to human health. To date, numerous research groups have focused on the study and characterization of herbal extracts to identify numerous plant metabolites, which have been found to exert remarkable effects on biological systems.

To a large extent, many diseases arise from the interruption or blockage of natural metabolic biological processes, resulting in the inability to maintain cellular homeostasis. In vitro and in vivo studies show how bioactive plant compounds possess the ability to activate cell signaling pathways that are altered in pathological situations or certain medical conditions. The elucidation of the mechanisms by which the bioactive compounds of plants act continues to be approached as a directional axis in research projects. In this sense, there is a wide area of opportunity to explore the impact of phytochemicals on human health, physical exercise, and athletic performance. In addition, phytochemicals currently seem to have high potential in the treatment of various diseases, proving to be a viable alternative to currently available medicines.

This reprint collates several publications from the international scientific community on the role of phytochemicals in human health, whether in cases of diseases, such as cancer, or special conditions such as physical exercise.

José Antonio Morales-González and Nancy Vargas Mendoza
Editors

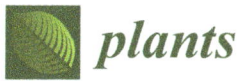

Review

Phytochemicals in Skeletal Muscle Health: Effects of Curcumin (from *Curcuma longa* Linn) and Sulforaphane (from *Brassicaceae*) on Muscle Function, Recovery and Therapy of Muscle Atrophy

Nancy Vargas-Mendoza [1,†], Eduardo Madrigal-Santillán [1,†], Isela Álvarez-González [2], Eduardo Madrigal-Bujaidar [2], Liliana Anguiano-Robledo [3], José Leopoldo Aguilar-Faisal [1], Mauricio Morales-Martínez [4], Luis Delgado-Olivares [5], Elda Victoria Rodríguez-Negrete [6], Ángel Morales-González [7,*] and José A. Morales-González [1,*]

1. Laboratorio de Medicina de Conservación, Escuela Superior de Medicina, Instituto Politécnico Nacional, Plan de San Luis y Díaz Mirón, Col. Casco de Santo Tomás, Del. Miguel Hidalgo, Mexico City 11340, Mexico
2. Escuela Nacional de Ciencias Biológicas, Instituto Politécnico Nacional, Unidad Profesional A. López Mateos, Av. Wilfrido Massieu. Col., Zacatenco, Mexico City 07738, Mexico
3. Laboratorio de Farmacología Molecular, Escuela Superior de Medicina, Instituto Politécnico Nacional, Plan de San Luis y Díaz Mirón, Col. Casco de Santo Tomás, Del. Miguel Hidalgo, Mexico City 11340, Mexico
4. Licenciatura en Nutrición, Universidad Intercontinental, Insurgentes Sur 4303, Santa Úrsula Xitla, Alcaldía Tlalpan, Mexico City 14420, Mexico
5. Centro de Investigación Interdisciplinario, Área Académica de Nutrición, Instituto de Ciencias de la Salud, Universidad Autónoma del Estado de Hidalgo, Circuito Actopan-Tilcuauttla, s/n, Ex Hacienda la Concepción, San Agustín Tlaxiaca, Hidalgo 2160, Mexico
6. Servicio de Gastroenterología, Hospital de Especialidades Centro Medico Nacional Siglo 21, Mexico City 06720, Mexico
7. Escuela Superior de Cómputo, Instituto Politécnico Nacional, Av. Juan de Dios Bátiz s/n Esquina Miguel Othón de Mendizabal, Unidad Profesional Adolfo López Mateos, Mexico City 07738, Mexico
* Correspondence: anmorales@ipn.mx (Á.M.-G.); jmorales101@yahoo.com.mx (J.A.M.-G.); Tel.: +52-55-5729-6300 (Á.M-G & J.A.M.-G.)
† These authors contributed equally to this work.

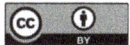

Abstract: The mobility of the human body depends on, among other things, muscle health, which can be affected by several situations, such as aging, increased oxidative stress, malnutrition, cancer, and the lack or excess of physical exercise, among others. Genetic, metabolic, hormonal, and nutritional factors are intricately involved in maintaining the balance that allows proper muscle function and fiber recovery; therefore, the breakdown of the balance among these elements can trigger muscle atrophy. The study from the nutrigenomic perspective of nutritional factors has drawn wide attention recently; one of these is the use of certain compounds derived from foods and plants known as phytochemicals, to which various biological activities have been described and attributed in terms of benefiting health in many respects. This work addresses the effect that the phytochemicals curcumin from *Curcuma longa* Linn and sulforaphane from *Brassicaceae* species have shown to exert on muscle function, recovery, and the prevention of muscle atrophy, and describes the impact on muscle health in general. In the same manner, there are future perspectives in research on novel compounds as potential agents in the prevention or treatment of medical conditions that affect muscle health.

Keywords: phytochemicals; curcumin; sulforaphane; skeletal muscle

1. Introduction

The mobility of the human body is supported by the skeletal muscle, which is a highly plastic organ that fulfills vital metabolic and endocrine functions and participates in the respiratory process and in the body's physical posture. The functionality of the skeletal muscle is determined by, among other things, its contractile capacity, in which an extensive network of molecular mechanisms that regulate the signaling pathways responsible for protein synthesis and degradation is intricately involved, promoting the balance between hypertrophic and atrophic signals. Under healthy conditions, an equilibrium between protein synthesis and degradation is maintained, but there are several situations that break the balance, favoring proteolysis in the fibers and producing muscle atrophy [1]. Physiological situations such as aging itself or numerous chronic diseases such as AIDS, cancer, kidney failure, chronic obstructive pulmonary disease, malnutrition, and immobility due to trauma, amputation, and neurodegenerative disease, etc., severely compromise the muscle health of humans. Muscle atrophy is the result of a decreased cross-sectional area (CSA) of muscle fibers, leading to the loss of muscle strength and contractile capacity [1,2]. Fundamentally, the synthesis of muscle mass occurs as a result of the conjunction of elements that involve the activation of signaling pathways and myogenesis. The phosphatidylinositol 3-kinase (PI3K)/serine threonine kinase (Akt) pathway is one of the most important anabolic signaling pathways that stimulates the target of rapamycin (mTOR) in mammals involved in the synthesis of muscle mass. Thus, the PI3K/Akt/mTOR pathway is the main one responsible for myofibrillar protein synthesis and is regulated by the hormones testosterone and insulin, the insulin-like growth factor 1 (IGF-1), leucin, and exercise. The activation of the PI3K/Akt/mTOR pathway will be crucial for enhancing hypertrophy [3]. Myogenesis is triggered by muscle injury or by mechanical stimuli such as exercise, performed by satellite cells or muscle stem cells, which command a myogenic differentiation program that restores muscle tissue by forming new fibers. Contrariwise, muscle atrophy is influenced by proatrophic factors such as inflammation, oxidative stress, and mitochondrial damage; these factors play an important role in protein degradation through the ubiquitin proteasome system (UPS), which coordinates the main protein catabolic pathways upregulating the ubiquitin ligases atrogin-1, muscle RING finger1 (*MuRF-1*), and casitase-B-lineage lymphoma (Cbl-b) [2].

Oxidative stress and inflammation are closely related with chronic diseases and aging; for instance, the elevation of tumor necrosis factor alpha (TNF-α) along with the increase in the proinflammatory cytokines interleukin-6 (IL-6) and interleukin-1β (IL-1β) promote the nuclear factor kappa beta (NF-κB) transcription factor, leading to protein degradation and acting as an inducer of *MuRF-1* and atrogin-1 binding directly to the *MuRF-1* promoter [4]. NF-κB, along with other catabolic factors such as Forkhead box O (FoxO), p50 and p38 mitogen-activated protein kinase (p38-MAPK), enhance the transcription of E3 ubiquitin ligase genes including *MuRF-1* and *FBox* (*MAFbx*/atrogin-1) [5–7]. Autophagic-related genes can also be related with the activation of these pathways in protein breakdown by the UPS, such as microtubule-associated protein 1A/1B-light chain 3 (LC3) and the Bcl2/adenovirus E1B 19-kDa-interacting protein 3 (Bnip3) by means of the autophagic-lysosomal pathway [8,9]. Mostly, the impairment of the PI3K/Akt/mTOR pathway activates UPS; frequently, signaling activation initiates with the disruption of the binding of IGF-1 to its tyrosine kinase receptor GF-1R, this binding producing transphosphorylation of the receptor, and the phosphorylated tyrosines generate a docking site for the recruitment of the insulin receptor substrate 1 (IRS1) [10]. The phosphorylation of IRS1 is a key step in the regulation of IGF1 signaling. It has been reported that IRS1 degradation by inducing ubiquitin ligase Cbl-b and the activation of FoxO and FoxO-mediated ubiquitin ligases are also related with elevated oxidative stress and inflammation [11]

Moreover, myogenesis, which is regulated by the presence of myogenic factors such as myogenin, the myoblast determination protein (MyoD), myogenic factor 5 (Myf5), and myogenic regulatory factor 4, is involved in a redox-sensitive mechanism. During muscle regeneration, reactive oxygen species (ROS) and reactive nitrogen species (RNS) are considered crucial factors for satellite-cell biology through their modulating a wide range of the cellular processes involved [12]. However, excessive ROS/RNS might lead to an imbalance between antioxidant defenses and the ability to counteract the harmful effects on the cell, which is a major issue in the impairment of protein synthesis and myogenesis, favoring muscle atrophy. A strong association has been reported of the activation of the two main proteolytic systems, that is, the ubiquitin–proteosome and the lysosomal autophagy pathways, with increased oxidative stress related with protein degradation and age-dependent muscle atrophy [13]

The disruption of the anabolic mechanisms involved in regeneration and myogenesis reduces the capacity for mobility and independence, leading to frailty and poor quality of life; this entails repercussions, not only on the health of individuals, but also on the economic budgets allocated to health services at regional and global levels [14]. Muscle atrophy is a chronic condition characterized by loss of function and structural muscle damage in which there is an imbalance between proteolysis and muscle protein synthesis. Numerous reasons can be the cause of muscle deterioration, including aging, chronic diseases, starvation, sedentary lifestyle, lack of exercise, or overtraining without appropriate rest–recovery period. Although muscle atrophy is identified as a cause of immobility that contributes to frailty and poor quality of life, to date, not enough alternatives have been generated for the prevention or treatment of this condition. In recent years, widespread research has emerged on different therapeutic options that might aid in reducing the risk of developing muscle affectations. Some compounds that are derived from plants or foods, denominated phytochemicals, have attracted attention because their biological activity has been described as antioxidant, cardioprotector, antidiabetic, and anticancer [15]. In agreement with this, numerous in vivo/in vitro studies have found that phytochemicals such as polyphenols have been proven to encourage muscle recovery and could be used for the treatment of muscle atrophy [16]. This review describes in organized form the manner in which the phytochemicals curcumin (*Curcuma longa*) and sulforaphane (SFN) (*Brassicaceae*) have proven to exert an impact on the molecular mechanism signaling involved in muscle function at different levels. A growing body of evidence indicates that both curcumin and SFN trigger signaling intricate in-muscle protein synthesis while inhibiting protein degradation. Thus, they can be considered potential targets of the use of nutraceuticals in the treatment of muscle atrophy and recovery, possessing a positive impact on muscle health.

2. Curcumin

2.1. Botanical Description of Curcuma longa Linn

The rhizome *Curcuma longa* Linn (*C. longa*) belongs to the Zingiberaceae (ginger) family and is a perennial sterile plant commonly known as turmeric, which is cultivated and widely distributed in Asian nations. India and China have a long history in the use of *C. longa* in their traditional medicine, in cosmetics, and among spices in food. It is known as "The Golden Spice" in India. Turmeric is a tall herb with no stem and rootstock, reaching 1 m in height and flourishing in tropical and subtropical regions at temperatures ranging between 20 and 30 °C, requiring constant rainfall to grow and only reproducing through its rhizomes. The leaves are around 1 m in length, with long dark-green leaves on the upper surface and light-green leaves beneath; these leaves are oblong or lanceolate in shape, and take the appearance of spikes prior to that of leaves. The flowers are pale yellow in color and reddish on the top, while the flowering bract is green and intensely ferruginous purple in color. It has 2-meter-long pseudostems with 8–12 leaves proceeding from these. The ripe rhizomes have a rough and segmented skin; from the inside, they are yellowish-brown in color with a dull orange hue. Small pointed or conical tubers are 2.5–7.0 cm in length and 2.5 cm in diameter, sprouting from the main rhizome [17,18]. *C. longa* optimally grows in a humid environment, and exposure to sunlight facilitates the rhizome in achieving larger and better rhizomes, thus extending harvest times from January to March–April. Turmeric rhizomes require rich soil conditions, proper nutrients, and a small sand content; these grow ideally in irrigated and rain-fed areas in light-black ashen loam soil and in red-to-stiff loam soils. Turmeric is known to have originated in South and Southeast Asia in China, and in western India and Vietnam; it is currently cultivated in various Asian countries such as Nepal, Thailand, Malaysia, Cambodia, Madagascar, the Philippines, Indonesia, Bangladesh, and the state of West Bengal in India, as well as others.

From the grinding of the dry rhizome, a yellow powder is obtained that has a bitter and sweet taste; this powder is employed in traditional cuisine as a spice to provide color, flavor, and aroma, and it is frequently used as a food preservative or additive. In Chinese, Indian, Japanese, and Korean traditional medicine, turmeric has been utilized as a therapy for different affectations, due to its multiple benefits as an anti-inflammatory, anticancer compound, and analgesic; to treat skin disorders and wounds; and as an antidiabetic, liver protector, cardioprotector, neuroprotector, and antimicrobial with antiseptic effects, among many others [19]. These mentioned benefits are attributed to its components called curcuminoids, and curcumin comprises the most abundant and active bioactive compound (77%) (1,7-bis[4-hydroxy-3-methoxyphenyl]-1,6-heptadiene-3,5-dione), chemical structure $C_{21}H_{20}O_6$. Curcumin is a yellow-colored flavonoid with lipophilic characteristics and is water-insoluble.

2.2. Phytochemistry, Bioavailability, and Metabolism

The characterization of C. longa indicates that its nutritional profile is very complete, that it contains carbohydrates, fiber, some proteins, lipids, vitamin C, pyridoxine, calcium, potassium, magnesium, and phosphorus, and around 235 C. longa phytochemicals have been found, the majority of these of a phenolic and terpenoid nature. Curcuminoids comprise the most important phenolic compounds, as around 80% of the total. There are other minor components, such as sesquiterpenes, monoterpenes, diarylheptanoids, triterpenoids, diterpenes, sterols, and alkaloids [20,21]. Curcumin is a curcuminoid chemically identified as a member of the diarylheptanoids. It has a diketonic hydroxycarbon skeleton with a phenolic-conjugated group substituted for by methoxy groups through a 7-atom carbon chain with a 1,3-dicarbonyl function and various unsaturations. In solid phase, it is found in keto form, and in liquid phase as enol (Figure 1). It is a symmetrical structure without stereogenic centers; the skeleton is formed by two phenolic rings connected by a 7-carbon α,β-unsaturated diketone bond with an s hydroxyl group at par around the bond. Curcumin is insoluble in water at a neutral pH and is acidic; it is soluble in organic solvents such as methanol, ethanol, dimethylsulfoxide, and acetone due to its lipophilic nature [22].

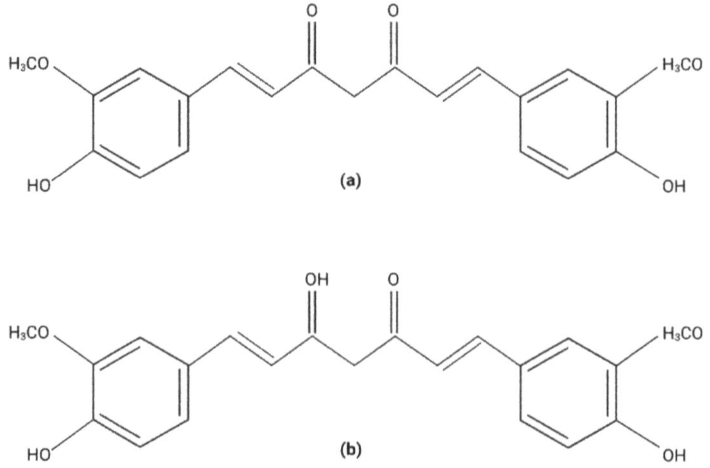

Figure 1. Curcumin chemical structure. (**a**) Ceto form. (**b**) Enol form. Created with BioRender.com.

Due to its low solubility and chemical characteristics, curcumin appears to be poorly absorbed; it has been reported as having a bioavailability range of between 0.47 and 1%. After the oral administration of 500 mg/kg of curcumin, the maximal concentration (C_{max}) in serum was 0.06 μm/mL, and time to reach maximal concentration (T_{max}) was 41.7 ± 5.4 min. Elimination half-times ($t_{1/2,\beta}$) were 28.1 ± 5.6 and 44.5 ± 7.5 min for curcumin (500 mg/kg, per os [p.o.]) and for curcumin (10 mg/kg, intravenously [i.v.]), respectively [23]. At doses of 10 and 12 g, the C_{max} reported was 2.30 ± 0.26 and 1.73 ± 0.19 mg/mL, respectively, while T_{max} and $t_{1/2}$ were 3.29 ± 0.43 and 6.77 ± 0.83 h, respectively Curcumin derivatives such as glucuronide and sulfate were detected in the plasma of human healthy volunteers at 0.25 and 72 h after the consumption of a single oral dose of a curcumin preparation [24]. Another study reported curcumin serum levels of 0.13–1.35 µg/mL at oral doses of 1–2 g/kg. It can be observed that, in spite of its low bioavailability, it is rapidly metabolized and eliminated; the data suggested that curcumin's low bioavailability can be due to its low water solubility and poor intestinal absorption, an affectation of the intestinal metabolism. The lipophilic nature of the molecule could affect the rate of absorption and, in addition, its rapid systemic metabolism and excretion are important factors [25]. Thus, to improve the bioavailability of curcumin, different strategies have been proven, such as the design of the formulation with nanoparticles, micelles, liposomes, analogues, lipid preparations, etc. [25–28].

The study conducted in humans demonstrated that a formulation of curcumin with a combination of cellulosic derivates, a hydrophilic carrier, and natural antioxidants (CHC) caused a 45.9-fold-higher absorption of curcuminoids compared with a standardized curcumin mixture; absorption was also significantly improved compared to a curcumin phytosome formulation, by 5.8-fold, and compared to a formulation with volatile oils of turmeric rhizome, by 34.9-fold. The CHC formulation significantly increased curcuminoids in blood in comparison with the other standardized unformulated curcumin preparations [27]. The new γ-cyclodextrin curcumin formulation (CW8) increased plasma concentrations of curcumin 39-fold compared with standardized unformulated curcumin extract, improving curcumin absorption significantly in healthy humans. Ciclodextrin formulations are better absorbed because it forms complexes with lipophilic compounds, improving aqueous solubility and dispersibility [28]. The novel CURCUGEN, a dispersible formulation with 50% curcuminoids—concentrated turmeric extract—demonstrated that the relative bioavailability of total tetrahydrocurcumin was 31 times higher compared to the standard curcumin reference product, curcuminoid 95% standardized extract (C-95). In addition, CURGUGEN had C_{max} and the area under de curve (AUC0-t) was 16.1 times higher and 39 times higher than that of C-95 [29]. Furthermore, Curcuwin Ultra+ (CU+), a novel formulation designed to protect curcuminoids from intestinal degradation, demonstrated a significant higher total systemic exposure and C_{max} for total curcuminoids compared with 95% turmeric extract (TUR 1800). Besides CU+ was 40% faster absorbed, it possesses superior bioavailability even at lower concentrations (250 and 500 mg) in comparison with higher doses of TUR 1800 (1900 mg) in healthy volunteers under fasting conditions [30]. The water-dispersible turmeric extract containing 60% curcuminoids (TurmXtra 60N), referred to as WDTE60N, using a concentration of 150 mg of curcuminoids, demonstrated a higher absorption and exposure for free curcumin, total curcumin, and total curcuminoids at 10-fold lower dose than standard turmeric extract 95% (STE95) (1500 mg) [31]. Additionally, other substances were utilized to enhance absorption, such as piperine, which increased curcumin bioavailability up to 2000% when administering 2 mg of curcumin plus 20 mg of piperine compared with curcumin alone in rats and humans, with no adverse effects [32]. Piperine improved the bioavailability of curcumin through the reduction of the velocity of its metabolism [33].

Once absorbed, curcumin is biotransformed during phase- and -II reactions by reduction and conjugation reactions in liver. Reduction is performed by NADPH-dependent reductase, alcohol dehydrogenases, and microsomal enzymes. Reduction is carried out in heptadione-chain double bonds to form di- tetra- and octahydrocurcumin. Glucuronidation is performed by the UDP-glucuronosyltransfererases hepatic UGT1A1 and intestinal UGT1A8 and UGT1A10. The isoforms UGT1A9, -1A8, and -2B7 demonstrated high activity for hexahydro-curcuminoids [34]. Sulfathion is produced by the phenol sulfotransferase isoenzymes SULT1A1 and SULT1A3 [26,35]. The major curcumin metabolites identified in vivo are curcumin-glucuronoside, dihydrocurcumin-glucuronoside, tetrahydrocurcumin-glucuronoside, and tetrahydrocurcumin (Figure 2) [36]. It was found that curcumin is converted into some active metabolites by colonic bacteria through the reactions of hydroxylation, demethylation, reduction, acetylation, and demethoxylation. Certain metabolites can recycle through the enterohepatic circulation and are eliminated in urine and feces, but curcumin derivatives are also found in organs such as the brain, liver, spleen, and lung [37].

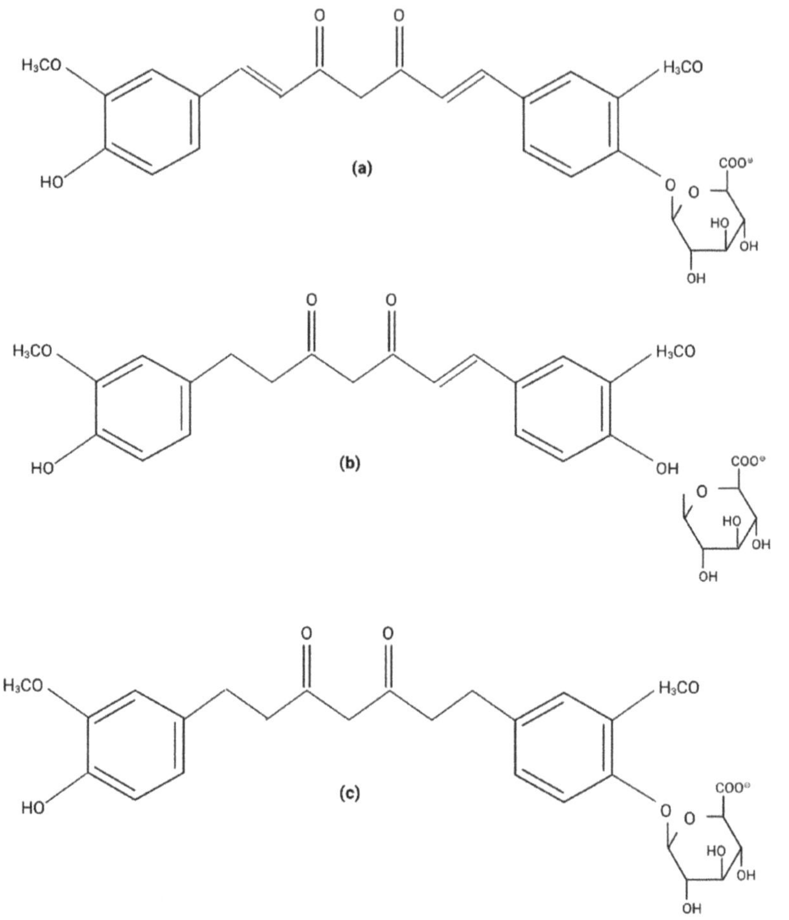

Figure 2. **Curcumin metabolites.** (a) Curcumin-glucurunoside. (b) Dihydrocurcumin-glucurunoside. (c) Tetrahydrocurcumin-glucurunoside.

2.3. Curcumin Effects on Muscle Health

2.3.1. Muscle Disorders

Numerous health benefits proven in countless trials have been attributed to curcumin; to date, there has been some evidence that proves these benefits for skeletal muscle (Table 1). For some years, it has been proposed that the use of curcumin may be a viable option for the prevention or therapy of muscle wasting [38]. In particular, in muscle wasting caused by sepsis, curcumin blocks the nuclear translocation of NF-kB subunit p25, as well as p65 DNA binding activity [39]. After traumatic injury, the systematic administration of curcumin induced myogenesis and muscle repair via the inhibition of NF-kB expression [40]. Indeed, curcumin can be considered an inhibitor of the NF-kB pathway, but it can also exert other anti-inflammatory actions within its mechanisms of action, such as inhibiting the activity of the p38 kinase, the induction of the response of heat shock proteins (HSP), and antioxidant activity [41,42].

Table 1. Studies evaluating the effect of curcumin in several models of muscle disorders.

Model	Supplementation	Curcumin Effects	Reference
In vivo: skeletal muscle wasting model in mice induced by LPS	Daily i.p. injection of curcumin (10–60 µg/kg) for 4 days	Inhibition of LPS-stimulated p38 activation and upregulation of atrogin-1/MAFbx in gastrocnemius and EDL muscles blocking loss of skeletal muscle mass	[43]
In vitro: human skeletal muscle cells In vivo: implant of MAC16 colon tumor in mice to induce muscle wasting	Curcumin c3 complex 2–5 µg/mL in muscle cells 100–250 mg/kg bw in mice	Inhibition of tyrosine release and chymotrypsin-like 20S proteasome activity muscle cells Prevention of weight loss at low doses (100 mg/kg bw) Promotion of body weight at high doses (250 mg/kg bw) Increase of muscle fiber size Inhibition of proteasome complex activity Reduced expression of ubiquitin ligases MAFbx and MURF-1	[44]
Individuals with CAS, randomized double-blind study	Oral curcumin dose 4000 mg/kg bw daily/8-weeks	Improved muscle mass, body composition, and handgrip strength Changes in absolute lymphocyte count	[45]
In vivo: skeletal muscle atrophy model in C57BL/6 J mice SZT-induced type 1 DM	Diet with or without curcumin 1500 mg/kg bw/day/2-weeks	Decrease in ubiquitination protein Reduced gene expression of muscle ubiquitin E3 ligase MAFbx and MURF-1 Inhibition of activation and concentration of NF-κB, IL-1β and TNF-α	[46]
In vivo: DEX muscle atrophy model in ICR mice	CLW 1 g/kg bw/day by gavage 1 week before DEX injection	CLW helped to suppress the decrease in handgrip strength Inhibition of decrease in muscle mass Inhibition of mRNA expression of myostatin, MURF-1 and atrogin-1 Improved antioxidant activity SOD, CAT, GPx and reduction of MDA levels	[47]
In vivo: COPD model in Sprague Dawley rats	Oral curcumin administration	Improved muscle fiber atrophy, myofibril disorganization, mitochondrial structure, and interstitial fibrosis Enhancement of mitochondrial enzyme activity, antioxidant enzymes MnSOD, GPx, and CAT Attenuation of MDA, IL-6, and TNF-α Increased mRNA expression of PGC-1α and SIRT-3	[48]
Healthy older adults: evaluation of macro and microvascular function, endothelial function, insulin and glucose metabolic response	Acute curcumin 1000 mg with and ONS vs. placebo	Improvement of MBV in m. tibialis anterior without potentiating m. vastus lateralis MBV, glucose uptake and endothelial or macrovascular function	[49]
In vivo: reloading and immobilization model in female C57BL/6J mice	Immobilization period: curcumin 1 mg/kg bw/24 h i.p./1 to 7 day Recovery period: curcumin 1 mg/kg bw/24 h i.p./day 8 to 14 day	Inhibition of proteolytic and signaling markers NF-κB, decrease of SIRT-1 Increase of fiber size of reloaded muscles Attenuated proteolysis via activation of deacetylation of SIRT-1 and decrease of atrophy signaling	[50]
In vivo: HU model in C57BLC mice	Administration of 5% fish oil and 1% curcumin in diet 10 days prior to HU	Improvement of muscle CSA and abundance of HSP70 Enhancement of anabolic signaling phosphorylation of Akt and p60S6K Reduced Nox2	[51]

Table 1. Cont.

Model	Supplementation	Curcumin Effects	Reference
In vivo: aging presarcopenia/sarcopenia in C57BL6J and C57BL10ScSn male mice	120 µg/kg of curcumin formulation in a volume of 100 µL s.c./6 months	Increase of survival in both strains without signs of liver toxicity Prevention of sarcopenia in soleus and presarcopenia in EDL Preservation of type 1 myofiber size, increase type 2A one in soleus muscle Improvement in satellite cell commitment and recruitment	[52]

i.p.: intraperitoneal; NF-κB: nuclear factor kappa B; LPS: lipopolysaccharide; EDL: extensor digitorium longus; MAFbx: atrogin-1/muscle atrophy F-box; MUFR-1: muscle RING finger-1; CAS: cancer anorexia–cachexia syndrome; SZT: streptozotocyne; DM: diabetes mellitus; DEX: dexamethasone; CLW: *Curcuma longa* water extract; SOD: superoxide dismutase, CAT: catalase; GPx: glutathione peroxidase; MDA: malondehyde; COPD: chronic obstructive pulmonary disease; IL-6: interleukin-6; PGC-1α: peroxisome proliferator-activated receptor-gamma coactivator; SIRT-3: sirtuin 3; ATO: arsenic trioxide; ONS: oral nutritional supplement; MBV: microvascular blood volume; WT: wild type; KO: knock out; SIRT-1: sirtuin 1; HU: hindlimb unloading; CSA: cross sectional area; Nox2: NADPH oxidase 2; s.c.: subcutaneous.

Several inflammatory conditions in skeletal muscle are related with the upregulation of the AKT and NF-κB and downstream genes such as atrogin-1/MAFbx or MuRF1, as well as TNF-α mediated by p38 MAPK related with the signaling pathways involved in muscle wasting. Jin and Li (2007) previously reported that the administration of curcumin over 4 days (10–60 µg/kg i.p.) attenuated muscle damage induced by lipopolysaccharide (LPS) stimulation in mouse gastrocnemius and extensor digitorum longus (EDL) muscles. Curcumin attenuated LPS-stimulated p38 activation and the upregulation of atrogin-1/MAFbx, inhibiting the loss of muscle mass [43]. However, it must be taken into consideration that this study did not come to express an absolute correlation between the expression of atrogin-1 and MAFbx and the muscle protein content, because an increase was reported of mRNA for atrogin-1, but not for MAFbx.

Muscles Affected by Chronic Diseases

Skeletal muscle loss in cancer cachexia appears to be the most relevant clinical issue; unfortunately, it is associated with a poor prognosis. Different models do suggest that muscle waste is the result of reduced protein synthesis and enhanced protein degradation by means of the active ubiquitin–proteosome pathway [53]. Curcumin has proved to interfere in proteosome degradation. In vivo studies found that the curcumin c3 complex at doses of 100 mg/kg body weight (bw) prevents the bw loss in muscle wasting induced in mice by implanting the MAC16 colon tumor. Elevated doses of curcumin c3 (250 mg/kg bw) improved bw gain up to 25% compared to the control. Moreover, there was an increase in muscle fiber size (30–65%) and in the weight of the gastrocnemius muscle (30–58%), and also an inhibition of the expression of muscle-specific ubiquitin ligases as well as the activity of the ubiquitin–proteosome complex; thus, curcumin is effective in preventing and reversing muscle waste, which renders it an optimal aid for the therapy against cachexia [44]. In a randomized, double-blind, placebo-controlled phase-IIa study, 20 patients with the cancer anorexia–cachexia syndrome in locally advanced or advanced head and neck cancer were treated with curcumin (4000 mg/day) or placebo for 8 weeks. The study reported important benefits in improving muscle mass and body composition compared with the placebo. Additionally, hand grip muscle strength and absolute lymphocyte count were favored. It is noteworthy that curcumin was well-tolerated in patients, which is important to bear in mind, due to the gastrointestinal symptoms these individuals tend to exhibit in the progression of and therapy for the disease [45].

Diabetes and other disabilities are related with chronic inflammation mediated by the NF-κB pathway, in which there are an important participation of the proinflammatory cytokines TNF-α and IL-1β. Together with chronic inflammation, elevated oxidative stress is also associated with muscle atrophy, especially in type 1 diabetes mellitus (DM).

Streptozotocin-induced type 1 DM in C57BL/6 J mice (200 mg kg^{-1} i.p.) significantly reduced bw, skeletal muscle weight, and CS. Treatment with curcumin (1500 mg kg^{-1} day^{-1}) for 2 weeks attenuated the gene expression of the ubiquitin E3 ligase atrogin-1/MAFbx and MuRF-1. Curcumin ameliorated inflammatory markers (cytokines TNF-α and IL-1β) and oxidative stress in type 1 DM. These results indicate that curcumin may be helpful in the management of muscle atrophy in patients with type 1 DM [46]. Other models with dexamethasone, which is a promoter of proteolysis by activating the ubiquitin proteosome system and ROS, point out that the *Curcuma longa*-L. water extract administered in ICR mice at 1 mg/kg/bw day decreased myostatin, MuRF-1, and Atrogin-1 levels along with MDA, and was additionally associated with an increase of antioxidant enzymes that reduced ROS, suggesting that the *Curcuma longa*-L. water extract may be a natural product for preventing skeletal muscle atrophy by regulating muscle atrophy target genes and stimulating an antioxidant response [47].

Chronic obstructive pulmonary disease (COPD) induced by cigarette smoke exposure in combination with LPD in a rodent model demonstrated that curcumin treatment ameliorated damage in airways and improved interstitial fibrosis, myofibril disorganization, inflammation, fiber atrophy, and mitochondrial damage in the skeletal muscle of COPD rats [48]. The mitochondria play a key role in energy production and in the regulation of oxidative stress; in consequence, mitochondrial damage contributes to the development of skeletal muscle dysfunction and the inflammatory response [54]. In the previously mentioned study, a treatment with curcumin significantly improved the mitochondrial enzyme activities of cytochrome c oxidase, succinate dehydrogenase, Na$^+$/K$^+$-ATPase, and Ca^{2+}-ATPase in skeletal muscle. On the other hand, oxidative stress was attenuated by reducing the levels of MDA and enhancing the antioxidant enzymes MnSOD and GPx. In addition, the inflammatory markers IL-6 and TNF-α were reduced. Curcumin promoted the upregulation of the PGC-1α/SIRT3 signaling pathway by increasing mRNA and the protein expression of PGC-1α and SIRT3 of the skeletal muscle of COPD rats [48]. The peroxisome-proliferator-activated receptor gamma coactivator 1 alpha (PGC-1α) is a transcriptional regulator that controls the expressions of the genes involved in mitochondrial biogenesis, energy metabolism, and oxidative stress [55]. The silent-mating-type information regulation 2 homolog 3 (SIRT3) is a downstream gene located in the mitochondrial matrix that participates in mitochondrial fatty acid oxidation and is also active in efficient electron flow in the electron transport chain (ETC) for energy metabolism [56]. It is crucial to mention the role that curcumin might play in the activation of the PGC-1α/SIRT3 signaling pathway; these findings suggest that curcumin could play a pivotal role in the recovery of skeletal muscle in chronic pulmonary disease (COPD).

As with cancer, diabetes, or COPD, chronic kidney disease (CDK) is characterized by a catabolic environment with high levels of oxidative stress and mitochondrial dysfunction, which render these individuals highly susceptible to experiencing muscle atrophy, poor tolerance to exercise, further poor prognosis, low quality of life, and an increase in mortality [57]. Previously, the benefits that apparently accompany curcumin in preventing or reversing muscle atrophy were mentioned, but the complete mechanisms of action remained unclear. Recent findings point out that curcumin treatment (100 mg/kg/bw day) over 12 weeks in a wild-type and muscle-specific glycogen synthase kinase3β (GSK-3β) knockout (KO) CKD mouse model alleviated mitochondrial dysfunction and oxidative damage by inhibiting GSK-3β activity in skeletal muscle [58]. GSK-3β is thought to participate in the regulation of protein metabolism and in mitochondrial function in skeletal muscle [59,60]. In fact, the suppression of GSK-3β is found to be beneficial for PGC-1α signaling and mitochondrial function by increasing the expression of PGC-1α in C2CL2 muscle cells [60]. The genetic and pharmacological inactivation of GSK-3β raises the mitochondrial DNA (mtDNA) copy number, the expression of oxidative phosphorylation (PhoOx) protein levels, and the activity of the enzymatic machinery involved in fatty acid oxidation and the Krebs cycle, enhancing mitochondrial biogenesis during the myogenic process [61]. The researchers observed that curcumin could improve mitochondrial function by optimizing the activity of the electron transport chain and mitochondrial respiration, ATP synthesis, the reduction of the membrane potential, and the attenuation of oxidative mitochondrial stress via the suppression of GSK-3β activity in skeletal muscle [58].

Muscles Affected by Toxics

Curcumin could comprise a novel strategy for the treatment of several types of skeletal muscle damage caused by toxic substances such as arsenic. In a model using arsenic trioxide (ATO) to induce muscle damage in ducks, curcumin treatment was able to reduce the oxidative stress manifested by the augmented total antioxidant capacity, SOD, and reduced MDA. Curcumin promoted mitochondrial biogenesis by activating the PGC-1α, NRF1/2, and TFAM pathways. Likewise, curcumin treatment helped to regulate proapoptotic genes (p53, Bax, Caspase-3, and Cytc) and mitophagy (PINK1, Parkin, LC3, and p62) by reducing mRNA protein levels. In turn, curcumin promoted mitochondrial function and integrity [62]. Acute curcumin (1000 mg) together with the oral nutrition supplementation (ONS) of proteins and carbohydrates enhanced the Musculus tibialis anterior microvascular blood volume, and also increased glucose uptake and insulin in the presence of ONS in healthy older adults, which may have an impact on promoting energy metabolism and muscle function [49].

Muscles Affected by Immobilization and Sarcopenia

Immobilization during long time periods might induce muscle atrophy, and the proteolytic ubiquitin–proteosome system and the mitochondrial apoptotic pathway play a pivotal role in its development. In the study of Vazeille et al. [63], in which the authors administered curcumin for 8 days to rats subjected to hind limb immobilization, the results indicated that curcumin did not reduce muscle atrophy at 8 days of immobilization, but instead improved muscle recovery and the CSA of immobilized muscles after 10 days. The authors observed that curcumin hampers proteasome chymotrypsin-like activity and the trend toward increased caspase-9-associated apoptosome activity at 8 days of immobilization. In addition, curcumin improved muscle recovery during reloading due to the reduction of the protein levels associated with immobilization (Smac/DIABLO) and the elevation of X-linked inhibitory apoptotic proteins after 10 days, enhancing muscle regeneration during the first steps. Recently, the use of curcumin (1 mg/kg/bw i.p.) and resveratrol (20 mg/kg/bw i.p.) elicited important changes in the number of muscle satellite cells, as well as progenitor muscle cell numbers, activating the quiescent cells in limb muscles of mice (C57BL/6J, 10 weeks) subjected to reloading for 7 days subsequent to a 7-day period of hind limb immobilization [50]. Curcumin alone promoted the growth of CSA and the recovery of muscle fibers, and increased the activity of sirtuin 1. Treatment with both curcumin and resveratrol promoted the numbers of subtypes of satellite cells in the unloaded limb muscle, but not in the reloaded muscle. Therefore, the benefits may not be equal in the reloaded phase; however, the target phytochemicals could have potential clinical advantages during muscle regeneration. Certain other pathways involved in immobilization-induced atrophy have improved when curcumin is administered. For instance, the reduction of proteolytic and signaling markers (NF-kB p50) was reported; conversely, sirtuin-1 and hybrid fiber size attenuated in the gastrocnemius of mice subjected to reloading following 7 days of immobilization. It was hypothesized that curcumin would attenuate muscle proteolysis by the activation of histone deacetylase sirtuin-1, decreasing the atrophy signaling pathways [64].

Another study tested the combination of curcumin (1% diet) and fish oil (5% diet) to determine its effect on anabolic signals and protector stress proteins in C57BL/6 mice subjected to hind limb unloading. The results indicated that the intake of fish oil and curcumin for 10 days prior to hind limb unloading improved the CSA and enhanced the anabolic signaling of Akt phosphorylation, p70S6K phosphorylation, and the abundance of HSP70 while simultaneously reducing the NADPH oxidase-2-complex (Nox2), an indicator of oxidative stress, suggesting that such a mixture could aid in preventing muscle atrophy [65]. Recent available data highlight that the suppression of Nox2 would attenuate the disruption of HPS70, sarcolemnal oxide nitric synthase (nNOS), and Nrf2, consequently mitigating unloading-induced muscle atrophy [51].

Curcumin is also being associated with the prevention of age-related sarcopenia. Gorza et al. [52] evaluated the effect of curcumin treatment at 120 µg/kg in a volume of 100 µL in 18-month-old C57BL6J and C57BL10ScSn male mice. In this study, the researchers observed that curcumin was able to significantly increase survival in both strains, preventing sarcopenia and pre-sarcopenia, preserving type-1 myofibers, and increasing type-2A ones, positively influencing the satellite cells by preserving adult levels of myofiber maturation in old, regenerating soleus muscle.

2.3.2. Physical Exercise and Skeletal Muscle

Little evidence has been produced by studies conducted under exercise conditions to prove the effects of curcumin on protecting muscle from exercise-induced damage. Recently, it was reported that curcumin exerts a positive impact on performance during exercise and may enhance recovery. A new formulation of curcumin, Next-Generation Ultrasol Curcumin (NGUC), which is more bioavailable, was evaluated in a rodent exhaustive treadmill exercise protocol. Animals that received NGUC at doses of 100 and 200 mg/kg/bw improved endurance capacity and hand grip strength; at the same time, indicators of fatigue (lactic acid, LDH), muscle damage (creatine kinase) (CK), oxidative stress (MDA), and inflammation were attenuated. In particular, IL-1β, IL-6, and TNF-α proteins in muscle were effectively reduced in the exercise group at doses of 200 mg/kg of NGUC. The study indicated that NGUC reduced mTOR phosphorylation similarly to that of the PGC-1α protein level and diminished MAFbx and MuRF1 protein levels. In conclusion, curcumin promoted muscle recovery and exercise performance, attenuating muscle damage and activating anti-inflammatory, antioxidant, and muscle-mass regulatory signaling in a dose-dependent manner [66]. In another eccentric exercise model, curcumin was administered over 20 days via oral gavage at doses of 200 mg/kg bw dissolved in corn oil. On day 21, the rats were subjected to a treadmill run and sacrificed; the analysis of blood and muscle tissue demonstrated that curcumin attenuated the muscle damage induced by the eccentric exercise. However, a difference was not observed in the antioxidant response because there were no significant differences in SOD and glutathione and MDA levels. Thus, it can be concluded that curcumin protected against muscle damage but did not necessarily exert an impact on oxidative stress and the antioxidant response [67].

In an exercise protocol, 6-week-old treadmill-running rats were exercised at 25 m/min for 45 min following a physical adaptation period. Animals were administered with 20 mg of curcuminoids daily during the 6-week exercise protocol. The results revealed significant improvement in run-to-exhaustion time and a reduction of MDA levels, NF-κB, and HSP70 in animals treated with curcuminoids. Furthermore, the protein levels of Sirt1, PGC-1α, Nrf2, and GLUT4 increased significantly, and the antioxidant–enzyme activities of GPx and SOD were higher, similar to those of the glutathione content compared with non-treated animals. In conclusion, curcumin protected skeletal muscle from the damage induced by exhaustive exercise, inhibiting NF-κB and promoting Nrf2 signaling pathways [68]. In another model of heart failure with a low ejection fraction (HFrEF)—a mouse model with ligation-induced coronary artery characterized by intolerance to exercise—the application of subcutaneous osmotic minipump curcumin (50 mg·kg^{-1}·day^{-1} for 8 weeks) was evaluated. It was found that animals treated with curcumin significantly improved in maximal speed, running distance to exhaustion, and limb grip force. It could also be observed that reduced force and rapid fatigue in soleus and extensor digitorium longus muscles were reduced. Likewise, curcumin enhanced Nrf2, SOD, hemoxygenase-1 (HO-1), MyoD, and myogenin; these results indicated a positive impact on reducing oxidative stress, promoting exercise performance, and better tolerance to exercise in HFrEF mice [69].

The underlying mechanism of curcumin regarding muscle health is summarized in Figure 3.

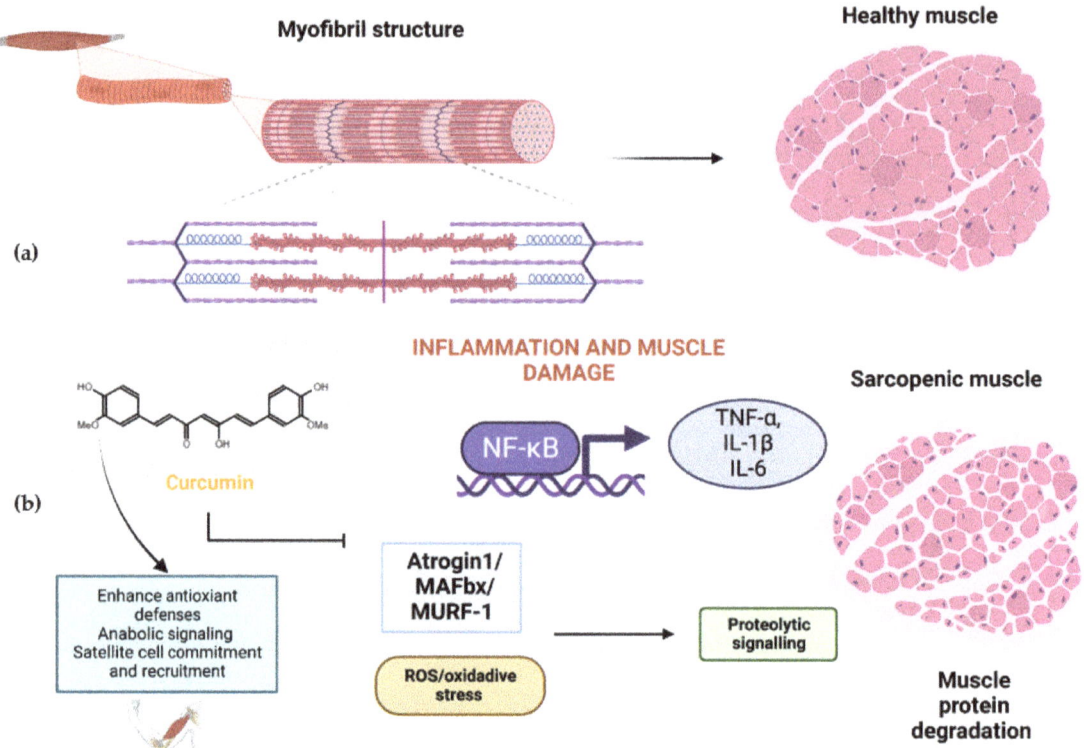

Figure 3. (**a**) Myofibril structure in healthy muscles. (**b**) Effects of curcumin on human skeletal muscle. Curcumin inhibits inflammation and muscle damage by hampering NF-kB and the proinflammatory interleukins TNF-α, IL-1β, and IL-6, as well as the proteasome complex system for protein muscle degradation integrated by ubiquitin ligases atrogin 1, muscle atrophy F-box (MAFbx), and muscle RING finger-1 (MUFR-1). Curcumin reduces oxidative-stress-enhancing antioxidant cell defenses and promotes anabolic signaling, myofibril integrity, mitochondrial function, and satellite cell commitment and recruitment for muscle repair. Created with BioRender.com.

3. Sulforaphane

3.1. Botanical Description

Brassicaceae or Cruciferae is a family that includes various cruciferous vegetables, such as broccoli, cauliflower, cabbage, kohlrabi, mustard, and brussels sprouts. Broccoli (*Brassica oleracea* L. var. *italica* Plenk) is 45.7–76.2 cm in height, with a 30–60-cm spread. The stem arises from the roots and is surrounded by leaves; mature broccoli flowers are small with four yellow petals [70]. Broccoli contains fruits in siliqua with rounded pink seeds. Broccoli has green leaves and a green flowerhead (the edible inflorescence) that bears green, purple, yellow, or white flowers. Broccoli leaves have petioles with elongated limbs with grey-green leaves and wavy deep lobes. Broccoli may be grown as an annual, as a biennial (flowers in the second year), or as a perennial crop, depending on the type of broccoli and the region. It is a harvest-time seasonal bloomer and needs full sun and a medium amount of water to grow. It is a cool-weather vegetable that is grown for a harvest of large, tight terminal heads of green flower buds at the ends of thick, edible stems [71]. *Brassica oleracea* is thought to be the phylogenetic parent of broccoli; it is a species native to Atlantic coastal

Europe, and it occurs along the coasts of the United Kingdom, Germany, France, and Spain. Brassica species have been cultivated for at least 2000 years [72].

Broccoli is highlighted because of its content of the bioactive compound sulforaphane (SFN). Several studies have been conducted with regard to the consumption of cruciferous vegetables and their multiple benefits to health, supporting that the bioactive compounds that they possess are responsible for their previously mentioned biological activities. The majority of studies support the potential anticancer, antidiabetic, and cardioprotector effects, and its help in losing body weight (bw). Since 1992, Zhang et al. [73] reported that SFN and its sulfide and sulfone analogues induced the activities of the phase II detoxification enzymes NQO1 and GST in several mouse tissues, in that it is known that SFN is the most biologically active component deriving from broccoli with anticarcinogenic action.

3.2. Phytochemistry and Bootability and Metabolism

Glucosinolates (GSL) are the major biologically active compounds within *Brassicaceae* species; they are the precursors of isothiocyanates (ITC), which are produced by myrosinase during slicing, harvesting, and chewing by enzymatic degradation [74]. GSL are thiglucosides that share a β-D-thioglucose, a sulfonated oxime group, and a side chain derived from some essential amino acids (such as phenylalanine, tryptophan, and methionine) as their basic structure [75] (Figure 4). In the human digestive tract, GSL can be transformed by the intestinal microflora myrosinase isoform. SFN is the most studied among the GSL, which currently entertains the major evidence of beneficial effects. The SFN chemical structure comprises 4-methylsulfinybutyl isothiocyanate; young broccoli contains approximately 1153 mg/100 mg of SFN and the mature vegetable contains 44–171 mg/100 mg dry weight (dw). The edible portion of mature broccoli contains 507–684 µg/g SFN dw [76]. SFN is lipophilic in nature, of a low molecular weight, and is a thermo-sensitive molecule [77].

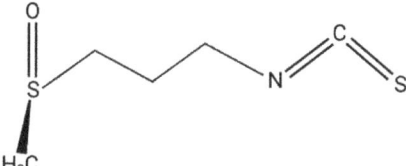

Figure 4. Sulforaphane, basic chemical structure. Created with BioRender.com.

The bioavailability of SFN depends on certain factors, such as mode of preparation. For the cooking of broccoli, for example, it has been reported that on quickly steaming the broccoli sprouts following a myrosinase treatment, the vegetable contains 11 and 5 times higher amounts of SFN than freeze-dried and untreated steamed broccoli. After the oral administration of 2.5 mg/g bw of the broccoli sprout preparations (quickly steaming and unsteaming), SFN was rapidly absorbed and distributed throughout the tissues. The SFN-rich preparation presented the highest peak of a plasma SF concentration of 337 ng/mL, which is 6.0 times and 2.6 times higher compared than that of the other two preparations [78]. The oral administration of SFN 2.8 µmol/kg or 0.5 mg/kg presents 80% bioavailability, whereas doses of 28 µmol/kg or 5 mg/kg demonstrated only around 20% bioavailability [79]. In another study, a peak concentration was found of SFN metabolites of 1.91 ± 0.24 µM after 1 h with an oral dose of 200 µmol. The same oral dose of 200 µmol reported a peak concentration of SFN metabolites of 0.7 ± 0.2 µM after 3 h [80]. The consumption of 200 g of crushed broccoli indicated that higher bioavailability was found (37%) in men who ate raw broccoli vs. men who consumed cooked broccoli (bioavailability, 3.4%). It was found that the time of absorption was delayed in cooked broccoli (peak plasma time = 6 h) compared with raw broccoli (1.6 h); nevertheless, their excretion half-lives were similar, that is, 2.5 and 2.4 for raw and cooked broccoli, respectively [81].

After the conversion of glucosinolates by myrosinase, SFN is metabolized within the body by conjugation in the presence of glutathione. The reaction produces N-acetylcysteine derivatives in the form of mercapturic acids, termed dithiocarbamates (DTC), or conjugates of SFN through the mercapturic acid pathway. First, SFN is conjugated with glutathione in a glutathione transferase GST catalyzed reaction. Afterward, sulforaphane-N-acetylcysteine (SFR-NAC) is systematized via cleavage reactions catalyzed by γ-glutamyl transpeptidase, cysteinyl glycinase, and N-acetyltransferase [75]. Following the oral consumption of 200 μmol of SFN from broccoli sprouts, 70–90% of DTC metabolites were identified in urine [82]. According to the pharmacokinetic assessment of the relation of dithiocarbamates (DTC)/isothiocyanates (ITC) in human volunteers who received 200 μmol of broccoli sprout isothiocyanates (SFN at a major proportion and less iberin and erucin), it was found that SFN was rapidly absorbed (concentration 0.943–2.27 μmol/l) in plasma, serum, and erythrocytes 1 h after intake, with a reported half-life of 1.77 $\pm$ 0.13 h and an excretion time at 8 h (58.3 $\pm$ 2.8% of the dose). Renal clearance was 369 $\pm$ 53 mL/min [83].

3.3. Sulforaphane Effects on Muscle Health

3.3.1. Sulforaphane and Biological Activity

SFN is considered the most powerful nutraceutical contained in cruciferous vegetables, due to its multiple biological activities on and benefits to human health described in a growing body of evidence. The anticarcinogenic activity of SFN is a very efficient activator of the E2 factor-related factor (Nrf2) and the signaling pathway involved in the antioxidant and cytoprotector response in response to stress stimuli [84–86]. The activation of Nrf2 is closely involved in the repression of NF-KB inflammatory signaling and downstream proinflammatory cytokines and their mediators [87]. Nrf2 is a member of the cap 'n' collar (CNC) family of basic region–leucine zipper (bZIP) transcription factors. In humans, Nrf2 is a 66-kDa and 606-amino-acid protein divided into Nrf2-ECH homology regions and seven Neh domains; it is coded by the *NFE2L2* gene. These factors regulate more than 250 genes implicated in cell defense and in the redox response [88].

Under homeostatic circumstances, Nrf2 remains attached in the cytosol to the suppressor regulator Kelch-like erythroid cell-derived protein with CNC homology-associated protein 1 (Keap1) through the ETGE and DLG motifs in the Neh2 domain, forming a dimer with Keap1 in Kelch domains, leading to the ubiquitination of seven lysines and the consequent degradation in the 26S complex [89]. Keap1 is a redox-sensitive regulator and dissociates from Nrf2 with electrophilics such as ROS/NOS. Thus, Nrf2 is released and translocated into the nucleus to bind the specific DNA sequence of the antioxidant response element (ARE) within small musculo-aponeurotic fibrosarcoma proteins (sMaf) [90]. Bonding with the ARE sequence promotes the expression of a wide range of genes involved in cytoprotection and the antioxidant response, such as the phase II detoxifying enzymes NAD(P)H quinone oxidoreductase 1 (NQO1) and glutathione S-transferase (GST), heme oxygenase 1 (HO-1), and enzymes involved in the synthesis and metabolism of glutathione. In agreement with the latter, Nrf2 modulation has become a target for elucidating the mechanism of several aliments related with redox balance [91]. It has been found that different synthetic or natural compounds are potential Nrf2 activators; SFN efficiently activates the Nrf2/Keap1/ARE signaling pathway. It has been discovered that more than 500 genes are activated by SFN through the Nrf2/ARE signaling pathway; for that reason, SFN is considered a potent nutrigenomic compound. SFN can induce Nrf2 translocation and nuclear accumulation and can phosphorylate Nrf2 through the activation of MAPK, protein kinase B (PKB/Akt), and protein kinase C (PKC) [92,93].

From the nutrigenomic perspective, certain molecules, including some phytochemicals, are effective Nrf2 activators or inducers according to their CD value, which is an indicator of the amount of specific compound required to double NQO1 activity in murine hepatoma cells (hepg2). NQO1 is one of the most important protector enzymes and it has been employed to evaluate the phytochemicals involved in chemopreventive and anticancer activity [94]. The nutrigenomic effect of certain bioactive compounds can be determined by measuring the CD value; SFN exhibited the highest potential, taking into account that the lesser the amount of the concentration required to activate Nrf2, the more efficient an activator the compound is considered to be. SFN requires 0.2 µM and curcumin, 2.7 µM; this may help towards understanding why both SFN and curcumin have achieved very promising results in numerous trials. Among other effective phytochemicals reported, we find andrographolides, silymarin, quercetin, beta-carotene, genistein, lutein, resveratrol, and zeaxanthin [95]. Substantial evidence from pre-clinical and clinical reports supports that SFN deriving from cruciferous vegetables such as broccoli possesses enormous chemoprotective potential and more benefits to health upon its use [96].

In addition to the activation of the antioxidant response, SFN is capable of modulating the inflammatory response by inhibiting the binding of NF-κB to DNA. Furthermore, it constrains the activation of I-κB and the translocation of NF-κB, thereby reducing inflammation. Suppression of the activation of the NF-κB signaling pathway blocks the release of inflammatory mediators such as TNF-α IL-1β, IL-6, nitric oxide (NO), and prostaglandin E2 (PGE2). The attenuated activity can be observed in inflammatory enzymes such as cyclooxygenase-2 (COX-2) and inducible NO synthase (iNOS).

3.3.2. Muscle Disorders

The cumulative studies conducted of SFN on skeletal muscle are presented in Table 2. Since SFN is described as one of the major bioactivators of the Nrf2/Keap1/ARE signaling pathway, some studies report that it protects skeletal muscle from damage in different models; however, evidence of this remains scarce. Duchenne muscular dystrophy is a muscle disorder associated with elevated oxidative stress and inflammation. The investigation was conducted by Sun et al., who utilized a rodent Duchenne muscular dystrophy model. The animals were treated with SFN by gavage (2 mg·kg body wt^{-1}·day^{-1} for 8 weeks. SFN treatment augmented muscle mass, strength, and running capacity related with the enhancement of subsarcolemmal integrity, central nucleation, and myofibrillar variability. Likewise, the GSH/GSSG ratio was favorable; the muscle markers of damage and oxidative stress, LDH, CPK, and MDA, were significantly reduced [97]. Afterward, in a very similar model, it was evidenced that SFN activated Nrf2 and targeted the expression of the HO-1 enzyme; in parallel, the central inflammatory-signaling command by NF-κB was inhibited with the reported reduction of NF-κB (p65), and the phosphorylated IκB kinase-α augmented inhibitor κB-α expression, proinflammatory cytokines TNF-α, IL-1β, and IL-6, and the inflammatory cytokine CD45, as long as the infiltration of immune cells into mdx mouse skeletal muscle lasted. In summary, SFN activates the antioxidant response and blunts inflammatory signaling; therefore, it may be a potential tool with clinical benefits in the therapy of individuals with muscular dystrophy [98].

Table 2. Studies evaluating the effect of sulforaphane in several models of muscle disorders and exercise.

Model	Supplementation	Sulforaphane Effects	Reference
In vivo: Duchenne muscular dystrophy in mdx mice	SFN 2 mg/kg bw/day by gavage/8 weeks	Increased expression and activity of NQO1 and HO-1 in dependent manner of Nrf2 Increase in skeletal muscle mass, muscle force, running distance and GSH-to-GSSG ratio Decreased activities of CK and LDH Reduction in MDA levels, myocardial and gastrocnemius hypertrophy Improved fiber size ability, inflammation and sarcolemma integrity	[97]

Table 2. Cont.

Model	Supplementation	Sulforaphane Effects	Reference
In vivo: muscle dystrophy in mdx mice	SFN 2 mg/kg bw/day by gavage/4 weeks	Increased expression and activity of HO-1 IN dependent manner of Nrf2 Decreased inflammation, cell infiltrate, proinflammatory cytokine CD45 and inflammatory cytokines TNF-α and IL-1β Reduced expression of NF-κB(p65) and phosphorylated IκB kinase-α Increased IκB-α expression in Nrf2-dependent manner	[98]
In vitro: porcine satellite cells	SFN at 5, 10, and 15 μM	Inhibition of HDAC activity and disturbed mRNA levels of HDAC family members Elevation of acetylated histone H3 and H4 Upregulation of protein and mRNA levels of SMAD7 Increased the acetylation level of histone H4 in the SMAD7 promoter Increased PSC proliferation	[99]
In vivo: male Wistar rats Acute exhaustive exercise	SFN pre-training 25 mg/kg bw i.p.	Enhanced Nrf2 expression and the downstream target genes NQO1, GST, and GR in vastus lateralis muscle Promoted antioxidant enzyme activity Increased TAC Reduced LDH and CK activities	[100]
In vivo: Male WT mice (Nrf2+/+) and Nrf2-KO (Nrf2−/−) on C57BL/6 Exhaustive incremental treadmill test	SFN pre-training treatment 4 times for 3 days (72, 48, 24, and 3 h) 25 mg/kg bw i.p.	Upregulation of Nrf2 signaling and gene expression of HO-1, NQO1, CAT, and γ-GCS in Nrf2+/+ mice skeletal muscle Reduction of TBARS Augmented AMPKα and mtDNA copies Augmented running distance Decreased LDH and CK activities	[101]
Young man performed 6 sets of 5 eccentric exercises with the nondominant arm in elbow flexion 70% MVC	SFN 30 mg/day/2 weeks	Attenuated DOMS and ROM 2 days after exercise Augmented NQO1 mRNA expression in PBMCs Reduction of serum MDA levels 2 days after exercise	[102]
In vivo: male C57BL/6 mice Exhaustive running exercise	SFN 50/mg b/2 h prior to exhaustive running test	Reduction of cytokines TNF-α, IL-1β, and IL-6 Reduction of damage blood biomarkers AST, ALT, and LDH Enhanced mRNA expression of Nrf2 and the downstream enzymes HO-1, SOD1, CAT, and GPx1 in liver tissue	[103]

SFN: sulforaphane; NOQ1: NADPH quinone oxidoreductase 1; HO-1: hem oxygenase 1; Nrf2: E2-factor-related factor; GSH: reduced glutathione; GSSG: oxidized glutathione; CK: creatin kinase; LDH: lactate dehydrogenase; TNFα: factor de necrosis tumoral α; IL-1β: interleukin 1β; NF-κB: nuclear factor kappa B; IκB: inhibitor of kappa B HDAC: histone deacetylase; SMAD7: smad family member 7; PSC: porcine satellite cells; NQO1: NADPH quinone oxidoreductase-1; GST: glutathione S-transferase; GR: glutathione reductase; TAC: total antioxidant activity; CPK: creatin phosphor-kinase; WT: wild type; KO: knock out; mtDNA: mitochondrial DNA; DOMS: delayed onset muscle soreness; ROM: range of motion; MVC: maximum voluntary contraction; PBMCs: peripheral blood mononuclear cells; HO-1: hem oxygenase-1; SOD1: superoxide dismutase 1; CAT: catalase; GPx: glutathione peroxidase.

Beyond the scope of whether SFN would modulate antioxidant and inflammatory responses, new research conducted by Zhan et al. [99] reported that SFN can control the growth of porcine satellite cells (PSC) and that it epigenetically increased the expression of SMAD7, a family member of regulators involved in myogenesis and muscle regeneration that inhibits transforming growth factor beta (TGF-β) signaling. SFN at 5, 10, and 15 μM boosted PSC proliferation by modifying the mRNA expression of myogenic regulatory factors. Moreover, SFN repressed histone deacetylase (HDAC) activity and disturbed mRNA levels of HDAC family members, favoring an abundance of histone H3 and H4 in

PSC. SFN improved the level of acetylation of histone H4 in the SMAD7 promoter; at the same time, SFN reduced the expression of microRNA. These results indicate that SFN may be a powerful stimulator of skeletal muscle growth. Previous work demonstrated that SFN (5 µM, 10 µM, and 15 µM) avoids oxidative stress and apoptosis in PS; further, SFN acts as an HDAC and DNA methyltransferase (DNMT) inhibitor. The most relevant issue was related to the inhibition of myostatin expression and the markedly lesser expression of the negative feedback inhibitors of myostatin signaling [104]. Myostatin is a member of the TGF-β family and is considered a potent inhibitor of skeletal muscle growth; it can hamper cell activation and the cell renewal of satellite cells [105]. Hence, SFN can be a nutraceutical that can inhibit the myostatin signaling pathway, promoting muscle anabolism.

3.3.3. Physical Exercise and Skeletal Muscle

Cumulative evidence supports that the practice of regular physical exercise provides great benefits to health and that, in general, it prevents the development of chronic diseases, improves immune function, and prevents obesity. Nevertheless, extended exercise sessions along with inadequate recovery periods may cause muscle damage. Throughout exercise, the increased oxygen consumption induces an elevated production of ROS within the myofibers, which is counteracted by antioxidant defenses; nonetheless, overtraining may surpass the ability to constrain exercise-induced oxidative stress [106]. The prolonged periods of fatigue induced by intense training or competitive seasons, along with inappropriate recovery post-exercise/competition episodes, contributes to the development of overtraining syndrome (OTS). Consequently, excessive ROS and OTS are closely related with muscle fatigue and low physical performance [107]. Muscle fatigue can be defined as a decline in maximal force production in response to contractile activity [108]. Detrimental skeletal muscle force could also be explained by the predominance of the oxidized state of muscle fibers continuously exposed to elevated ROS, especially H_2O_2 [109]. In contrast, unfatigued muscle fibers are maintained in a reduced state. Furthermore, inflammation is also a result of the inability to restrain the sustaining of redox imbalance. In exhaustive exercise, inflammatory cells such as macrophages and neutrophils infiltrate into muscle fibers. The released cytokines, chemokines, and damage-associated molecular patterns (DAMP) are increased in damaged tissue, which promotes the migration of leukocytes [110].

SFN is considered the most powerful nutraceutical contained in cruciferous vegetables due to the multiple biological activities described in this efficient activator of the Nrf2 pathway. SFN may prevent damage to skeletal muscle during very hard physical workouts. Previously, SFN was reported at doses of 25 mg/kg/bw i.p. in male Wistar rats that performed a single bout of exercise until exhaustion on a rodent treadmill (+7% slope and 24% slope). The 3-day SFN treatment increased the expression and activity of glutathione S-transferase (GST), glutathione reductase (GR), and NQO1; the expression of Nrf2 augmented significantly, as did total antioxidant capacity. On the other hand, a decrease was found in LDH and CK activity. These results suggest that the SFN pre-treatment may exert a protective effect against muscle damage induced by exhaustive training, the mechanism of action appearing to be that SFN triggers the antioxidant pathway [100]. Afterward, wild-type mice (Nrf2+/+) and Nrf2-null mice (Nrf2−/−) C57BL/6J were subjected to a progressive continuous all-out test. The administration of SFN (25 mg/kg/bw i.p.) significantly improved the run distance, which was directly related with the upregulation of the Nrf2 target genes *NQO1*, *OH-1*, *CAT*, and *γ-GCS* in the gastrocnemius muscle and soleus of SFN-treated Nrf2+/+ mice. Of note, CK and LDH as muscle damage markers significantly decreased, and the lactate content remained low in the same group. Indicators of oxidative damage, such as TBARS, were reduced as well. Additionally, a higher number of mtDNA was also reported, but intriguingly, there were no significant differences in PGC-1α and Sirt1, though AMPKα increased. The authors suggested that SFN exerts a protective effect on active skeletal muscles, preventing fatigue, attenuating oxidative damage, and improving aerobic capacity through the upregulation of the antioxidant response during exhaustive exercise [101].

The studies reporting the use of SFN in terms of exercise and muscle recovery on humans are very limited. Notwithstanding this, lately the manner in which SFN could impact muscle soreness was explored in young men who performed six sets of five eccentric exercises with the nondominant arm in elbow flexion with 70% maximal voluntary contraction by assessing the evaluation of delayed-onset muscle soreness (DMSO) and range of motion (ROM). After 2 weeks of SFN supplementation (30 mg/day), a marked reduction was observed in muscle soreness associated with a reduction of MDA serum levels, whereas the mRNA expression of NQO1 increased following 2 days of exercise, suggesting that SFN could aid in muscle recovery [102]. The study of Ruhee et al. [103] evaluated the oral consumption of SFN (50 mg/kg bw) 2 h prior to a running treadmill test. Acute exhaustive exercise elevated the damage markers alanine aminotransferase (ALT), aspartate aminotransferase (AST), and LDH. Moreover, a significant increase was observed in the mRNA expression of the proinflammatory cytokines IL-6, IL-1β, and TNF-α in the livers of the exercise group. However, SFN treatment remarkably reduced the biomarkers of tissue damage and cell death. Along with the latter, SFN upregulated Nrf2 signaling by increasing the mRNA expression of Nrf2, HO-1, and the antioxidant enzymes SOD1, CAT, and GPx1 in the liver of SFN-treated animals.

The underlying mechanisms of SFN with respect to muscle health are summarized in Figure 5.

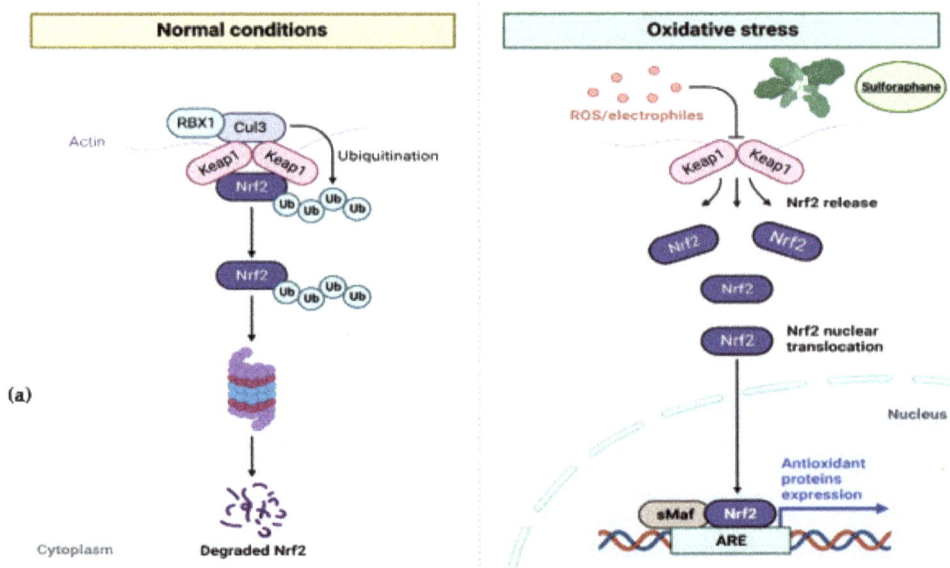

Figure 5. *Cont.*

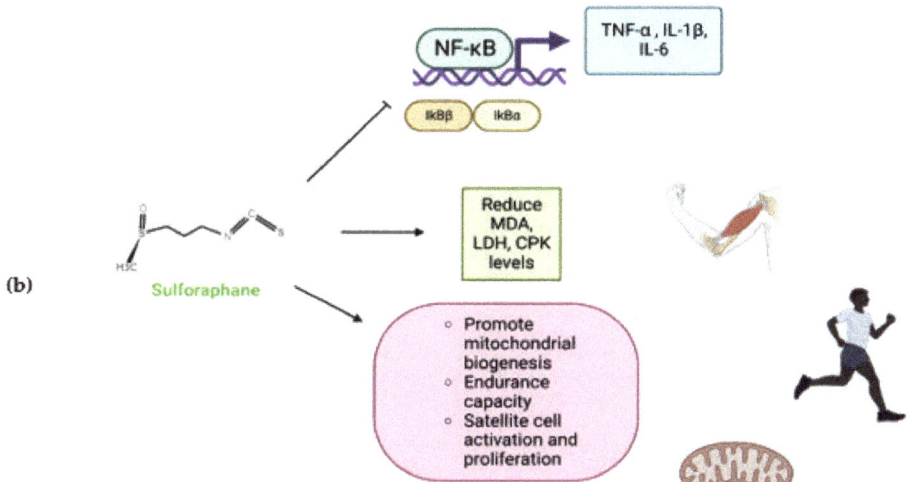

Figure 5. (**a**) Sulforaphane effects on Nrf2 signaling pathway. Sulforaphane promotes dissociation of Nrf2 from its negative regulator Keap1 leading to nuclear translocation and binding to the specific DNA sequence antioxidant response element (ARE) within small musculo-aponeurotic fibrosarcoma proteins (sMaf) inducing the antioxidant protein expression. (**b**) Effects of sulforaphane on skeletal muscle. Sulforaphane inhibits NF-κB inflammatory signaling and reduces muscle oxidative damage biomarkers such malonaldehyde (MDA), lactate dehydrogenase (LDH), and creatin phospho-kinase (CPK). Sulforaphane is capable of promoting mitochondrial biogenesis, improving aerobic endurance capacity, and enhancing satellite cell activation and proliferation. Created with BioRender.com.

4. Conclusions and Perspectives

The progressive deterioration of skeletal muscle mass can lead to the development of frailty and immobility in elderly individuals or in those suffering from chronic diseases such as cancer, diabetes, chronic kidney disease, AIDS, or severe trauma. The decrease in locomotion of the individual engenders dependency and a poor quality of life, in addition to generating a great burden for the economic budgets of health systems worldwide. Therefore, it is necessary to explore different medical alternatives to ascertain whether they are of aid in preventing deterioration or serve in the treatment of diseases that induce muscle damage or atrophy, promoting recovery and the maintenance of same. Since ancient times, the use of plants or foods has formed part of traditional medicine to improve human health. In this regard, it is known that there are endless species with specific therapeutic uses for certain conditions, which have been formally studied in order to find those responsible for their therapeutic effects. Based on this, it is known that there are active compounds in plants and foods with biological activity, denominated phytochemicals. Curcumin from *Curcuma longa* Linn and SFN from *Brassicaceae* species have been studied in several trials to prove their potential as nutraceuticals that are able to provide multiple benefits for human health.

In different models of muscle damage, including pathological or exhaustive exercise, curcumin and SFN have proven to be effective in preventing or reducing injuries to skeletal muscle mass by their investment in the promotion of the signaling pathways involved in cytoprotection and optimal antioxidant response. Both bioactive compounds efficiently blunt inflammation and help to recover skeletal muscle. In particular, curcumin has shown to prevent muscle atrophy by the suppression of protein synthesis, mostly by the downregulation of ubiquitin ligases and by the promotional, myogenetic, and mitochondrial qualities demonstrated in its in vitro and in vivo studies. A limitation of the use of phytochemicals lies in that the targeted studies employ supraphysiological amounts that are hardly achieved under normal circumstances with the foods containing them.

The issue of bioavailability must also be considered, as in the case of curcumin, but not with SFN, contained in broccoli, in which other factors are involved, such as preparing, cooking, etc. Finally, more studies should be conducted in humans because, although research on cell lines or in animal models is quite useful for understanding the molecular mechanisms by which active compounds act, it is necessary to understand their effects on human biological systems.

Author Contributions: N.V.-M. and J.A.M.-G. conceived and designed the study; N.V.-M., Á.M.-G., E.M.-S., M.M.-M., E.V.R.-N., E.M.-B., I.Á.-G., L.D.-O., L.A.-R. and J.L.A.-F. edited and wrote some portions of the paper, compiled the references, and analyzed the data; J.A.M.-G. Á.M.-G. and N.V.-M. wrote the manuscript. All authors have read and agreed to the published version of the manuscript.

Funding: Secretaría de Investigación y Posgrado, Instituto Politécnico Nacional: SIP-IPN:20220185.

Acknowledgments: Nancy Vargas-Mendoza is a scholarship holder for her postgraduate studies with the Consejo Nacional de Ciencia y Tecnologia (CONACyT) and the BEIFI program, Instituto Politécnico Nacional (IPN), Mexico.

Conflicts of Interest: The authors declare no conflict of interest.

References

1. Bonaldo, P.; Sandri, M. Cellular and molecular mechanisms of muscle atrophy. *Dis. Models Mech.* **2013**, *6*, 25–39. [CrossRef] [PubMed]
2. Schiaffino, S.; Dyar, K.A.; Ciciliot, S.; Blaauw, B.; Sandri, M. Mechanisms regulating skeletal muscle growth and atrophy. *FEBS J.* **2013**, *280*, 4294–4314. [CrossRef] [PubMed]
3. Glass, D.J. PI3 kinase regulation of skeletal muscle hypertrophy and atrophy. *Curr. Top. Microbiol. Immunol.* **2010**, *346*, 267–278. [CrossRef] [PubMed]
4. Li, H.; Malhotra, S.; Kumar, A. Nuclear factor-kappa B signaling in skeletal muscle atrophy. *J. Mol. Med.* **2008**, *86*, 1113–1126. [CrossRef]
5. Rom, O.; Reznick, A.Z. The role of E3 ubiquitin-ligases MuRF-1 and MAFbx in loss of skeletal muscle mass. *Free Radic. Biol. Med.* **2016**, *98*, 218–230. [CrossRef]
6. Hunter, R.B.; Stevenson, E.; Koncarevic, A.; Mitchell-Felton, H.; Essig, D.A.; Kandarian, S.C. Activation of an alternative NF-kappaB pathway in skeletal muscle during disuse atrophy. *FASEB J. Off. Publ. Fed. Am. Soc. Exp. Biol.* **2002**, *16*, 529–538. [CrossRef]
7. Bodine, S.C.; Baehr, L.M. Skeletal muscle atrophy and the E3 ubiquitin ligases MuRF1 and MAFbx/atrogin-1. *Am. J. Physiol. Endocrinol. Metab.* **2014**, *307*, E469–E484. [CrossRef]
8. Zhao, J.; Brault, J.J.; Schild, A.; Cao, P.; Sandri, M.; Schiaffino, S.; Lecker, S.H.; Goldberg, A.L. FoxO3 coordinately activates protein degradation by the autophagic/lysosomal and proteasomal pathways in atrophying muscle cells. *Cell Metab.* **2007**, *6*, 472–483. [CrossRef]
9. Mammucari, C.; Milan, G.; Romanello, V.; Masiero, E.; Rudolf, R.; Del Piccolo, P.; Burden, S.J.; Di Lisi, R.; Sandri, C.; Zhao, J.; et al. FoxO3 controls autophagy in skeletal muscle in vivo. *Cell Metab.* **2007**, *6*, 458–471. [CrossRef]
10. Zheng, L.F.; Chen, P.J.; Xiao, W.H. Signaling pathways controlling skeletal muscle mass. *Sheng Li Xue Bao (Acta Physiol. Sin.)* **2019**, *71*, 671–679.
11. Uchida, T.; Sakashita, Y.; Kitahata, K.; Yamashita, Y.; Tomida, C.; Kimori, Y.; Komatsu, A.; Hirasaka, K.; Ohno, A.; Nakao, R.; et al. Reactive oxygen species upregulate expression of muscle atrophy-associated ubiquitin ligase Cbl-b in rat L6 skeletal muscle cells. *Am. J. Physiol. Cell Physiol.* **2018**, *314*, C721–C731. [CrossRef]
12. Le Moal, E.; Pialoux, V.; Juban, G.; Groussard, C.; Zouhal, H.; Chazaud, B.; Mounier, R. Redox Control of Skeletal Muscle Regeneration. *Antioxid. Redox Signal.* **2017**, *27*, 276–310. [CrossRef] [PubMed]
13. Jang, Y.C.; Rodriguez, K.; Lustgarten, M.S.; Muller, F.L.; Bhattacharya, A.; Pierce, A.; Choi, J.J.; Lee, N.H.; Chaudhuri, A.; Richardson, A.G.; et al. Superoxide-mediated oxidative stress accelerates skeletal muscle atrophy by synchronous activation of proteolytic systems. *GeroScience* **2020**, *42*, 1579–1591. [CrossRef] [PubMed]
14. Beaudart, C.; Bonnefoy, M.; Gilbert, T.; Paillaud, E.; Raynaud-Simon, A.; Guérin, O.; Jeandel, C.; Le Sourd, B.; Haine, M.; Ferry, M.; et al. Which quality of life for the sarcopenic patient? *Geriatr. Et Psychol. Neuropsychiatr. Du Vieil.* **2021**, *19*, 245–252. [CrossRef] [PubMed]
15. Zhang, Y.J.; Gan, R.Y.; Li, S.; Zhou, Y.; Li, A.N.; Xu, D.P.; Li, H.B. Antioxidant Phytochemicals for the Prevention and Treatment of Chronic Diseases. *Molecules* **2015**, *20*, 21138–21156. [CrossRef]
16. Nikawa, T.; Ulla, A.; Sakakibara, I. Polyphenols and Their Effects on Muscle Atrophy and Muscle Health. *Molecules* **2021**, *26*, 4887. [CrossRef]
17. Royal Botanic Gardens, K. Plants of the World Online, *Curcuma longa* L. Available online: http://www.plantsoftheworldonline.org/ (accessed on 14 July 2022).

18. Fuloria, S.; Mehta, J.; Chandel, A.; Sekar, M.; Rani, N.; Begum, M.Y.; Subramaniyan, V.; Chidambaram, K.; Thangavelu, L.; Nordin, R.; et al. A Comprehensive Review on the Therapeutic Potential of *Curcuma longa* Linn. in Relation to its Major Active Constituent Curcumin. *Front. Pharmacol.* **2022**, *13*, 820806. [CrossRef]
19. Prasad, S.; Gupta, S.C.; Tyagi, A.K.; Aggarwal, B.B. Curcumin, a component of golden spice: From bedside to bench and back. *Biotechnol. Adv.* **2014**, *32*, 1053–1064. [CrossRef]
20. Nisar, T.; Iqbal, M.; Raza, A.; Safdar, M.; Iftikhar, F.; Waheed, M. Estimation of Total Phenolics and Free Radical Scavenging of Turmeric (*Curcuma longa*). *Environ. Sci.* **2015**, *15*, 1272–1277. [CrossRef]
21. Sun, W.; Wang, S.; Zhao, W.; Wu, C.; Guo, S.; Gao, H.; Tao, H.; Lu, J.; Wang, Y.; Chen, X. Chemical constituents and biological research on plants in the genus Curcuma. *Crit. Rev. Food Sci. Nutr.* **2017**, *57*, 1451–1523. [CrossRef]
22. Esatbeyoglu, T.; Huebbe, P.; Ernst, I.M.; Chin, D.; Wagner, A.E.; Rimbach, G. Curcumin–from molecule to biological function. *Angew. Chem.* **2012**, *51*, 5308–5332. [CrossRef] [PubMed]
23. Yang, K.-Y.; Lin, L.-C.; Tseng, T.-Y.; Wang, S.-C.; Tsai, T.-H. Oral bioavailability of curcumin in rat and the herbal analysis from *Curcuma longa* by LC–MS/MS. *J. Chromatogr. B* **2007**, *853*, 183–189. [CrossRef]
24. Vareed, S.K.; Kakarala, M.; Ruffin, M.T.; Crowell, J.A.; Normolle, D.P.; Djuric, Z.; Brenner, D.E. Pharmacokinetics of Curcumin Conjugate Metabolites in Healthy Human Subjects. *Cancer Epidemiol. Biomark. Prev.* **2008**, *17*, 1411–1417. [CrossRef] [PubMed]
25. Toden, S.; Goel, A. The Holy Grail of Curcumin and its Efficacy in Various Diseases: Is Bioavailability Truly a Big Concern? *J. Restor. Med.* **2017**, *6*, 27–36. [CrossRef] [PubMed]
26. Dei Cas, M.; Ghidoni, R. Dietary Curcumin: Correlation between Bioavailability and Health Potential. *Nutrients* **2019**, *11*, 2147. [CrossRef]
27. Jäger, R.; Lowery, R.P.; Calvanese, A.V.; Joy, J.M.; Purpura, M.; Wilson, J.M. Comparative absorption of curcumin formulations. *Nutr. J.* **2014**, *13*, 11. [CrossRef] [PubMed]
28. Purpura, M.; Lowery, R.P.; Wilson, J.M.; Mannan, H.; Münch, G.; Razmovski-Naumovski, V. Analysis of different innovative formulations of curcumin for improved relative oral bioavailability in human subjects. *Eur. J. Nutr.* **2018**, *57*, 929–938. [CrossRef]
29. Panda, S.K.; Nirvanashetty, S.; Missamma, M.; Jackson-Michel, S. The enhanced bioavailability of free curcumin and bioactive-metabolite tetrahydrocurcumin from a dispersible, oleoresin-based turmeric formulation. *Medicine* **2021**, *100*, e26601. [CrossRef]
30. Kothaplly, S.; Alukapally, S.; Nagula, N.; Maddela, R. Superior Bioavailability of a Novel Curcumin Formulation in Healthy Humans Under Fasting Conditions. *Adv. Ther.* **2022**, *39*, 2128–2138. [CrossRef]
31. Thanawala, S.; Shah, R.; Alluri, K.V.; Somepalli, V.; Vaze, S.; Upadhyay, V. Comparative bioavailability of curcuminoids from a water-dispersible high curcuminoid turmeric extract against a generic turmeric extract: A randomized, cross-over, comparative, pharmacokinetic study. *J. Pharm. Pharmacol.* **2021**, *73*, 816–823. [CrossRef]
32. Shoba, G.; Joy, D.; Joseph, T.; Majeed, M.; Rajendran, R.; Srinivas, P.S. Influence of piperine on the pharmacokinetics of curcumin in animals and human volunteers. *Planta Med.* **1998**, *64*, 353–356. [CrossRef]
33. Anand, P.; Kunnumakkara, A.B.; Newman, R.A.; Aggarwal, B.B. Bioavailability of curcumin: Problems and promises. *Mol. Pharm.* **2007**, *4*, 807–818. [CrossRef] [PubMed]
34. Hoehle, S.I.; Pfeiffer, E.; Metzler, M. Glucuronidation of curcuminoids by human microsomal and recombinant UDP-glucuronosyltransferases. *Mol. Nutr. Food Res.* **2007**, *51*, 932–938. [CrossRef]
35. Schneider, C.; Gordon, O.N.; Edwards, R.L.; Luis, P.B. Degradation of Curcumin: From Mechanism to Biological Implications. *J. Agric. Food Chem.* **2015**, *63*, 7606–7614. [CrossRef] [PubMed]
36. Pan, M.H.; Huang, T.M.; Lin, J.K. Biotransformation of curcumin through reduction and glucuronidation in mice. *Drug Metab. Dispos. Biol. Fate Chem.* **1999**, *27*, 486–494. [PubMed]
37. Ravindranath, V.; Chandrasekhara, N. Metabolism of curcumin—Studies with [3H] curcumin. *Toxicology* **1981**, *22*, 337–344. [CrossRef]
38. Alamdari, N.; O'Neal, P.; Hasselgren, P.O. Curcumin and muscle wasting: A new role for an old drug? *Nutrition* **2009**, *25*, 125–129. [CrossRef]
39. Poylin, V.; Fareed, M.U.; O'Neal, P.; Alamdari, N.; Reilly, N.; Menconi, M.; Hasselgren, P.O. The NF-kappaB inhibitor curcumin blocks sepsis-induced muscle proteolysis. *Mediat. Inflamm.* **2008**, *2008*, 317851. [CrossRef]
40. Thaloor, D.; Miller, K.J.; Gephart, J.; Mitchell, P.O.; Pavlath, G.K. Systemic administration of the NF-kappaB inhibitor curcumin stimulates muscle regeneration after traumatic injury. *Am. J. Physiol.* **1999**, *277*, C320–C329. [CrossRef]
41. Chattopadhyay, I.; Bandyopadhyay, U.; Biswas, K.; Maity, P.; Banerjee, R.K. Indomethacin inactivates gastric peroxidase to induce reactive-oxygen-mediated gastric mucosal injury and curcumin protects it by preventing peroxidase inactivation and scavenging reactive oxygen. *Free Radic. Biol. Med.* **2006**, *40*, 1397–1408. [CrossRef]
42. Thiemermann, C. The spice of life: Curcumin reduces the mortality associated with experimental sepsis. *Crit. Care Med.* **2006**, *34*, 2009–2011. [CrossRef] [PubMed]
43. Jin, B.; Li, Y.-P. Curcumin prevents lipopolysaccharide-induced atrogin-1/MAFbx upregulation and muscle mass loss. *J. Cell. Biochem.* **2007**, *100*, 960–969. [CrossRef] [PubMed]
44. Siddiqui, R.A.; Hassan, S.; Harvey, K.A.; Rasool, T.; Das, T.; Mukerji, P.; DeMichele, S. Attenuation of proteolysis and muscle wasting by curcumin c3 complex in MAC16 colon tumour-bearing mice. *Br. J. Nutr.* **2009**, *102*, 967–975. [CrossRef]

45. Thambamroong, T.; Seetalarom, K.; Saichaemchan, S.; Pumsutas, Y.; Prasongsook, N. Efficacy of Curcumin on Treating Cancer Anorexia-Cachexia Syndrome in Locally or Advanced Head and Neck Cancer: A Double-Blind, Placebo-Controlled Randomised Phase IIa Trial (CurChexia). *J. Nutr. Metab.* **2022**, *2022*, 5425619. [CrossRef]
46. Ono, T.; Takada, S.; Kinugawa, S.; Tsutsui, H. Curcumin ameliorates skeletal muscle atrophy in type 1 diabetic mice by inhibiting protein ubiquitination. *Exp. Physiol.* **2015**, *100*, 1052–1063. [CrossRef]
47. Kim, S.; Kim, K.; Park, J.; Jun, W. *Curcuma longa* L. Water Extract Improves Dexamethasone-Induced Sarcopenia by Modulating the Muscle-Related Gene and Oxidative Stress in Mice. *Antioxidants* **2021**, *10*, 1000. [CrossRef]
48. Zhang, M.; Tang, J.; Li, Y.; Xie, Y.; Shan, H.; Chen, M.; Zhang, J.; Yang, X.; Zhang, Q.; Yang, X. Curcumin attenuates skeletal muscle mitochondrial impairment in COPD rats: PGC-1α/SIRT3 pathway involved. *Chem. Biol. Interact.* **2017**, *277*, 168–175. [CrossRef] [PubMed]
49. Deane, C.S.; Din, U.S.U.; Sian, T.S.; Smith, K.; Gates, A.; Lund, J.N.; Williams, J.P.; Rueda, R.; Pereira, S.L.; Atherton, P.J.; et al. Curcumin Enhances Fed-State Muscle Microvascular Perfusion but Not Leg Glucose Uptake in Older Adults. *Nutrients* **2022**, *14*, 1313. [CrossRef] [PubMed]
50. Mañas-García, L.; Guitart, M.; Duran, X.; Barreiro, E. Satellite Cells and Markers of Muscle Regeneration during Unloading and Reloading: Effects of Treatment with Resveratrol and Curcumin. *Nutrients* **2020**, *12*, 1870. [CrossRef]
51. Lawler, J.M.; Hord, J.M.; Ryan, P.; Holly, D.; Janini Gomes, M.; Rodriguez, D.; Guzzoni, V.; Garcia-Villatoro, E.; Green, C.; Lee, Y.; et al. Nox2 Inhibition Regulates Stress Response and Mitigates Skeletal Muscle Fiber Atrophy during Simulated Microgravity. *Int. J. Mol. Sci.* **2021**, *22*, 3252. [CrossRef]
52. Gorza, L.; Germinario, E.; Tibaudo, L.; Vitadello, M.; Tusa, C.; Guerra, I.; Bondì, M.; Salmaso, S.; Caliceti, P.; Vitiello, L.; et al. Chronic Systemic Curcumin Administration Antagonizes Murine Sarcopenia and Presarcopenia. *Int. J. Mol. Sci.* **2021**, *22*, 1789. [CrossRef] [PubMed]
53. Johns, N.; Stephens, N.A.; Fearon, K.C. Muscle wasting in cancer. *Int. J. Biochem. Cell Biol.* **2013**, *45*, 2215–2229. [CrossRef] [PubMed]
54. López-Armada, M.J.; Riveiro-Naveira, R.R.; Vaamonde-García, C.; Valcárcel-Ares, M.N. Mitochondrial dysfunction and the inflammatory response. *Mitochondrion* **2013**, *13*, 106–118. [CrossRef] [PubMed]
55. Houten, S.M.; Auwerx, J. PGC-1α: Turbocharging mitochondria. *Cell* **2004**, *119*, 5–7. [CrossRef] [PubMed]
56. Rato, L.; Duarte, A.I.; Tomás, G.D.; Santos, M.S.; Moreira, P.I.; Socorro, S.; Cavaco, J.E.; Alves, M.G.; Oliveira, P.F. Pre-diabetes alters testicular PGC1-α/SIRT3 axis modulating mitochondrial bioenergetics and oxidative stress. *Biochim. Biophys. Acta (BBA) Bioenerg.* **2014**, *1837*, 335–344. [CrossRef] [PubMed]
57. Moorthi, R.N.; Avin, K.G. Clinical relevance of sarcopenia in chronic kidney disease. *Curr. Opin. Nephrol. Hypertens.* **2017**, *26*, 219–228. [CrossRef] [PubMed]
58. Wang, D.; Yang, Y.; Zou, X.; Zheng, Z.; Zhang, J. Curcumin ameliorates CKD-induced mitochondrial dysfunction and oxidative stress through inhibiting GSK-3β activity. *J. Nutr. Biochem.* **2020**, *83*, 108404. [CrossRef]
59. Yang, K.; Chen, Z.; Gao, J.; Shi, W.; Li, L.; Jiang, S.; Hu, H.; Liu, Z.; Xu, D.; Wu, L. The Key Roles of GSK-3β in Regulating Mitochondrial Activity. *Cell. Physiol. Biochem.* **2017**, *44*, 1445–1459. [CrossRef]
60. Theeuwes, W.F.; Gosker, H.R.; Langen, R.C.J.; Verhees, K.J.P.; Pansters, N.A.M.; Schols, A.M.W.J.; Remels, A.H.V. Inactivation of glycogen synthase kinase-3β (GSK-3β) enhances skeletal muscle oxidative metabolism. *Biochim. Biophys. Acta (BBA) Mol. Basis Dis.* **2017**, *1863*, 3075–3086. [CrossRef] [PubMed]
61. Theeuwes, W.F.; Gosker, H.R.; Langen, R.C.J.; Pansters, N.A.M.; Schols, A.; Remels, A.H.V. Inactivation of glycogen synthase kinase 3β (GSK-3β) enhances mitochondrial biogenesis during myogenesis. *Biochim. Biophys. Acta. Mol. Basis Dis.* **2018**, *1864*, 2913–2926. [CrossRef]
62. Lan, J.; Tang, L.; Wu, S.; Huang, R.; Zhong, G.; Jiang, X.; Tang, Z.; Hu, L. Curcumin alleviates arsenic-induced injury in duck skeletal muscle via regulating the PINK1/Parkin pathway and protecting mitochondrial function. *Toxicol. Appl. Pharmacol.* **2022**, *434*, 115820. [CrossRef] [PubMed]
63. Vazeille, E.; Slimani, L.; Claustre, A.; Magne, H.; Labas, R.; Béchet, D.; Taillandier, D.; Dardevet, D.; Astruc, T.; Attaix, D.; et al. Curcumin treatment prevents increased proteasome and apoptosome activities in rat skeletal muscle during reloading and improves subsequent recovery. *J. Nutr. Biochem.* **2012**, *23*, 245–251. [CrossRef]
64. Mañas-García, L.; Bargalló, N.; Gea, J.; Barreiro, E. Muscle Phenotype, Proteolysis, and Atrophy Signaling During Reloading in Mice: Effects of Curcumin on the Gastrocnemius. *Nutrients* **2020**, *12*, 388. [CrossRef] [PubMed]
65. Lawler, J.M.; Garcia-Villatoro, E.L.; Guzzoni, V.; Hord, J.M.; Botchlett, R.; Holly, D.; Lawler, M.S.; Janini Gomes, M.; Ryan, P.; Rodriguez, D.; et al. Effect of combined fish oil & Curcumin on murine skeletal muscle morphology and stress response proteins during mechanical unloading. *Nutr. Res.* **2019**, *65*, 17–28. [CrossRef]
66. Sahin, E.; Orhan, C.; Erten, F.; Er, B.; Acharya, M.; Morde, A.A.; Padigaru, M.; Sahin, K. Next-Generation Ultrasol Curcumin Boosts Muscle Endurance and Reduces Muscle Damage in Treadmill-Exhausted Rats. *Antioxidants* **2021**, *10*, 1692. [CrossRef] [PubMed]
67. Boz, I.; Belviranli, M.; Okudan, N. Curcumin Modulates Muscle Damage but not Oxidative Stress and Antioxidant Defense Following Eccentric Exercise in Rats. *Int. J. Vitam. Nutr. Res. Int. Z. Fur Vitam. Und Ernahrungsforschung. J. Int. Vitaminol. Nutr.* **2014**, *84*, 163–172. [CrossRef] [PubMed]

68. Sahin, K.; Pala, R.; Tuzcu, M.; Ozdemir, O.; Orhan, C.; Sahin, N.; Juturu, V. Curcumin prevents muscle damage by regulating NF-κB and Nrf2 pathways and improves performance: An in vivo model. *J. Inflamm. Res.* **2016**, *9*, 147–154. [CrossRef] [PubMed]
69. Wafi, A.M.; Hong, J.; Rudebush, T.L.; Yu, L.; Hackfort, B.; Wang, H.; Schultz, H.D.; Zucker, I.H.; Gao, L. Curcumin improves exercise performance of mice with coronary artery ligation-induced HFrEF: Nrf2 and antioxidant mechanisms in skeletal muscle. *J. Appl. Physiol.* **2019**, *126*, 477–486. [CrossRef]
70. Online, B. Characteristics of Brocolli. Available online: https://www.botanical-online.com/en/natural-products/broccoli (accessed on 20 July 2022).
71. Garden, M.B. Brassica Oleracea (Italica Group). Available online: https://www.missouribotanicalgarden.org/PlantFinder/PlantFinderDetails.aspx?taxonid=268653&isprofile=0& (accessed on 20 July 2022).
72. Brinckmann, J. Broccoli *Brassica oleracea* var. *italica*, Family: Brassicaceae. *HerbalGram* **2022**, *131*, 6–13. Available online: https://www.herbalgram.org/resources/herbalgram/issues/131/table-of-contents/hg131-herbprofile-broccoli/ (accessed on 20 July 2022).
73. Zhang, Y.; Talalay, P.; Cho, C.G.; Posner, G.H. A major inducer of anticarcinogenic protective enzymes from broccoli: Isolation and elucidation of structure. *Proc. Natl. Acad. Sci. USA* **1992**, *89*, 2399–2403. [CrossRef]
74. Dinkova-Kostova, A.T.; Kostov, R.V. Glucosinolates and isothiocyanates in health and disease. *Trends Mol. Med.* **2012**, *18*, 337–347. [CrossRef]
75. Vanduchova, A.; Anzenbacher, P.; Anzenbacherova, E. Isothiocyanate from Broccoli, Sulforaphane, and Its Properties. *J. Med. Food* **2019**, *22*, 121–126. [CrossRef]
76. Nakagawa, K.; Umeda, T.; Higuchi, O.; Tsuzuki, T.; Suzuki, T.; Miyazawa, T. Evaporative Light-Scattering Analysis of Sulforaphane in Broccoli Samples: Quality of Broccoli Products Regarding Sulforaphane Contents. *J. Agric. Food Chem.* **2006**, *54*, 2479–2483. [CrossRef] [PubMed]
77. Jin, Y.; Wang, M.; Rosen, R.T.; Ho, C.-T. Thermal Degradation of Sulforaphane in Aqueous Solution. *J. Agric. Food Chem.* **1999**, *47*, 3121–3123. [CrossRef] [PubMed]
78. Li, Y.; Zhang, T.; Li, X.; Zou, P.; Schwartz, S.J.; Sun, D. Kinetics of sulforaphane in mice after consumption of sulforaphane-enriched broccoli sprout preparation. *Mol. Nutr. Food Res.* **2013**, *57*, 2128–2136. [CrossRef] [PubMed]
79. Hanlon, N.; Coldham, N.; Gielbert, A.; Kuhnert, N.; Sauer, M.J.; King, L.J.; Ioannides, C. Absolute bioavailability and dose-dependent pharmacokinetic behaviour of dietary doses of the chemopreventive isothiocyanate sulforaphane in rat. *Br. J. Nutr.* **2008**, *99*, 559–564. [CrossRef]
80. Atwell, L.L.; Hsu, A.; Wong, C.P.; Stevens, J.F.; Bella, D.; Yu, T.-W.; Pereira, C.B.; Löhr, C.V.; Christensen, J.M.; Dashwood, R.H.; et al. Absorption and chemopreventive targets of sulforaphane in humans following consumption of broccoli sprouts or a myrosinase-treated broccoli sprout extract. *Mol. Nutr. Food Res.* **2015**, *59*, 424–433. [CrossRef]
81. Vermeulen, M.; Klöpping-Ketelaars, I.W.A.A.; van den Berg, R.; Vaes, W.H.J. Bioavailability and Kinetics of Sulforaphane in Humans after Consumption of Cooked versus Raw Broccoli. *J. Agric. Food Chem.* **2008**, *56*, 10505–10509. [CrossRef]
82. Fahey, J.W.; Wade, K.L.; Wehage, S.L.; Holtzclaw, W.D.; Liu, H.; Talalay, P.; Fuchs, E.; Stephenson, K.K. Stabilized sulforaphane for clinical use: Phytochemical delivery efficiency. *Mol. Nutr. Food Res.* **2017**, *61*, 1600766. [CrossRef]
83. Ye, L.; Dinkova-Kostova, A.T.; Wade, K.L.; Zhang, Y.; Shapiro, T.A.; Talalay, P. Quantitative determination of dithiocarbamates in human plasma, serum, erythrocytes and urine: Pharmacokinetics of broccoli sprout isothiocyanates in humans. *Clin. Chim. Acta* **2002**, *316*, 43–53. [CrossRef]
84. Su, X.; Jiang, X.; Meng, L.; Dong, X.; Shen, Y.; Xin, Y. Anticancer Activity of Sulforaphane: The Epigenetic Mechanisms and the Nrf2 Signaling Pathway. *Oxidative Med. Cell. Longev.* **2018**, *2018*, 5438179. [CrossRef]
85. Wang, X.; Chen, X.; Zhou, W.; Men, H.; Bao, T.; Sun, Y.; Wang, Q.; Tan, Y.; Keller, B.B.; Tong, Q.; et al. Ferroptosis is essential for diabetic cardiomyopathy and is prevented by sulforaphane via AMPK/NRF2 pathways. *Acta Pharm. Sinica. B* **2022**, *12*, 708–722. [CrossRef] [PubMed]
86. Subedi, L.; Lee, J.H.; Yumnam, S.; Ji, E.; Kim, S.Y. Anti-Inflammatory Effect of Sulforaphane on LPS-Activated Microglia Potentially through JNK/AP-1/NF-κB Inhibition and Nrf2/HO-1 Activation. *Cells* **2019**, *8*, 194. [CrossRef] [PubMed]
87. Ruhee, R.T.; Suzuki, K. The Integrative Role of Sulforaphane in Preventing Inflammation, Oxidative Stress and Fatigue: A Review of a Potential Protective Phytochemical. *Antioxidants* **2020**, *9*, 521. [CrossRef] [PubMed]
88. Moi, P.; Chan, K.; Asunis, I.; Cao, A.; Kan, Y.W. Isolation of NF-E2-related factor 2 (Nrf2), a NF-E2-like basic leucine zipper transcriptional activator that binds to the tandem NF-E2/AP1 repeat of the beta-globin locus control region. *Proc. Natl. Acad. Sci. USA* **1994**, *91*, 9926–9930. [CrossRef]
89. Itoh, K.; Wakabayashi, N.; Katoh, Y.; Ishii, T.; Igarashi, K.; Engel, J.D.; Yamamoto, M. Keap1 represses nuclear activation of antioxidant responsive elements by Nrf2 through binding to the amino-terminal Neh2 domain. *Genes Dev.* **1999**, *13*, 76–86. [CrossRef]
90. Itoh, K.; Igarashi, K.; Hayashi, N.; Nishizawa, M.; Yamamoto, M. Cloning and characterization of a novel erythroid cell-derived CNC family transcription factor heterodimerizing with the small Maf family proteins. *Mol. Cell. Biol.* **1995**, *15*, 4184–4193. [CrossRef]
91. Tu, W.; Wang, H.; Li, S.; Liu, Q.; Sha, H. The anti-inflammatory and anti-oxidant mechanisms of the Keap1/Nrf2/ARE signaling pathway in chronic diseases. *Aging Dis.* **2019**, *10*, 637–651. [CrossRef]

92. Sun, Z.; Huang, Z.; Zhang, D.D. Phosphorylation of Nrf2 at Multiple Sites by MAP Kinases Has a Limited Contribution in Modulating the Nrf2-Dependent Antioxidant Response. *PLoS ONE* **2009**, *4*, e6588. [CrossRef]
93. Hu, R.; Xu, C.; Shen, G.; Jain, M.R.; Khor, T.O.; Gopalkrishnan, A.; Lin, W.; Reddy, B.; Chan, J.Y.; Kong, A.N. Gene expression profiles induced by cancer chemopreventive isothiocyanate sulforaphane in the liver of C57BL/6J mice and C57BL/6J/Nrf2 (−/−) mice. *Cancer Lett.* **2006**, *243*, 170–192. [CrossRef]
94. Houghton, C.A.; Fassett, R.G.; Coombes, J.S. Sulforaphane: Translational research from laboratory bench to clinic. *Nutr. Rev.* **2013**, *71*, 709–726. [CrossRef]
95. Houghton, C.A.; Fassett, R.G.; Coombes, J.S. Sulforaphane and Other Nutrigenomic Nrf2 Activators: Can the Clinician's Expectation Be Matched by the Reality? *Oxidative Med. Cell. Longev.* **2016**, *2016*, 7857186. [CrossRef] [PubMed]
96. Yang, L.; Palliyaguru, D.L.; Kensler, T.W. Frugal chemoprevention: Targeting Nrf2 with foods rich in sulforaphane. *Semin. Oncol.* **2016**, *43*, 146–153. [CrossRef] [PubMed]
97. Sun, C.; Yang, C.; Xue, R.; Li, S.; Zhang, T.; Pan, L.; Ma, X.; Wang, L.; Li, D. Sulforaphane alleviates muscular dystrophy in mdx mice by activation of Nrf2. *J. Appl. Physiol.* **2015**, *118*, 224–237. [CrossRef] [PubMed]
98. Sun, C.C.; Li, S.J.; Yang, C.L.; Xue, R.L.; Xi, Y.Y.; Wang, L.; Zhao, Q.L.; Li, D.J. Sulforaphane Attenuates Muscle Inflammation in Dystrophin-deficient mdx Mice via NF-E2-related Factor 2 (Nrf2)-mediated Inhibition of NF-κB Signaling Pathway. *J. Biol. Chem.* **2015**, *290*, 17784–17795. [CrossRef] [PubMed]
99. Zhang, R.; Neuhoff, C.; Yang, Q.; Cinar, M.U.; Uddin, M.J.; Tholen, E.; Schellander, K.; Tesfaye, D. Sulforaphane Enhanced Proliferation of Porcine Satellite Cells via Epigenetic Augmentation of SMAD7. *Animals* **2022**, *12*, 1365. [CrossRef] [PubMed]
100. Malaguti, M.; Angeloni, C.; Garatachea, N.; Baldini, M.; Leoncini, E.; Collado, P.S.; Teti, G.; Falconi, M.; Gonzalez-Gallego, J.; Hrelia, S. Sulforaphane treatment protects skeletal muscle against damage induced by exhaustive exercise in rats. *J. Appl. Physiol.* **2009**, *107*, 1028–1036. [CrossRef]
101. Oh, S.; Komine, S.; Warabi, E.; Akiyama, K.; Ishii, A.; Ishige, K.; Mizokami, Y.; Kuga, K.; Horie, M.; Miwa, Y.; et al. Nuclear factor (erythroid derived 2)-like 2 activation increases exercise endurance capacity via redox modulation in skeletal muscles. *Sci. Rep.* **2017**, *7*, 12902. [CrossRef]
102. Komine, S.; Miura, I.; Miyashita, N.; Oh, S.; Tokinoya, K.; Shoda, J.; Ohmori, H. Effect of a sulforaphane supplement on muscle soreness and damage induced by eccentric exercise in young adults: A pilot study. *Physiol. Rep.* **2021**, *9*, e15130. [CrossRef]
103. Ruhee, R.T.; Ma, S.; Suzuki, K. Protective Effects of Sulforaphane on Exercise-Induced Organ Damage via Inducing Antioxidant Defense Responses. *Antioxidants* **2020**, *9*, 136. [CrossRef]
104. Fan, H.; Zhang, R.; Tesfaye, D.; Tholen, E.; Looft, C.; Hölker, M.; Schellander, K.; Cinar, M.U. Sulforaphane causes a major epigenetic repression of myostatin in porcine satellite cells. *Epigenetics* **2012**, *7*, 1379–1390. [CrossRef]
105. McCroskery, S.; Thomas, M.; Maxwell, L.; Sharma, M.; Kambadur, R. Myostatin negatively regulates satellite cell activation and self-renewal. *J. Cell Biol.* **2003**, *162*, 1135–1147. [CrossRef] [PubMed]
106. Cheng, A.J.; Yamada, T.; Rassier, D.E.; Andersson, D.C.; Westerblad, H.; Lanner, J.T. Reactive oxygen/nitrogen species and contractile function in skeletal muscle during fatigue and recovery. *J. Physiol.* **2016**, *594*, 5149–5160. [CrossRef] [PubMed]
107. Cheng, A.J.; Jude, B.; Lanner, J.T. Intramuscular mechanisms of overtraining. *Redox Biol.* **2020**, *35*, 101480. [CrossRef] [PubMed]
108. Wan, J.-j.; Qin, Z.; Wang, P.-y.; Sun, Y.; Liu, X. Muscle fatigue: General understanding and treatment. *Exp. Mol. Med.* **2017**, *49*, e384. [CrossRef] [PubMed]
109. Andrade, F.H.; Reid, M.B.; Allen, D.G.; Westerblad, H. Effect of hydrogen peroxide and dithiothreitol on contractile function of single skeletal muscle fibres from the mouse. *J. Physiol.* **1998**, *509*, 565–575. [CrossRef]
110. Suzuki, K.; Tominaga, T.; Ruhee, R.T.; Ma, S. Characterization and Modulation of Systemic Inflammatory Response to Exhaustive Exercise in Relation to Oxidative Stress. *Antioxidants* **2020**, *9*, 401. [CrossRef]

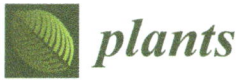

Review

The Protective Role of Cranberries and Blueberries in Oral Cancer

César Esquivel-Chirino [1,*], Mario Augusto Bolaños-Carrillo [2], Daniela Carmona-Ruiz [3], Ambar Lopéz-Macay [4], Fernando Hernández-Sánchez [5], Delina Montés-Sánchez [6], Montserrat Escuadra-Landeros [7], Luis Alberto Gaitán-Cepeda [8], Silvia Maldonado-Frías [9], Beatriz Raquel Yáñez-Ocampo [10], José Luis Ventura-Gallegos [11], Hugo Laparra-Escareño [12], Claudia Patricia Mejía-Velázquez [13] and Alejandro Zentella-Dehesa [11,14]

1. Área de Básicas Médicas, División de Estudios Profesionales, Facultad de Odontología, Universidad Nacional Autónoma de México, Ciudad de México 04510, Mexico
2. Área de Ciencias Naturales, Departamento de Bachillerato, Universidad del Valle de México, Campus Guadalajara Sur, Guadalajara 045601, Mexico; mario_bolanos@my.uvm.edu.mx
3. Área de Ortodoncia, División de Estudios Profesionales, Facultad de Odontología, Universidad Nacional Autónoma de México, Ciudad de México 04510, Mexico
4. Laboratorio de Liquído Sinovial, Instituto Nacional de Rehabilitación LGII, Ciudad de México 14389, Mexico
5. Departamento de Virología y Micología, Instituto Nacional de Enfermedades Respiratorias "Ismael Cosío Villegas", Ciudad de México 04502, Mexico
6. Investigación Biomédica Básica, Licenciatura en Estomatología, Benemérita Universidad Autónoma de Puebla, Puebla 75770, Mexico
7. Facultad de Odontología, Universidad Intercontinental, Ciudad de México 14420, Mexico
8. Departamento de Medicina y Patología Oral Clínica, División de Estudios de Posgrado e Investigación, Facultad de Odontología, Universidad Nacional Autónoma de México, Ciudad de México 04510, Mexico
9. Laboratorio de Bioingeniería de Tejidos, División de Estudios de Posgrado e Investigación, Facultad de Odontología, Universidad Nacional Autónoma de México, Ciudad de México 04360, Mexico; sylvymaf@comunidad.unam.mx
10. Especialidad en Periodoncia e Implantología, División de Estudios de Posgrado e Investigación, Facultad de Odontología, Universidad Nacional Autónoma de México, Ciudad de México 04510, Mexico
11. Departamento de Medicina Genómica y Toxicología Ambiental, Instituto de Investigaciones Biomédicas, UNAM, Ciudad de México 04510, Mexico
12. Departamento de Cirugía, Sección de Cirugía Vascular y Terapia, Instituto de Ciencias Médicas y Nutrición Salvador Zubirán, Ciudad de México 14080, Mexico
13. Departamento de Patología, Medicina Bucal y Maxilofacial, Facultad de Odontología, Universidad Nacional Autónoma de México, Ciudad de México 04510, Mexico
14. Unidad de Bioquímica, Instituto de Ciencias Médicas y Nutrición Salvador Zubirán, Ciudad de México 14080, Mexico
* Correspondence: seminarioinvestigacion@fo.odonto.unam.mx; Tel.: +52-55-5109-8656

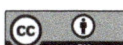

Citation: Esquivel-Chirino, C.; Bolaños-Carrillo, M.A.; Carmona-Ruiz, D.; Lopéz-Macay, A.; Hernández-Sánchez, F.; Montés-Sánchez, D.; Escuadra-Landeros, M.; Gaitán-Cepeda, L.A.; Maldonado-Frías, S.; Yáñez-Ocampo, B.R.; et al. The Protective Role of Cranberries and Blueberries in Oral Cancer. *Plants* **2023**, *12*, 2330. https://doi.org/10.3390/plants12122330

Academic Editor: Milena Popova

Received: 17 May 2023
Revised: 8 June 2023
Accepted: 10 June 2023
Published: 15 June 2023

Copyright: © 2023 by the authors. Licensee MDPI, Basel, Switzerland. This article is an open access article distributed under the terms and conditions of the Creative Commons Attribution (CC BY) license (https://creativecommons.org/licenses/by/4.0/).

Abstract: Background: Oral cancer has a high prevalence worldwide, and this disease is caused by genetic, immunological, and environmental factors. The main risk factors associated with oral cancer are smoking and alcohol. Results: There are various strategies to reduce risk factors, including prevention programs as well as the consumption of an adequate diet that includes phytochemical compounds derived from cranberries (*Vaccinium macrocarpon* A.) and blueberries (*Vaccinium corymbosum* L.); these compounds exhibit antitumor properties. Results: The main outcome of this review is as follows: the properties of phytochemicals derived from cranberries were evaluated for protection against risk factors associated with oral cancer. Conclusions: The secondary metabolites of cranberries promote biological effects that provide protection against smoking and alcoholism. An alternative for the prevention of oral cancer can be the consumption of these cranberries and blueberries.

Keywords: oral cancer; oral squamous carcinoma cell (OSCC); phytochemicals; berries; flavonoids; flavanols; cranberries; blueberries

1. Background

Cancer is a disease characterized by the proliferation of tumor cells, followed by the invasion of distant organs (metastasis), and can cause serious health complications, often leading to the death of the patient [1–5]. According to statistics from 2020, approximately 10 million people in the world died from cancer, and one in every six deaths was attributed to this disease. A significant percentage of cases correspond to oral cancer, which affects anatomical regions, such as the base of the tongue, lip, gingiva, tonsil, floor of the mouth, and uvula [6–8]. Oral cancer accounts for 85% of neoplasms in the oral cavity [9].

Approximately 90% of oral cancers correspond to oral squamous cell carcinoma, while the remaining 10% are classified as melanomas, sarcomas, minor salivary gland carcinomas, or metastatic carcinomas [10]. Oral cancer survival is reported to average five years [11,12]. The cause of oral cancer involves several factors, including genetic, environmental, immunological, and viral infections, and contact mainly with tobacco and alcohol consumption [6]. An inadequate daily diet, especially a low consumption of fruits and vegetables, is another important factor associated with cancer progression [13,14]. A balanced diet should include compounds derived from plant and fruit extracts, such as phytochemicals, phenolics, and flavonoids, to obtain their antioxidant and protective properties against various risk factors, as well as their antitumor effects [15–17]. Furthermore, the use of phytochemicals has been identified as a possible protective factor against oral cancer, particularly in fruits of the *Ericaceae* family, such as cranberries and blueberries [18].

Berries contain phytochemical compounds with biological activity, such as flavanols, ellagitannins, gallotannins, proanthocyanidins, and anthocyanins [15–17]. The antioxidant and antitumor properties of berry phytochemicals have been shown in vitro and in vivo in oral cancer models [17–21]. The aim of this work is to investigate the antioxidant activities of berry and cranberry phytochemicals in protecting the oral mucosa against oral cancer risk factors.

2. Materials and Methods

A comprehensive literature search was conducted from March 2000 to March 2023. Keyword searches were conducted in databases, such as PubMed, EBSCO, Wiley, and SpringerLink, using terms, such as "oral cancer,", "berries", "oral cancer and berries", "phytochemicals and oral cancer", and "cranberries and oral cancer." Articles were selected if they contained information about phytochemicals and cancer. Studies that mentioned effects on other types of cancer were also included. The exclusion criteria were articles that were not written in English and articles from popular science journals and dissertations.

3. Introduction

3.1. Head and Neck Cancer

This neoplasm involves the oral cavity, larynx, oropharynx, and paranasal sinuses (Figure 1) [21,22].

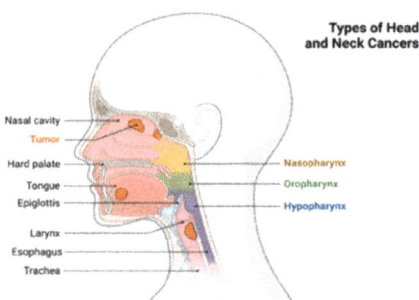

Figure 1. Head and neck cancer distribution. Created with BioRender.com (accessed on 10 March 2022).

3.2. Oral Cancer

Oral cancer is defined as a malignant neoplasm that can manifest in any part of the oral cavity [21]. The most frequent anatomical sites for oral cancer are the tongue (including the base and anterior part), gums, tonsils, oropharynx, lips, floor of the mouth, soft and hard palate, oral mucosa, and salivary glands (Figure 2) [22].

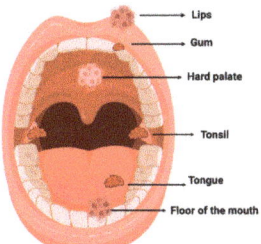

Figure 2. Distribution of oral cancer. Created with BioRender.com (accessed on 10 March 2022).

3.3. Epidemiology

Oral cancer represents the sixth-highest prevalence of malignant neoplasms in the developed world; however, it is the eighth most-prevalent malignant neoplasm in less-developed countries [23]. During 2020, 377,713 new cases of oral cancer were diagnosed worldwide, and of those cases, 177,757 resulted in death [24,25]. A retrospective study conducted between 1990 and 2019 reported that Asia had the highest number of oral cancer cases, followed by North America, South America, and Europe [26]. Oral cancer is 3.6 times more frequent among men than women, with higher mortality rates in underdeveloped countries [27].

3.4. Etiology and Risk Factors

The cause of oral cancer involves multiple factors; however, the main risk factors are tobacco and alcohol consumption [7,28]. Several risk factors have been identified for oral cancer, including viral infections, especially human papillomavirus (HPV), immunosuppression, genetic predisposition, poor oral hygiene, and an inadequate diet [26,27,29]. Another important factor associated with oral cancer is chronic inflammatory processes, such as periodontal disease [30,31].

3.4.1. Tobacco

The use of tobacco products is the principal cause of more than 8 million cancer deaths worldwide [32]. Tobacco products have different carcinogenic properties [33]. People who smoke have a predisposition to oral cancer that is between seven and ten times higher than that of nonsmokers, although the level of exposure depends on the frequency and duration of smoking [34–37]. The most common carcinogens in tobacco are benzopyrenes, 4-(methylnitrosamine)-1-(3-pyridyl)-1-butanone, and N′-nitrosornornicotine (NNN) [38,39]. The metabolites of these compounds present in tobacco induce mutations that affect DNA replication and the genes involved in the control of cell growth, favoring damage to the oral mucosa and malignant transformation [40,41]. In Asia, a form of smokeless tobacco called Guthka is consumed, which is a mixture of betel nut (*Areca catechu*), tobacco, and spices. This preparation is popular among the young population due to its stimulating, relaxing effects [42]. However, betel nut contains tannins and alkaloids, such as arecoline, which have negative effects on health and have been associated with oral cancer [30,42]. Tobacco products have carcinogenic and genotoxic effects on epithelial cells and are related to pancreatic cancer, cardiovascular disease, periodontal conditions, and asthma [31]. In addition, tobacco consumption can contribute to the development of esophageal carcinoma [43]. Tobacco products generate reactive oxygen species (ROS), change pH, and cause mucosal irritation, activating T cells as well as macrophages, which promote prostaglandin production and hyperplasia [40]. These types of irritants and subsequent inflammation are important promoter events in the progression to malignant transformation.

3.4.2. Alcohol

Alcohol consumption is a recognized factor in the development of oral and oropharyngeal cancer [12,40]. The main metabolite of alcohol is acetaldehyde, which is involved in DNA synthesis and repair and induces, among many other effects, the exchange of sister chromatids and mutations [40,41]. Alcohol acts as a local irritant chemical when in contact with the oral mucosa. Therefore, by dissolving and damaging the lipids of the epithelium, alcohol consumption increases the permeability of the oral mucosa [44]. Frequent alcohol consumption is associated with impaired innate and acquired immunity, which increases the susceptibility of the oral cavity to infections and neoplasms [45]. Alcohol is metabolized by enzymes, such as dehydrogenase, cytochrome P-4502 E1, and catalases, generating acetaldehyde. This metabolite has carcinogenic and genotoxic properties [46]. In addition, the consumption of alcohol activates inflammatory processes since inflammatory white cells are recruited and various interleukins are produced, which causes the formation of ROS [47]. It has been reported that the consumption of 10 g or more of alcohol per day has been related to a 15% increased risk of having oral cancer and a 10% increased risk of having pharyngeal cancer [48]. Oral squamous cell carcinoma is related to polymorphisms of the ALDH2 gene [49]. Alcohol and tobacco use increase the risk of oral cancer up to five-fold [50–52].

3.4.3. Viral Infections

The major viral infections associated with oral cancer include human herpesvirus and human papillomavirus (HPV) [53,54]. These viruses cause genetic instability through mutations, aberrations, and DNA damage [55].

Human Papillomavirus

HPV is the virus most frequently associated with cases of oral cancer [56]. HPV genotypes 16 and 18 are the most frequently associated with oral cancer. HPV encodes two oncoproteins, E6 and E7, which bind to p53 and Rb proteins, causing the loss of regulation of DNA replication, repair, and apoptosis [57].

Epstein–Barr Virus

This virus presents double-stranded DNA with oncogenic potential and has been considered the causal agent of several neoplasms, including squamous oral cell carcinoma (OSCC) [58]. In 1997, this virus was recognized as the cause of nasopharyngeal carcinoma and has also been associated with Hodgkin lymphoma, NK cell lymphoma, and gastric carcinoma [59]. People infected with Epstein–Barr virus have a 2.5-fold increased probability of acquiring OSCC. However, the direct association between OSCC and Epstein–Barr virus is not completely clear [60].

3.4.4. Oral Health

Poor oral hygiene can affect the oral microbiota by allowing bacteria to evade the host immune response and increase their growth, which can cause a shift from symbiosis to dysbiosis [61]. In addition, an increased amount of endogenous nitrosamine, a major carcinogen, is produced, which may pose a risk for oral cancer initiation [50]. A report found that, in patients with inadequate mouth hygiene, there was a seven-fold increased risk of developing oral cancer [51]. In addition, tooth fractures, tooth decay, and poorly fitting dentures can cause chronic irritation of the oral mucosa, which, in combination with other factors, such as smoking or drinking alcohol, may promote the occurrence of oral cancer [62]. Another relevant factor is the use of mouthwashes containing alcohol as a solvent or preservative in combination with tobacco or alcohol consumption [63,64].

However, there are no conclusive data to suggest an increased risk of oral cancer from the use of these mouthwashes alone.

3.4.5. Diet and Nutrition

Several studies have found that low fruit and vegetable consumption may contribute to the increased risk of developing oral cancer [65]. A high body mass index (BMI) has been implicated in an elevated risk of developing oral cancer [66]. It is important to analyze the relationship between food consumption and the risk of oral cancer. To date, it is considered that an adequate diet should include the consumption of phytochemicals, phenolics, and flavonoids that have antioxidant and antitumor properties [16–18]. In addition, the consumption of phytochemicals has been reported to have protective effects against risk factors associated with oral cancer [18]. Therefore, it is recommended to consume foods that contain a significant concentration of phytochemicals, such as berries, the consumption of which has been related to a reduction in oxidative stress and inflammation [16].

3.5. Premalignant Lesions

One area of opportunity remains the early detection of oral cancer. Therefore, the development of programs and strategies for the early detection of premalignant lesions may improve patient survival and prognosis [67]. Therefore, a detailed patient history and a thorough clinical examination are essential [16]. Oral cancer patients have no symptoms in the early stages, leading to diagnosis in advanced stages [61]. Prevention programs should guide oral health professionals to search for and identify precancerous lesions. The most common premalignant lesions are leukoplakia, erythroplakia, and oral lichen planus [68].

3.5.1. Leucoplakia

Leucoplakia is characterized by white spots or plaques that are not scraped off. In the clinical diagnosis, leukoplakia must be differentiated from other lesions, such as lichen planus, candidiasis, friction keratosis, smoker's keratosis, nicotinic and uremic stomatitis, leukoedema, and hairy leukoplakia [68]. Leucoplakia has been reported to have a malignant transformation rate between 1 and 5%; however, studies suggest that it may have a chance of dysplasia or invasive carcinoma [69,70].

3.5.2. Erythroplasia

Erythroplasia is characterized by the presence of a red patch or spot. It is considered a high-risk lesion for malignancy and must be differentiated from erythematous candidiasis, erythema migrans, lichen planus lesions, lupus, and other erosive lesions [71,72]. In contrast to leukoplakia, erythroplakia is more than 90% likely to have dysplasia or carcinoma in situ [73].

3.5.3. Lichen Planus

Lichen planus is an inflammatory disease from an unclear cause that presents as white reticular lesions that may be associated with atrophic, erosive, ulcerative, and plaque-like areas [74]. The pathophysiology of lichen planus begins with an autoimmune response mediated by T lymphocytes that causes alterations in the basal cells of the epithelium, generating an inflammatory infiltrate in the basement membrane and leading to subsequent complications [75].

3.6. Histological Aspects of Oral Cancer

Oral cancer presents various degrees of histological differentiation. Histologic features include (1) loss of basement membrane and stratum basal structure, (2) increased number of mitoses, and (3) invasion of the underlying connective tissue [75,76]. Oral cancer is the result of genetic and epigenetic changes that lead to histological changes, all associated with a malignant transformation of the epithelium [77,78]. It is an invasive neoplasm that has a poor prognosis and can develop metastases in distant organs. Oral cancer metastases spread primarily through the submandibular, cervical, and jugular lymph nodes. Distant metastasis spreads to the jaw and finally to the lungs, which compromises the health of the patient and has a higher risk of death [17–20]. Investigating and identifying the major mechanisms involved in oral carcinogenesis is therefore important.

3.7. Carcinogenesis of Oral Cancer

Carcinogenesis is a process that involves the alteration of molecular function, changes in cell morphology, and epithelial, connective tissue, and immune function. As a result of this process, cells acquire new functions that allow them to survive and proliferate [79]. Carcinogenesis comprises three phases: initiation, promotion, and progression. During initiation, endogenous and exogenous factors generate molecular defects, such as mutations, chromosomal abnormalities, and epigenetic alterations [80]. The initiation phase continues through the promotion phase, which is characterized by the selective proliferation of tumor cells with stem cell characteristics. Then, the progression phase continues, in which tumor cells act on their tumor microenvironment to create conditions that favor cell proliferation and survival [81]. In the carcinogenesis of oral cancer, oncogenes and tumor suppressor genes and their associated epigenetic alterations play an important role [82].

3.7.1. Oncogenes and Tumor Suppressor Genes

Proto-oncogenes encode the proteins that regulate cell division and differentiation and activate oncogenes through DNA mutations and the inactivation of tumor suppressor genes [83]. Various oncogenes have been implicated in oral cancer development, including the epidermal growth factor receptor (EGFR/c-erb 1), members of the Ras gene family, c-myc, int-2, hst-1, PRAD-1, and bcl-1 [84]. Gain-function mutations of these oncogenes facilitate the appearance of neoplastic transformation. On the other hand, tumor suppressor genes participate in oral carcinogenesis and their alteration indicates the onset of a neoplastic transformation. Tumor suppressor genes associated with oral cancer include: (1) cell cycle genes (TP53, CDKN2A, and Rb1), (2) genes related to the tumor microenvironment, (3) adhesion molecules, and (4) DNA repair genes and genes associated with apoptosis [84].

3.7.2. Epigenetic Alterations

DNA methylation mechanisms and histone code modifications may contribute to tumor development and neoplastic transformation [85]. Aberrant hypermethylation of the promoter regions of tumor suppressor genes disrupts the binding of a transcription factor, causing the genes to be silenced and promoting uncontrolled cell proliferation. The p16 protein, whose gene is located at the CDKN2A locus, is no longer expressed in 50–75% of oral cancer patients [86]. The absence of its expression is related to the methylation of the promoter of this gene, which affects the expressions of p15 and p14, two inhibitors of cyclin/CDK complexes. Gene silencing has also been detected in patients with oral cancer associated with DNA repair, apoptosis, the Wnt signaling pathway, and E-cadherin [86].

Histones are structural proteins that form a complex with DNA, and the acetylation or methylation of these proteins induces conformational changes in DNA that regulate transcription [87–89].

4. Treatment

Oral cancer treatment focuses on eradicating the tumor, preserving or restoring the shape and function of the mouth, preventing recurrence, and reducing the mortality rate while increasing the quality of life of the patient [21–23,90]. The main treatment option is the surgical resection of the tumor in combination with radiation therapy and chemotherapy, and it is most effective when oral cancer is detected early on. The success of treatments is significantly improved when performed by a multidisciplinary team, including maxillofacial surgeons, oral pathologists, oncologists, plastic surgeons, dentists, physiotherapists, radiologists, psychologists, and nutritionists [91].

Prevention and Antioxidants

To diagnose premalignant lesions in the oral cavity in a timely manner, it is necessary to make an accurate diagnosis, as these lesions are usually not detected at an early stage. However, it is essential to identify the risk factors associated with the development of oral cancer. Preventing and controlling oral cancer is a global challenge; therefore, it is necessary to establish prevention programs to reduce the incidence of cases [92]. Oral cancer-prevention measures include self-examination, regular visits to the dentist, and eliminating risk factors. In these prevention programs, it is recommended to include a diet rich in foods with anti-inflammatory or antioxidant value. Optimal nutritional intake is a fundamental element for the preservation of health in general. It has been identified that some foods, such as fruits and vegetables, which are frequently found in the diet can have this type of protective effect [93,94]. Reports in recent years have investigated the beneficial effects of berries with special antioxidant properties in oral cancer [95]. In addition, in recent years, it has been suggested that a diet rich in fruit and vegetable phytochemicals can help reduce the risk of oral cancer [96,97].

5. Phytochemical Compounds

The phytochemicals or secondary metabolites of plants form a group of compounds that, although they are not considered essential nutrients, have beneficial properties for health when they are included in the diet. These compounds provide anti-inflammatory and antioxidant properties [15–17,98,99]. Approximately 10,000 plant-derived compounds are known in the world; however, only 200 plant species are considered safe for human consumption [98–100]. The Western diet, characterized by a high consumption of refined sugars, saturated fats, and red meat, combined with the inadequate consumption of fruits and vegetables and other risk factors, is associated with a higher incidence of oral and pharyngeal cancers [101]. Therefore, the consumption of phytochemical compounds through the diet can represent a strategy to reduce the negative effects of cancer risk factors associated with oral cancer and can be found in the *Ericaceae family*, especially in berries [94] (Figures 3 and 4).

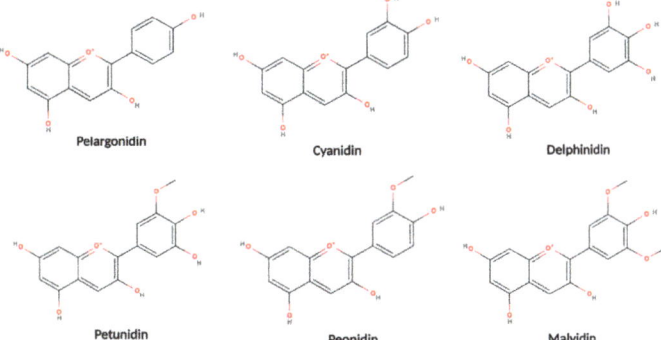

Figure 3. Representative chemical structures of blueberries and cranberries (created with the MolView program).

5.1. Family Ericaceae

The *Ericaceae* family is a family of plants composed of at least 4250 species distributed in 124 genera and nine subfamilies [102]. Within this family is the subfamily *Vaccinioidae*, which includes many important blueberry species, such as cranberries (*Vaccinium macrocarpon* A.), blueberries (*Vaccinium corymbosum* L.), European blueberries or bilberries (*Vaccinium myrtillus* L.), among others [103]. These fruits contain a high concentration of phytochemical compounds; in particular, blueberries have twice the antioxidant capacity of red pomegranate [98]. In the last two decades, the therapeutic use of berry-derived compounds in the treatment of cancer has increased due to the association between the development of cancer and the consumption of fruits and vegetables [99,100,104]. In the studies conducted by Greenwald, new approaches have been discovered based on the interactions between the components of the diet, nutrients, genes, and environmental and dietary factors for the benefit of health [105]. It is important to note that the compounds responsible for biological activity in the *Ericaceae* family are anthocyanins, flavonoids, anthocyanidins, flavanols, flavan-3-ols, proanthocyanidins, phenolic acids, and triterpenoids [101,102,106–108].

5.2. Anthocyanidins

Anthocyanidins belong to the flavonoid family and anthocyanidins are the largest group of water-soluble pigments in the plant kingdom. The main sources of these phytochemicals are blueberries, cherries, raspberries, strawberries, etc., which usually give the characteristic color to this type of fruit [109]. These anthocyanins exhibit a wide range of biological properties, including antioxidant, anti-inflammatory, antimicrobial, and antitumor activities [110]. The ability of anthocyanins to (1) inhibit cell proliferation, (2) induce apoptosis by the intrinsic and extrinsic pathways, (3) suppress angiogenesis, (4) suppress angiogenesis through inhibition, (5) inhibit matrix metalloproteinase (MMP) expression, and (6) suppress plasminogen activator urokinase has been reported in in vitro and in vivo studies of hydrogen peroxide and tumor necrosis factor (TNF) induced by the expression of vascular epidermal growth factor (VEGF) in epidermal keratinocytes [111–116].

5.3. Anthocyanins

The purple, red, and blue colors in vegetables are due to anthocyanins. Fruits, such as purple cabbage, grapes, and blueberries, are an available food source with this property. Anthocyanins are the product of glycosidic replacement in anthocyanidins. Within the group of anthocyanins are delphinidin, malvidin, petunidin, cyanidin, and peonidin, together with their fractions of glucose, galactose, and arabinose. These anthocyanins are found in berries. They have been reported to present antitumor activity against oral cancer [99,117–125]. The anthocyanins of black rice (*Oryza sativa*) have anticancer properties, such as the inhibition of metastasis of the oral cancer cell line (CAL-27), through the downregulation of matrix metalloproteinases [126]. In addition, a similar effect was observed in other oral cancer cell lines using a lyophilized extract of *Rubus idaeus*, which showed a concentration-dependent inhibition of both the migration and invasion of the oral cancer cell line SCC-9 and SAS [127]. Blueberry anthocyanins may induce G2/M cell cycle arrest in oral cancer cell line KB [128]. In addition, anthocyanins also increase the levels of caspase 9 and cytochrome c in KB cells, which indicates the induction of apoptosis, and simultaneously increase the amount of p53, which in most neoplasms has lost its function due to mutation [128]. Moreover, certain strawberry-derived anthocyanins, including cyanidin-3-glucoside (C3G), pelargonidin, and pelargonidin-3-glucoside (P3G), have been shown to inhibit tumor growth in oral cancer cell lines in the colon and prostate [129].

5.4. Flavan-3-ols and Proanthocyanidins

Flavan-3-ols represent one of the most complex subclasses of flavonoids, which range from monomers to oligomeric and polymeric proanthocyanidins, also named condensed tannins [130]. In studies on esophageal adenocarcinoma, the antiproliferative effect of protoanthocyanidins was observed, showing their ability to stop the cell cycle, induce apoptosis, or trigger autophagy as an alternative mechanism involving PI3K (phosphoinositide-3-kinase), AKT (Protein kinase B) and the mammalian target of rapamycin (mTOR) signaling [131]. Catechin, epicatechin, and polymeric pro-anthocyanidins are found in cranberries. It is known that this type of compound can delay the onset of tumors in transgenic mice that spontaneously develop tumors [20].

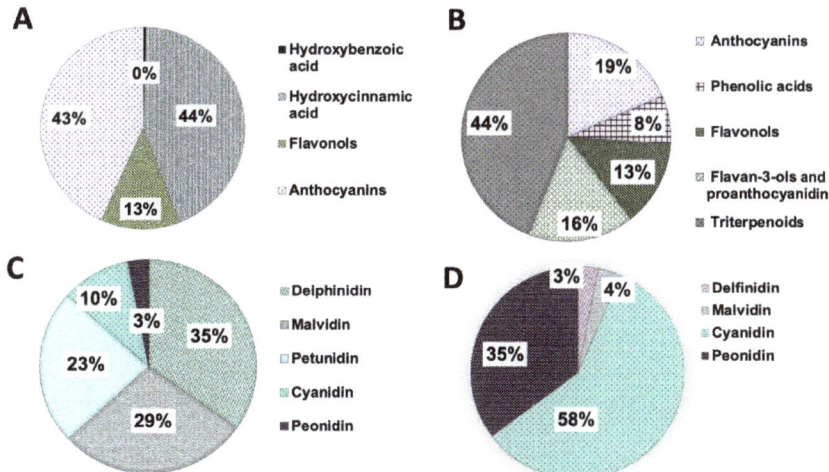

Figure 4. Percentage of some secondary metabolites in blueberries (fresh weight) and cranberries (dry matter) (**A**,**B**) and their anthocyanins (**C**) and derivatives (**D**). The percentages are calculated using the mean between the lowest and highest values identified in the literature for blueberries in mg/kg of fresh weight and in the case of the lingonberries in mg/100 g of dry matter, as referenced in the literature [98,99,132,133]. The values of each secondary metabolite depend on the size of the fruit, the state of maturation and, other postharvest conditions.

5.5. Phenolic Acids

Phenolic acids belong to a broad family of phenolic molecules, which are subdivided into hydroxybenzoic and hydroxycinnamic acids. Each of these compounds has shown antioxidant, antiproliferative, and anti-inflammatory activities [20]. Cranberries and blueberries contain phenolic compounds with antitumor potential [104].

5.6. Triterpenoids

Triterpenes are natural alkenes that are composed of 30 carbon atoms and are made of six isoprene units. These are usually found in a linear fashion, mainly in the form of squalene derivatives, tetracyclic and pentacyclic, containing four and five cycles, respectively, as well as those with two or three cycles [106,107]. In cranberries, ursolic, oleanolic, and betulinic acids are found in greater proportions [99]. These acids have antitumor, anti-inflammatory and antioxidant activities [122]. The compounds responsible for the biological activity in the *Ericaceae* family are anthocyanins, flavonoids, anthocyanidins, flavanols, flavan-3-ols, proanthocyanidins, phenolic acids, and triterpenoids, as shown in Table 1.

Table 1. Secondary metabolites present in cranberry and blueberry extracts. * Note 1: dm—dry matter; fw—fresh weight. Note 2: The concentration of each secondary metabolite depends on the size of the fruit, the state of maturation, the postharvest conditions, and the environmental and storage conditions.

Secondary Metabolite	Average Concentration in the Extract *	Reference:
Vaccinium corymbosum L. (blueberries)		
Phenolic acids		
Hydroxybenzoic acid	1.5 mg/kg fw	[132]
Hydroxycinnamic acid	135 mg/kg fw	[132]
Flavonoids		[132]

Table 1. *Cont.*

Secondary Metabolite	Average Concentration in the Extract *	Reference:
Flavonols	38.7 mg/kg fw	[132]
Anthocyanins	134 mg/kg fw	[132]
Vaccinium macrocarpon A. (lingonberries)		
Anthocyanins	695–1716 mg/100 g dm	[99]
Phenolic acids	327–649 mg/100 g dm	[99]
Flavonols	643–1088 mg/100 g dm	[99]
Flavan-3-ols and proanthocyanidins	860–1283 mg/100 g dm	[99]
Triterpenoids	2528–3201.5 mg/kg dm	[99]

6. Berries and Cancer

Berries are rich in minerals, vitamins, fatty acids, fiber, and polyphenolic compounds, including pterostilbene, malvidin, and malvidin-3-galactosidase [20,130]. Cranberries and blueberries have been shown to have antitumor properties in vitro, in vivo, and in clinical studies [117–119]. This activity is due to the presence of compounds, such as phenolic acids, flavonoids, anthocyanins, procyanidins, ascorbic acid, quercetin, kaempferol, catechin, epicatechin, p-coumaric acid, gallic acid, caffeic acid, ferulic acid, hydroxycinnamic acid, and chlorogenic acid, which are able to inhibit proinflammatory molecules, decrease oxidative stress, prevent DNA damage, inhibit tumor cell proliferation, and enhance tumor cell apoptosis Table 2 [120,121]. Chlorogenic acid, which is found in a variety of fruits, including blueberries, has been studied for its potential health benefits, particularly for its antioxidant and potential antitumor properties. The effects of coffee consumption on antitumor activity are complex and multifaceted. This is because coffee contains a variety of compounds that have been studied for their potential health effects [134]. Despite its high antioxidant content, the processing and heating of coffee may reduce its antitumor activity [135]. Further investigations are needed to understand the specific mechanisms by which coffee exerts its potential antitumor effects. Seeram determined that the polyphenolic compounds present in cranberry were responsible for the antiproliferative effects found in oral, prostate, and colon cancer cells, not the sugars [118]. These findings have been extended to other widely consumed berries. These include blackberries, black raspberries, blueberries, red raspberries, and strawberries [119]. Protoanthocyanidins derived from V. macrocarpon were reported to be the relevant bioactives involved in the reduction in urinary tract infections after cranberry juice consumption due to the inhibition of the adhesion of *E. coli fimbriae* to uroepithelial cells [136]. Furthermore, when these protoanthocyanidins were used in tumor explants of colon or prostate cancer cells, a decrease in the growth rate was observed in vivo [137]. Therefore, it is important to apply this knowledge to models of oral cancer and to strengthen epidemiological studies that assess the benefit of berries to reduce the incidence of oral cancer.

6.1. Mechanism of Action of Berries in Cancer

The mechanism of action of berry-derived phytochemicals can induce various effects on tumor cells, such as the inhibition of the nuclear transcription factor (NF-κB), inhibition of the MAP kinase pathway, interference with the production of detoxification enzymes, interference with the beta-catenin modulation of apoptosis, and modulation of the PI3K/AKT/mTOR pathway [138,139]. Studies have reported that polyphenols have an action on the NF-κB pathway, with effects on the Mitogen-activated protein kinase (MAP kinase pathway), the cAMP-dependent protein kinase (PKA) pathway, apoptosis, and the generation of oxidative stress, processes that depend on the consumption of berries in the diet [139,140]. The physicochemical and biotransformation properties of berry polyphenols by liver enzymes and the intestinal microbiota exert different effects on tumor cells in in vitro and animal models [141,142]. Resveratrol is the most widely characterized example of polyphenols regarding its cellular effects. This compound, found in red grapes, can have effects on tumor cells, in addition to inducing cell cycle arrest in oral cancer lines, and it can induce DNA damage and increase cell death in several cancer models [143,144]. Resveratrol appears to influence autophagy, as an alternative mechanism, and apoptosis, affecting oral cancer cell resistance to cisplatin through the AMPK and PI3K/AKT/mTOR pathways [145,146]. In esophageal adenocarcinoma, the anti-proliferative effects of resveratrol proanthocyanidins were observed, in addition to their ability to arrest the cell cycle [147]. Blackberries have also been reported to inhibit oxidative stress in rat esophageal squamous cell carcinogenesis models and the hydrogen peroxide-activated NF-kB/MAPK pathway [148]. In a study, a potential mechanism of oral cancer inhibition was identified through black raspberries via the glycolysis and AMPK pathways [149]. The authors suggested administering blackberries to animals to prevent oral cancer. Black raspberry phytochemicals can negatively modulate these pathways and thus compromise tumor cell growth (Figure 5) [149]. Berry flavonoids and polyphenols have been associated with effects on inflammation, apoptosis, autophagy, and the inhibition of the PI3K/Akt/mTOR pathway, among others, in cancer models [149]. The effects on the immune system of berries have shown effects on cancer metabolism in mice against the cell cycle, activation of MAP kinase signaling, DNA repair, leukocyte extravasation, and modulation of the inflammatory response [150].

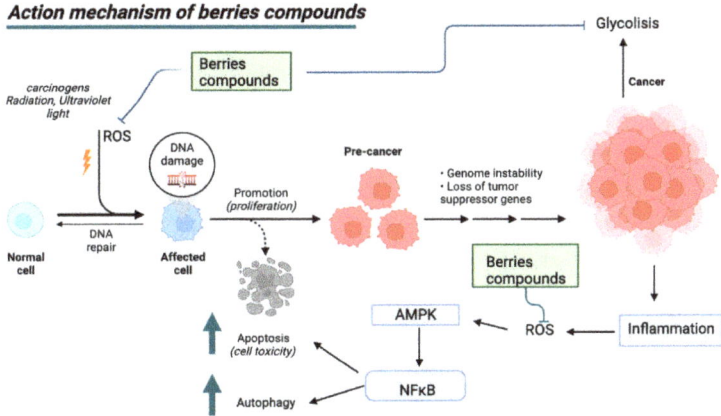

Figure 5. Mechanism of action of berries in cancer. Created with BioRender.com (accessed on 10 March 2022).

6.2. Mechanism of Action of Berry-Derived Phytochemicals in Oral Cancer

The fruits of the species *Vaccinium* ssp. represent an excellent natural food resource rich in phenolic compounds, flavonoids, polyphenols, anthocyanins, procyanidins, chlorogenic acid, ascorbic acid, quercetin, kaempferol, catechin, epicatechin, p-coumaric acid, gallic acid, caffeic acid, ferulic acid, and hydroxycinnamic acid, among others [110]. The consumption of both fresh and processed products can be an alternative to prevent oral squamous cell cancer [151].

6.3. Consumption of Cranberries and Blueberries in Protection against Risk Factors for Oral Cancer

Preventive measures to protect against oral cancer are classified into three categories: primary, secondary, and tertiary [152]. Among these measures is chemoprevention, which consists of the administration of an agent to prevent the appearance of cancer [153]. These agents can be drugs or natural products that are easy to administer, with little or low toxicity, and that do not cause long-term sequelae. Blueberries are interesting candidates because they contain many phytochemicals with antitumor potential [154]. These phytochemicals can be effective in the short and long terms, and they can be consumed fresh or processed. The main source of phytochemicals in cranberries and blueberries is anthocyanins, which account for more than 60% of the total polyphenols in their ripe state. This means approximately 387–487 mg/100 g anthocyanins in their fresh form [155]. To take advantage of these effects, it is recommended to drink a 250 mL cup of fresh cranberry or processed juices daily for at least 28–36 days, both in the morning and afternoon [156–159]. However, it is important to note that the processed juice should not contain ascorbic acid, as it reduces the number of phenolic compounds present in the juice and its biological efficacy by up to 10% [160]. Cranberries and blueberries are rich in phytochemicals with anticancer potential, such as anthocyanins and flavanols [161]. These phytochemicals can be consumed both fresh and processed to exert their potential long-term protective effects against oral cancer. Other important components in blueberries, especially cranberries, are flavan-3-ol and triterpenoids. These phytochemicals can also contribute to the treatment of oral premalignant lesions and the reduction in other factors that promote oral carcinogenesis. It is important to mention that the effects of climate change on secondary metabolism cover many aspects, ranging from the molecular level to the overall effects on organisms resulting from changing concentrations of phytochemical compounds. To obtain the essential information needed to understand how plants perform under changing climatic conditions, a thorough analysis of the existing knowledge on the effects of climate change components on berry secondary metabolites is crucial. Further research is needed to better understand the complex effects of multiple environmental factors on berry secondary metabolites [162]. However, there are still a relatively small number of studies investigating the metabolome in berries. Berries, as a group of fruits, have remarkable resilience in the preservation of their inherent qualities. Cranberries are widely recognized for their ability to retain their distinctive biochemical characteristics [163].

6.3.1. Cranberries and Blueberries and Their Protection against Tobacco-Induced Oral Cancer

A variety of oral lesions, including leukoplakia, erythroplakia, oral submucosal fibrosis, and oral cancer, have been implicated in tobacco use [164]. This is due to the presence of over sixty carcinogens in the smoke of cigarettes, as well as, at minimum, sixteen in uncombusted tobacco [91]. This includes tobacco-specific nitrosamines, such as 4-(methylnitrosamine)-1-(3-pyridyl)-1-butanone (NNK) and N'-nitrosonornicotine (NNN); polycyclic aromatic hydrocarbons, such as benzo[α] pyrene; and aromatic amines, such as 4-aminobiphenyl, which have been shown to cause cancer [165]. Strategies to use chemopreventive agents to counteract or inhibit the effects of tobacco use on oral carcinogenesis can be very useful in preventing this disease. One example of these agents is blueberry extracts, which have been shown in an in vivo study to inhibit the initiation and progression of carcinomas through the inhibition of the TGF-β and PI3K/AKT pathways [166,167]. Furthermore, supplementation suppressed the activation of NF-κB, preventing the translocation of this transcription factor [168]. Furthermore, these extracts have been shown to modulate the expression of oncomiR miR-21 and the tumor suppressor let-7 [167]. A study on a mouse model showed that black raspberry extracts inhibit the binding of the carcinogen dibenzo [α, l] pyrene-DNA, which is crucial for the repair of lesions caused by this carcinogen in DNA [169]. Protocatechuic acid, found in blueberries, has also been shown to be responsible for some of the benefits of anthocyanin consumption, including the inhibition of mutagenic effects as well as the generation of DNA adducts of the tobacco smoke carcinogen dibenzopyrene [94].

6.3.2. Cranberries and Blueberries and Their Protection against Alcohol-Induced Oral Cancer

Alcohol consumption, such as tobacco smoking, has been recognized as an important contributor to the development of oral cancer for over fifty years. It has been associated with approximately 75% of cancers affecting the superior aerodigestive tract and causes changes in the cellular structure of the oral epithelium [170]. Mechanisms through which the consumption of alcohol causes carcinogenic damage are not fully understood; however, they may include the genotoxic effect of acetaldehyde on the oral mucosa, an increase in the concentration of estrogens, the role of a solvent producing other carcinogens, such as those from tobacco, the generation of ROS and nitric oxide synthases (NOS), and alterations in folate metabolism [171]. It is believed that the consumption of blueberries may have chemopreventive effects on oral cancer induced by alcohol consumption due to its content of phytochemicals, such as quercetin and resveratrol [172]. Anthocyanins, which are one of the major components of blueberries, have interesting anticancer properties that are useful for the prevention of oral cancer [116]. One of these compounds, malvidin (malvidin-3-glucoside), showed inhibitory activity against (Signal transducer and activator of transcription 3) STAT-3 within the oral cancer cell line (SCC131) by suppressing the phosphorylation and nuclear translocation of this factor, which resulted in cell cycle arrest and mitochondrial-mediated apoptosis [120]. In addition, blueberry extract has been shown to inhibit The Janus-Kinase signal transducer and the transcription activation pathway (JAK/STAT-3) signaling by modulating the downstream sites affecting cell proliferation and apoptosis in a hamster model of oral oncogenesis [120]. Therefore, due to the action of this phytochemical, it is possible to inhibit oral carcinogenesis by alcohol, which is an important inducing factor of this type of cancer that can contribute to the large number of people who regularly consume this substance [173,174]. Other studies have shown the chemopreventive capacity of grape wine in cells of the oral mucosa. Although regular consumption in moderate doses produces metabolites, such as acetaldehyde, which is the main producer of DNA adducts, it has been shown that grape wine has the ability to mitigate the deleterious actions of alcohol and reduce the chances of developing oral cancer [124,175]. This is due to the presence of phenolic compounds, such as those found in cranberries, which activate the p53 tumor suppressor gene to induce cell cycle arrest as well as apoptosis in cells of the oral cavity [119].

6.4. Consumption of Cranberries and Blueberries Protects against the Effects of Bacteria and Poor Oral Hygiene

The oral cavity is a special place where there are more than 250 varieties of microorganisms called commensals, which have a crucial role in maintaining the individual status of organisms [176]. Many of these species, according to epidemiological studies, are closely related to oral cancer. Among the most important are *Fusobacterium nucleatum* and *Porphyromonas gingivalis*, among others, which have been related to different types of carcinomas and oral tumor processes [177]. Additionally, some papillomaviruses, oral fungi, such as *Candida albicans*, and parasites have been linked to oropharyngeal cancer [178]. *Candida albicans* infection has been implicated in the initiation and progression of oral cancer through the activation of proto-oncogenes, induction of DNA damage, and overexpression of oncogenic pathways [179]. Inflammatory signaling in the oral mucosa can also be modulated by the phytochemicals of blueberries, especially red berries. The crude extracts and their fractions enriched with other species of red fruits (*Vaccinium myrtillus* L. and *Malpighia punicifolica* L.) exert antiadhesion activity against *Candida* spp. when used at concentrations > 1.25 mg/mL [180]. This mechanism is related to the action of type-A cranberry proanthocyanidins, which do not have a relevant effect on *Candida* spp. but do so on the adhesion of this on the oral mucosa [181,182]. Thus, for carcinogenic implantation functions to occur, phenomena, such as microbial dysbiosis, colonization, and translocation, must occur, which produce an excessive inflammatory response, host immunosuppression, enhancement of malignant transformation, anti-apoptotic effects, and the secretion of carcinogens [178]. Therefore, the consumption of blueberries and cranberries may be a potential source to prevent these types of infections [183]. An example of this is the effect of proanthocyanidins (PACs) in both blueberries and cranberries to reduce the deleterious effects of the *Porphyromonas gingivalis* species on the cells of the oral mucosa [184]. This is achieved by protecting against the damage produced by said bacteria in the keratinocytic gingival barrier, inhibiting its translocation, reducing the proteolytic degradation of tight epithelial junctions, and reducing the secretion of IL-6 and IL-8, among others, in an in vitro model of the gingival keratinocyte barrier against *P. gingivalis* [185]. In addition, PACs from cranberries have also been associated with antimicrobial, anti-adhesion, antioxidant, and anti-inflammatory properties, which is why they can be potentially useful in the prevention of periodontal disease that affects dental tissues [186]. This is achieved through the inhibition of both bacterial and host-derived proteolytic enzymes, as well as host inflammation and osteoclast differentiation and activity [186].

6.5. Cranberries and Blueberries and Their Protection against Oral Cancer Induced by Viral Infections

Two infectious factors associated with the onset and development of oral cancer are human papillomavirus (HPV) and Epstein–Barr virus (EBV) [187,188]. For example, the polyphenolic and flavonoid components (also found in cranberries and blueberries) in the *Polygonatum odoratum* plant have been shown in recent studies to have antibacterial, antifungal, antioxidant, anti-inflammatory, and anticancer activities. A study has shown that extracts of this plant significantly affect human lymphoblastoid carriers of the Epstein–Barr virus genome through the induction of apoptosis, cell cycle arrest, inhibition of cell proliferation, migration, and colonization [189]. Moreover, this extract suppresses proteins that are essential to cell proliferation, colonization, and migration, including cyclin D, cyclooxygenase 2 (COX-2), matrix metalloproteinase-9 (MMP-9), and vascular endothelial growth factor A (VEGF-A) [188]. This makes these components of interest in the prevention of oral cancer mediated by this virus.

Table 2. Effects of cranberry extracts and phytochemicals against oral cancer.

Cranberry Type	Type of Study Conducted (In Vitro/In Vivo/Clinical Study)	Evidence against Oral Cancer	Reference
Vaccinium corymbosum L. (blueberries)	In vitro	The methanolic extract of blueberries inhibits cell proliferation in the oral cancer line KB.	[128,188]
	In vivo/In vitro	Dietary administration of blueberry produces significant effects on the SCC131 cancer cell line through the inhibition of TGF-β and NF-κB, as well as act against invasion and angiogenesis at doses higher than 200 mg/kg.	[20,167]
	In vitro	The phytochemical pterostilbene present in blueberries induces apoptotic cell death and, through autophagy in cisplatin-resistant human oral cancer cells (CAR cells), which is related to the AKT pathway, are mediated by the suppression of MDR1.	[100]
Vaccinium macrocarpon A. (lingonberries)	In vitro	The methanol extract of the cranberries inhibits cellular proliferation in the line of oral cancer KB.	[128,188]
	In vivo/In vitro	The extract composed of proanthocyanidins (C-PAC) derived from cranberries inhibits the growth of resistant and acid-sensitive esophageal adenocarcinoma (EAC) cells, both in cell lines and xenotransplant mice, inducing caspase-independent cell death, mainly by the autophagic pathway.	[131]
	In vitro	The hydroethanolic extract of cranberries produces an antiproliferative effect on the caspase-independent KB cell line, mainly by the autophagic route.	[190]
	In vitro	Cranberry extract produces an inhibitory effect on the proliferation of OSCC lines cAL27 and SCC25 at an optimal concentration of 40 µg/mL, producing the upstream regulation of caspases 2 and 8, and effects cell adhesion, cell morphology, and the cell cycle.	[191]

7. Limitations and Perspectives of the Consumption of Cranberries and Blueberries for Protection against Oral Cancer

Diet is a complex issue influenced by cultural and resource-related factors. Scientific research aimed at understanding the molecular mechanisms underlying the reduced risk of cancer associated with certain dietary habits has revealed that isolating individual compounds fails to capture the broad range of benefits observed in epidemiological studies. Allium vegetables, including garlic, onions, chives, shallots, and leeks, present an intriguing case. This diverse group of plants comprises over 500 species and contains numerous bioactive compounds, particularly sulfur compounds, such as allicin, S-allylcysteine, diallysulfides, and others. Assessing the impact of allium consumption remains challenging due to the likely influence of various environmental and dietary variables on its potential cancer-preventive effects. However, several phytochemicals found in allium vegetables have demonstrated their ability to reduce cancer risk at different stages of cancer development, including initiation, promotion, and progression. Similar findings have also been observed in the context of berries and fruits. The scientific evidence supports the notion that lifestyle modifications, particularly dietary changes, can enhance cancer-prevention efforts. However, it is important to avoid overstating the significance of individual components, and further studies are warranted to expand our understanding [192].

Limitations

Oral cancer is a multifaceted disease involving various factors that trigger the carcinogenic process. Strategies incorporating antioxidants and phytochemicals from cranberries can help prevent these factors by modifying molecular mechanisms and inducing apoptosis in tumor cells. However, it is crucial to consider the source of blueberries (natural or processed) as the latter may degrade phytochemicals, reducing their protective effects. Furthermore, there is a lack of clinical research investigating the impact of cranberries and blueberries on oral cancer through traditional consumption methods (juice and fresh) among smokers and regular alcohol consumers to determine their protective effects. The effectiveness of cranberry supplementation also depends on the stage of carcinogenesis, with varying benefits depending on tumor development levels. Despite the existing evidence, scientific studies supporting the use of these fruits for oral cancer prevention and treatment are limited. Additional research is needed to recommend their consumption, particularly in advanced stages of oral tumor diseases, such as metastasis, where the effects remain unknown. Blueberries contain phytochemicals, such as anthocyanins, quercetin, and ellagic acid, which similarly reduce the diet-related risk factors associated with oral cancer, akin to black raspberries. It is important to be aware of these limitations in the interpretation of the available published scientific evidence on the association between berries and oral cancer reduction.

Perspectives: conducting rigorous clinical trials with carefully designed protocols and representative samples is a promising approach to berry research for reducing oral cancer risk factors. To develop precise treatment strategies, it is critical to understand the specific mechanisms by which the bioactive compounds in berries exert their beneficial effects. In addition, there is great promise for increasing efficacy and improving outcomes by exploring combinations of berries with other treatments. Elucidating the mechanisms of action and exploring berry combinations with other treatments to improve outcomes are future perspectives in this field.

8. Conclusions

Studies performed in vitro, in vivo, and in clinical research have shown that the phytochemicals and polyphenolic compounds found in blueberries, cranberries, and other berries have antitumor properties. Polyphenolic compounds found in cranberries are responsible for the antiproliferative effects on oral cancer cells in in vitro and in vivo models. Berries' mechanisms of action in oral cancer include: (i) the inhibition of inflammation through interference with the nuclear transcription factor NF-κB, (ii) effects on proliferation by interfering with the MAP kinase pathway, (iii) reduction in resistance by interfering with the expression of detoxification enzymes, (iv) interference with the β-catenin signaling pathway, (v) modulation of apoptosis, and (vi) modulation of the antiapoptotic and anabolic pathways of PI3K/AKT/mTOR. The use of protective strategies is based on the consumption of functional foods, nutraceuticals, or supplements based on fruits, such as berries of the species *Vaccinium* ssp. It can be of great interest to reduce the effects of the risk factors associated with oral cancer.

Author Contributions: Conceptualization, C.E.-C., M.A.B.-C. and A.Z.-D.; investigation, M.E.-L., A.L.-M., D.M.-S., F.H.-S., D.C.-R., B.R.Y.-O. and J.L.V.-G.; writing—original draft preparation, S.M.-F., L.A.G.-C., F.H.-S., A.L.-M., D.M.-S. writing—review and editing, H.L.-E., J.L.V.-G. and C.P.M.-V.; visualization, A.Z.-D. and J.L.V.-G. All authors have read and agreed to the published version of the manuscript.

Funding: This research received no external funding.

Informed Consent Statement: Not applicable.

Data Availability Statement: Not applicable.

Conflicts of Interest: The authors declare no conflict of interest.

Abbreviations

OSCC	Oral squamous carcinoma cell
HPV	Human papillomavirus
EBV	Epstein–Barr virus
NNN	N′-nitrosonornicotine
NNK	4-(methylnitrosamine)-1-(3-pyridyl)-1-butanone
ROS	Reactive oxygen species
BMI	Body mass index
EGFR/c-erb	Epidermal growth factor receptor
TNF	tumor necrosis factor
MMP	matrix metalloproteinase
CAL-27	oral cancer cell line
C3G	cyanidin-3-glucoside
PACs	Proanthocyanidins
COX-2	Cyclooxygenase 2
MMP-9	Matrix metalloproteinase-9
VEGF-A	Vascular endothelial growth factor A
NF-κB	Nuclear transcription factor
NOSs	Nitric oxide synthases
P3G	pelargonidin-3-glucoside
SCC131	oral cancer cell line 131
PI3K	phosphoinositide-3-kinase
AKT	Protein kinase B
mTOR	the mammalian target of rapamycin
MAP	Mitogen-activated protein kinase
PKA	cAMP-dependent protein kinaseB
AMPK	the AMP-activated protein kinase
TGF-β	Transforming growth factor-β
STAT-3	Signal transducer and activator of transcription 3
JAK/STAT	The Janus-Kinase signal transducer and the transcription activation pathway

References

1. Hammer, W. What Is Cancer? Available online: https://www.aacr.org/patients-caregivers/about-cancer/what-is-cancer/ (accessed on 8 July 2022).
2. Head and Neck Cancers—NCI. Available online: https://www.cancer.gov/types/head-and-neck/head-neck-fact-sheet (accessed on 12 July 2022).

3. Latest Global Cancer Data: Cancer Burden Rises to 19.3 Million New Cases and 10.0 Million Cancer Deaths in 2020—IARC. Available online: https://www.iarc.who.int/news-events/latest-global-cancer-data-cancer-burden-rises-to-19-3-million-new-cases-and-10-0-million-cancer-deaths-in-2020/ (accessed on 12 July 2022).
4. Module 5: What Is Cancer? Available online: https://www.tn.gov/health/health-program-areas/tcr/cancer-reporting-facility-training/module5.html (accessed on 8 July 2022).
5. Research Areas—Global Health—NCI. Available online: https://www.cancer.gov/research/areas/global-health (accessed on 8 July 2022).
6. Cancer Tomorrow. Available online: https://gco.iarc.fr/tomorrow/en (accessed on 8 July 2022).
7. Conway, D.I.; Purkayastha, M.; Chestnutt, I.G. The changing epidemiology of oral cancer: Definitions, trends, and risk factors. *Br. Dent. J.* **2018**, *225*, 867–873. [CrossRef]
8. Westra, W.H.; Lewis, J.S. Update from the 4th Edition of the World Health Organization Classification of Head and Neck Tumours: Oropharynx. *Head Neck Pathol.* **2017**, *11*, 41–47. [CrossRef] [PubMed]
9. Mouth and Oral Cancer Statistics. Available online: https://www.wcrf.org/cancer-trends/mouth-and-oral-cancer-statistics/ (accessed on 7 August 2022).
10. Li, C.C.; Shen, Z.; Bavarian, R.; Yang, F.; Bhattacharya, A. Oral Cancer: Genetics and the Role of Precision Medicine. *Dent. Clin. N. Am.* **2018**, *62*, 29–46. [CrossRef] [PubMed]
11. Oral Cavity & Oropharyngeal Cancer Key Statistics 2021. Available online: https://www.cancer.org/cancer/oral-cavity-and-oropharyngeal-cancer/about/key-statistics.html (accessed on 7 August 2022).
12. Watters, C.; Brar, S.; Pepper, T. Oral Mucosa Cancer. In *StatPearls*; StatPearls Publishing: Treasure Island, FL, USA, 2022.
13. Pavia, M.; Pileggi, C.; Nobile, C.G.A.; Angelillo, I.F. Association between fruit and vegetable consumption and oral cancer: A meta-analysis of observational studies. *Am. J. Clin. Nutr.* **2006**, *83*, 1126–1134. [CrossRef]
14. Cancer Treatment | SEER Training. Available online: https://training.seer.cancer.gov/treatment/ (accessed on 7 August 2022).
15. Porro, C.; La Torre, M.E.; Tartaglia, N.; Benameur, T.; Santini, M.; Ambrosi, A.; Messina, G.; Cibelli, G.; Fiorelli, A.; Polito, R.; et al. The Potential Role of Nutrition in Lung Cancer Establishment and Progression. *Life* **2022**, *12*, 270. [CrossRef] [PubMed]
16. Khedkar, R.; Singh, K.; Sharma, V.; Thakur, M. Physicochemical Properties and Antioxidant Potential of Curry Leaf Chutney Powder: A Traditional Functional Food Adjunct. In *Bioactive Components: A Sustainable System for Good Health and Well-Being*; Springer: Berlin/Heidelberg, Germany, 2022; pp. 595–609.
17. George, B.P.; Chandran, R.; Abrahamse, H. Role of Phytochemicals in Cancer Chemoprevention: Insights. *Antioxidants* **2021**, *10*, 1455. [CrossRef]
18. Brewczyński, A.; Jabłońska, B.; Kentnowski, M.; Mrowiec, S.; Składowski, K.; Rutkowski, T. The Association between Carotenoids and Head and Neck Cancer Risk. *Nutrients* **2021**, *14*, 88. [CrossRef]
19. Stoner, G.D.; Wang, L.S.; Casto, B.C. Laboratory and clinical studies of cancer chemoprevention by antioxidants in berries. *Carcinogenesis* **2008**, *29*, 1665–1674. [CrossRef]
20. Prakash, S.; Radha; Kumar, M.; Kumari, N.; Thakur, M.; Rathour, S.; Pundir, A.; Sharma, A.K.; Bangar, S.P.; Dhumal, S.; et al. Plant-Based Antioxidant Extracts and Compounds in the Management of Oral Cancer. *Antioxidants* **2021**, *10*, 1358. [CrossRef] [PubMed]
21. Johnson, D.E.; Burtness, B.; Leemans, C.R.; Lui, V.W.Y.; Bauman, J.E.; Grandis, J.R. Head and neck squamous cell carcinoma. *Nat. Rev. Dis. Prim.* **2020**, *6*, 92. [CrossRef]
22. Ellington, T.D. Trends in Incidence of Cancers of the Oral Cavity and Pharynx—United States 2007–2016. *MMWR Morb. Mortal. Wkly. Rep.* **2020**, *69*, 433–438. [CrossRef] [PubMed]
23. Jose, M.; Rajagopal, V.; Thankam, F.G. Chapter 9—Oral tissue regeneration: Current status and future perspectives. In *Regenerated Organs*; Sharma, C.P., Ed.; Academic Press: Cambridge, MA, USA, 2021; pp. 169–187.
24. Cancer Today. Available online: https://gco.iarc.fr/today/fact-sheets-cancers (accessed on 7 August 2022).
25. Ali, K. Oral Cancer—The Fight Must Go on against All Odds... *Evid.-Based Dent.* **2022**, *23*, 4–5. [CrossRef]
26. Zhang, S.-Z.; Xie, L.; Shang, Z.-J. Burden of Oral Cancer on the 10 Most Populous Countries from 1990 to 2019: Estimates from the Global Burden of Disease Study 2019. *Int. J. Environ. Res. Public Health* **2022**, *19*, 875. [CrossRef] [PubMed]
27. Gupta, B.; Johnson, N.W.; Kumar, N. Global Epidemiology of Head and Neck Cancers: A Continuing Challenge. *Oncology* **2016**, *91*, 13–23. [CrossRef]
28. McKeon, M.G.; Gallant, J.-N.; Kim, Y.J.; Das, S.R. It Takes Two to Tango: A Review of Oncogenic Virus and Host Microbiome Associated Inflammation in Head and Neck Cancer. *Cancers* **2022**, *14*, 3120. [CrossRef] [PubMed]
29. Irani, S. New Insights into Oral Cancer-Risk Factors and Prevention: A Review of Literature. *Int. J. Prev. Med.* **2020**, *11*, 202. [CrossRef]
30. Cancer Net. Oral and Oropharyngeal Cancer—Risk Factors and Prevention. 2012. Available online: https://www.cancer.net/cancer-types/oral-and-oropharyngeal-cancer/risk-factors-and-prevention (accessed on 7 August 2022).
31. Kavarthapu, A.; Gurumoorthy, K. Linking chronic periodontitis and oral cancer: A review. *Oral Oncol.* **2021**, *121*, 105375. [CrossRef]
32. Tabaco. Available online: https://www.who.int/es/news-room/fact-sheets/detail/tobacco (accessed on 27 October 2022).

33. Valavanidis, A.; Vlachogianni, T.; Fiotakis, K. Tobacco smoke: Involvement of reactive oxygen species and stable free radicals in mechanisms of oxidative damage, carcinogenesis and synergistic effects with other respirable particles. *Int. J. Environ. Res. Public Health* **2009**, *6*, 445–462. [CrossRef] [PubMed]
34. Goodchild, M.; Nargis, N.; Tursan d'Espaignet, E. Global economic cost of smoking-attributable diseases. *Tob. Control* **2018**, *27*, 58–64. [CrossRef]
35. Zhang, Y.; He, J.; He, B.; Huang, R.; Li, M. Effect of tobacco on periodontal disease and oral cancer. *Tob. Induc. Dis.* **2019**, *17*, 40. [CrossRef]
36. Pelucchi, C.; Gallus, S.; Garavello, W.; Bosetti, C.; La Vecchia, C. Cancer risk associated with alcohol and tobacco use: Focus on upper aero-digestive tract and liver. *Alcohol. Res. Health* **2006**, *29*, 193–198. [PubMed]
37. Pérez-Ortuño, R.; Martínez-Sánchez, J.M.; Fu, M.; Fernández, E.; Pascual, J.A. Evaluation of tobacco specific nitrosamines exposure by quantification of 4-(methylnitrosamino)-1-(3-pyridyl)-1-butanone (NNK) in human hair of non-smokers. *Sci. Rep.* **2016**, *6*, 25043. [CrossRef] [PubMed]
38. Zhang, S.; Wang, M.; Villalta, P.W.; Lindgren, B.R.; Upadhyaya, P.; Lao, Y.; Hecht, S.S. Analysis of pyridyloxobutyl and pyridylhydroxybutyl DNA adducts in extrahepatic tissues of F344 rats treated chronically with 4-(methylnitrosamino)-1-(3-pyridyl)-1-butanone and enantiomers of 4-(methylnitrosamino)-1-(3-pyridyl)-1-butanol. *Chem. Res. Toxicol.* **2009**, *22*, 926–936. [CrossRef] [PubMed]
39. Ronai, Z.A.; Gradia, S.; Peterson, L.A.; Hecht, S.S. G to A transitions and G to T transversions in codon 12 of the Ki-ras oncogene isolated from mouse lung tumors induced by 4-(methylnitrosamino)-1-(3-pyridyl)-1-butanone (NNK) and related DNA methylating and pyridyloxobutylating agents. *Carcinogenesis* **1993**, *14*, 2419–2422. [CrossRef]
40. Balbo, S.; Johnson, C.S.; Kovi, R.C.; James-Yi, S.A.; O'Sullivan, M.G.; Wang, M.; Le, C.T.; Khariwala, S.S.; Upadhyaya, P.; Hecht, S.S. Carcinogenicity and DNA adduct formation of 4-(methylnitrosamino)-1-(3-pyridyl)-1-butanone and enantiomers of its metabolite 4-(methylnitrosamino)-1-(3-pyridyl)-1-butanol in F-344 rats. *Carcinogenesis* **2014**, *35*, 2798–2806. [CrossRef]
41. Watters, C.; Brar, S.; Pepper, T. Oral Mucosa Cancer. In *StatPearls*; StatPearls Publishing LLC.: Treasure Island, FL, USA, 2023.
42. Niaz, K.; Maqbool, F.; Khan, F.; Bahadar, H.; Ismail Hassan, F.; Abdollahi, M. Smokeless tobacco (paan and gutkha) consumption, prevalence, and contribution to oral cancer. *Epidemiol. Health* **2017**, *39*, e2017009. [CrossRef]
43. Rossini, A.R.; Hashimoto, C.L.; Iriya, K.; Zerbini, C.; Baba, E.R.; Moraes-Filho, J.P. Dietary habits, ethanol and tobacco consumption as predictive factors in the development of esophageal carcinoma in patients with head and neck neoplasms. *Dis. Esophagus* **2008**, *21*, 316–321. [CrossRef]
44. Feng, L.; Wang, L. Effects of alcohol on the morphological and structural changes in oral mucosa. *Pak. J. Med. Sci.* **2013**, *29*, 1046–1049. [CrossRef]
45. González-López, L.L.; Morales-González, Á.; Sosa-Gómez, A.; Madrigal-Santillán, E.O.; Anguiano-Robledo, L.; Madrigal-Bujaidar, E.; Álvarez-González, I.; Delgado-Olivares, L.; Valadez-Vega, C.; Esquivel-Chirino, C.; et al. Damage to Oral Mucosae Induced by Weekend Alcohol Consumption: The Role of Gender and Alcohol Concentration. *Appl. Sci.* **2022**, *12*, 3464. [CrossRef]
46. Jiang, Y.; Zhang, T.; Kusumanchi, P.; Han, S.; Yang, Z.; Liangpunsakul, S. Alcohol Metabolizing Enzymes, Microsomal Ethanol Oxidizing System, Cytochrome P450 2E1, Catalase, and Aldehyde Dehydrogenase in Alcohol-Associated Liver Disease. *Biomedicines* **2020**, *8*, 50. [CrossRef]
47. Wu, D.; Cederbaum, A.I. Alcohol, oxidative stress, and free radical damage. *Alcohol. Res. Health* **2003**, *27*, 277–284.
48. Maeng, J.-S. Food, nutrition, physical activity and cancer: A global perspective and analysis of the research. *Bull. Food Technol.* **2012**, *25*, 2–26.
49. Rumgay, H.; Shield, K.; Charvat, H.; Ferrari, P.; Sornpaisarn, B.; Obot, I.; Islami, F.; Lemmens, V.; Rehm, J.; Soerjomataram, I. Global burden of cancer in 2020 attributable to alcohol consumption: A population-based study. *Lancet Oncol.* **2021**, *22*, 1071–1080. [CrossRef] [PubMed]
50. Piemonte, E.D.; Lazos, J.P.; Gilligan, G.M.; Panico, R.L.; Werner, L.C.; Yang, Y.H.; Warnakulasuriya, S. Chronic mechanical irritation enhances the effect of tobacco and alcohol on the risk of oral squamous cell carcinoma: A case-control study in Argentina. *Clin. Oral Investig.* **2022**, *26*, 6317–6326. [CrossRef] [PubMed]
51. Lissoni, A.; Agliardi, E.; Peri, A.; Marchioni, R.; Abati, S. Oral microbiome and mucosal trauma as risk factors for oral cancer: Beyond alcohol and tobacco. A literature review. *J. Biol. Regul. Homeost. Agents* **2020**, *34*, 11–18.
52. Alnuaimi, A.D.; Wiesenfeld, D.; O'Brien-Simpson, N.M.; Reynolds, E.C.; McCullough, M.J. Oral Candida colonization in oral cancer patients and its relationship with traditional risk factors of oral cancer: A matched case-control study. *Oral Oncol.* **2015**, *51*, 139–145. [CrossRef]
53. Di Cosola, M.; Cazzolla, A.P.; Charitos, I.A.; Ballini, A.; Inchingolo, F.; Santacroce, L. *Candida albicans* and Oral Carcinogenesis. A Brief Review. *J. Fungi* **2021**, *7*, 476. [CrossRef]
54. Jain, M. Assesment of Correlation of Herpes Simplex Virus-1 with Oral Cancer and Precancer—A Comparative Study. *J. Clin. Diagn. Res.* **2016**, *10*, Zc14–Zc17. [CrossRef]
55. Dylawerska, A.; Barczak, W.; Wegner, A.; Golusinski, W.; Suchorska, W.M. Association of DNA repair genes polymorphisms and mutations with increased risk of head and neck cancer: A review. *Med. Oncol.* **2017**, *34*, 197. [CrossRef]
56. Giraldi, L.; Collatuzzo, G.; Hashim, D.; Franceschi, S.; Herrero, R.; Chen, C.; Schwartz, S.M.; Smith, E.; Kelsey, K.; McClean, M.; et al. Infection with Human Papilloma Virus (HPV) and risk of subsites within the oral cancer. *Cancer Epidemiol.* **2021**, *75*, 102020. [CrossRef]

57. Kim, Y.; Joo, Y.H.; Kim, M.S.; Lee, Y.S. Prevalence of high-risk human papillomavirus and its genotype distribution in head and neck squamous cell carcinomas. *J. Pathol. Transl. Med.* **2020**, *54*, 411–418. [CrossRef] [PubMed]
58. Melo, B.A.C.; Vilar, L.G.; Oliveira, N.R.; Lima, P.O.; Pinheiro, M.B.; Domingueti, C.P.; Pereira, M.C. Human papillomavirus infection and oral squamous cell carcinoma—A systematic review. *Braz. J. Otorhinolaryngol.* **2021**, *87*, 346–352. [CrossRef] [PubMed]
59. Kim, W.Y.; Montes-Mojarro, I.A.; Fend, F.; Quintanilla-Martinez, L. Epstein-Barr Virus-Associated T and NK-Cell Lymphoproliferative Diseases. *Front. Pediatr.* **2019**, *7*, 71. [CrossRef]
60. Núñez-Acurio, D.; Bravo, D.; Aguayo, F. Epstein-Barr Virus-Oral Bacterial Link in the Development of Oral Squamous Cell Carcinoma. *Pathogens* **2020**, *9*, 1059. [CrossRef] [PubMed]
61. Thomas, C.; Minty, M.; Vinel, A.; Canceill, T.; Loubières, P.; Burcelin, R.; Kaddech, M.; Blasco-Baque, V.; Laurencin-Dalicieux, S. Oral Microbiota: A Major Player in the Diagnosis of Systemic Diseases. *Diagnostics* **2021**, *11*, 1376. [CrossRef]
62. Singhvi, H.R.; Malik, A.; Chaturvedi, P. The Role of Chronic Mucosal Trauma in Oral Cancer: A Review of Literature. *Indian J. Med. Paediatr. Oncol.* **2017**, *38*, 44–50. [CrossRef]
63. Aceves Argemí, R.; González Navarro, B.; Ochoa García-Seisdedos, P.; Estrugo Devesa, A.; López-López, J. Mouthwash With Alcohol and Oral Carcinogenesis: Systematic Review and Meta-analysis. *J. Evid. Based Dent. Pract.* **2020**, *20*, 101407. [CrossRef]
64. Carr, E.; Aslam-Pervez, B. Does the use of alcohol mouthwash increase the risk of developing oral cancer? *Evid. Based Dent.* **2022**, *23*, 28–29. [CrossRef]
65. Key, T.J.; Bradbury, K.E.; Perez-Cornago, A.; Sinha, R.; Tsilidis, K.K.; Tsugane, S. Diet, nutrition, and cancer risk: What do we know and what is the way forward? *BMJ* **2020**, *368*, m511. [CrossRef]
66. Bhaskaran, K.; Douglas, I.; Forbes, H.; dos-Santos-Silva, I.; Leon, D.A.; Smeeth, L. Body-mass index and risk of 22 specific cancers: A population-based cohort study of 5·24 million UK adults. *Lancet* **2014**, *384*, 755–765. [CrossRef]
67. Jafari, A.; Najafi, S.; Moradi, F.; Kharazifard, M.; Khami, M. Delay in the diagnosis and treatment of oral cancer. *J. Dent. (Shiraz)* **2013**, *14*, 146–150. [PubMed]
68. Maymone, M.B.C.; Greer, R.O.; Kesecker, J.; Sahitya, P.C.; Burdine, L.K.; Cheng, A.D.; Maymone, A.C.; Vashi, N.A. Premalignant and malignant oral mucosal lesions: Clinical and pathological findings. *J. Am. Acad. Dermatol.* **2019**, *81*, 59–71. [CrossRef] [PubMed]
69. Wils, L.J.; Poell, J.B.; Brink, A.; Evren, I.; Brouns, E.R.; De Visscher, J.G.A.M.; Bloemena, E.; Brakenhoff, R.H. Elucidating the Genetic Landscape of Oral Leukoplakia to Predict Malignant Transformation. *Clin. Cancer Res.* **2023**, *29*, 602–613. [CrossRef] [PubMed]
70. Chaturvedi, A.K.; Udaltsova, N.; Engels, E.A.; Katzel, J.A.; Yanik, E.L.; Katki, H.A.; Lingen, M.W.; Silverberg, M.J. Oral Leukoplakia and Risk of Progression to Oral Cancer: A Population-Based Cohort Study. *J. Natl. Cancer Inst.* **2020**, *112*, 1047–1054. [CrossRef] [PubMed]
71. Parakh, M.K.; Ulaganambi, S.; Ashifa, N.; Premkumar, R.; Jain, A.L. Oral potentially malignant disorders: Clinical diagnosis and current screening aids: A narrative review. *Eur. J. Cancer Prev.* **2020**, *29*, 65–72. [CrossRef] [PubMed]
72. Ganesh, D.; Sreenivasan, P.; Öhman, J.; Wallström, M.; Braz-Silva, P.H.; Giglio, D.; Kjeller, G.; Hasséus, B. Potentially Malignant Oral Disorders and Cancer Transformation. *Anticancer Res.* **2018**, *38*, 3223–3229. [CrossRef]
73. Woo, S.B. Oral Epithelial Dysplasia and Premalignancy. *Head Neck Pathol.* **2019**, *13*, 423–439. [CrossRef]
74. Gupta, S.; Jawanda, M.K. Oral Lichen Planus: An Update on Etiology, Pathogenesis, Clinical Presentation, Diagnosis and Management. *Indian J. Dermatol.* **2015**, *60*, 222–229. [CrossRef]
75. Dionne, K.R.; Warnakulasuriya, S.; Zain, R.B.; Cheong, S.C. Potentially malignant disorders of the oral cavity: Current practice and future directions in the clinic and laboratory. *Int. J. Cancer* **2015**, *136*, 503–515. [CrossRef]
76. Nosratzehi, T. Oral Lichen Planus: An Overview of Potential Risk Factors, Biomarkers and Treatments. *Asian Pac. J. Cancer Prev.* **2018**, *19*, 1161–1167. [CrossRef]
77. Nagaraju, K.; Prasad, S.; Ashok, L. Diagnostic efficiency of toluidine blue with Lugol's iodine in oral premalignant and malignant lesions. *Indian J. Dent. Res.* **2010**, *21*, 218–223. [CrossRef] [PubMed]
78. Bittar, R.F.; Ferraro, H.P.; Ribas, M.H.; Lehn, C.N. Predictive factors of occult neck metastasis in patients with oral squamous cell carcinoma. *Braz. J. Otorhinolaryngol.* **2016**, *82*, 543–547. [CrossRef]
79. Lin, N.C.; Hsien, S.I.; Hsu, J.T.; Chen, M.Y.C. Impact on patients with oral squamous cell carcinoma in different anatomical subsites: A single-center study in Taiwan. *Sci. Rep.* **2021**, *11*, 15446. [CrossRef] [PubMed]
80. Basu, A.K. DNA Damage, Mutagenesis and Cancer. *Int. J. Mol. Sci.* **2018**, *19*, 970. [CrossRef]
81. Georgaki, M.; Theofilou, V.I.; Pettas, E.; Stoufi, E.; Younis, R.H.; Kolokotronis, A.; Sauk, J.J.; Nikitakis, N.G. Understanding the complex pathogenesis of oral cancer: A comprehensive review. *Oral Surg. Oral Med. Oral Pathol. Oral Radiol.* **2021**, *132*, 566–579. [CrossRef]
82. Gasche, J.A.; Goel, A. Epigenetic mechanisms in oral carcinogenesis. *Future Oncol.* **2012**, *8*, 1407–1425. [CrossRef] [PubMed]
83. Sasahira, T.; Kirita, T. Hallmarks of Cancer-Related Newly Prognostic Factors of Oral Squamous Cell Carcinoma. *Int. J. Mol. Sci.* **2018**, *19*, 2413. [CrossRef]
84. Usman, S.; Jamal, A.; Teh, M.T.; Waseem, A. Major Molecular Signaling Pathways in Oral Cancer Associated With Therapeutic Resistance. *Front. Oral Health* **2020**, *1*, 603160. [CrossRef]

85. Irimie, A.I.; Braicu, C.; Sonea, L.; Zimta, A.A.; Cojocneanu-Petric, R.; Tonchev, K.; Mehterov, N.; Diudea, D.; Buduru, S.; Berindan-Neagoe, I. A Looking-Glass of Non-coding RNAs in oral cancer. *Int. J. Mol. Sci.* **2017**, *18*, 2620. [CrossRef]
86. Gabusi, A.; Gissi, D.B.; Grillini, S.; Stefanini, M.; Tarsitano, A.; Marchetti, C.; Foschini, M.P.; Montebugnoli, L.; Morandi, L. Shared epigenetic alterations between oral cancer and periodontitis: A preliminary study. *Oral Dis.* **2022**, *29*, 2052–2060. [CrossRef]
87. Flausino, C.S.; Daniel, F.I.; Modolo, F. DNA methylation in oral squamous cell carcinoma: From its role in carcinogenesis to potential inhibitor drugs. *Crit. Rev. Oncol. Hematol.* **2021**, *164*, 103399. [CrossRef] [PubMed]
88. Hussain, T.; Nguyen, Q.T. Molecular imaging for cancer diagnosis and surgery. *Adv. Drug Deliv. Rev.* **2014**, *66*, 90–100. [CrossRef] [PubMed]
89. Kaur, J.; Jacobs, R.; Huang, Y.; Salvo, N.; Politis, C. Salivary biomarkers for oral cancer and pre-cancer screening: A review. *Clin. Oral Investig.* **2018**, *22*, 633–640. [CrossRef] [PubMed]
90. Shah, J.P.; Gil, Z. Current concepts in management of oral cancer--surgery. *Oral Oncol.* **2009**, *45*, 394–401. [CrossRef] [PubMed]
91. Vonk, J.; de Wit, J.G.; Voskuil, F.J.; Witjes, M.J.H. Improving oral cavity cancer diagnosis and treatment with fluorescence molecular imaging. *Oral Dis.* **2021**, *27*, 21–26. [CrossRef]
92. González-Moles, M.; Aguilar-Ruiz, M.; Ramos-García, P. Challenges in the Early Diagnosis of Oral Cancer, Evidence Gaps and Strategies for Improvement: A Scoping Review of Systematic Reviews. *Cancers* **2022**, *14*, 4967. [CrossRef]
93. Ali Khani, J.; Fatemeh, J. Oral Cancer: Epidemiology, Prevention, Early Detection, and Treatment. In *Oral Cancer*; Gokul, S., Ed.; IntechOpen: Rijeka, Croatia, 2021; Chapter 1. [CrossRef]
94. May, S.; Parry, C.; Parry, L. Berry chemoprevention: Do berries decrease the window of opportunity for tumorigenesis. *Food Front.* **2020**, *1*, 260–275. [CrossRef]
95. Golovinskaia, O.; Wang, C.K. Review of Functional and Pharmacological Activities of Berries. *Molecules* **2021**, *26*, 3904. [CrossRef]
96. Kristo, A.S.; Klimis-Zacas, D.; Sikalidis, A.K. Protective Role of Dietary Berries in Cancer. *Antioxidants* **2016**, *5*, 37. [CrossRef]
97. Lee, T.-Y.; Tseng, Y.-H. The Potential of Phytochemicals in Oral Cancer Prevention and Therapy: A Review of the Evidence. *Biomolecules* **2020**, *10*, 1150. [CrossRef]
98. Michalska, A.; Łysiak, G. Bioactive Compounds of Blueberries: Post-Harvest Factors Influencing the Nutritional Value of Products. *Int. J. Mol. Sci.* **2015**, *16*, 18642–18663. [CrossRef] [PubMed]
99. Nemzer, B.V.; Al-Taher, F.; Yashin, A.; Revelsky, I.; Yashin, Y. Cranberry: Chemical Composition, Antioxidant Activity and Impact on Human Health: Overview. *Molecules* **2022**, *27*, 1503. [CrossRef] [PubMed]
100. Chang, H.P.; Lu, C.C.; Chiang, J.H.; Tsai, F.J.; Juan, Y.N.; Tsao, J.W.; Chiu, H.Y.; Yang, J.S. Pterostilbene modulates the suppression of multidrug resistance protein 1 and triggers autophagic and apoptotic mechanisms in cisplatin-resistant human oral cancer CAR cells via AKT signaling. *Int. J. Oncol.* **2018**, *52*, 1504–1514. [CrossRef] [PubMed]
101. Fan, Y.; Qiu, Y.; Wang, J.; Chen, Q.; Wang, S.; Wang, Y.; Li, Y.; Weng, Y.; Qian, J.; Chen, F.; et al. Association Between Dietary Fatty Acid Pattern and Risk of Oral Cancer. *Front. Nutr.* **2022**, *9*, 864098. [CrossRef] [PubMed]
102. Del Rio, D.; Rodriguez-Mateos, A.; Spencer, J.P.; Tognolini, M.; Borges, G.; Crozier, A. Dietary (poly)phenolics in human health: Structures, bioavailability, and evidence of protective effects against chronic diseases. *Antioxid. Redox Signal.* **2013**, *18*, 1818–1892. [CrossRef]
103. Martău, G.A.; Bernadette-Emőke, T.; Odocheanu, R.; Soporan, D.A.; Bochiș, M.; Simon, E.; Vodnar, D.C. Vaccinium Species (Ericaceae): Phytochemistry and Biological Properties of Medicinal Plants. *Molecules* **2023**, *28*, 1533. [CrossRef] [PubMed]
104. Mazza, G.J. Anthocyanins and heart health. *Ann. Dell'istituto Super. Sanita* **2007**, *43*, 369–374.
105. Greenwald, P.; Milner, J.A.; Clifford, C.K. Creating a New Paradigm in Nutrition Research within the National Cancer Institute. *J. Nutr.* **2000**, *130*, 3103–3105. [CrossRef]
106. Wei, H.; Li, H.; Wan, S.P.; Zeng, Q.T.; Cheng, L.X.; Jiang, L.L.; Peng, Y.D. Cardioprotective Effects of Malvidin against Isoproterenol-Induced Myocardial Infarction in Rats: A Mechanistic Study. *Med. Sci. Monit.* **2017**, *23*, 2007–2016. [CrossRef]
107. Bognar, E.; Sarszegi, Z.; Szabo, A.; Debreceni, B.; Kalman, N.; Tucsek, Z.; Sumegi, B.; Gallyas, F., Jr. Antioxidant and anti-inflammatory effects in RAW264.7 macrophages of malvidin, a major red wine polyphenol. *PLoS ONE* **2013**, *8*, e65355. [CrossRef]
108. Kim, Y.S.; Kim, E.K.; Tang, Y.; Hwang, J.W.; Natarajan, S.B.; Kim, W.S.; Moon, S.H.; Jeon, B.T.; Park, P.J. Antioxidant and anticancer effects of extracts from fermented *Haliotis discus hannai* with *Cordyceps militaris* mycelia. *Food Sci. Biotechnol.* **2016**, *25*, 1775–1782. [CrossRef]
109. Gao, L.; Mazza, G. Quantitation and Distribution of Simple and Acylated Anthocyanins and Other Phenolics in Blueberries. *J. Food Sci.* **1994**, *59*, 1057–1059. [CrossRef]
110. Russo, G.I.; Campisi, D.; Di Mauro, M.; Regis, F.; Reale, G.; Marranzano, M.; Ragusa, R.; Solinas, T.; Madonia, M.; Cimino, S.; et al. Dietary Consumption of Phenolic Acids and Prostate Cancer: A Case-Control Study in Sicily, Southern Italy. *Molecules* **2017**, *22*, 2159. [CrossRef]
111. Mohammed, H.A.; Khan, R.A. Anthocyanins: Traditional Uses, Structural and Functional Variations, Approaches to Increase Yields and Products' Quality, Hepatoprotection, Liver Longevity, and Commercial Products. *Int. J. Mol. Sci.* **2022**, *23*, 2149. [CrossRef] [PubMed]
112. Panchal, S.K.; John, O.D.; Mathai, M.L.; Brown, L. Anthocyanins in Chronic Diseases: The Power of Purple. *Nutrients* **2022**, *14*, 2161. [CrossRef]
113. Hair, R.; Sakaki, J.R.; Chun, O.K. Anthocyanins, Microbiome and Health Benefits in Aging. *Molecules* **2021**, *26*, 537. [CrossRef] [PubMed]

114. Ma, Z.; Du, B.; Li, J.; Yang, Y.; Zhu, F. An Insight into Anti-Inflammatory Activities and Inflammation Related Diseases of Anthocyanins: A Review of Both In Vivo and In Vitro Investigations. *Int. J. Mol. Sci.* **2021**, *22*, 11076. [CrossRef]
115. Oliveira, H.; Correia, P.; Pereira, A.R.; Araújo, P.; Mateus, N.; de Freitas, V.; Oliveira, J.; Fernandes, I. Exploring the Applications of the Photoprotective Properties of Anthocyanins in Biological Systems. *Int. J. Mol. Sci.* **2020**, *21*, 7464. [CrossRef]
116. Lin, B.W.; Gong, C.C.; Song, H.F.; Cui, Y.Y. Effects of anthocyanins on the prevention and treatment of cancer. *Br. J. Pharmacol.* **2017**, *174*, 1226–1243. [CrossRef]
117. Milner, J.A. Foods and health promotion: The case for cranberry. *Crit. Rev. Food Sci. Nutr.* **2002**, *42*, 265–266. [CrossRef]
118. Seeram, N.P.; Adams, L.S.; Hardy, M.L.; Heber, D. Total cranberry extract versus its phytochemical constituents: Antiproliferative and synergistic effects against human tumor cell lines. *J. Agric. Food Chem.* **2004**, *52*, 2512–2517. [CrossRef] [PubMed]
119. Seeram, N.P.; Adams, L.S.; Zhang, Y.; Lee, R.; Sand, D.; Scheuller, H.S.; Heber, D. Blackberry, black raspberry, blueberry, cranberry, red raspberry, and strawberry extracts inhibit growth and stimulate apoptosis of human cancer cells in vitro. *J. Agric. Food Chem.* **2006**, *54*, 9329–9339. [CrossRef]
120. Baba, A.B.; Nivetha, R.; Chattopadhyay, I.; Nagini, S. Blueberry and malvidin inhibit cell cycle progression and induce mitochondrial-mediated apoptosis by abrogating the JAK/STAT-3 signalling pathway. *Food Chem. Toxicol.* **2017**, *109*, 534–543. [CrossRef] [PubMed]
121. Rothwell, J.A.; Perez-Jimenez, J.; Neveu, V.; Medina-Remón, A.; M'Hiri, N.; García-Lobato, P.; Manach, C.; Knox, C.; Eisner, R.; Wishart, D.S.; et al. Phenol-Explorer 3.0: A major update of the Phenol-Explorer database to incorporate data on the effects of food processing on polyphenol content. *Database* **2013**, *2013*, bat070. [CrossRef] [PubMed]
122. Chudzik, M.; Korzonek-Szlacheta, I.; Król, W. Triterpenes as potentially cytotoxic compounds. *Molecules* **2015**, *20*, 1610–1625. [CrossRef] [PubMed]
123. Khoo, H.E.; Azlan, A.; Tang, S.T.; Lim, S.M. Anthocyanidins and anthocyanins: Colored pigments as food, pharmaceutical ingredients, and the potential health benefits. *Food Nutr. Res.* **2017**, *61*, 1361779. [CrossRef] [PubMed]
124. Mattioli, R.; Francioso, A.; Mosca, L.; Silva, P. Anthocyanins: A Comprehensive Review of Their Chemical Properties and Health Effects on Cardiovascular and Neurodegenerative Diseases. *Molecules* **2020**, *25*, 3809. [CrossRef]
125. Ullah, A.; Munir, S.; Badshah, S.L.; Khan, N.; Ghani, L.; Poulson, B.G.; Emwas, A.H.; Jaremko, M. Important Flavonoids and Their Role as a Therapeutic Agent. *Molecules* **2020**, *25*, 5243. [CrossRef]
126. Fan, M.J.; Wang, I.C.; Hsiao, Y.T.; Lin, H.Y.; Tang, N.Y.; Hung, T.C.; Quan, C.; Lien, J.C.; Chung, J.G. Anthocyanins from black rice (*Oryza sativa* L.) demonstrate antimetastatic properties by reducing MMPs and NF-κB expressions in human oral cancer CAL 27 cells. *Nutr. Cancer* **2015**, *67*, 327–338. [CrossRef]
127. Huang, Y.W.; Chuang, C.Y.; Hsieh, Y.S.; Chen, P.N.; Yang, S.F.; Shih Hsuan, L.; Chen, Y.Y.; Lin, C.W.; Chang, Y.C. Rubus idaeus extract suppresses migration and invasion of human oral cancer by inhibiting MMP-2 through modulation of the Erk1/2 signaling pathway. *Environ. Toxicol.* **2017**, *32*, 1037–1046. [CrossRef]
128. Qi, C.; Li, S.; Jia, Y.; Wang, L. Blueberry anthocyanins induce G2/M cell cycle arrest and apoptosis of oral cancer KB cells through down-regulation methylation of p53. *Yi Chuan* **2014**, *36*, 566–573. [PubMed]
129. Chen, J.L.; Lai, C.Y.; Ying, T.H.; Lin, C.W.; Wang, P.H.; Yu, F.J.; Liu, C.J.; Hsieh, Y.H. Modulating the ERK1/2-MMP1 Axis through Corosolic Acid Inhibits Metastasis of Human Oral Squamous Cell Carcinoma Cells. *Int. J. Mol. Sci.* **2021**, *22*, 8641. [CrossRef] [PubMed]
130. Maarten, J.M.C.; James, W.B. *The Number of Known Plants Species in the World and Its Annual Increase*; Magnolia Press: Waco, TX, USA, 2016; Volume 261, p. 201. [CrossRef]
131. Kresty, L.A.; Weh, K.M.; Zeyzus-Johns, B.; Perez, L.N.; Howell, A.B. Cranberry proanthocyanidins inhibit esophageal adenocarcinoma in vitro and in vivo through pleiotropic cell death induction and PI3K/AKT/mTOR inactivation. *Oncotarget* **2015**, *6*, 33438–33455. [CrossRef]
132. Miller, K.; Feucht, W.; Schmid, M. Bioactive Compounds of Strawberry and Blueberry and Their Potential Health Effects Based on Human Intervention Studies: A Brief Overview. *Nutrients* **2019**, *11*, 1510. [CrossRef] [PubMed]
133. Su, X.; Zhang, J.; Wang, H.; Xu, J.; He, J.; Liu, L.; Zhang, T.; Chen, R.; Kang, J. Phenolic Acid Profiling, Antioxidant, and Anti-Inflammatory Activities, and miRNA Regulation in the Polyphenols of 16 Blueberry Samples from China. *Molecules* **2017**, *22*, 312. [CrossRef]
134. Butt, M.S.; Sultan, M.T. Coffee and its consumption: Benefits and risks. *Crit. Rev. Food Sci. Nutr.* **2011**, *51*, 363–373. [CrossRef]
135. Gökcen, B.B.; Şanlier, N. Coffee consumption and disease correlations. *Crit. Rev. Food Sci. Nutr.* **2019**, *59*, 336–348. [CrossRef]
136. Howell, A.B.; Vorsa, N.; Der Marderosian, A.; Foo, L.Y. Inhibition of the adherence of P-fimbriated *Escherichia coli* to uroepithelial-cell surfaces by proanthocyanidin extracts from cranberries. *N. Engl. J. Med.* **1998**, *339*, 1085–1086. [CrossRef]
137. Ferguson, P.J.; Kurowska, E.M.; Freeman, D.J.; Chambers, A.F.; Koropatnick, J. In vivo inhibition of growth of human tumor lines by flavonoid fractions from cranberry extract. *Nutr. Cancer* **2006**, *56*, 86–94. [CrossRef]
138. Al-Ishaq, R.K.; Overy, A.J.; Büsselberg, D. Phytochemicals and Gastrointestinal Cancer: Cellular Mechanisms and Effects to Change Cancer Progression. *Biomolecules* **2020**, *10*, 105. [CrossRef]
139. de Moura, C.F.; Noguti, J.; de Jesus, G.P.; Ribeiro, F.A.; Garcia, F.A.; Gollucke, A.P.; Aguiar, O., Jr.; Ribeiro, D.A. Polyphenols as a chemopreventive agent in oral carcinogenesis: Putative mechanisms of action using in-vitro and in-vivo test systems. *Eur. J. Cancer Prev.* **2013**, *22*, 467–472. [CrossRef] [PubMed]

140. Chen, C.Y.; Kao, C.L.; Liu, C.M. The Cancer Prevention, Anti-Inflammatory and Anti-Oxidation of Bioactive Phytochemicals Targeting the TLR4 Signaling Pathway. *Int. J. Mol. Sci.* **2018**, *19*, 2729. [CrossRef] [PubMed]
141. Chen, J.; Shu, Y.; Chen, Y.; Ge, Z.; Zhang, C.; Cao, J.; Li, X.; Wang, Y.; Sun, C. Evaluation of Antioxidant Capacity and Gut Microbiota Modulatory Effects of Different Kinds of Berries. *Antioxidants* **2022**, *11*, 1020. [CrossRef] [PubMed]
142. Tu, P.; Chi, L.; Bian, X.; Gao, B.; Ru, H.; Lu, K. A Black Raspberry-Rich Diet Protects From Dextran Sulfate Sodium-Induced Intestinal Inflammation and Host Metabolic Perturbation in Association With Increased Aryl Hydrocarbon Receptor Ligands in the Gut Microbiota of Mice. *Front. Nutr.* **2022**, *9*, 842298. [CrossRef]
143. Singh, V.; Singh, R.; Kujur, P.K.; Singh, R.P. Combination of Resveratrol and Quercetin Causes Cell Growth Inhibition, DNA Damage, Cell Cycle Arrest, and Apoptosis in Oral Cancer Cells. *Assay Drug Dev. Technol.* **2020**, *18*, 226–238. [CrossRef]
144. Wang, P.; Shang, R.; Ma, Y.; Wang, D.; Zhao, W.; Chen, F.; Hu, X.; Zhao, X. Targeting microbiota-host interactions with resveratrol on cancer: Effects and potential mechanisms of action. *Crit. Rev. Food Sci. Nutr.* **2022**, *62*, 1–23. [CrossRef] [PubMed]
145. Chang, C.H.; Lee, C.Y.; Lu, C.C.; Tsai, F.J.; Hsu, Y.M.; Tsao, J.W.; Juan, Y.N.; Chiu, H.Y.; Yang, J.S.; Wang, C.C. Resveratrol-induced autophagy and apoptosis in cisplatin-resistant human oral cancer CAR cells: A key role of AMPK and Akt/mTOR signaling. *Int. J. Oncol.* **2017**, *50*, 873–882. [CrossRef]
146. Shi, P.; Li, B.; Chen, H.; Song, C.; Meng, J.; Xi, Z.; Zhang, Z. Iron Supply Affects Anthocyanin Content and Related Gene Expression in Berries of *Vitis vinifera cv.* Cabernet Sauvignon. *Molecules* **2017**, *22*, 283. [CrossRef]
147. Weh, K.M.; Zhang, Y.; Howard, C.L.; Howell, A.B.; Clarke, J.L.; Kresty, L.A. Cranberry Polyphenols in Esophageal Cancer Inhibition: New Insights. *Nutrients* **2022**, *14*, 969. [CrossRef]
148. Oghumu, S.; Casto, B.C.; Ahn-Jarvis, J.; Weghorst, L.C.; Maloney, J.; Geuy, P.; Horvath, K.Z.; Bollinger, C.E.; Warner, B.M.; Summersgill, K.F.; et al. Inhibition of Pro-inflammatory and Anti-apoptotic Biomarkers during Experimental Oral Cancer Chemoprevention by Dietary Black Raspberries. *Front. Immunol.* **2017**, *8*, 1325. [CrossRef]
149. Knobloch, T.J.; Ryan, N.M.; Bruschweiler-Li, L.; Wang, C.; Bernier, M.C.; Somogyi, A.; Yan, P.S.; Cooperstone, J.L.; Mo, X.; Brüschweiler, R.P.; et al. Metabolic Regulation of Glycolysis and AMP Activated Protein Kinase Pathways during Black Raspberry-Mediated Oral Cancer Chemoprevention. *Metabolites* **2019**, *9*, 140. [CrossRef] [PubMed]
150. Chiu, C.C.; Haung, J.W.; Chang, F.R.; Huang, K.J.; Huang, H.M.; Huang, H.W.; Chou, C.K.; Wu, Y.C.; Chang, H.W. Golden berry-derived 4β-hydroxywithanolide E for selectively killing oral cancer cells by generating ROS, DNA damage, and apoptotic pathways. *PLoS ONE* **2013**, *8*, e64739. [CrossRef] [PubMed]
151. Breitmaier, E. *Terpenes: Flavors, Fragrances, Pharmaca, Pheromones*; Wiley-Vch: Hoboken, NJ, USA, 2006.
152. D'Souza, S.; Addepalli, V. Preventive measures in oral cancer: An overview. *Biomed. Pharmacother.* **2018**, *107*, 72–80. [CrossRef] [PubMed]
153. Mangalath, U.; Aslam, S.A.; Abdul Khadar, A.H.; Francis, P.G.; Mikacha, M.S.; Kalathingal, J.H. Recent trends in prevention of oral cancer. *J. Int. Soc. Prev. Community Dent.* **2014**, *4*, S131–S138. [CrossRef] [PubMed]
154. Hwang, H.; Kim, Y.-J.; Shin, Y. Assessment of Physicochemical Quality, Antioxidant Content and Activity, and Inhibition of Cholinesterase between Unripe and Ripe Blueberry Fruit. *Foods* **2020**, *9*, 690. [CrossRef]
155. Nile, S.H.; Park, S.W. Edible berries: Bioactive components and their effect on human health. *Nutrition* **2014**, *30*, 134–144. [CrossRef]
156. Kalt, W.; Lawand, C.; Ryan, D.A.J.; McDonald, J.E.; Donner, H.; Forney, C.F. Oxygen Radical Absorbing Capacity, Anthocyanin and Phenolic Content of Highbush Blueberries (*Vaccinium corymbosum* L.) during Ripening and Storage. *J. Am. Soc. Hortic. Sci. Jashs* **2003**, *128*, 917–923. [CrossRef]
157. Wu, X.; Beecher, G.R.; Holden, J.M.; Haytowitz, D.B.; Gebhardt, S.E.; Prior, R.L. Concentrations of anthocyanins in common foods in the United States and estimation of normal consumption. *J. Agric. Food Chem.* **2006**, *54*, 4069–4075. [CrossRef]
158. Kalt, W.; Blumberg, J.B.; McDonald, J.E.; Vinqvist-Tymchuk, M.R.; Fillmore, S.A.; Graf, B.A.; O'Leary, J.M.; Milbury, P.E. Identification of anthocyanins in the liver, eye, and brain of blueberry-fed pigs. *J. Agric. Food Chem.* **2008**, *56*, 705–712. [CrossRef]
159. Kalt, W.; McDonald, J.E.; Vinqvist-Tymchuk, M.R.; Liu, Y.; Fillmore, S.A.E. Human anthocyanin bioavailability: Effect of intake duration and dosing. *Food Funct.* **2017**, *8*, 4563–4569. [CrossRef]
160. Poei-Langston, M.S.; Wrolstad, R.E. Color Degradation in an Ascorbic Acid-Anthocyanin-Flavanol Model System. *J. Food Sci.* **1981**, *46*, 1218–1236. [CrossRef]
161. Neto, C.C. Cranberry and blueberry: Evidence for protective effects against cancer and vascular diseases. *Mol. Nutr. Food Res.* **2007**, *51*, 652–664. [CrossRef] [PubMed]
162. Qaderi, M.M.; Martel, A.B.; Strugnell, C.A. Environmental Factors Regulate Plant Secondary Metabolites. *Plants* **2023**, *12*, 447. [CrossRef] [PubMed]
163. D'Urso, G.; Piacente, S.; Pizza, C.; Montoro, P. Metabolomics of Healthy Berry Fruits. *Curr. Med. Chem.* **2018**, *25*, 4888–4902. [CrossRef] [PubMed]
164. Muthukrishnan, A.; Warnakulasuriya, S. Oral health consequences of smokeless tobacco use. *Indian J. Med. Res.* **2018**, *148*, 35–40. [CrossRef] [PubMed]
165. Hecht, S.S. Tobacco carcinogens, their biomarkers and tobacco-induced cancer. *Nat. Rev. Cancer* **2003**, *3*, 733–744. [CrossRef]
166. G, M.S.; Swetha, M.; Keerthana, C.K.; Rayginia, T.P.; Anto, R.J. Cancer Chemoprevention: A Strategic Approach Using Phytochemicals. *Front. Pharmacol.* **2021**, *12*, 809308. [CrossRef]

167. Baba, A.B.; Kowshik, J.; Krishnaraj, J.; Sophia, J.; Dixit, M.; Nagini, S. Blueberry inhibits invasion and angiogenesis in 7,12-dimethylbenz[a]anthracene (DMBA)-induced oral squamous cell carcinogenesis in hamsters via suppression of TGF-β and NF-κB signaling pathways. *J. Nutr. Biochem.* **2016**, *35*, 37–47. [CrossRef]
168. Gu, I.; Brownmiller, C.; Stebbins, N.B.; Mauromoustakos, A.; Howard, L.; Lee, S.-O. Berry Phenolic and Volatile Extracts Inhibit Pro-Inflammatory Cytokine Secretion in LPS-Stimulated RAW264.7 Cells through Suppression of NF-κB Signaling Pathway. *Antioxidants* **2020**, *9*, 871. [CrossRef]
169. El-Bayoumy, K.; Chen, K.M.; Zhang, S.M.; Sun, Y.W.; Amin, S.; Stoner, G.; Guttenplan, J.B. Carcinogenesis of the Oral Cavity: Environmental Causes and Potential Prevention by Black Raspberry. *Chem. Res. Toxicol.* **2017**, *30*, 126–144. [CrossRef]
170. Ogden, G.R. Alcohol and oral cancer. *Alcohol* **2005**, *35*, 169–173. [CrossRef] [PubMed]
171. Boffetta, P.; Hashibe, M. Alcohol and cancer. *Lancet Oncol.* **2006**, *7*, 149–156. [CrossRef] [PubMed]
172. Red Wine May Reduce Oral Cancer Risks. *J. Am. Dent. Assoc.* **2000**, *131*, 729–731. [CrossRef] [PubMed]
173. Bhandari, A.; Bhatta, N. Tobacco and its Relationship with Oral Health. *JNMA J. Nepal. Med. Assoc.* **2021**, *59*, 1204–1206. [CrossRef]
174. Varoni, E.M.; Lodi, G.; Iriti, M. Ethanol versus Phytochemicals in Wine: Oral Cancer Risk in a Light Drinking Perspective. *Int. J. Mol. Sci.* **2015**, *16*, 17029–17047. [CrossRef]
175. Stornetta, A.; Guidolin, V.; Balbo, S. Alcohol-Derived Acetaldehyde Exposure in the Oral Cavity. *Cancers* **2018**, *10*, 20. [CrossRef]
176. Sedghi, L.; DiMassa, V.; Harrington, A.; Lynch, S.V.; Kapila, Y.L. The oral microbiome: Role of key organisms and complex networks in oral health and disease. *Periodontology 2000* **2021**, *87*, 107–131. [CrossRef]
177. Binder Gallimidi, A.; Fischman, S.; Revach, B.; Bulvik, R.; Maliutina, A.; Rubinstein, A.M.; Nussbaum, G.; Elkin, M. Periodontal pathogens *Porphyromonas gingivalis* and *Fusobacterium nucleatum* promote tumor progression in an oral-specific chemical carcinogenesis model. *Oncotarget* **2015**, *6*, 22613–22623. [CrossRef]
178. Sun, J.; Tang, Q.; Yu, S.; Xie, M.; Xie, Y.; Chen, G.; Chen, L. Role of the oral microbiota in cancer evolution and progression. *Cancer Med.* **2020**, *9*, 6306–6321. [CrossRef]
179. Vadovics, M.; Ho, J.; Igaz, N.; Alföldi, R.; Rakk, D.; Veres, É.; Szücs, B.; Horváth, M.; Tóth, R.; Szücs, A.; et al. *Candida albicans* Enhances the Progression of Oral Squamous Cell Carcinoma In Vitro and In Vivo. *mBio* **2021**, *13*, e0314421. [CrossRef]
180. Dutreix, L.; Bernard, C.; Juin, C.; Imbert, C.; Girardot, M. Do raspberry extracts and fractions have antifungal or anti-adherent potential against *Candida* spp.? *Int. J. Antimicrob. Agents* **2018**, *52*, 947–953. [CrossRef]
181. Engku Nasrullah Satiman, E.A.F.; Ahmad, H.; Ramzi, A.B.; Abdul Wahab, R.; Kaderi, M.A.; Wan Harun, W.H.A.; Dashper, S.; McCullough, M.; Arzmi, M.H. The role of *Candida albicans* candidalysin ECE1 gene in oral carcinogenesis. *J. Oral Pathol. Med.* **2020**, *49*, 835–841. [CrossRef] [PubMed]
182. Girardot, M.; Guerineau, A.; Boudesocque, L.; Costa, D.; Bazinet, L.; Enguehard-Gueiffier, C.; Imbert, C. Promising results of cranberry in the prevention of oral Candida biofilms. *Pathog. Dis.* **2014**, *70*, 432–439. [CrossRef] [PubMed]
183. Hisano, M.; Bruschini, H.; Nicodemo, A.C.; Srougi, M. Cranberries and lower urinary tract infection prevention. *Clinics (Sao Paulo)* **2012**, *67*, 661–668. [CrossRef]
184. La, V.D.; Howell, A.B.; Grenier, D. Anti-Porphyromonas gingivalis and anti-inflammatory activities of A-type cranberry proanthocyanidins. *Antimicrob. Agents Chemother.* **2010**, *54*, 1778–1784. [CrossRef]
185. Vitkov, L.; Singh, J.; Schauer, C.; Minnich, B.; Krunić, J.; Oberthaler, H.; Gamsjaeger, S.; Herrmann, M.; Knopf, J.; Hannig, M. Breaking the Gingival Barrier in Periodontitis. *Int. J. Mol. Sci.* **2023**, *24*, 4544. [CrossRef]
186. Feghali, K.; Feldman, M.; La, V.D.; Santos, J.; Grenier, D. Cranberry proanthocyanidins: Natural weapons against periodontal diseases. *J. Agric. Food Chem.* **2012**, *60*, 5728–5735. [CrossRef]
187. Chaitanya, N.C.; Allam, N.S.; Gandhi Babu, D.B.; Waghray, S.; Badam, R.K.; Lavanya, R. Systematic meta-analysis on association of human papilloma virus and oral cancer. *J. Cancer Res. Ther.* **2016**, *12*, 969–974. [CrossRef]
188. Guidry, J.T.; Birdwell, C.E.; Scott, R.S. Epstein-Barr virus in the pathogenesis of oral cancers. *Oral Dis.* **2018**, *24*, 497–508. [CrossRef]
189. Khuayjarernpanishk, T.; Sookying, S.; Duangjai, A.; Saokaew, S.; Sanbua, A.; Bunteong, O.; Rungruangsri, N.; Suepsai, W.; Sodsai, P.; Soyliaid, J.; et al. Anticancer Activities of *Polygonum odoratum* Lour.: A Systematic Review. *Front. Pharmacol.* **2022**, *13*, 875016. [CrossRef]
190. Ankola, A.V.; Kumar, V.; Thakur, S.; Singhal, R.; Smitha, T.; Sankeshwari, R. Anticancer and antiproliferative efficacy of a standardized extract of *Vaccinium macrocarpon* on the highly differentiating oral cancer KB cell line athwart the cytotoxicity evaluation of the same on the normal fibroblast L929 cell line. *J. Oral Maxillofac. Pathol.* **2020**, *24*, 258–265. [CrossRef] [PubMed]
191. Chatelain, K.; Phippen, S.; McCabe, J.; Teeters, C.A.; O'Malley, S.; Kingsley, K. Cranberry and grape seed extracts inhibit the proliferative phenotype of oral squamous cell carcinomas. *Evid. Based Complement. Altern. Med.* **2011**, *2011*, 467691. [CrossRef] [PubMed]
192. Nicastro, H.L.; Ross, S.A.; Milner, J.A. Garlic and onions: Their cancer prevention properties. *Cancer Prev. Res. (Phila)* **2015**, *8*, 181–189. [CrossRef] [PubMed]

Disclaimer/Publisher's Note: The statements, opinions and data contained in all publications are solely those of the individual author(s) and contributor(s) and not of MDPI and/or the editor(s). MDPI and/or the editor(s) disclaim responsibility for any injury to people or property resulting from any ideas, methods, instructions or products referred to in the content.

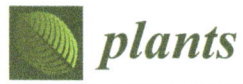

Review

Plant-Derived Nutraceuticals Involved in Body Weight Control by Modulating Gene Expression

Maria Vrânceanu [1], Simona-Codruța Hegheș [2,*], Anamaria Cozma-Petruț [3], Roxana Banc [3], Carmina Mariana Stroia [4], Viorica Raischi [5], Doina Miere [3], Daniela-Saveta Popa [1] and Lorena Filip [3]

1. Department of Toxicology, "Iuliu Hațieganu" University of Medicine and Pharmacy, 6 Pasteur Street, 400349 Cluj-Napoca, Romania; marievranceanu@gmail.com (M.V.); dpopa@umfcluj.ro (D.-S.P.)
2. Department of Drug Analysis, "Iuliu Hațieganu" University of Medicine and Pharmacy, 6 Pasteur Street, 400349 Cluj-Napoca, Romania
3. Department of Bromatology, Hygiene, Nutrition, "Iuliu Hațieganu" University of Medicine and Pharmacy, 6 Pasteur Street, 400349 Cluj-Napoca, Romania; anamaria.cozma@umfcluj.ro (A.C.-P.); roxana.banc@umfcluj.ro (R.B.); dmiere@umfcluj.ro (D.M.); lfilip@umfcluj.ro (L.F.)
4. Department of Pharmacy, Oradea University, 1 Universității Street, 410087 Oradea, Romania; carmina.marian@yahoo.com
5. Laboratory of Physiology of Stress, Adaptation and General Sanocreatology, Institute of Physiology and Sanocreatology, 1 Academiei Street, 2028 Chișinău, Moldova; vioricalana@gmail.com
* Correspondence: cmaier@umfcluj.ro; Tel.: +40-745-535-256

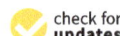

Citation: Vrânceanu, M.; Hegheș, S.-C.; Cozma-Petruț, A.; Banc, R.; Stroia, C.M.; Raischi, V.; Miere, D.; Popa, D.-S.; Filip, L. Plant-Derived Nutraceuticals Involved in Body Weight Control by Modulating Gene Expression. *Plants* **2023**, *12*, 2273. https://doi.org/10.3390/plants12122273

Academic Editors: Nancy Vargas Mendoza and José Antonio Morales-González

Received: 11 May 2023
Revised: 9 June 2023
Accepted: 9 June 2023
Published: 11 June 2023

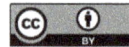

Copyright: © 2023 by the authors. Licensee MDPI, Basel, Switzerland. This article is an open access article distributed under the terms and conditions of the Creative Commons Attribution (CC BY) license (https:// creativecommons.org/licenses/by/ 4.0/).

Abstract: Obesity is the most prevalent health problem in the Western world, with pathological body weight gain associated with numerous co-morbidities that can be the main cause of death. There are several factors that can contribute to the development of obesity, such as diet, sedentary lifestyle, and genetic make-up. Genetic predispositions play an important role in obesity, but genetic variations alone cannot fully explain the explosion of obesity, which is why studies have turned to epigenetics. The latest scientific evidence suggests that both genetics and environmental factors contribute to the rise in obesity. Certain variables, such as diet and exercise, have the ability to alter gene expression without affecting the DNA sequence, a phenomenon known as epigenetics. Epigenetic changes are reversible, and reversibility makes these changes attractive targets for therapeutic interventions. While anti-obesity drugs have been proposed to this end in recent decades, their numerous side effects make them not very attractive. On the other hand, the use of nutraceuticals for weight loss is increasing, and studies have shown that some of these products, such as resveratrol, curcumin, epigallocatechin-3-gallate, ginger, capsaicin, and caffeine, can alter gene expression, restoring the normal epigenetic profile and aiding weight loss.

Keywords: obesity; nutraceuticals; epigenetics; gene expression; weight loss

1. Introduction

Despite the degree of malnutrition existing on the planet, according to the World Health Organization (WHO), obesity is one of the main public health problems in the world. In fact, we are facing a real global epidemic, which is spreading in many countries and which, in the absence of immediate action, could cause very serious health problems in the coming years. There are 375 million women and 266 million men who are overweight or obese in the world, and the US is at the top of obesity rankings. Among the most developed countries, Japan is the one in which the inhabitants have the lowest body mass index. In Europe, the most in line are Swiss women and Bosnian men. Globally, 2.3% of men and 5% of women are considered severely obese, that is, with a BMI above 35. Continuing at the current rate, 18% of men and 21% of women will suffer from severe obesity by 2025 [1].

Obesity is a condition characterized by excessive body weight due to the accumulation of adipose tissue, which develops due to the interaction of various factors, including genetic, endocrine-metabolic, and environmental factors. Therefore, it is a very common chronic condition that can negatively affect the state of health because it increases the risk of developing other diseases and worsens the person's quality of life [2].

Indeed, obesity has a wide range of health impacts. Obese individuals are in fact at greater risk for the development of various disorders, including metabolic diseases such as diabetes and dyslipidemia (high levels of cholesterol and triglycerides), cardiovascular diseases such as stroke and heart attack, respiratory diseases, joint problems, gynecological disorders (menstrual irregularities, polycystic ovary syndrome, pregnancy complications), infertility, sexual disorders (impotence), predisposition to the development of diseases of the digestive system (e.g., gastroesophageal reflux, gallbladder stones), and mood disorders (e.g., depression) [3]. Finally, it should be remembered that the presence of obesity increases the risk of developing certain tumors, such as endometrial cancer (a type of uterine cancer), colorectal, gallbladder, and breast cancer [4]. This is why it is essential to understand basic cellular and molecular mechanisms in order to identify new therapeutic targets against obesity.

On a psychological level, obesity can completely turn a person's life upside down; those who are obese are often isolated and subjected to social stigmatization, which makes any type of sociability difficult. In particular, overweight children tend to develop a difficult relationship with their bodies and with their peers, resulting in isolation, which often translates into further sedentary habits [5].

The recent "Human Obesity Gene Map" [6] lists 11 single gene mutations, 50 related loci to the relevant Mendelian syndromes in obesity, 244 transgenic or "knockout" animal models, and 127 gene candidates, of which just under 20% are replicates in more than five studies; a total of 253 "quantitative trait loci" for different phenotypes related to obesity are related to 61 genomes, and of these only about 20% are supported by more than one study [7]. Even if GWAS studies have identified hundreds of loci associated with BMI, this correlation can explain only 3–5% of BMI variance in the population [8].

The inability to correlate obesity to specific genes in a marked way has prompted research towards epigenetic studies. In fact, the genes not being sufficient to explain what happens in the phenotype, other forms of variation such as epigenetic markers must be taken into consideration. It is already known that obesity can be prevented through changes in lifestyle, nutrition, exercise, and other variables which can altering DNA transcription and consequent gene expression [9]. This is an epigenetic process and reflects the body's interaction with the environment and its dynamic and adjustable molecular changes. This is why when we talk about obesity it is important to understand how lifestyle changes and different therapies can change gene expression and lead to favorable results regarding body mass index (BMI).

Recent years have seen the design of drugs to reduce BMI, and the nutraceutical market for weight loss has grown. Considering the many side effects that weight loss drugs have, nutraceuticals seem to be a much more suitable choice due to absence of toxicity. This review provides an overview of the intricate interplay between epigenetics and the most studied nutraceuticals, such as resveratrol, curcumin, epigallocatechin-3-gallate (EGCG), ginger, capsaicin, and caffeine, in the context of obesity management.

2. Methods

For this narrative review, we have summarized the articles that could be relevant, using the academic databases Pubmed and ScienceDirect for this purpose. Because we focused on the impact of nutraceuticals in epigenetics modulation in the obesity literature, a search was performed with the following search terms: obesity, monogenic obesity, polygenic obesity, epigenetic of obesity, nutraceuticals, resveratrol, curcumin, epigallocatechin gallate, ginger, capsaicin, and caffeine, which were used during the literature survey individually or in combination. We searched for clinical studies, original research, and reviews published in the English language until January of 2023. Due to the numerous published articles on epigenetics of obesity and nutraceuticals included in the study, as well as the limited number of references allowed, we focused on the most impactful and relevant papers supporting the hypothesis of obesity gene modulation by nutraceuticals.

3. Aspect of Genetic Obesity

From a genetic point of view, obesity is commonly classified into subgroups according to the presumed etiology: monogenic obesity, extremely severe but not accompanied by developmental delay; syndromic obesity, involving obese subjects with dysmorphia, mental retardation, and developmental anomalies; and polygenic obesity, also called common obesity [10]. However, the forms of obesity transmitted hereditarily are very rare and represent a small part of all cases of obesity present in the population. Syndromic obesity is caused by chromosomal rearrangements such as WAGR syndrome, Prader-Willi syndrome, Bardet-Biedl syndrome, SIM1 syndrome, Down syndrome, etc. [11].

The most frequent causes of monogenic obesity are mutations in the genes leptin (LEP), leptin receptor (LEPR), melanocortin 4 receptor (MC4R), proopiomelanocortin (POMC), proprotein convertase subtilisin/kexin type 1 (PCSK1), and neurotrophic receptor tyrosine kinase 2 (NTRK2) [12].

3.1. Common or Polygenic Obesity

Common obesity, defined by a BMI > 30 kg/m^2, is a continuous quantitative trait. The genetics of quantitative traits in humans have historically made use of observational studies on pairs of twins. The first studies on the heritability of common obesity date back to the late 1970s, including one important study that observed more than 15,000 pairs of twin brothers, roughly 6000 of whom were monozygotic and 7500 of whom were dizygotic. This was a longitudinal study that followed a large group of war veterans over time (25 years), studying both concordance and heritability with the Falconer method for studying twins; the results showed that BMI, weight, and high were highly correlated across time.

In the last two decades, genome-wide association studies (GWAS) for obesity phenotype have shown a correlation between polymorphism in FTO and BMI, identifying two other polymorphisms associated with the phenotype that map in the proximity of the MC4R gene. It is interesting to note that in these cases a cumulative effect of two susceptibility variants was identified; subjects with risk-conferring alleles in both FTO and MC4R have a higher BMI compared to subjects with only one risk allele (FTO or MC4R) [13].

Several other studies have identified different susceptibility variants in different genomic regions and for different study populations, according to which dozens of genetic susceptibility variants are known, each of which provides a very modest contribution to the formation of the phenotype. Furthermore, studies of genes regulating glycolipid metabolism and thermogenesis revealed that a specific polymorphism (Pro12Ala) in the peroxisome proliferative activated receptor gamma (PPARγ) gene is associated with lower BMI and increased insulin sensitivity [14]. Similarly, recent meta-analyses involving up to 7000 subjects have demonstrated a significant association between BMI and two other polymorphisms, the Trp64Arg SNP in the β3-adrenergic receptor (ADRB3) gene [15] and the insertion/deletion (I/D) in the Uncoupling protein-2 (UCP-2) gene [16]. In contrast, the results regarding the impact of the 2G866A SNP in the UCP-2 gene on obesity remain inconclusive.

Therefore, polygenic obesity results from the complex interaction between genes and the surrounding environment, physical activity, diet, and gender [17].

3.2. The Role of Epigenetics in Obesity

As we have seen, the excessive increase in obesity in recent decades is impossible to explain only through genetics, which is why studies have turned to epigenetics. Certain variables, for example nutrition and physical exercises have the ability to modify gene expression without affecting the DNA sequence, a phenomenon known as epigenetics. The term "epigenetics" was introduced in 1942 by the biologist Conrad Hal Waddington, referring to certain inherited changes not accompanied by changes in the DNA sequence itself.

The most important and studied epigenetic mechanisms are DNA methylation, histone modification, and non-coding RNAs (ncRNAs), which can be transmitted transgenerationally through mitotic or meiotic cell division [18]. Epigenetic programming of parental gametes, the fetus, and early postnatal development can be influenced by environmental factors; therefore, even gene expression can be altered in response to environmental exposures. The animal model of agouti mouse with the agouti viable yellow (A^{vy}) mutation is a classic example of obesity that can be modulated through epigenetic mechanism [19]. The *Agouti* gene in mice controls the color of hair, and is under the control of a specific promoter in exon 2. During hair follicle cell development, the gene switches ON at a specific time and produces an agouti coat with a yellow stripe in the dark hair. The mutant A^{vy} form of this gene makes the mice yellow and predisposes them to obesity, diabetes, and cancer. However, when the mutant pregnant mice are fed food enriched with extra methyl groups, non-obese brown pups resulted that were longer lived [3,20].

Following this example, later results showed that the mutant *Agouti* gene in the obese yellow mice is unmethylated and turned on, while in the brown mice the gene is methylated and shut down. The color of the agouti mice acts as a sensor for the DNA methylation status in the color gene. The agouti mice model allows us to understand how environmental factors and maternal diet affect the epigenome and regulate gene expression.

3.2.1. DNA Methylation

However, one of the main mechanisms responsible for this process is DNA methylation capable of activating or deactivating a determined gene, thereby suppressing or activating the relative function [21]. DNA methylation changes can be dynamic in the sense that they can be modified under the influence of environmental factors or can be stable and transmitted to the next generations [22]. In mammals, 98% of DNA methylation occurs in a CpG dinucleotide context in somatic cells and above a quarter appears in a non-CpG context in embryonic stem cells. DNA methyltransferases (DNMTs), DNA demethylases, and the ten–eleven translocation (TET) proteins are involved in the regulation of DNA methylation. In mammals, five family members have been described: DNMT, DNMT1, DNMT2, DNMT3a, DNMT3b, and DNMT3L, of which only DNMT1, DNMT3a, and DNMT3b possess DNMT activity. DNMT1 maintains DNA methylation, while DNMT3a and DNMT3b can establish new DNA methylation. Removal of DNA methylation is mediated by TET proteins (TET1, TET2, and TET3) [23].

Certain human exome sequencing studies have identified de novo mutations in DNMT3A in subjects with autism spectrum disorder. Mice with whole-body DNMT3A haploinsufficiency show obesity in adults life associated with the autism phenotype [24]

DNA methylation can be strongly influenced by diet. Certain nutrients, such as folate, methionine, choline, vitamin B12, and pyridoxal phosphate can influence DNA methylation status, in this manner playing an important role in the modulation of gene expression, in particular of genes connected to main metabolic regulations such as energy balance and body composition [25]. Regarding the correlation between genes involved in polygenic obesity and methylation, several studies confirm the link between the methylation state of certain genes and obesity. A recent cohort study found a negative association between hypomethylation of the LEP gene promoter, obesity, lipid profile modification, and low insulin sensitivity [26]. In another cross-sectional study involving obese pre-bariatric adult subjects, LEP gene methylation was negatively correlated with BMI, while ADIPOQ adiponectin methylation resulted in a positive association [27]. The association between obesity and methylation of the LEP and ADIPOQ genes has been confirmed by several studies [28–30].

Methylation of PGC1A (peroxisome proliferator-activated receptor γ coactivator 1 alpha), a transcription factor critical in energy expenditure, and of IGF-2 (insulin-like growth factor 2), was disrupted in high fat diet (HFD), gestational diabetes, and obesity, with caloric restriction restoring the methylation state [31].

The NPY gene stimulates food intake, while the POMC gene promotes satiety. hypermethylation of POMC and hypomethylation of NPY was found in obese people [32]. Certain genes involved in inflammation and oxidative stress, such as TNF, TFAM (mitochondrial transcription factor A), and Il6, showed aberrant methylation levels in obese people [33]. In subjects with obesity and metabolic diseases, a hypermethylation of the IRS1 promoter and of the PIK3R1 gene was noted in obese individuals [34].

3.2.2. Histone Modifications

Histones are well-conserved proteins involved in DNA packaging into chromatin. The most common and well-known histone modifications are acetylation, methylation, phosphorylation, O-GlcNAcylation, adenosine diphosphate (ADP) ribosylation, and lactylation. Modifications to the histone tails change the chromatin structure and regulate enhancer and promoter activities [35,36]. Acetylation opens the chromatin structure, favoring the binding of factors necessary for gene transcription; hyperacetylation is associated with an active transcription state, while histone deacetylation is associated with compacted and condensed chromatin, causing transcriptional repression. Histone acetylation and deacetylation are catalyzed by histone acetyltransferases (HATs) and HDACs, respectively. HATs catalyze the transfer of the acetyl group from acetyl-CoA onto a lysine residue, which can be reversed by HDACs [37].

Histone methylation can occur at the level of lysine and arginine residues [38]. Histone methylations may confer either active or repressive transcription depending on their positions and methylation states. H3K4, H3K36, and H3K79 methylations are markers of active transcription, whereas H3K9, H3K27, and H4K20 methylations are associated with suppressive transcription. These histone methylations are regulated by histone methyltransferases (HMTs, 'writers') and histone demethylases (HDMs, 'erasers'). The methylation reaction can be reversed via multiple mechanisms [39]. PPARγ and C/EBPα are considered the most important regulators of adipogenesis, both in culture and in vivo, followed by C/EBPβ and C/EBPδ (which are essential for adipose tissue development), preadipocyte factor-1 (Pref-1), and adipocyte protein 2 (aP2). All these genes are regulated by histone modification during adipocyte differentiation [40]. In addition, histone modifications are involved in the control of the appetite-regulated genes POMC and NPY. Investigation of histone tail modifications on hypothalamic chromatin extracts from 16-day-old rats showed decreased acetylation of lysine 9 in histone 3 (H3K9) for the POMC gene and increased acetylation for the same residue for the NPY gene, modifications correlated with altered expression of the genes and obesity [19,41]. In the liver of obese mice fed an HFD, an increase of H3 lysine 9 and 18 acetylation was observed at TNFα and Ccl2 (monocyte chemotactic protein 1). On the other hand, weight loss interventions increased H4 acetylation at the GLU4 gene, increasing its expression [42]. All these findings show that histone modification can play an important role in obesity [43].

3.2.3. Non-Coding RNAs

MicroRNAs (miRNA) are small non-coding RNA molecules with an average length of 22 nucleotides. Despite their small size, they are able to control gene expression by exploiting the perfect or similar complementarity they have with other RNA molecules [44]. Recent findings have shown that miRNAs regulate adipogenesis and are involved in obesity development. The miRNAs involved in adipogenesis are *miR-30*, *miR-26b*, *miR-199a*, and *miR-148a*. In obese subjects fed a high fat diet, researchers have found high levels of this miRNA. In obese adults, *miR-17-5p* and *miR-132* were more highly expressed in the visceral adipose tissues and were correlated with impaired glucose, high BMI, and dyslipidemia [45].

miR-26b is involved in the adipogenesis process, and studies regarding the proliferation of human preadipocytes that overexpress *miR-26b* exhibited increased triglyceride content in the adipocytes and upregulation of PPAR-γ expression during differentiation [46,47].

miR-200a, *miR-200b*, and *miR-429* are upregulated in the hypothalami of obese and leptin deficient ob/ob mice. Treatment with leptin downregulates these miRNAs, and hipotalamic silencing of *miR-200a* increases expression of LEPR and ISR-2 (insulin receptor substrate 2), suggesting that this miRNA can be a target for obesity treatment [48].

In the last decades, a large number of miRNAs differently expressed in obese people have been discovered involved in fat metabolism, adipogenesis, hypoxia, insulin signaling, inflammation, and cell differentiation and development. A comprehensive list of miRNAs related to obesity and metabolic diseases was published by Landrier et al. [45].

4. Nutraceuticals

The term "nutraceutical" was coined by Stephen L. De Felice, who used it for the first time in a 1989 publication; it comes from the union of the words "nutrition" and "pharmaceutical" [49]. Since then, it has been used to indicate the science that studies the individual components of foods that have health benefits [50]. Our ancestors already understood that eating certain types of food had consequences on the body. "Let food be your medicine and your medicine be food" is a phrase attributed to Hippocrates, the father of scientific medicine, who already 400 years before the birth of Christ understood the link between nutrition and well-being. Today the food nutrients that have the power to bring benefits to our body are studied biologically and chemically, and through nutraceuticals it is possible to know how they act in our body.

Regarding weight loss, nutraceuticals have many ways to act; as nutrient absorption regulators (ginseng, green tea, chitosan, psyllium, inulin, guar gum), appetite regulators (whey proteins and chlorogenic acid), energy expenditure modulators (curcumin and L-carnitine), and on the fat metabolism (resveratrol and flaxseed) [51].

Nutraceuticals are not involved in primary metabolism, and usually have health-promoting bioactivities. According to computational chemistry data, there are about 400,000 bioactive compounds of pharmaceutical interest [52]. Obesity is a very complex diseases involving the coexistence of different signals, including epigenetic changes [53]. For this reason, an ideal nutraceuticals formula should be able to act on all possible pathways regarding obesity, which we can expect to be very challenging.

In this review, we describe nutraceuticals that have been shown to be helpful in obesity by modulating gene expression. We focus on the most studied substances in this area, such as resveratrol, curcumin, ginger, EGCG, capsaicin, and caffeine, as shown in Figure 1. The most important epigenetic mechanisms through which these nutraceuticals act beneficially in obesity are summarized in Table S1.

4.1. Resveratrol

Resveratrol (3,5,4'-trihydroxystilbene) is part of a large group of phytochemicals, including flavonoids and lignans, and is produced by plants in response to attack by pathogens such as bacteria or fungi as well as to injury [54]. Sources of resveratrol in food include grapes (*Vitis vinifera* L.), raspberries (*Rubus idaeus* L.), blueberries (*Vaccinium corymbosum* L.), peanuts (*Arachis hypogaea* L.), and mulberries (*Morus alba* Hort. ex Loudon L.) [55,56]. Resveratrol presents two geometric isomers, cis-(Z) and trans-(E). The *trans* form can undergo isomerization to the cis form when exposed to ultraviolet radiation [57]. In prevalence and biological activity, the dominant form is cis [58,59]. Resveratrol was first isolated in 1940 from the roots of white hellebore (*Veratrum album* L.) [60] and subsequently from knotweed in 1963 (*Polygonum cuspidatum* Sieb. et Zucc.), which is one of the richest sources of resveratrol in nature and plays an important role in ancient Chinese and Japanese medicine [61]. Resveratrol has been demonstrated in translational models to have anti-obesity and metabolic reprogramming properties [62,63]. It has been shown to be beneficial in animal studies for reducing body weight, insulin resistance, adipose tissue size, and weight [64,65].

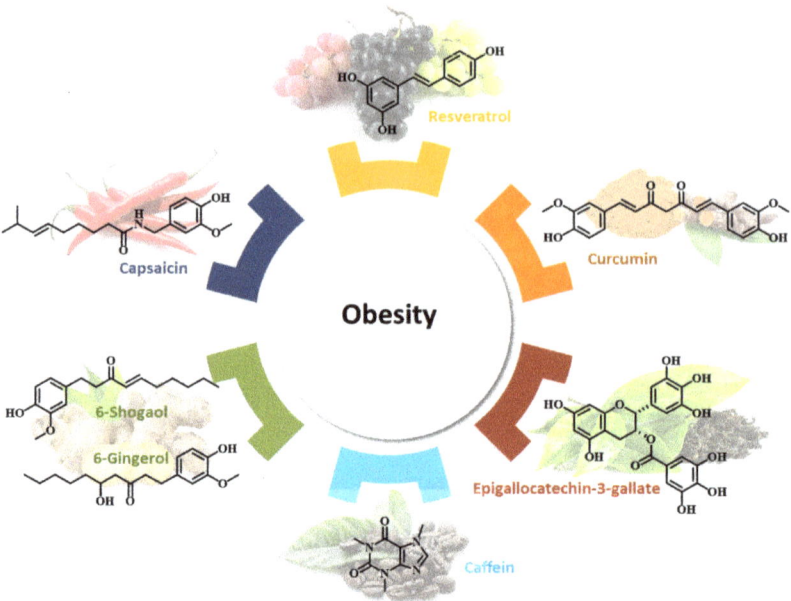

Figure 1. The main natural compounds involved in obesity management.

The mechanisms through which resveratrol exerts its beneficial effects seem to be related to gene expression modulation and changes that mimics calorie restriction [66]. In patients with obesity, intracellular targets such as the deacetylating enzyme sirtuin-1 (SIRT-1), adenosine monophosphate-activated protein kinase (AMPK), and peroxisome proliferator-activated receptor γ coactivator-1α (PGC-1α) are altered [67]. In this context, resveratrol can activate the SIRT-1 gene, which plays an important role in mitochondrial activity modulation, glucose homeostasis, and other metabolic conditions related to obesity [68].

Numerous studies have analyzed the effect of resveratrol on adipogenesis using both in vivo and in vitro models, finding that resveratrol has an inhibitory effect on this process. Thus, the incubation of pre-adipocyte cells in vitro with different concentrations of resveratrol (1, 10, and 25 μM) for 24 h showed a lower expression of acetyl-CoA carboxylase (ACC), a decrease in the content of triacylglycerol, and inhibition of lipoprotein lipase [69]. Authors have found that resveratrol is able to reduce adipogenesis by downregulating the expression of CCAAT-enhancer-binding protein (C/EBPα), sterol regulatory element-binding protein 1c (SREBP-1c), and PPARγ after the incubation of pre-adipocytes with >10 μM resveratrol concentration [70]. Other authors confirmed these findings using (10–40 μM) resveratrol dosage and incubation times of 2, 4, and 6 days; the best result was achieved at 40 μM resveratrol dosage and 6 days incubation time, when 40% of pre-adipocyte differentiation was inhibited [71].

Several studies have demonstrated that resveratrol can increase expression of the thermogenesis markers UCP1 and BMP7; followed by reduction of fat accumulation, increased oxygen consumption and due to these processes exhibits an important effect on thermogenesis and the browning process [72]. Fibronectin type III domain-containing protein 5 (FNDC5) can promote conversion of white adipose tissue (WAT) to brown adipose tissue (BAT) by increased UCP1 expression [73], and it was demonstrated that resveratrol can increase FNDC5 expression in the subcutaneous adipose tissue from mice and humans [74].

In another study, oral administration of resveratrol in mice fed with a standard diet improved glycemic and lipidic profile and enhanced thermogenesis by increasing UCP1 expression in BAT. The authors suggested that increased expression of UCP1 was associated with increased expression of SIRT-1, PTEN, and BMP7 in the same BAT [72].

In addition, resveratrol fights against obesity by enhancing catecholamine production, suppressing pro-inflammatory M1 macrophages and activation of anti-inflammatory M2 macrophages in WAT [75]. In mice fed HFD resveratrol by activation of PI3K/SIRT1 and Nrf2 signaling pathways, the inhibition of transcriptional regulators (e.g., EP300 gene) decreased fat mass and body weight, modulated insulin and glucose metabolism, and restored immune dysfunction [76,77]. Being able to protect against sarcopenic obesity through the PKA/liver kinase B1 (LKB1)/AMPK pathway, resveratrol improves mitochondrial function and reduces oxidative stress [78].

Administration of resveratrol in rat model with diet-induced obesity has been shown to reduce body weight, subcutaneous adipose tissue (SAT) masses, and WAT. Regarding the effects in microRNA expression after resveratrol administration, *miR-211-3p*, *miR-1224*, and *miR-539-5p* were increased and *miR-511-3p* was decreased. The target genes were PPAR-γ, SP1 transcription factor (SP1), and hormone-sensitive lipase (HSL), which are involved in FA (fatty acids) metabolism in adipose tissue [79]. The SP1 gene is a target of *miR-1224* and *miR-539-5p*, both of which are involved in SP1 regulation. The synergistic action of SREBP-1 and SP1 induces the expression of FAS, which promotes de novo lipogenesis [80]. The expression of SP1 and SREBP-1 was downregulated by resveratrol due to upregulation of *miR-539-5p*.

Resveratrol can act as a prebiotic as well, being metabolized by gut microbiota, and produces metabolites such as lunularin and dihydroresveratrol [81]. In mice fed HFD, resveratrol intake of 200 mg/kg/day had anti-obesity effects by improving gut dysbiosis, *Bacteroidetes/Firmicutes* ratio, increasing the abundance of *Lactobacillus* and *Bifidobacterium*, and inhibiting the growth of *Enterococcus faecalis* [65,82].

A positive correlation was found between body weight and *Enterococcus faecalis* and a negative one with *Lactobacillus*, *Bifidobacterium*, and *Bacteroidetes/Firmicutes* ratio. Resveratrol intake in these mice increased FIAF and decreased LPL gene expression, suppressing fatty acid biosynthesis in the liver [82].

The recommended doses of resveratrol are 250–1000 mg orally daily for up to three months. Overall, it is well tolerated in healthy individuals; however, adverse effects, including nephrotoxicity and gastrointestinal symptoms such as nausea, diarrhea, and abdominal discomfort, have been reported in human subjects. In doses higher than 1000 mg/day, it has been reported that resveratrol modifies the activity of cytochrome P450 isoenzymes, leading to interactions with other medications. [83,84].

Due to all the effects described above, resveratrol can be used as a therapeutic agent against obesity. Of course, due to data scarcity, further studies remain needed to evaluate the long-term effects of resveratrol, especially in vivo and in human trials.

4.2. Curcumin

Curcuma longa L. is a perennial and rhizomatous herbaceous plant which belongs to the family of Zingiberaceae, as ginger (*Zingiber officinale* Rosc.) does. The most important component of nutritional and phytotherapeutic interest is the root, constituted by a cylindrical, branched, aromatic rhizome of orange-yellow color. In traditional Indian, Thai, and Middle Eastern cuisine it is used in food as a spice. The term curcumin usually refers to 1,7-bis(4-hydroxy-3-methoxyphenyl)-1,6-heptadiene-3,5-dione, a compound known as "curcumin I", although the plant contains more than 100 chemical compounds. The two other best-known compounds are curcumin II (demethoxycurcumin, 1-(4-hydroxy-3-methoxyphenyl)-7-(4-hydroxyphenyl)-1,6-heptadiene-3,5-dione) and curcumin III (bisdemethoxycurcumin, 1,7-bis(4-hydroxyphenyl)-1,6-heptadiene-3,5-dione) [85]. The yellow color is due to "curcumin I" and the curcuminoids bisdemethoxycurcumin and demethoxycurcumin, generally used as a natural dye and in the food industry [86]. Turmerone (ar-turmerone), β-turmerone, α-turmerone, β-bisabolene, β-sesquiphellandrene, α-zingiberene, curcumol, and curcumenol are the principal essential oils of curcumin [87]. Curcumin has several biological activities, and functions as an antioxidative, anti-inflammatory, anti-cancer, and anti-obesity agent.

Regarding obesity, it has been shown that curcumin can interfere with adipocyte differentiation [88] and alter the adipocyte life cycle. Curcumin has anti-adipogenic functions and can suppress the 3T3-L1 adipogenesis in murine cell models and in human primary preadipocytes by stimulating the Wnt signaling cascade [89–91]. During adipocyte differentiation, curcumin blocks mitotic clonal expansion by inhibition of transcription factors such as C/EBPα, Krüppel-like factor 5(KLF5) and PPARγ [91,92]. Adipocyte protein 2 (aP2) is a mature adipocyte marker, and in the 3T3-L1 cells it was found that curcumin decreases aP2 microRNA expression, increases expression of certain Wnt pathways targets such as c-Myc and cyclin D1, and reduces mitogen-activated protein kinase (MAPK) phosphorylation, which is associated with differentiation of 3T3-L1 cells into adipocytes [92].

In several clinical trials, oral curcumin intake decreased the plasma lipid levels induced by HFD, an aspect correlated with AMPK and PPARα activation (both of which inhibit acetyl-CoA carboxylase (ACC)), followed by a decrease in lipid accumulation and FA synthesis [93,94]. In animals with hyperlipidemia induced by a high glucose diet (HGD), curcumin intake resulted in reducing total cholesterol, triglycerides, fatty acids [95,96]. and transaminase levels, along with insulin resistance improvements [97,98]. Therefore, in obese subjects, curcumin can reduce inflammation and insulin resistance by inhibiting activation of signal transducers and activation of transcription 3 (STAT3) in human adipocytes [99].

In the C57BL/6 mice on a regular low-fat chow diet receiving curcumin gavage (50–100 mg/kg body weight per day) for 50 days, a browning of WAT was observed, which is associated with an increase of gene expression involved in thermogenesis and mitochondrial biogenesis. Curcumin can increase body temperature, energy expenditure, and UCP1 expression in the BAT [100].

After oral administration, curcumin is distributed throughout the intestines, where it affects the GM composition [101]. Studies on animal models have shown that curcumin intake improve the richness of intestinal microbiota and has significant effects on family members such as *Bacteroidaceae*, *Prevotellaceae*, and *Rikenellaceae* [102]. In addition, curcumin improves the composition of gut microbiota in colitis mice [103]. In a menopausal rat model, curcumin administered 100 mg/kg per day had a weight-loss effect by improving gut dysbiosis and promoting species such as *Anaerotruncus*, *Exiguobacterium*, *Helicobacter*, *Shewanella*, and *Serratia* [104]. Islam et al. [105] found that administration of curcumin for 14 weeks in a human-equivalent dose of 2 g daily as supplementation in a HFD was correlated with reduced adiposity and relative abundance of *Lactococcus*, *Turicibacter*, and *Parasutterella* genera. Scientists believe that curcumin has protective effects in dietary obesity due to downregulation of inflammation in adipose tissue. Curcumin seems to attenuate the high-fat and high-cholesterol Western-type diet (WD)-induced chronic inflammation and associated metabolic diseases, including obesity. Furthermore, by reducing the dysfunction of the intestinal barrier, curcumin modulates chronic inflammatory diseases despite its low bioavailability. The Western diet is characterized by high fat and refined carbohydrates intake, which induce metabolic diseases and inflammation. Curcumin pretreatment in this case is associated with reduced IL-1β-induced activation of p38 MAPK in intestinal epithelial cells (IECs) [106].

To discover new therapeutic targets against obesity, it is necessary to understand the mechanism of adipogenic differentiation. Adipogenic differentiation is repressed by activation of Wtn pathway, and certain microRNAs intervene in the regulation of preadipocyte differentiation and proliferation. An important component of the Wtn signaling cascade is TCF7L2, which together with free β-catenin (β-cat) molecules forms the complex transcription factor β-cat/TCF, a key effector of Wtn [107]. TCF7L2 is one of the most studied genes involved in the development of type 2 diabetes [90,108]. Silencing of TCF7L2 leads to impaired adipogenesis, disruption of Wnt signaling, and upregulation of axis inhibition protein 2 (Axin2) mRNA [109]. Tian et al. found that curcumin treatment attenuated *miR-17-5p* expression and stimulated TCF7L2 expression in 3T3-L1 cells [107].

Turmeric is safe when used short-term, having been approved by the US Food and Drug Administration (FDA) as "Generally Recognized as Safe". For example, a maximum of 8 g of curcumin per day is safe when used for up to 2 months. Administration of up to 3 g per day appears to be safe when used for up to 3 months. Turmeric can be used in doses of up to 1.5 g daily for up to 9 months. Generally, turmeric does not cause serious side effects; however, when taken in large doses or for extended periods it may cause gastrointestinal symptoms such as diarrhea, nausea, and stomach upset [83,110].

Unfortunately, for now it is unknown how curcumin treatment represses adipogenesis in vivo and reduces body weight gain. As can be seen, curcumin is a promising compound in obesity prevention and reduction, and there are many preparations containing this nutraceutical. However, more comprehensive human studies are necessary in order to understand how exactly to use it in obesity management.

4.3. Ginger

Zingiber officinale Roscoe is a perennial herbaceous plant native to Asia and India. In the first century it was introduced to the Mediterranean area, and in the third to Japan. In England and America, it arrived in the eleventh century. Today, it is mostly cultivated in Africa and Asia. Ginger is a spice and flavoring agent for food, being used in cuisine in different forms such as fresh, dry, oil, paste, and emulsion [111]. Ginger is rich in bioactive phenolic compounds such as gingerols, shogaols, paradol, and zingerones. Ginger has been used since antiquity in Ayurvedic, Chinese, and Yunani medicine to treat nausea, rheumatoid arthritis, muscular aches, indigestion, sore throats, constipation, and fever, and is a stimulant and carminative of the gastrointestinal tract [112,113]. The health potential of ginger has been intensively studied, and different regulatory authorities consider it a safe nutraceutical [114].

Recently, the anti-obesity effects of ginger and its compounds have been taken into consideration, and the results from in vitro and in vivo studies support this idea [115–120], although research in humans remains limited. Ginger seems to be able to influence body composition and weight through several mechanisms, such as inhibition of adipocyte differentiation and lipid accumulation [117] and through increasing thermogenesis, lipolysis, and energy expenditure [115,120].

Ginger can interfere with adipogenesis of 3T3-L1 cells. It is known that the 3T3-L1 cell line is the most reliable model for research on adipogenesis [121]. In several studies it has been shown that 6-gingerol ((S)-5-hydroxy-1-(4-hydroxy-3-methoxyphenyl)-3-decanone), one of the most abundant components in ginger root, was able to inhibit adipogenesis via different mechanisms. In one study, 6-gingerol diminished the insulin-stimulated serine phosphorylation of Akt (Ser473) and GSK3 (Ser9) and suppressed adipogenesis by down-regulation of C/EBP and PPARγ followed by subsequent inhibition of the expression of relevant markers for lipid accumulation, aP2, and FAS. In addition, 6-gingerol can suppress differentiation of 3T3-L1 cells by attenuating the Akt/GSK3 pathway [122].

Li et al. found that 6-gingerol can inhibit adipogenesis by down-regulation of C/EBP-α and PPAR-γ followed by inhibition of FAS and Acetyl-CoA carboxylase (ACC) expression and activation of the canonical pathway Wnt/β-catenin, the activation of which is responsible for dephosphorylation and nuclear translocation of β-catenin. 6-gingerol increases the mRNA and protein levels of dishevelled segment polarity protein 2 (DVL2) and Low-Density Lipoprotein Receptor-Related Protein 6 (LRP6), an important component of Wnt, suggesting that up-regulation of several components of the Wnt/β-catenin pathway results in inhibition of adipogenic differentiation [123].

6-Shogaol [1-(4-hydroxy-methoxyphenyl)-4-decen-one], another important constituent in ginger, has the ability to inhibit adipogenesis of 3T3-L1 preadipocytes at 40 μM and to decrease expression of adipogenic/lipogenic markers levels such as PPAR-γ, FAS and C/EBPα. By increasing glycerol release, 6-shogaol decreases intracellular lipid accumulation [124]. This compound decreases the phosphorylation of IRS-1, PI3K, and AKT, suggesting that 6-shogaol exerts its antiobesity effect through the PI3K/AKT pathway [125].

The antiobesity effects of 6-gingerol and 6-shogaol seems to be associated with their anti-inflammatory properties. These compounds can downregulate mRNA levels of tumor necrosis factor alpha (TNFα) and interleukin-6 (IL-6) in the adipose tissue of rats fed HFD [126,127]. Studies have shown that both compounds are able to inhibit TNF-mediated downregulation of adiponectin expression in adipocytes by functioning as PPARγ agonists. 6-gingerol inhibits the phosphorylation of anti-phospho-c-Jun-NH2-terminal kinase (JNK) and activates the upstream kinase of JNK. These aspects are very important and suggest that the ginger compounds might have important implications in diabetes prevention via improvement of adipocyte dysfunction [128]. To date, several studies have demonstrated the beneficial effects of ginger compounds in regulation of glycolytic enzyme, limitation of gluconeogenesis, and insulin sensitivity improvement in diabetic animal models [129,130].

6-gingerol protects pancreatic cells from oxidative stress and shows significant anti-inflammatory properties in amelioration of insulin resistance in fructose-induced adipose tissue, probably by suppressing adipose macrophage. By controlling inflammation and inhibition of TNFα and IL6 expression, 6-gingerol exerts a hypoglycemic effect [131–133].

Another ginger compound, 12-dehydrogingerdione, has anti-inflammatory and antioxidant properties, and stimulated nitric oxide (NO) production and suppressed mRNA levels of cytokines IL-6, IL-8 in RAW 264.7. In addition, ginger extract can reduce the intestinal absorption of carbohydrates with antihyperglycemic effect [134–136].

In a recent study, it has been shown that ginger supplementation (5% ginger flour intake for 7 weeks) can ameliorate metabolic parameters induced by HFD. C57BL/6 mice fed a HFD ginger supplementation showed body weight loss and improvements in lipid and glucose profiles. By upregulation of the genes involved in fatty acid oxidation, such as fibroblast growth factor 21 (FGF21), carnitine palmitoyltransferase 1 (CPT1), and acyl-CoA oxidase 1 (ACOX1), ginger supplementation determined a reduction in the accumulation of hepatic lipids. In addition, an upregulation of antioxidant enzymes involved in the first line of defense against oxidative damage, such as nuclear factor erythroid 2-related factor (NRF), 1/2 superoxide dismutase (SOD), and glutathione peroxidase (GPX), was observed [137].

Adipocyte size was reduced by ginger supplementation, which was accompanied by PPAR and aP2 attenuation. In contrast, CPT1 gene expression was upregulated by ginger administration [138].

It has been demonstrated that ginger can reduce body weight, with positive effects on HDL cholesterol level and increase of peroxisomal catalase level [139]. In addition, ginger can decrease appetite by its modulatory effect on 5-hydroxytryptamine [120].

Regarding the effect on thermogenesis and energy expenditure, ginger seems to have an agonistic effect on transient receptor potential vanilloid Type 1 (TRPV1). This is a temperature sensor able to activate the sympathetic nerve system and norepinephrine (NE) release, with a resulting increase of uncoupling protein-1 (UCP-1) expression, thermogenesis followed by cAMP high production, increased activity of hormone sensitive lipase (HSL), and lipolysis [140].

Uncoupling protein 1 genes play an important role in body weight regulation and energy homeostasis, being associated with resistance to weight loss, reduced resting energy expenditure, and increased weight gain over time [141]. Ginger supplementation significantly decreased body weight, waist circumferences, hip circumference (HC), and waist-to-height ratio (WHtR) in the G allele carriers of UCP1 (-3826A>G polymorphism and Arg alleles carriers for ADRB3 (Trp64Arg) polymorphism [142].

In rats fed HFD and supplemented with high-hydrostatic pressure ginger extract (HPG) and hot water extract of ginger (WEG), a reduction of *miR-21* expression was observed followed by amelioration of adipogenic gene expression. *miR-132* levels were decreased in HPG supplemented rats, followed by a decrease in expression of inflammation-related genes such as Il6, MCP-1, and TNFα [143].

Ginger supplementation can modulate the composition of gut microbiota and the abundance of microbial taxa [144,145]. Short-term ginger juice supplementation increased the *Firmicutes/Bacteroidetes* ratio and the abundance of *Proteobacteria* in healthy adults and decreased pro-inflammatory *Ruminococcus* [146]. All these data suggest that ginger is able to decrease body weight and adipose tissue by modulating gene expression involved in these processes and could be useful as a nutraceutical for the prevention of obesity and inflammation.

Ginger can be taken orally in doses of 0.5–3 g per day for up to 12 weeks. While generally considered safe for most people when consumed in moderate amounts, excessive or prolonged use may have potential adverse effects. Doses higher than 5 g per day increase the risk of mild side effects, such as heartburn, diarrhea, belching, and general stomach discomfort. Cases of arrhythmias and low blood pressure have been cited as well. By increasing bile acid secretion, ginger can aggravate gallstone formation [83,147].

4.4. Epigallocatechin-3-Gallate (EGCG)

EGCG is the most abundant catechin in green tea (*Camellia sinensis* L.) and is found in smaller quantities in other foods such as carob (*Ceratonia siliqua* L.) flour, blackberries (*Rubus plicatus* L. Weihe & Nees), apples (*Malus domestica* (Suckow) Borkh.), raspberries (*Rubus idaeus* L.), prunes (*Prunus domestica* L.), pistachios (*Pistacia vera* L.), peaches (*Prunus persica* (L.) Batsch), and avocados (*Persea americana* Mill.) [50].

During the manufacturing process, tea leaves are heated to inactivate the enzymes, rolled, and dried. The process prevents oxidation of the constituents and stabilizes tea compounds during storage. Green tea is rich in polyphenolic compounds called catechins, such as epicatechin, epigallocatechin, EGCG, epicatechin gallate (ECG), and other polyphenols in low quantities, such as kaempferol, myricetin, quercetin, certain alkaloids, theobromine, and caffeine. In brewed green tea, catechins account for 30–42% of the dry weight. A green tea beverage (250 mL hot water and 2.5 g leaves) contains about 260 mg of catechins, of which about 96 mg is EGCG [148,149].

EGCG is a polyphenol with anti-inflammatory, antioxidant, and anti-obesity actions. As anti-obesity agent, it decreases weight gain and adipose tissue weight by decreasing calorie intake and AMPK activation in the liver, white adipose tissue, and skeletal muscle, reducing the absorption of lipids, cholesterol, triacylglycerols (TAGs), and leptins, stimulating energy expenditure and fat oxidation, and increasing the level of high-density lipoproteins and fecal excretion of lipids [150–152].

In HFD mice, 100 mg/kg daily EGCG supplementation decreased the expression of the genes ACC1, SCD1, FAS, PPARγ, C/EBPB, and SREBP1, all of which are involved in de novo synthesis of fatty acids, and increased the expression of the genes HSL, ATGL, PPARα, ACO2, and MCAD, which are associated with lipolysis and lipid oxidation in epididymal adipose tissues. An increase in the expression level of the genes PGC1α and aP2, which are associated with thermogenesis and fatty acid transfer, was observed as well [152]. Likewise, in mice fed HFD, treatment of EGCG increased the expression of genes involved in fat oxidation, such as MCAD, PPARGα, UCP3, and NRF1 [153]. It is well known that UCP3 gene mutations are associated with increased risk of morbid obesity, dyslipidemia, and diabetes [154]. In the skeletal muscle of subjects characterized by obesity and insulin resistance, the gene expression of NRF1 and UCP3 are decreased. MCAD gene deficiency is associated with the most common fatty acid oxidation disorder, and enhancing its expression can increase fat oxidation [155]. By increasing expression of these genes, EGCG enhances basal metabolism and lipid oxidation and decreases body weight in HFD-fed mice. Similar results were obtained in obese Beagle dogs, in which supplementation with green tea extract increased PPARα, GLUT4, and LPL expression, followed by insulin sensitivity and lipid profile improvement, suggesting that EGCG is able to reverse obesity-related metabolic disturbances [156].

Numerous epidemiological studies have demonstrated that circadian misalignment in human can be associated with metabolic syndrome, including obesity, hypertension, and insulin resistance [157]. In a mouse model, mutations in the genes CLOCK, Per2, Bmal1, and RORα were associated with various metabolic disorders, suggesting the importance of clock genes in metabolic regulation [158,159]. In C57BL/6J mice fed a high-fat high-fructose diet (HFHFD), supplementation with EGCG showed beneficial effects on circadian misalignment, obesity, insulin resistance, and lipid metabolism by normalizing the expression of the clock genes CLOCK and Bmal1 and by regulating the levels of SIRT1 and PGC1α.

Moreover, EGCG decreased fatty acid synthesis in the liver, increased BAT energy expenditure, and prevented adipocyte hypertrophy [160]. In an HFD-fed dog model, ECCG administration in both low doses (0.25 g/kg BW) and high doses (0.50 g/kg BW) decreased BW gain and suppressed liver inflammation by decreasing the expression of the COX-2 and iNOS genes involved in the inflammatory process [161].

In the skeletal muscle of diabetic rats, oral gavage of 100 mg EGCG for 3 month decreased expression of dynamin-related protein 1 (DRP1 and Beclin1 due to down-regulation of the ROS/ERK/JNK-p53 pathway and amelioration of excessive muscle autophagy [162].

In a randomized double-blind crossover study with obese women without comorbidities, administration of 738 mg green tea resulted in decreased expression of *miR-1297*, *miR-373-3p*, *miR-192-5p*, *miR-1266-5p*, and *miR-595* compared with a control group. These microRNAs are involved in the regulation of genes associated with the Coactivator Associated Arginine Methyltransferase 1 (CARM1), Transforming growth factor beta (TGF-beta), Bone morphogenetic proteins (BMPS), and ribosomal S6 kinase (RSK) pathways. This study showed the beneficial effects of green tea intake by suppressing the expression of microRNAs that target genes mainly involved in adipogenesis and carcinogenesis [163].

Liu et al. found that EGCG regulated the gut microbiome profile in HFD-fed mice by reversing the abundance of Bacteroides and Parasutterella species decreased by HFD, and also reduced *Allobaculum*, *Roseburia*, norank_*Erysipelotrichaceae*, norank_*Lachnospiraceae*, unclassified_f_*Ruminococcaceae*, *Anaerotruncus*, *Odoribacter*, *Enterorhadu*, and *Lachnospiraceae*_UCG_006 and induced the enrichment of *Akkermansia* [164]. In another study, EGCG treatment increased the abundance of the beneficial bacteria *Bacteroides*, *Christensenellaceae* and *Bifidobacterium* and inhibited the pathogenic *Fusobacterium varium*, *Enterobacteriaceae*, and *Bilophila* [165]. Beneficial effects on body weight were observed when adults consumed up to 460 mg/day, while doses higher than 800 mg/kg were responsible for adverse effects [83]. While EGCG is generally considered safe when consumed in moderate amounts through dietary sources, there have been concerns regarding its toxicity at high doses or in concentrated forms. Human and animal experiments suggest the liver is the primary target for toxicity [166,167].

All these data suggest that EGCG as a nutraceutical could be a therapeutic agent in obesity treatment and prevention via moderate intake. However, further investigations are needed, especially in humans, to confirm these hypotheses.

4.5. Capsaicin

Capsaicin is a chemical compound present in different concentrations in plants of the genus *Capsicum*, knows as chili pepper, the main source of capsaicinoids in nature. These chemical compounds are produced by plants as secondary metabolites as a way of defense to deter predators [168] and are responsible for the fruit's burning sensation and spicy flavor [169]. The natural capsaicinoids are capsaicin (C), dihydrocapsaicin (DHC), homodihydrocapsaicin (HDHC), nordihydrocapsaicin (NDHC), and homocapsaicin (HC). The concentration of capsaicinoids in a pepper varies from species to species and from variety to variety, and act and stimulate differently [170]. Natural capsaicinoids are capable of exerting multiple pharmacological and physiological effects, and in clinical practice can be used for pain relief, cancer prevention, and weight loss [171].

The most abundant capsaicinoid in peppers is capsaicin (trans-8-methyl-N-vanillyl-6-nonenamide), discovered in 1846 by Tresh; its chemical structure was determined in 1919 by Nelson [172,173]. Over the years, several studies have demonstrated that from a pharmacological point of view capsaicin is one of the most important constituents currently used for treatment of pain syndromes and diabetic neuropathy [173].

In particular, capsaicin acts by binding to receptors present on the peripheral nerve endings, the so-called vanilloid receptors type 1 or TRPV1, mainly localized on polymodal sensory nerve fibers of type C. These play a fundamental role in hyperalgesia and allodynia. The analgesic effect of capsaicin following binding to these receptors is thought to involve the entry of calcium into the cell until the channel is closed; although until recently it was not clear how the loss of sensitivity was determined by the entry of calcium ions, we now know that it is related to a decrease in phosphatidylinositol 4,5-bisphosphate PIP2, which contributes to the desensitization of TRPV1 receptors [174]. TRPV1 is excited by capsaicin, and through the afferent nerves it contains, the resulting signal is transmitted to the spinal cord. The excitation of efferent nerves by the central nervous system causes an increased release of catecholamines (norepinephrine, epinephrine and dopamine) at the adrenal level. In turn, catecholamines bind β-adrenergic receptors, increasing thermogenic activity. At the gastrointestinal level, TRPV1 activation by capsaicin increases thermogenesis and activates UCP1 in BAT. Taking into account the exposed mechanisms, it is clear that capsaicin increases thermogenesis and energy expenditure via TRPV1 activation, as shown in Figure 2.

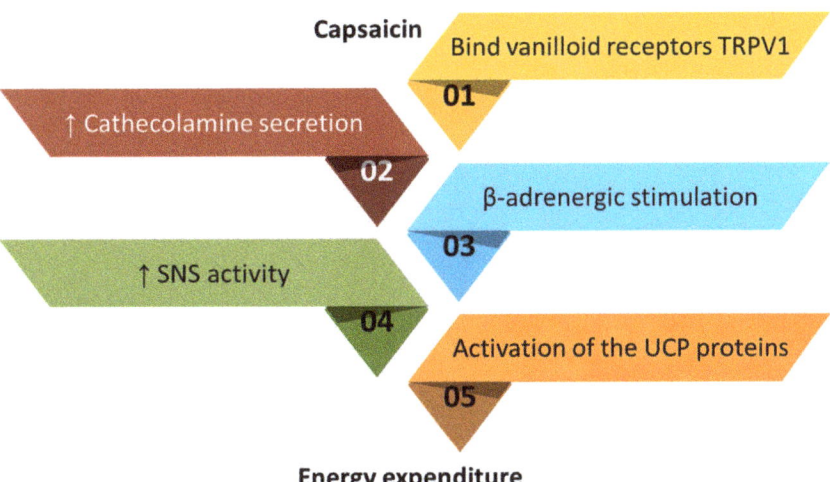

Figure 2. The mechanism of action of capsaicin. TRPV1 is excited by capsaicin, and the resulting signal is transmitted to the spinal cord through the afferent nerves it contains. The excitation of efferent nerves by the central nervous system causes an increased release of catecholamines (norepinephrine, epinephrine, and dopamine) at the adrenal level. In turn, catecholamines bind b-adrenergic receptors, increasing thermogenic activity. At gastrointestinal level, TRPV1 activation by capsaicin increases thermogenesis and activates UCP1 in BAT. Taking into account the exposed mechanisms, it is clear that capsaicin increases thermogenesis and energy expenditure via TRPV1 activation.

Capsaicin has shown anti-obesity effects, being able to induce body weight reduction, improve lipolysis in adipocytes, increase energy expenditure, increase satiety, and decrease the desire to eat [175]. The anti-obesity action of capsaicin might be linked to the activation of both UCP proteins and of the sympathetic nervous system. Both properties carry out an inducing activity towards the metabolism, increasing thermogenesis (Figure 2). For example, treatment for 12 weeks with 6 mg/day of oral capsinoids has been associated with the loss of abdominal fat and is conditioned by the presence or absence of certain genetic polymorphisms, in this case TRPV1 Val585Ile and UCP2 -866 G/A, which may be predictive of the type of therapeutic response [176]. TRPV1 has an important role in body metabolic health, including lipid and glucose metabolism, and its activation by capsaicin stimulates insulin secretion, increases GLP-1 level, and regulates glucose homeostasis [177–179]. In obese mice, capsaicin inactivated nuclear factor-κB (NF-κB) and activated PPARγ in a receptor-independent manner, with suppression of inflammatory response modulating the adipocyte function of adipose tissues macrophages, which are independent on TRPV1 [180].

Several studies have demonstrated that capsaicin inhibits the expression of leptin, PPARγ, and C/EBP-α while up-regulating adiponectin at the protein level, and in this manner efficiently induces apoptosis and adipogenesis to inhibit 3T3-L1 preadipocytes in vitro [181,182].

In C57BL/6 male obese mice fed HFD for 10 weeks, capsaicin supplementation improved glucose intolerance, decreased leptin and insulin concentrations, decreased TRPV-1 expression in adipose tissue, and increased adiponectin expression, accompanied with increased expression of PPARα and PGC-1α in the liver [183]. In C57BL/6J mice, capsinoid supplementation decreased BW gain and fat accumulation, increased energy expenditure by lipolysis activation, and increased cyclic adenosine monophosphate (cAMP) levels and PKA activity in BAT [184]. In addition, capsaicin can improve cholesterol level and counter the harmful effects of HFD in mice by increasing the expression of the thermogenic genes UCP-1, SIRT-1, BMP8b, and PGC-1α and by enhancing the respiratory exchange ratio [185].

Another study found that in HFD rats capsaicin treatment increased expression of oxidation and thermogenic genes in WAT. It was observed that expression of aldo-keto reductase (AKR1B7)-encoding mRNA was decreased in adipose tissues of obese mice and capsaicin treatment reversed expression. In humans, AKR1B1 is involved in development of diabetic complications. In the same study, capsaicin was able to decrease FABP4 and TNFα expression, and UCP2 expression level decreased upon HFD was normalized by capsaicin supplementation [186]

Baboota et al. [187] demonstrated that 3T3-L1 adipocytes treated with 1 μM of capsaicin increased the expression of PGC 1α, UCP1, BDNF, PRMD16, PPARα, FOXC2, NCOA1, DIO2, and SIRT1, which are associated with browning of white adipocytes through a TRPV1-dependent mechanism.

Treatment with nonivamide, a capsaicin analogue, increased expression of the anti-adipogenic microRNAs mmu-let-7a-5p, mmu-let-7d-5p, and mmu-let7b-3p, which are associated with decreased PPARγ levels and anti-obesity effects [188].

In a recent study in HFD-fed mice, capsaicin supplementation was associated with weight loss and altered gut microbiota composition. Capsaicin increased the numbers of *Akkermansia, Bacteroides, Prevotella, Allobaculum, Odoribacter*, and *Coprococcus* and decreased the numbers of *Escherichia, Desulfovibrio, Sutterella*, and *Helicobacter*. In addition, capsaicin increased the abundance of SCFAs along with acetate and propionate concentrations, with positive effects in treatment and prevention of obesity [189].

Capsaicin is safe for short-term use. With long-term use side effects may occur, including stomach irritation, sweating, and runny nose [83]. It has been shown in various studies in which animals have been given high doses to have carcinogenic, neurotoxic, and genotoxic effects [190]. In humans, high consumption of chilis has been reported to be a risk factor for cancer of the upper gastrointestinal tract, possibly due to the irritating effect of capsaicinoids [191].

To summarize, capsaicin plays an important role in human health at the metabolic level, especially in obese people. It is a spice with a long culinary history, and as such its use to treat obesity is more feasible compared to other medical interventions. Nevertheless, a better understanding of its mechanisms of action is necessary, and additional research is required to determine the optimal dose and duration of capsaicinoids for weight loss.

4.6. Caffeine

1,3,7-trimethylxanthine, or caffeine, is an alkaloid found naturally in more than 60 plant species, including coffee beans (*Coffea arabica* L.), cocoa beans (*Theobroma cacao* L.), tea leaves (*Camellia sinensis* (L.) Kuntze), kola nuts (*Cola acuminata* (P.Beauv.) Schott & Endl., *Cola nitida* (Vent.) Schott & Endl.), guarana berries (*Paullinia cupana* Kunth), yerba mate (*Ilex paraguariensis* A.St.-Hil.), and guayusa (*Ilex guayusa* Loes.) [192,193].

Numerous epidemiological studies have linked caffeine consumption to health benefits in moderate coffee drinkers, including reduction of mortality [194,195], protection against cancer development [196], decreased risk of type 2 diabetes [197], controlling Parkinson's disease [198], slowing the progression of dementia [199], and slowing the progression of many forms of liver disease [200]. In the sporting world caffeine is ubiquitous due to its ergogenic aids [201], and use of caffeine supplements has been shown to improve performance in such different aspects of exercise as muscular strength, muscular endurance, jumping, sprinting, and movement speed. In addition, caffeine ingestion before exercise in the morning seems to promote weight loss according to published studies [202]. Regarding the effect of caffeine on weight loss, several studies have demonstrated that caffeine intake promotes a decreasing in weight, BMI, and body fat [203].

Caffeine supplementation results in reduced food intake and increased energy expenditure by inhibition of phosphodiesterase-induced degradation of intracellular cAMP, increasing cAMP-dependent protein kinase (PKA), and inhibition of PI3K/AKT activity [204]. In another study, increased energy expenditure and reduced number of adipocytes were related to FAS activity inhibition and decreased expression of PPARγ [205]. Caffeine was able to reduce lipid accumulation by increasing lipolysis in adipocytes and inhibiting insulin-stimulated glucose uptake [206].

Another study showed that caffeine supplementation inhibited the expression of C/EBPβ, C/EBPα, and PPARγ in 3T3-L1 preadipocytes during differentiation by regulating the expression of G1-S cell cycle markers [207].

In HFSD-fed rats, caffeine treatments (0.1%) equivalent to four cups of coffee in humans modulated the mRNA expression of pyruvate kinase (PKM), microsomal triglyceride transfer protein (MTTP), and FASN in the liver, resulting in reduced de novo fatty synthesis [205]. Velickovic et al. found that caffeine treatment increased UCP1 expression in mMSC culture and upregulated gene expression of PPARγ, FABP4, adiponectin, the beige markers CD137, CITED1, and P2RX5, and the brown-selective genes PRDM16, LHX8, PGC-1α, AR-ß3, and COX8b, following by conversion of white/beige cells into brown adipocytes and an increase in lipolysis [208].

Mitani et al. showed that incubation of 3T3-L1 adipocytes with caffeine for 24 h miniaturized lipid droplets and decreased accumulation by inhibiting expression of PPARγ and CCAAT/enhancer binding protein (C/EBP) α. Interestingly, the expression levels of C/EBPβ and C/EBPδ were not observed at the level of mRNA, only at the protein level. The same authors found that caffeine inhibited expression of SERPIN1 in Caco-2 cells and decreased secretion of the proinflammatory cytokines Il-8 and PAI-1 [209].

It has been demonstrated that caffeine ingestion improves hyperglycemia in KK-Ay type 2 diabetic mice, enhances insulin sensitivity, significantly decreases the expression of the inflammatory cytokines TNFα, MCP-1, and IL-6, and decreases the mRNA levels of the macrophage marker F4/80 in adipose tissue, suggesting that caffeine is able to lower the production of the inflammatory adipocytokines and decrease inflammation. In addition, caffeine intake improved dyslipidemia, fatty liver and total cholesterol serum level with decreasing in SREBP-1 and FAS genes expression. An increase in IRS- 2 expression was observed as well, which is correlated with an improvement in insulin resistance at the hepatic level [210].

Regarding the effects of caffeine on gut microbiota, studies have shown an improvement in *Firmicutes/Bacteroidetes* ratio and increase in *Bifidobacterium* spp. in humans [211]., High fecal levels of *Bacteroides-Prevotella-Porphyromonas*, which are correlated with better metabolic status, have been observed in high coffee consumers [212,213].

Caffeine is administered orally in doses of 50–260 mg daily. It is safe for most healthy adults when used in doses up to 400 mg per day, the equivalent of about 4 cups of coffee. When used over a long period of time or in doses over 400 mg per day, caffeine can cause insomnia, nervousness, restlessness, nausea, increased heart rate, and other side effects. Higher doses can cause headaches, anxiety, and chest pain [83]. Caffeine overdose may cause hypokalemia, hyponatremia, impaired iron and zinc absorption, rhabdomyolysis, and circulatory collapse [167].

In light of all the evidence, it is clear that that caffeine consumption or supplementation can promote weight reduction; however, additional studies are necessary to explain all the mechanisms correlated with fat loss, improved BMI, and appetite reduction.

5. Conclusions

Obesity is rising all around the world. It is clear that fat accumulation is caused by several factors, such as genetic, epigenetic, and lifestyle factors, and the use of nutraceuticals for the treatment of this condition is constantly increasing. In fact, many products have been publicized and studied to investigate their effectiveness in the control and loss of body weight. Among these products, nutraceuticals enjoy great success among the population compared to anti-obesity drugs, in particular thanks to their low toxicity, competitive pricing, and lack of requirement for a medical prescription.

The mechanisms by which nutraceuticals can contribute to weight management are varied, including anti-inflammatory activities, inhibition of the sense of hunger, inhibition of fatty acid biosynthesis and/or intestinal fatty acid and cholesterol absorption levels, modulation of several pathways involved in carbohydrate digestion, fatty acid storage, insulin production and cellular glucose uptake, increase in energy expenditure, inhibition of adipocyte differentiation, lipolysis activation, and increasing of satiating effect. Through their potential to modify gene expression, certain nutraceuticals can assume the role of true epigenetic drugs, and their future potential must be explored through future clinical trials in humans. While it should not be forgotten that the effects of nutraceuticals are not such as to be able to mask a patient's noncompliance with dietary and behavioral prescriptions, they can encourage adherence by accelerating achievement of the desired results.

Supplementary Materials: The following supporting information can be downloaded at: https://www.mdpi.com/article/10.3390/plants12122273/s1, Table S1: Epigenetic modifications induced by nutraceuticals in relation to obesity.

Author Contributions: Conceptualization, M.V., L.F. and D.-S.P.; resources, M.V. and S.-C.H.; writing—original draft preparation, M.V., S.-C.H., L.F., C.M.S., A.C.-P. and R.B.; writing—review and editing, M.V., S.-C.H., L.F., V.R. and D.-S.P.; visualization, A.C.-P. and R.B.; supervision, D.-S.P. and D.M.; project administration, M.V., S.-C.H. and L.F.; funding acquisition, M.V. and S.-C.H. All authors have read and agreed to the published version of the manuscript.

Funding: This research received no external funding.

Data Availability Statement: Not applicable.

Conflicts of Interest: The authors declare no conflict of interest.

References

1. Di Cesare, M.; Bentham, J.; Stevens, G.A.; Zhou, B.; Danaei, G.; Lu, Y.; Bixby, H.; Cowan, M.J.; Riley, L.M.; Hajifathalian, K.; et al. Trends in adult body-mass index in 200 countries from 1975 to 2014: A pooled analysis of 1698 population-based measurement studies with 19.2 million participants. *Lancet* **2016**, *387*, 1377–1396. [CrossRef]
2. Pérez, L.M.; Pareja-Galeano, H.; Sanchis-Gomar, F.; Emanuele, E.; Lucia, A.; Gálvez, B.G. 'Adipaging': Ageing and obesity share biological hallmarks related to a dysfunctional adipose tissue. *J. Physiol.* **2016**, *594*, 3187–3207. [CrossRef]
3. Pantalone, K.M.; Hobbs, T.M.; Chagin, K.M.; Kong, S.X.; Wells, B.J.; Kattan, M.W.; Bouchard, J.; Sakurada, B.; Milinovich, A.; Weng, W.; et al. Prevalence and recognition of obesity and its associated comorbidities: Cross-sectional analysis of electronic health record data from a large US integrated health system. *BMJ Open* **2017**, *7*, e017583. [CrossRef]
4. Avgerinos, K.I.; Spyrou, N.; Mantzoros, C.S.; Dalamaga, M. Obesity and cancer risk: Emerging biological mechanisms and perspectives. *Metabolism* **2019**, *92*, 121–135. [CrossRef]
5. Sarwer, D.B.; Polonsky, H.M. The Psychosocial Burden of Obesity. *Endocrinol. Metab. Clin. North Am.* **2016**, *45*, 677–688. [CrossRef]
6. Rankinen, T.; Zuberi, A.; Chagnon, Y.C.; Weisnagel, S.J.; Argyropoulos, G.; Walts, B.; Perusse, L.; Bouchard, C. The human obesity gene map: The 2005 update. *Obesity* **2006**, *14*, 529–644. [CrossRef]

7. Saunders, C.L.; Chiodini, B.D.; Sham, P.; Lewis, C.M.; Abkevich, V.; Adeyemo, A.A.; De Andrade, M.; Arya, R.; Berenson, G.S.; Blangero, J.; et al. Meta-analysis of genome-wide linkage studies in BMI and obesity. *Obesity* **2007**, *15*, 2263–2275. [CrossRef]
8. Yengo, L.; Sidorenko, J.; Kemper, K.E.; Zheng, Z.; Wood, A.R.; Weedon, M.N.; Frayling, T.M.; Hirschhorn, J.; Yang, J.; Visscher, P.M.; et al. Meta-analysis of genome-wide association studies for height and body mass index in ~700,000 individuals of European ancestry. *Hum. Mol. Genet.* **2018**, *27*, 3641–3649. [CrossRef]
9. Park, Y.J.; Han, S.M.; Huh, J.Y.; Kim, J.B. Emerging roles of epigenetic regulation in obesity and metabolic disease. *J. Biol. Chem.* **2021**, *297*, 101296. [CrossRef]
10. Thaker, V.V. Genetic and epigenetic causes of obesity. *Adolesc. Med. State Art. Rev.* **2017**, *28*, 379–405. [CrossRef]
11. Mahmoud, R.; Kimonis, V.; Butler, M.G. Genetics of Obesity in Humans: A Clinical Review. *Int. J. Mol. Sci.* **2022**, *23*, 11005. [CrossRef]
12. Sohn, Y.B. Genetic obesity: An update with emerging therapeutic approaches. *Ann. Pediatr. Endocrinol. Metab.* **2022**, *27*, 169–175. [CrossRef]
13. Loos, R.J.F.; Lindgren, C.M.; Li, S.; Wheeler, E.; Zhao, J.H.; Prokopenko, I.; Inouye, M.; Freathy, R.M.; Attwood, A.P.; Beckmann, J.S.; et al. Common variants near MC4R are associated with fat mass, weight and risk of obesity. *Nat. Genet.* **2008**, *40*, 768–775. [CrossRef]
14. González Sanchez, J.; SeRrano Rios, M.; FPernández Perez, C.; Laakso, M.; Martínez Larrad, M. Effect of the Pro12Ala polymorphism of the peroxisome proliferator-activated receptor gamma-2 gene on adiposity, insulin sensitivity and lipid profile in the Spanish population. *Eur. J. Endocrinol.* **2002**, *147*, 495–501. [CrossRef]
15. Hsueh, W.-C.; Cole, S.A.; Shuldiner, A.R.; Beamer, B.A.; Blangero, J.; Hixson, J.E.; MacCluer, J.W.; Mitchell, B.D. Interactions between variants in the β3-adrenergic receptor and peroxisome proliferator–Activated receptor-γ2 genes and obesity. *Diabetes Care* **2001**, *24*, 672–677. [CrossRef]
16. Hashemi, M.; Rezaei, H.; Kaykhaei, M.-A.; Taheri, M. A 45-bp insertion/deletion polymorphism of UCP2 gene is associated with metabolic syndrome. *J. Diabetes Metab. Disord.* **2014**, *13*, 12. [CrossRef]
17. Tyrrell, J.; Wood, A.R.; Ames, R.M.; Yaghootkar, H.; Beaumont, R.N.; Jones, S.E.; Tuke, M.A.; Ruth, K.S.; Freathy, R.M.; Smith, G.D.; et al. Gene–obesogenic environment interactions in the UK Biobank study. *Int. J. Epidemiol.* **2017**, *46*, 559–575. [CrossRef]
18. Dhurandhar, E.J.; Keith, S.W. The aetiology of obesity beyond eating more and exercising less. *Best Pract. Res. Clin. Gastroenterol.* **2014**, *28*, 533–544. [CrossRef]
19. Lopomo, A.; Burgio, E.; Migliore, L. Epigenetics of Obesity. *Prog. Mol. Biol. Transl. Sci.* **2016**, *140*, 151–184. [CrossRef]
20. Bernal, A.J.; Murphy, S.K.; Jirtle, R.L. Mouse Models of Epigenetic Inheritance. In *Handbook of Epigenetics: The New Molecular and Medical Genetics*; Tollefsbol, T., Ed.; Academic Press: Cambridge, MA, USA, 2011; pp. 233–249, ISBN 9780123757098.
21. Samblas, M.; Milagro, F.I.; Martínez, A. DNA methylation markers in obesity, metabolic syndrome, and weight loss. *Epigenetics* **2019**, *14*, 421–444. [CrossRef]
22. Abdul, Q.A.; Yu, B.P.; Chung, H.Y.; Jung, H.A.; Choi, J.S. Epigenetic modifications of gene expression by lifestyle and environment. *Arch. Pharmacal Res.* **2017**, *40*, 1219–1237. [CrossRef]
23. Horvath, S.; Raj, K. DNA methylation-based biomarkers and the epigenetic clock theory of ageing. *Nat. Rev. Genet.* **2018**, *19*, 371–384. [CrossRef]
24. Satterstrom, F.K.; Walters, R.K.; Singh, T.; Wigdor, E.M.; Lescai, F.; Demontis, D.; Kosmicki, J.A.; Grove, J.; Stevens, C.; Bybjerg-Grauholm, J.; et al. Autism spectrum disorder and attention deficit hyperactivity disorder have a similar burden of rare protein-truncating variants. *Nat. Neurosci.* **2019**, *22*, 1961–1965. [CrossRef] [PubMed]
25. Franzago, M.; Santurbano, D.; Vitacolonna, E.; Stuppia, L. Genes and Diet in the Prevention of Chronic Diseases in Future Generations. *Int. J. Mol. Sci.* **2020**, *21*, 2633. [CrossRef]
26. Sadashiv; Modi, A.; Khokhar, M.; Sharma, P.; Joshi, R.; Mishra, S.S.; Bharshankar, R.N.; Tiwari, S.; Singh, P.K.; Bhosale, V.V.; et al. Leptin DNA Methylation and Its Association with Metabolic Risk Factors in a Northwest Indian Obese Population. *J. Obes. Metab. Syndr.* **2021**, *30*, 304–311. [CrossRef] [PubMed]
27. Houde, A.-A.; Légaré, C.; Biron, S.; Lescelleur, O.; Biertho, L.; Marceau, S.; Tchernof, A.; Vohl, M.-C.; Hivert, M.-F.; Bouchard, L. Leptin and adiponectin DNA methylation levels in adipose tissues and blood cells are associated with BMI, waist girth and LDL-cholesterol levels in severely obese men and women. *BMC Med. Genet.* **2015**, *16*, 29. [CrossRef] [PubMed]
28. Kim, A.Y.; Park, Y.J.; Pan, X.; Shin, K.C.; Kwak, S.-H.; Bassas, A.F.; Sallam, R.M.; Park, K.S.; Alfadda, A.A.; Xu, A.; et al. Obesity-induced DNA hypermethylation of the adiponectin gene mediates insulin resistance. *Nat. Commun.* **2015**, *6*, 7585. [CrossRef]
29. Ott, R.; Stupin, J.H.; Melchior, K.; Schellong, K.; Ziska, T.; Dudenhausen, J.W.; Henrich, W.; Rancourt, R.C.; Plagemann, A. Alterations of adiponectin gene expression and DNA methylation in adipose tissues and blood cells are associated with gestational diabetes and neonatal outcome. *Clin. Epigenetics* **2018**, *10*, 13. [CrossRef]
30. Houshmand-Oeregaard, A.; Hansen, N.S.; Hjort, L.; Kelstrup, L.; Broholm, C.; Mathiesen, E.R.; Clausen, T.D.; Damm, P.; Vaag, A. Differential adipokine DNA methylation and gene expression in subcutaneous adipose tissue from adult offspring of women with diabetes in pregnancy. *Clin. Epigenetics* **2017**, *9*, 37. [CrossRef]
31. Perkins, E.; Murphy, S.K.; Murtha, A.P.; Schildkraut, J.; Jirtle, R.L.; Demark-Wahnefried, W.; Forman, M.R.; Kurtzberg, J.; Overcash, F.; Huang, Z.; et al. Insulin-like growth factor 2/H19 methylation at birth and risk of overweight and obesity in children. *J. Pediatr.* **2012**, *161*, 31–39. [CrossRef]

32. Crujeiras, A.B.; Campion, J.; Díaz-Lagares, A.; Milagro, F.I.; Goyenechea, E.; Abete, I.; Casanueva, F.F.; Martínez, J.A. Association of weight regain with specific methylation levels in the NPY and POMC promoters in leukocytes of obese men: A translational study. *Regul. Pept.* **2013**, *186*, 1–6. [CrossRef] [PubMed]
33. Ali, M.M.; Naquiallah, D.; Qureshi, M.; Mirza, M.I.; Hassan, C.; Masrur, M.; Bianco, F.M.; Frederick, P.; Cristoforo, G.P.; Gangemi, A.; et al. DNA methylation profile of genes involved in inflammation and autoimmunity correlates with vascular function in morbidly obese adults. *Epigenetics* **2022**, *17*, 93–109. [CrossRef] [PubMed]
34. Rohde, K.; Klös, M.; Hopp, L.; Liu, X.; Keller, M.; Stumvoll, M.; Dietrich, A.; Schön, M.R.; Gärtner, D.; Lohmann, T.; et al. IRS1 DNA promoter methylation and expression in human adipose tissue are related to fat distribution and metabolic traits. *Sci. Rep.* **2017**, *7*, 12369. [CrossRef]
35. Bannister, A.J.; Kouzarides, T. Regulation of chromatin by histone modifications. *Cell Res.* **2011**, *21*, 381–395. [CrossRef] [PubMed]
36. Gujral, P.; Mahajan, V.; Lissaman, A.C.; Ponnampalam, A.P. Histone acetylation and the role of histone deacetylases in normal cyclic endometrium. *Reprod. Biol. Endocrinol.* **2020**, *18*, 84. [CrossRef] [PubMed]
37. Albini, S.; Zakharova, V.; Ait-Si-Ali, S. Histone Modifications. In *Epigenetics and Regeneration*; Palacios, D., Ed.; Academic Press: Cambridge, MA, USA, 2019; Volume 11, pp. 47–72, ISBN 9780128148792.
38. Husmann, D.; Gozani, O. Histone lysine methyltransferases in biology and disease. *Nat. Struct. Mol. Biol.* **2019**, *26*, 880–889. [CrossRef]
39. Bhat, K.P.; Ümit Kaniskan, H.; Jin, J.; Gozani, O. Epigenetics and beyond: Targeting writers of protein lysine methylation to treat disease. *Nat. Rev. Drug Discov.* **2021**, *20*, 265–286. [CrossRef]
40. Lee, J.-E.; Schmidt, H.; Lai, B.; Ge, K. Transcriptional and Epigenomic Regulation of Adipogenesis. *Mol. Cell. Biol.* **2019**, *39*, e00601-18. [CrossRef]
41. Mikula, M.; Majewska, A.; Ledwon, J.K.; Dzwonek, A.; Ostrowski, J. Obesity increases histone H3 lysine 9 and 18 acetylation at Tnfa and Ccl2 genes in mouse liver. *Int. J. Mol. Med.* **2014**, *34*, 1647–1654. [CrossRef]
42. Wheatley, K.E.; Nogueira, L.M.; Perkins, S.N.; Hursting, S.D. Differential effects of calorie restriction and exercise on the adipose transcriptome in diet-induced obese mice. *J. Obes.* **2011**, *2011*, 265417. [CrossRef]
43. Funato, H.; Oda, S.; Yokofujita, J.; Igarashi, H.; Kuroda, M. Fasting and high-fat diet alter histone deacetylase expression in the medial hypothalamus. *PLoS ONE* **2011**, *6*, e18950. [CrossRef]
44. O'Brien, J.; Hayder, H.; Zayed, Y.; Peng, C. Overview of MicroRNA biogenesis, mechanisms of actions, and circulation. *Front. Endocrinol.* **2018**, *9*, 402. [CrossRef] [PubMed]
45. Jean-François, L.; Derghal, A.; Mounien, L. MicroRNAs in Obesity and Related Metabolic Disorders. *Cells* **2019**, *8*, 859. [CrossRef]
46. Song, G.; Xu, G.; Ji, C.; Shi, C.; Shen, Y.; Chen, L.; Zhu, L.; Yang, L.; Zhao, Y.; Guo, X. The role of microRNA-26b in human adipocyte differentiation and proliferation. *Gene* **2014**, *533*, 481–487. [CrossRef] [PubMed]
47. Xu, G.; Ji, C.; Song, G.; Shi, C.; Shen, Y.; Chen, L.; Yang, L.; Zhao, Y.; Guo, X. Obesity-associated microRNA-26b regulates the proliferation of human preadipocytes via arrest of the G1/S transition. *Mol. Med. Rep.* **2015**, *12*, 3648–3654. [CrossRef]
48. Pan, S.; Yang, X.; Jia, Y.; Li, R.; Zhao, R. Microvesicle-shuttled mir-130b reduces fat deposition in recipient primary cultured porcine adipocytes by inhibiting PPAR-γ expression. *J. Cell. Physiol.* **2014**, *229*, 631–639. [CrossRef]
49. Puri, V.; Nagpal, M.; Singh, I.; Singh, M.; Dhingra, G.A.; Huanbutta, K.; Dheer, D.; Sharma, A.; Sangnim, T. A Comprehensive Review on Nutraceuticals: Therapy Support and Formulation Challenges. *Nutrients* **2022**, *14*, 4637. [CrossRef]
50. Vrânceanu, M.; Galimberti, D.; Banc, R.; Dragoş, O.; Cozma-Petruţ, A.; Hegheş, S.-C.; Voştinaru, O.; Cuciureanu, M.; Stroia, C.M.; Miere, D.; et al. The Anticancer Potential of Plant-Derived Nutraceuticals via the Modulation of Gene Expression. *Plants* **2022**, *11*, 2524. [CrossRef]
51. Bertuccioli, A.; Cardinali, M.; Biagi, M.; Moricoli, S.; Morganti, I.; Zonzini, G.B.; Rigillo, G. Nutraceuticals and Herbal Food Supplements for Weight Loss: Is There a Prebiotic Role in the Mechanism of Action? *Microorganisms* **2021**, *9*, 2427. [CrossRef]
52. Sorokina, M.; Steinbeck, C. Review on natural products databases: Where to find data in 2020. *J. Cheminform.* **2020**, *12*, 20. [CrossRef]
53. Ammendola, S.; Scotto D'abusco, A. Nutraceuticals and the Network of Obesity Modulators. *Nutrients* **2022**, *14*, 5099. [CrossRef] [PubMed]
54. Fraga, C.G.; Croft, K.D.; Kennedy, D.O.; Tomás-Barberán, F.A. The effects of polyphenols and other bioactives on human health. *Food Funct.* **2019**, *10*, 514–528. [CrossRef] [PubMed]
55. Tian, B.; Liu, J. Resveratrol: A review of plant sources, synthesis, stability, modification and food application. *J. Sci. Food Agric.* **2020**, *100*, 1392–1404. [CrossRef] [PubMed]
56. Vestergaard, M.; Ingmer, H. Antibacterial and antifungal properties of resveratrol. *Int. J. Antimicrob. Agents* **2019**, *53*, 716–723. [CrossRef]
57. Lamuela-Raventos, R.M.; Romero-Perez, A.I.; Waterhouse, A.L.; de la Torre-Boronat, M.C. Direct HPLC Analysis of cis- and trans-Resveratrol and Piceid Isomers in Spanish Red Vitis vinifera Wines. *J. Agric. Food Chem.* **1995**, *43*, 281–283. [CrossRef]
58. Akinwumi, B.C.; Bordun, K.-A.M.; Anderson, H.D. Biological Activities of Stilbenoids. *Int. J. Mol. Sci.* **2018**, *19*, 792. [CrossRef]

59. Anisimova, N.Y.U.; Kiselevsky, M.V.; Sosnov, A.V.; Sadovnikov, S.V.; Stankov, I.N.; Gakh, A.A. Trans-, cis-, and dihydro-resveratrol: A comparative study. *Chem. Cent. J.* **2011**, *5*, 88. [CrossRef]
60. Delmas, D.; Cornebise, C.; Courtaut, F.; Xiao, J.; Aires, V. New Highlights of Resveratrol: A Review of Properties against Ocular Diseases. *Int. J. Mol. Sci.* **2021**, *22*, 1295. [CrossRef]
61. Zhang, H.; Li, C.; Kwok, S.-T.; Zhang, Q.-W.; Chan, S.-W. A Review of the Pharmacological Effects of the Dried Root of *Polygonum cuspidatum* (Hu Zhang) and Its Constituents. *Evid. -Based Complement. Altern. Med.* **2013**, *2013*, 208349. [CrossRef]
62. Craveiro, M.; Cretenet, G.; Mongellaz, C.; Matias, M.I.; Caron, O.; de Lima, M.C.P.; Zimmermann, V.S.; Solary, E.; Dardalhon, V.; Dulić, V.; et al. Resveratrol stimulates the metabolic reprogramming of human $CD4^+T$ cells to enhance effector function. *Sci. Signal* **2017**, *10*, eaal3024. [CrossRef]
63. Hou, C.-Y.; Tain, Y.-L.; Yu, H.-R.; Huang, L.-T. The Effects of Resveratrol in the Treatment of Metabolic Syndrome. *Int. J. Mol. Sci.* **2019**, *20*, 535. [CrossRef]
64. Dyck, G.J.B.; Raj, P.; Zieroth, S.; Dyck, J.R.B.; Ezekowitz, J.A. The Effects of Resveratrol in Patients with Cardiovascular Disease and Heart Failure: A Narrative Review. *Int. J. Mol. Sci.* **2019**, *20*, 904. [CrossRef]
65. Zhou, L.; Xiao, X.; Zhang, Q.; Zheng, J.; Deng, M. Deciphering the Anti-obesity Benefits of Resveratrol: The "Gut Microbiota-Adipose Tissue" Axis. *Front. Endocrinol.* **2019**, *10*, 413. [CrossRef]
66. Scapagnini, G.; Davinelli, S.; Kaneko, T.; Koverech, G.; Koverech, A.; Calabrese, E.J.; Calabrese, V. Dose response biology of resveratrol in obesity. *J. Cell Commun. Signal* **2014**, *8*, 385–391. [CrossRef] [PubMed]
67. Timmers, S.; Konings, E.; Bilet, L.; Houtkooper, R.H.; van de Weijer, T.; Goossens, G.H.; Hoeks, J.; van der Krieken, S.; Ryu, D.; Kersten, S.; et al. Calorie restriction-like effects of 30 days of resveratrol supplementation on energy metabolism and metabolic profile in obese humans. *Cell Metab.* **2011**, *14*, 612–622. [CrossRef] [PubMed]
68. Mongioì, L.M.; La Vignera, S.; Cannarella, R.; Cimino, L.; Compagnone, M.; Condorelli, R.A.; Calogero, A.E. The Role of Resveratrol Administration in Human Obesity. *Int. J. Mol. Sci.* **2021**, *22*, 4362. [CrossRef] [PubMed]
69. Lasa, A.; Churruca, I.; Eseberri, I.; Andrés-Lacueva, C.; Portillo, M.P. Delipidating effect of resveratrol metabolites in 3T3-L1 adipocytes. *Mol. Nutr. Food Res.* **2012**, *56*, 1559–1568. [CrossRef] [PubMed]
70. Aguirre, L.; Fernández-Quintela, A.; Arias, N.; Portillo, M.P. Resveratrol: Anti-Obesity Mechanisms of Action. *Molecules* **2014**, *19*, 18632–18655. [CrossRef]
71. Kang, N.E.; Ha, A.W.; Kim, J.Y.; Kim, W.K. Resveratrol inhibits the protein expression of transcription factors related adipocyte differentiation and the activity of matrix metalloproteinase in mouse fibroblast 3T3-L1 preadipocytes. *Nutr. Res. Pract.* **2012**, *6*, 499–504. [CrossRef]
72. Andrade, J.M.O.; Frade, A.C.M.; Guimarães, J.B.; Freitas, K.M.; Lopes, M.T.P.; Guimaraes, A.L.S.; De Paula, A.M.B.; Coimbra, C.C.; Santos, S.H.S. Resveratrol increases brown adipose tissue thermogenesis markers by increasing SIRT1 and energy expenditure and decreasing fat accumulation in adipose tissue of mice fed a standard diet. *Eur. J. Nutr.* **2014**, *53*, 1503–1510. [CrossRef]
73. Boström, P.; Wu, J.; Jedrychowski, M.P.; Korde, A.; Ye, L.; Lo, J.C.; Rasbach, K.A.; Boström, E.A.; Choi, J.H.; Long, J.Z.; et al. A PGC1-α-dependent myokine that drives brown-fat-like development of white fat and thermogenesis. *Nature* **2012**, *481*, 463–468. [CrossRef] [PubMed]
74. Andrade, J.M.O.; Barcala-Jorge, A.S.; Batista-Jorge, G.C.; Paraíso, A.F.; de Freitas, K.M.; Lelis, D.D.F.; Guimarães, A.L.S.; de Paula, A.M.B.; Santos, S.H.S. Effect of resveratrol on expression of genes involved thermogenesis in mice and humans. *Biomed. Pharmacother.* **2019**, *112*, 108634. [CrossRef] [PubMed]
75. Parmar, A.; Mula, R.V.; Azhar, Y.; Shashidharamurthy, R.; Rayalam, S. Resveratrol Increases Catecholamine Synthesis in Macrophages: Implications on Obesity. *FASEB J.* **2016**, *30*, lb346. [CrossRef]
76. Nishimura, Y.; Sasagawa, S.; Ariyoshi, M.; Ichikawa, Y.; Shimada, Y.; Kawaguchi, K.; Kawase, R.; Yamamoto, R.; Uehara, T.; Yanai, T.; et al. Systems pharmacology of adiposity reveals inhibition of EP300 as a common therapeutic mechanism of caloric restriction and resveratrol for obesity. *Front. Pharmacol.* **2015**, *6*, 199. [CrossRef]
77. Wang, B.; Sun, J.; Li, L.; Zheng, J.; Shi, Y.; Le, G. Regulatory effects of resveratrol on glucose metabolism and T-lymphocyte subsets in the development of high-fat diet-induced obesity in C57BL/6 mice. *Food Funct.* **2014**, *5*, 1452–1463. [CrossRef]
78. Huang, Y.; Zhu, X.; Chen, K.; Lang, H.; Zhang, Y.; Hou, P.; Ran, L.; Zhou, M.; Zheng, J.; Yi, L.; et al. Resveratrol prevents sarcopenic obesity by reversing mitochondrial dysfunction and oxidative stress via the PKA/LKB1/AMPK pathway. *Aging* **2019**, *11*, 2217–2240. [CrossRef]
79. Gracia, A.; Miranda, J.; Fernández-Quintela, A.; Eseberri, I.; Garcia-Lacarte, M.; Milagro, F.I.; Martínez, J.A.; Aguirre, L.; Portillo, M.P. Involvement of miR-539-5p in the inhibition of de novo lipogenesis induced by resveratrol in white adipose tissue. *Food Funct.* **2016**, *7*, 1680–1688. [CrossRef]
80. Magaña, M.M.; Koo, S.-H.; Towle, H.C.; Osborne, T.F. Different sterol regulatory element-binding protein-1 isoforms utilize distinct co-regulatory factors to activate the promoter for fatty acid synthase. *J. Biol. Chem.* **2000**, *275*, 4726–4733. [CrossRef]
81. Chaplin, A.; Carpéné, C.; Mercader, J. Resveratrol, Metabolic Syndrome, and Gut Microbiota. *Nutrients* **2018**, *10*, 1651. [CrossRef]
82. Qiao, Y.; Sun, J.; Xia, S.; Tang, X.; Shi, Y.; Le, G. Effects of resveratrol on gut microbiota and fat storage in a mouse model with high-fat-induced obesity. *Food Funct.* **2014**, *5*, 1241–1249. [CrossRef]
83. WebMD's Comprehensive Database for Vitamins and Supplements Information from A to Z. Available online: https://www.webmd.com/vitamins/index (accessed on 10 May 2023).

84. Shaito, A.; Posadino, A.M.; Younes, N.; Hasan, H.; Halabi, S.; Alhababi, D.; Al-Mohannadi, A.; Abdel-Rahman, W.M.; Eid, A.H.; Nasrallah, G.K.; et al. Potential Adverse Effects of Resveratrol: A Literature Review. *Int. J. Mol. Sci.* **2020**, *21*, 2084. [CrossRef]
85. Sharifi-Rad, J.; El Rayess, Y.; Rizk, A.A.; Sadaka, C.; Zgheib, R.; Zam, W.; Sestito, S.; Rapposelli, S.; Neffe-Skocińska, K.; Zielińska, D.; et al. Turmeric and Its Major Compound Curcumin on Health: Bioactive Effects and Safety Profiles for Food, Pharmaceutical, Biotechnological and Medicinal Applications. *Front. Pharmacol.* **2020**, *11*, 01021. [CrossRef] [PubMed]
86. Hwang, K.-W.; Son, D.; Jo, H.-W.; Kim, C.H.; Seong, K.C.; Moon, J.-K. Levels of curcuminoid and essential oil compositions in turmerics (*Curcuma longa* L.) grown in Korea. *Appl. Biol. Chem.* **2016**, *59*, 209–215. [CrossRef]
87. Dosoky, N.; Setzer, W. Chemical Composition and Biological Activities of Essential Oils of *Curcuma* Species. *Nutrients* **2018**, *10*, 1196. [CrossRef] [PubMed]
88. Mohamed, G.A.; Ibrahim, S.R.M.; Elkhayat, E.S.; El Dine, R.S. Natural anti-obesity agents. *Bull. Fac. Pharm. Cairo Univ.* **2014**, *52*, 269–284. [CrossRef]
89. Jin, T. Mechanisms underlying the metabolic beneficial effect of curcumin intervention: Beyond anti-inflammation and anti-oxidative stress. *Obes. Med.* **2019**, *13*, 1–5. [CrossRef]
90. Jin, T. Current Understanding on Role of the Wnt Signaling Pathway Effector TCF7L2 in Glucose Homeostasis. *Endocr. Rev.* **2016**, *37*, 254–277. [CrossRef] [PubMed]
91. Kim, C.Y.; Le, T.T.; Chen, C.; Cheng, J.-X.; Kim, K.-H. Curcumin inhibits adipocyte differentiation through modulation of mitotic clonal expansion. *J. Nutr. Biochem.* **2011**, *22*, 910–920. [CrossRef]
92. Ahn, J.; Lee, H.; Kim, S.; Ha, T. Curcumin-induced suppression of adipogenic differentiation is accompanied by activation of Wnt/β-catenin signaling. *Am. J. Physiol. Cell Physiol.* **2010**, *298*, C1510–C1516. [CrossRef]
93. Rahmani, S.; Asgary, S.; Askari, G.; Keshvari, M.; Hatamipour, M.; Feizi, A.; Sahebkar, A. Treatment of Non-alcoholic Fatty Liver Disease with Curcumin: A Randomized Placebo-controlled Trial. *Phytother. Res.* **2016**, *30*, 1540–1548. [CrossRef]
94. Faghihzadeh, F.; Adibi, P.; Hekmatdoost, A. The effects of resveratrol supplementation on cardiovascular risk factors in patients with non-alcoholic fatty liver disease: A randomised, double-blind, placebo-controlled study. *Br. J. Nutr.* **2015**, *114*, 796–803. [CrossRef]
95. Baziar, N.; Parohan, M. The effects of curcumin supplementation on body mass index, body weight, and waist circumference in patients with nonalcoholic fatty liver disease: A systematic review and dose–response meta-analysis of randomized controlled trials. *Phytother. Res.* **2020**, *34*, 464–474. [CrossRef]
96. Jalali, M.; Mahmoodi, M.; Mosallanezhad, Z.; Jalali, R.; Imanieh, M.H.; Moosavian, S.P. The effects of curcumin supplementation on liver function, metabolic profile and body composition in patients with non-alcoholic fatty liver disease: A systematic review and meta-analysis of randomized controlled trials. *Complement. Ther. Med.* **2020**, *48*, 102283. [CrossRef]
97. Den Hartogh, D.J.; Gabriel, A.; Tsiani, E. Antidiabetic Properties of Curcumin I: Evidence from In Vitro Studies. *Nutrients* **2020**, *12*, 118. [CrossRef] [PubMed]
98. Pivari, F.; Mingione, A.; Brasacchio, C.; Soldati, L. Curcumin and Type 2 Diabetes Mellitus: Prevention and Treatment. *Nutrients* **2019**, *11*, 1837. [CrossRef]
99. Hu, W.; Lv, J.; Han, M.; Yang, Z.; Li, T.; Jiang, S.; Yang, Y. STAT3: The art of multi-tasking of metabolic and immune functions in obesity. *Prog. Lipid Res.* **2018**, *70*, 17–28. [CrossRef] [PubMed]
100. Wang, S.; Wang, X.; Ye, Z.; Xu, C.; Zhang, M.; Ruan, B.; Wei, M.; Jiang, Y.; Zhang, Y.; Wang, L.; et al. Curcumin promotes browning of white adipose tissue in a norepinephrine-dependent way. *Biochem. Biophys. Res. Commun.* **2015**, *466*, 247–253. [CrossRef] [PubMed]
101. Shabbir, U.; Rubab, M.; Daliri, E.B.-M.; Chelliah, R.; Javed, A.; Oh, D.-H. Curcumin, Quercetin, Catechins and Metabolic Diseases: The Role of Gut Microbiota. *Nutrients* **2021**, *13*, 206. [CrossRef]
102. Shen, L.; Liu, L.; Ji, H.-F. Regulative effects of curcumin spice administration on gut microbiota and its pharmacological implications. *Food Nutr. Res.* **2017**, *61*, 1361780. [CrossRef]
103. Zhong, Y.-B.; Kang, Z.-P.; Wang, M.-X.; Long, J.; Wang, H.-Y.; Huang, J.-Q.; Wei, S.-Y.; Zhou, W.; Zhao, H.-M.; Liu, D.-Y. Curcumin ameliorated dextran sulfate sodium-induced colitis via regulating the homeostasis of DCs and Treg and improving the composition of the gut microbiota. *J. Funct. Foods* **2021**, *86*, 104716. [CrossRef]
104. Zhang, Z.; Chen, Y.; Xiang, L.; Wang, Z.; Xiao, G.G.; Hu, J. Effect of Curcumin on the Diversity of Gut Microbiota in Ovariectomized Rats. *Nutrients* **2017**, *9*, 1146. [CrossRef]
105. Islam, T.; Koboziev, I.; Albracht-Schulte, K.; Mistretta, B.; Scoggin, S.; Yosofvand, M.; Moussa, H.; Zabet-Moghaddam, M.; Ramalingam, L.; Gunaratne, P.H.; et al. Curcumin Reduces Adipose Tissue Inflammation and Alters Gut Microbiota in Diet-Induced Obese Male Mice. *Mol. Nutr. Food Res.* **2021**, *65*, e2100274. [CrossRef]
106. Wang, J.; Ghosh, S.S.; Ghosh, S. Curcumin improves intestinal barrier function: Modulation of intracellular signaling, and organization of tight junctions. *Am. J. Physiol. Physiol.* **2017**, *312*, C438–C445. [CrossRef]
107. Tian, L.; Song, Z.; Shao, W.; Du, W.W.; Zhao, L.R.; Zeng, K.; Yang, B.B.; Jin, T. Curcumin represses mouse 3T3-L1 cell adipogenic differentiation via inhibiting miR-17-5p and stimulating the Wnt signalling pathway effector Tcf7l2. *Cell Death Dis.* **2017**, *8*, e2559. [CrossRef] [PubMed]
108. Grant, S.F.A.; Thorleifsson, G.; Reynisdottir, I.; Benediktsson, R.; Manolescu, A.; Sainz, J.; Helgason, A.; Stefansson, H.; Emilsson, V.; Helgadottir, A.; et al. Variant of transcription factor 7-like 2 (*TCF7L2*) gene confers risk of type 2 diabetes. *Nat. Genet.* **2006**, *38*, 320–323. [CrossRef] [PubMed]

109. Chen, X.; Ayala, I.; Shannon, C.; Fourcaudot, M.; Acharya, N.K.; Jenkinson, C.P.; Heikkinen, S.; Norton, L. The diabetes gene and wnt pathway effector TCF7L2 regulates adipocyte development and function. *Diabetes* **2018**, *67*, 554–568. [CrossRef]
110. Hewlings, S.J.; Kalman, D.S. Curcumin: A Review of Its Effects on Human Health. *Foods* **2017**, *6*, 92–98. [CrossRef] [PubMed]
111. Bartley, J.P.; Jacobs, A.L. Effects of drying on flavour compounds in Australian-grown ginger (*Zingiber officinale*)—Bartley—2000—Journal of the Science of Food and Agriculture—Wiley Online Library. *J. Sci. Food Agric.* **2000**, *80*, 209–215. [CrossRef]
112. Masuda, Y.; Kikuzaki, H.; Hisamoto, M.; Nakatani, N. Antioxidant properties of gingerol related compounds from ginger. *Biofactors* **2004**, *21*, 293–296. [CrossRef]
113. Shukla, Y.; Singh, M. Cancer preventive properties of ginger: A brief review. *Food Chem. Toxicol.* **2007**, *45*, 683–690. [CrossRef]
114. Wei, C.-K.; Tsai, Y.-H.; Korinek, M.; Hung, P.-H.; El-Shazly, M.; Cheng, Y.-B.; Wu, Y.-C.; Hsieh, T.-J.; Chang, F.-R. 6-Paradol and 6-Shogaol, the Pungent Compounds of Ginger, Promote Glucose Utilization in Adipocytes and Myotubes, and 6-Paradol Reduces Blood Glucose in High-Fat Diet-Fed Mice. *Int. J. Mol. Sci.* **2017**, *18*, 168. [CrossRef] [PubMed]
115. Pulbutr, P.; Thunchomnang, K.; Lawa, K.; Mangkhalathon, A.; Saenubol, P. Lipolytic effects of zingerone in adipocytes isolated from normal diet-fed rats and high fat diet-fed rats. *Int. J. Pharmacol.* **2011**, *7*, 629–634. [CrossRef]
116. Malik, Z.A.; Sharmaa, P.L. Attenuation of High-fat Diet Induced Body Weight Gain, Adiposity and Biochemical Anomalies after Chronic Administration of Ginger (*Zingiber officinale*) in Wistar Rats. *Int. J. Pharmacol.* **2011**, *7*, 801–812. [CrossRef]
117. Ahn, E.-K.; Oh, J.S. Inhibitory effect of galanolactone isolated from *Zingiber officinale* roscoe extract on adipogenesis in 3T3-L1 cells. *J. Korean Soc. Appl. Biol. Chem.* **2012**, *55*, 63–68. [CrossRef]
118. Mahmoud, R.H.; Elnour, W.A. Comparative evaluation of the efficacy of ginger and orlistat on obesity management, pancreatic lipase and liver peroxisomal catalase enzyme in male albino rats. *Eur. Rev. Med. Pharmacol. Sci.* **2013**, *17*, 75–83.
119. Saravanan, G.; Ponmurugan, P.; Deepa, M.A.; Senthilkumar, B. Anti-obesity action of gingerol: Effect on lipid profile, insulin, leptin, amylase and lipase in male obese rats induced by a high-fat diet. *J. Sci. Food Agric.* **2014**, *94*, 2972–2977. [CrossRef]
120. Mansour, M.S.; Ni, Y.-M.; Roberts, A.L.; Kelleman, M.; RoyChoudhury, A.; St-Onge, M.-P. Ginger consumption enhances the thermic effect of food and promotes feelings of satiety without affecting metabolic and hormonal parameters in overweight men: A pilot study. *Metabolism* **2012**, *61*, 1347–1352. [CrossRef]
121. Roberts, L.D.; Virtue, S.; Vidal-Puig, A.; Nicholls, A.W.; Griffin, J.L. Metabolic phenotyping of a model of adipocyte differentiation. *Physiol. Genom.* **2009**, *39*, 109. [CrossRef]
122. Tzeng, T.-F.; Liu, I.-M. 6-Gingerol prevents adipogenesis and the accumulation of cytoplasmic lipid droplets in 3T3-L1 cells. *Phytomedicine* **2013**, *20*, 481–487. [CrossRef]
123. Li, C.; Zhou, L. Inhibitory effect 6-gingerol on adipogenesis through activation of the Wnt/β-catenin signaling pathway in 3T3-L1 adipocytes. *Toxicol. Vitr.* **2015**, *30*, 394–401. [CrossRef]
124. Suk, S.; Seo, S.G.; Yu, J.G.; Yang, H.; Jeong, E.; Jang, Y.J.; Yaghmoor, S.S.; Ahmed, Y.; Yousef, J.M.; Abualnaja, K.O.; et al. A Bioactive Constituent of Ginger, 6-Shogaol, Prevents Adipogenesis and Stimulates Lipolysis in 3T3-L1 Adipocytes. *J. Food Biochem.* **2016**, *40*, 84–90. [CrossRef]
125. Jiao, W.; Mi, S.; Sang, Y.; Jin, Q.; Chitrakar, B.; Wang, X.; Wang, S. Integrated network pharmacology and cellular assay for the investigation of an anti-obesity effect of 6-shogaol. *Food Chem.* **2022**, *374*, 131755. [CrossRef] [PubMed]
126. Nammi, S.; Sreemantula, S.; Roufogalis, B.D. Protective effects of ethanolic extract of *Zingiber officinale* rhizome on the development of metabolic syndrome in high-fat diet-fed rats. *Basic Clin. Pharmacol. Toxicol.* **2009**, *104*, 366–373. [CrossRef]
127. Brahma Naidu, P.; Uddandrao, V.V.S.; Ravindar Naik, R.; Suresh, P.; Meriga, B.; Begum, M.S.; Pandiyan, R.; Saravanan, G. Ameliorative potential of gingerol: Promising modulation of inflammatory factors and lipid marker enzymes expressions in HFD induced obesity in rats. *Mol. Cell. Endocrinol.* **2016**, *419*, 139–147. [CrossRef] [PubMed]
128. Isa, Y.; Miyakawa, Y.; Yanagisawa, M.; Goto, T.; Kang, M.-S.; Kawada, T.; Morimitsu, Y.; Kubota, K.; Tsuda, T. 6-Shogaol and 6-gingerol, the pungent of ginger, inhibit TNF-α mediated downregulation of adiponectin expression via different mechanisms in 3T3-L1 adipocytes. *Biochem. Biophys. Res. Commun.* **2008**, *373*, 429–434. [CrossRef]
129. Akhani, S.P.; Vishwakarma, S.L.; Goyal, R.K. Anti-diabetic activity of *Zingiber officinale* in streptozotocin-induced type I diabetic rats. *J. Pharm. Pharmacol.* **2004**, *56*, 101–105. [CrossRef] [PubMed]
130. Al-Amin, Z.M.; Thomson, M.; Al-Qattan, K.K.; Peltonen-Shalaby, R.; Ali, M. Anti-diabetic and hypolipidaemic properties of ginger (*Zingiber officinale*) in streptozotocin-induced diabetic rats. *Br. J. Nutr.* **2006**, *96*, 660–666. [CrossRef]
131. Son, M.J.; Miura, Y.; Yagasaki, K. Mechanisms for antidiabetic effect of gingerol in cultured cells and obese diabetic model mice. *Cytotechnology* **2015**, *67*, 641–652. [CrossRef]
132. Wang, J.; Gao, H.; Ke, D.; Zuo, G.; Yang, Y.; Yamahara, J.; Li, Y. Improvement of Liquid Fructose-Induced Adipose Tissue Insulin Resistance by Ginger Treatment in Rats Is Associated with Suppression of Adipose Macrophage-Related Proinflammatory Cytokines. *Evid.-Based Complement. Altern. Med.* **2013**, *2013*, 590376. [CrossRef]
133. Chakraborty, D.; Mukherjee, A.; Sikdar, S.; Paul, A.; Ghosh, S.; Khuda-Bukhsh, A.R. 6-Gingerol isolated from ginger attenuates sodium arsenite induced oxidative stress and plays a corrective role in improving insulin signaling in mice. *Toxicol. Lett.* **2012**, *210*, 34–43. [CrossRef]

134. Priya Rani, M.; Padmakumari, K.P.; Sankarikutty, B.; Lijo Cherian, O.; Nisha, V.M.; Raghu, K.G. Inhibitory potential of ginger extracts against enzymes linked to type 2 diabetes, inflammation and induced oxidative stress. *Int. J. Food Sci. Nutr.* **2011**, *62*, 106–110. [CrossRef] [PubMed]
135. Pagano, E.; Souto, E.B.; Durazzo, A.; Sharifi-Rad, J.; Lucarini, M.; Souto, S.B.; Salehi, B.; Zam, W.; Montanaro, V.; Lucariello, G.; et al. Ginger (*Zingiber officinale* Roscoe) as a nutraceutical: Focus on the metabolic, analgesic, and antiinflammatory effects. *Phytother. Res.* **2020**, *35*, 2403–2417. [CrossRef] [PubMed]
136. Dugasani, S.; Pichika, M.R.; Nadarajah, V.D.; Balijepalli, M.K.; Tandra, S.; Korlakunta, J.N. Comparative antioxidant and anti-inflammatory effects of [6]-gingerol, [8]-gingerol, [10]-gingerol and [6]-shogaol. *J. Ethnopharmacol.* **2010**, *127*, 515–520. [CrossRef] [PubMed]
137. Morvaridzadeh, M.; Sadeghi, E.; Agah, S.; Fazelian, S.; Rahimlou, M.; Kern, F.G.; Heshmati, S.; Omidi, A.; Persad, E.; Heshmati, J. Effect of ginger (*Zingiber officinale*) supplementation on oxidative stress parameters: A systematic review and meta-analysis. *J. Food Biochem.* **2021**, *45*, e13612. [CrossRef] [PubMed]
138. Seo, S.H.; Fang, F.; Kang, I. Ginger (*Zingiber officinale*) Attenuates Obesity and Adipose Tissue Remodeling in High-Fat Diet-Fed C57BL/6 Mice. *Int. J. Environ. Res. Public Health* **2021**, *18*, 631. [CrossRef]
139. Salaramoli, S.; Mehri, S.; Yarmohammadi, F.; Hashemy, S.I.; Hosseinzadeh, H. The effects of ginger and its constituents in the prevention of metabolic syndrome: A review. *Iran. J. Basic Med. Sci.* **2022**, *25*, 664. [CrossRef]
140. Ebrahimzadeh Attari, V.; Malek Mahdavi, A.; Javadivala, Z.; Mahluji, S.; Zununi Vahed, S.; Ostadrahimi, A. A systematic review of the anti-obesity and weight lowering effect of ginger (*Zingiber officinale* Roscoe) and its mechanisms of action. *Phytotherapy Res.* **2018**, *32*, 577–585. [CrossRef]
141. Bonet, M.L.; Mercader, J.; Palou, A. A nutritional perspective on UCP1-dependent thermogenesis. *Biochimie* **2017**, *134*, 99–117. [CrossRef]
142. Ebrahimzadeh Attari, V.; Asghari Jafarabadi, M.; Zemestani, M.; Ostadrahimi, A. Effect of *Zingiber officinale* Supplementation on Obesity Management with Respect to the Uncoupling Protein 1-3826A>G and ß3-adrenergic Receptor Trp64Arg Polymorphism. *Phytother. Res.* **2015**, *29*, 1032–1039. [CrossRef]
143. Kim, S.; Lee, M.-S.; Jung, S.; Son, H.-Y.; Park, S.; Kang, B.; Kim, S.-Y.; Kim, I.-H.; Kim, C.-T.; Kim, Y. Ginger Extract Ameliorates Obesity and Inflammation via Regulating MicroRNA-21/132 Expression and AMPK Activation in White Adipose Tissue. *Nutrients* **2018**, *10*, 1567. [CrossRef]
144. Wang, J.; Wang, P.; Li, D.; Hu, X.; Chen, F. Beneficial effects of ginger on prevention of obesity through modulation of gut microbiota in mice. *Eur. J. Nutr.* **2020**, *59*, 699–718. [CrossRef]
145. Wang, P.; Wang, R.; Zhu, Y.; Sang, S. Interindividual Variability in Metabolism of [6]-Shogaol by Gut Microbiota. *J. Agric. Food Chem.* **2017**, *65*, 9618–9625. [CrossRef] [PubMed]
146. Wang, X.; Zhang, D.; Jiang, H.; Zhang, S.; Pang, X.; Gao, S.; Zhang, H.; Zhang, S.; Xiao, Q.; Chen, L.; et al. Gut Microbiota Variation with Short-Term Intake of Ginger Juice on Human Health. *Front. Microbiol.* **2021**, *11*, 576061. [CrossRef]
147. Modi, M.; Modi, K. *Ginger Root*; StatPearls: Tampa, FL, USA, 2022.
148. Balentine, D.A.; Wiseman, S.A.; Bouwens, L.C.M. The chemistry of tea flavonoids. *Crit. Rev. Food Sci. Nutr.* **1997**, *37*, 693–704. [CrossRef]
149. Sang, S.; Lambert, J.D.; Ho, C.-T.; Yang, C.S. The chemistry and biotransformation of tea constituents. *Pharmacol. Res.* **2011**, *64*, 87–99. [CrossRef]
150. Yang, C.S.; Zhang, J.; Zhang, L.; Huang, J.; Wang, Y. Mechanisms of Body Weight Reduction and Metabolic Syndrome Alleviation by Tea. *Mol. Nutr. Food Res.* **2016**, *60*, 160–174. [CrossRef] [PubMed]
151. Liao, S.; Kao, Y.-H.; Hiipakka, R.A. Green tea: Biochemical and biological basis for health benefits. *Vitam. Horm.* **2001**, *62*, 1–94. [CrossRef] [PubMed]
152. Li, F.; Gao, C.; Yan, P.; Zhang, M.; Wang, Y.; Hu, Y.; Wu, X.; Wang, X.; Sheng, J.; Li, F.; et al. EGCG Reduces Obesity and White Adipose Tissue Gain Partly Through AMPK Activation in Mice. *Front. Pharmacol.* **2018**, *9*, 1366. [CrossRef]
153. Sae-Tan, S.; Grove, K.A.; Kennett, M.J.; Lambert, J.D. (−)-Epigallocatechin-3-Gallate Increases the Expression of Genes Related to Fat Oxidation in the Skeletal Muscle of High Fat-Fed Mice. *Food Funct.* **2011**, *2011*, 111–116. [CrossRef]
154. Pravednikova, A.E.; Shevchenko, S.Y.; Kerchev, V.V.; Skhirtladze, M.R.; Larina, S.N.; Kachaev, Z.M.; Egorov, A.D.; Shidlovskii, Y.V. Association of uncoupling protein (Ucp) gene polymorphisms with cardiometabolic diseases. *Mol. Med.* **2020**, *26*, 51. [CrossRef]
155. Mason, E.; Hindmarch, C.C.T.; Dunham-Snary, K.J. Medium-chain Acyl-COA dehydrogenase deficiency: Pathogenesis, diagnosis, and treatment. *Endocrinol. Diabetes Metab.* **2023**, *6*, e385. [CrossRef]
156. Serisier, S.; Leray, V.; Poudroux, W.; Magot, T.; Ouguerram, K.; Nguyen, P. Effects of green tea on insulin sensitivity, lipid profile and expression of PPARα and PPARγ and their target genes in obese dogs. *Br. J. Nutr.* **2008**, *99*, 1208–1216. [CrossRef]
157. Škrlec, I.; Talapko, J.; Džijan, S.; Cesar, V.; Lazić, N.; Lepeduš, H. The Association between Circadian Clock Gene Polymorphisms and Metabolic Syndrome: A Systematic Review and Meta-Analysis. *Biology* **2021**, *11*, 20. [CrossRef]
158. Zhou, B.; Zhang, Y.; Zhang, F.; Xia, Y.; Liu, J.; Huang, R.; Wang, Y.; Hu, Y.; Wu, J.; Dai, C.; et al. CLOCK/BMAL1 regulates circadian change of mouse hepatic insulin sensitivity by SIRT1. *Hepatology* **2014**, *59*, 2196–2206. [CrossRef]

159. Grimaldi, B.; Bellet, M.M.; Katada, S.; Astarita, G.; Hirayama, J.; Amin, R.H.; Granneman, J.G.; Piomelli, D.; Leff, T.; Sassone-Corsi, P. PER2 Controls Lipid Metabolism by Direct Regulation of PPARγ. *Cell Metab.* **2010**, *12*, 509–520. [CrossRef] [PubMed]
160. Mi, Y.; Qi, G.; Fan, R.; Ji, X.; Liu, Z.; Liu, X. EGCG ameliorates diet-induced metabolic syndrome associating with the circadian clock. *Biochim. Biophys. Acta (BBA)—Mol. Basis Dis.* **2017**, *1863*, 1575–1589. [CrossRef] [PubMed]
161. Rahman, S.U.; Huang, Y.; Zhu, L.; Chu, X.; Junejo, S.A.; Zhang, Y.; Khan, I.M.; Li, Y.; Feng, S.; Wu, J.; et al. Tea polyphenols attenuate liver inflammation by modulating obesity-related genes and down-regulating COX-2 and iNOS expression in high fat-fed dogs. *BMC Veter Res.* **2020**, *16*, 234. [CrossRef] [PubMed]
162. Casanova, E.; Salvadó, J.; Crescenti, A.; Gibert-Ramos, A. Epigallocatechin Gallate Modulates Muscle Homeostasis in Type 2 Diabetes and Obesity by Targeting Energetic and Redox Pathways: A Narrative Review. *Int. J. Mol. Sci.* **2019**, *20*, 532. [CrossRef] [PubMed]
163. Bastos, R.V.S.; Dorna, M.S.; Chiuso-Minicucci, F.; Felix, T.F.; Fernandes, A.A.H.; Azevedo, P.S.; Franco, E.T.; Polegato, B.F.; Rogero, M.M.; Mota, G.A.F.; et al. Acute green tea intake attenuates circulating microRNA expression induced by a high-fat, high-saturated meal in obese women: A randomized crossover study. *J. Nutr. Biochem.* **2023**, *112*, 109203. [CrossRef]
164. Liu, X.; Zhao, K.; Jing, N.; Kong, Q.; Yang, X. Epigallocatechin Gallate (EGCG) Promotes the Immune Function of Ileum in High Fat Diet Fed Mice by Regulating Gut Microbiome Profiling and Immunoglobulin Production. *Front. Nutr.* **2021**, *8*, 720439. [CrossRef] [PubMed]
165. Liu, Z.; de Bruijn, W.J.C.; Bruins, M.E.; Vincken, J.-P. Reciprocal Interactions between Epigallocatechin-3-gallate (EGCG) and Human Gut Microbiota In Vitro. *J. Agric. Food Chem.* **2020**, *68*, 9804–9815. [CrossRef] [PubMed]
166. Hu, J.; Webster, D.; Cao, J.; Shao, A. The safety of green tea and green tea extract consumption in adults—Results of a systematic review. *Regul. Toxicol. Pharmacol.* **2018**, *95*, 412–433. [CrossRef]
167. Guldiken, B.; Catalkaya, G.; Ozkan, G.; Ceylan, F.D.; Capanoglu, E. Toxicological effects of commonly used herbs and spices. In *Toxicology: Oxidative Stress and Dietary Antioxidants*; Patel, V.B., Preedy, V.R., Eds.; Academic Press: Cambridge, MA, USA, 2021; pp. 201–213, ISBN 9780128190920.
168. Tewksbury, J.J.; Nabhan, G.P. Directed deterrence by capsaicin in chillies. *Nature* **2001**, *412*, 403–404. [CrossRef] [PubMed]
169. Chinn, M.S.; Sharma-Shivappa, R.R.; Cotter, J.L. Solvent extraction and quantification of capsaicinoids from Capsicum chinense. *Food Bioprod. Process.* **2011**, *89*, 340–345. [CrossRef]
170. Antonio, A.S.; Wiedemann, L.S.M.; Veiga Junior, V.F. The genus *Capsicum*: A phytochemical review of bioactive secondary metabolites. *RSC Adv.* **2018**, *8*, 25767–25784. [CrossRef] [PubMed]
171. Luo, X.-J.; Peng, J.; Li, Y.-J. Recent advances in the study on capsaicinoids and capsinoids. *Eur. J. Pharmacol.* **2011**, *650*, 1–7. [CrossRef] [PubMed]
172. Al Othman, Z.A.; Ahmed, Y.B.H.; Habila, M.A.; Ghafar, A.A. Determination of capsaicin and dihydrocapsaicin in capsicum fruit samples using high performance liquid chromatography. *Molecules* **2011**, *16*, 8919–8929. [CrossRef]
173. Hayman, M.; Kam, P.C.A. Capsaicin: A review of its pharmacology and clinical applications. *Curr. Anaesth. Crit. Care* **2008**, *19*, 338–343. [CrossRef]
174. Smutzer, G.; Devassy, R.K. Integrating TRPV1 Receptor Function with Capsaicin Psychophysics. *Adv. Pharmacol. Sci.* **2016**, *2016*, 1512457. [CrossRef]
175. Zheng, J.; Zheng, S.; Feng, Q.; Zhang, Q.; Xiao, X. Dietary capsaicin and its anti-obesity potency: From mechanism to clinical implications. *Biosci. Rep.* **2017**, *37*, BSR20170286. [CrossRef]
176. Snitker, S.; Fujishima, Y.; Shen, H.; Ott, S.; Pi-Sunyer, X.; Furuhata, Y.; Sato, H.; Takahashi, M. Effects of novel capsinoid treatment on fatness and energy metabolism in humans: Possible pharmacogenetic implications. *Am. J. Clin. Nutr.* **2009**, *89*, 45–50. [CrossRef]
177. Chen, J.; Li, L.; Li, Y.; Liang, X.; Sun, Q.; Yu, H.; Zhong, J.; Ni, Y.; Chen, J.; Zhao, Z.; et al. Activation of TRPV1 channel by dietary capsaicin improves visceral fat remodeling through connexin43-mediated Ca^{2+} Influx. *Cardiovasc. Diabetol.* **2015**, *14*, 22. [CrossRef]
178. Gram, D.X.; Ahrén, B.; Nagy, I.; Olsen, U.B.; Brand, C.L.; Sundler, F.; Tabanera, R.; Svendsen, O.; Carr, R.D.; Santha, P.; et al. Capsaicin-sensitive sensory fibers in the islets of Langerhans contribute to defective insulin secretion in Zucker diabetic rat, an animal model for some aspects of human type 2 diabetes. *Eur. J. Neurosci.* **2007**, *25*, 213–223. [CrossRef]
179. Wang, P.; Yan, Z.; Zhong, J.; Chen, J.; Ni, Y.; Li, L.; Ma, L.; Zhao, Z.; Liu, D.; Zhu, Z. Transient receptor potential vanilloid 1 activation enhances gut glucagon-like peptide-1 secretion and improves glucose homeostasis. *Diabetes* **2012**, *61*, 2155–2165. [CrossRef]
180. Kang, J.-H.; Kim, C.-S.; Han, I.-S.; Kawada, T.; Yu, R. Capsaicin, a spicy component of hot peppers, modulates adipokine gene expression and protein release from obese-mouse adipose tissues and isolated adipocytes, and suppresses the inflammatory responses of adipose tissue macrophages. *FEBS Lett.* **2007**, *581*, 4389–4396. [CrossRef] [PubMed]
181. Hsu, C.-L.; Yen, G.-C. Effects of capsaicin on induction of apoptosis and inhibition of adipogenesis in 3T3-L1 cells. *J. Agric. Food Chem.* **2007**, *55*, 1730–1736. [CrossRef] [PubMed]
182. Zhang, L.L.; Liu, D.Y.; Ma, L.Q.; Luo, Z.D.; Cao, T.B.; Zhong, J.; Yan, Z.C.; Wang, L.J.; Zhao, Z.G.; Zhu, S.J.; et al. Activation of transient receptor potential vanilloid type-1 channel prevents adipogenesis and obesity. *Circ. Res.* **2007**, *100*, 1063–1070. [CrossRef] [PubMed]

183. Kang, J.-H.; Tsuyoshi, G.; Han, I.-S.; Kawada, T.; Kim, Y.M.; Yu, R. Dietary capsaicin reduces obesity-induced insulin resistance and hepatic steatosis in obese mice fed a high-fat diet. *Obesity* **2010**, *18*, 780–787. [CrossRef]
184. Ohyama, K.; Nogusa, Y.; Suzuki, K.; Shinoda, K.; Kajimura, S.; Bannai, M. A combination of exercise and capsinoid supplementation additively suppresses diet-induced obesity by increasing energy expenditure in mice. *Am. J. Physiol. Endocrinol. Metab.* **2015**, *308*, E315–E323. [CrossRef]
185. Baskaran, P.; Krishnan, V.; Fettel, K.; Gao, P.; Zhu, Z.; Ren, J.; Thyagarajan, B. TRPV1 activation counters diet-induced obesity through sirtuin-1 activation and PRDM-16 deacetylation in brown adipose tissue. *Int. J. Obes.* **2017**, *41*, 739–749. [CrossRef] [PubMed]
186. Joo, J.I.; Kim, D.H.; Choi, J.-W.; Yun, J.W. Proteomic analysis for antiobesity potential of capsaicin on white adipose tissue in rats fed with a high fat diet. *J. Proteome Res.* **2010**, *9*, 2977–2987. [CrossRef] [PubMed]
187. Baboota, R.K.; Singh, D.P.; Sarma, S.M.; Kaur, J.; Sandhir, R.; Boparai, R.K.; Kondepudi, K.K.; Bishnoi, M. Capsaicin induces "brite" phenotype in differentiating 3T3-L1 preadipocytes. *PLoS ONE* **2014**, *9*, e103093. [CrossRef] [PubMed]
188. Rohm, B.; Holik, A.K.; Kretschy, N.; Somoza, M.M.; Ley, J.P.; Widder, S.; Krammer, G.E.; Marko, D.; Somoza, V. Nonivamide enhances miRNA let-7d expression and decreases adipogenesis PPARγ expression in 3T3-L1 cells. *J. Cell. Biochem.* **2015**, *116*, 1153–1163. [CrossRef] [PubMed]
189. Wang, Y.; Tang, C.; Tang, Y.; Yin, H.; Liu, X. Capsaicin has an anti-obesity effect through alterations in gut microbiota populations and short-chain fatty acid concentrations. *Food Nutr. Res.* **2020**, *64*, 3525. [CrossRef]
190. Adetunji, T.L.; Olawale, F.; Olisah, C.; Adetunji, A.E.; Aremu, A.O. Capsaicin: A Two-Decade Systematic Review of Global Research Output and Recent Advances Against Human Cancer. *Front. Oncol.* **2022**, *12*, 908487. [CrossRef]
191. Scientific Committee on Food SCF/CS/FLAV/FLAVOUR/8 ADD1 Final Opinion of the Scientific Committee on Food on Capsaicin. 2002. Available online: https://ec.europa.eu/food/fs/sc/scf/out120_en.pdf (accessed on 28 April 2023).
192. Bonita, J.S.; Mandarano, M.; Shuta, D.; Vinson, J. Coffee and cardiovascular disease: In vitro, cellular, animal, and human studies. *Pharmacol. Res.* **2007**, *55*, 187–198. [CrossRef]
193. Heckman, M.A.; Weil, J.; de Mejia, E.G. Caffeine (1,3,7-trimethylxanthine) in foods: A comprehensive review on consumption, functionality, safety, and regulatory matters. *J. Food Sci.* **2010**, *75*, R77–R87. [CrossRef]
194. Poole, R.; Kennedy, O.J.; Roderick, P.; Fallowfield, J.A.; Hayes, P.C.; Parkes, J. Coffee consumption and health: Umbrella review of meta-analyses of multiple health outcomes. *BMJ* **2017**, *359*, j5024. [CrossRef]
195. Liu, D.; Li, Z.-H.; Shen, D.; Zhang, P.-D.; Song, M.W.-Q.; Zhang, M.W.-T.; Huang, Q.-M.; Chen, P.-L.; Zhang, X.-R.; Mao, C. Association of Sugar-Sweetened, Artificially Sweetened, and Unsweetened Coffee Consumption with All-Cause and Cause-Specific Mortality: A Large Prospective Cohort Study. *Ann. Intern. Med.* **2022**, *175*, 909–917. [CrossRef]
196. Zhao, L.-G.; Li, Z.-Y.; Feng, G.-S.; Ji, X.-W.; Tan, Y.-T.; Li, H.-L.; Gunter, M.J.; Xiang, Y.-B. Coffee drinking and cancer risk: An umbrella review of meta-analyses of observational studies. *BMC Cancer* **2020**, *20*, 101. [CrossRef]
197. Bhupathiraju, S.N.; Pan, A.; Manson, J.E.; Willett, W.C.; van Dam, R.M.; Hu, F.B. Changes in coffee intake and subsequent risk of type 2 diabetes: Three large cohorts of US men and women. *Diabetologia* **2014**, *57*, 1346–1354. [CrossRef] [PubMed]
198. Ren, X.; Chen, J.-F. Caffeine and Parkinson's Disease: Multiple Benefits and Emerging Mechanisms. *Front. Neurosci.* **2020**, *14*, 602697. [CrossRef] [PubMed]
199. Gardener, S.L.; Rainey-Smith, S.R.; Villemagne, V.L.; Fripp, J.; Doré, V.; Bourgeat, P.; Taddei, K.; Fowler, C.; Masters, C.L.; Maruff, P.; et al. Higher Coffee Consumption Is Associated with Slower Cognitive Decline and Less Cerebral Aβ-Amyloid Accumulation Over 126 Months: Data from the Australian Imaging, Biomarkers, and Lifestyle Study. *Front. Aging Neurosci.* **2021**, *13*, 744872. [CrossRef] [PubMed]
200. Wadhawan, M.; Anand, A.C. Coffee and Liver Disease. *J. Clin. Exp. Hepatol.* **2016**, *6*, 40–46. [CrossRef]
201. Pickering, C.; Grgic, J. Caffeine and Exercise: What Next? *Sports Med.* **2019**, *49*, 1007–1030. [CrossRef]
202. Ramírez-Maldonado, M.; Jurado-Fasoli, L.; del Coso, J.; Ruiz, J.R.; Amaro-Gahete, F.J. Caffeine increases maximal fat oxidation during a graded exercise test: Is there a diurnal variation? *J. Int. Soc. Sports Nutr.* **2021**, *18*, 5. [CrossRef]
203. Tabrizi, R.; Saneei, P.; Lankarani, K.B.; Akbari, M.; Kolahdooz, F.; Esmaillzadeh, A.; Nadi-Ravandi, S.; Mazoochi, M.; Asemi, Z. The effects of caffeine intake on weight loss: A systematic review and dos-response meta-analysis of randomized controlled trials. *Crit. Rev. Food Sci. Nutr.* **2019**, *59*, 2688–2696. [CrossRef]
204. Jacobson, K.A.; Gao, Z.-G. Adenosine receptors as therapeutic targets. *Nat. Rev. Drug Discov.* **2006**, *5*, 247–264. [CrossRef]
205. Zapata, F.J.; Rebollo-Hernanz, M.; Novakofski, J.E.; Nakamura, M.T.; de Mejia, E.G. Caffeine, but not other phytochemicals, in mate tea (Ilex paraguariensis St. Hilaire) attenuates high-fat-high-sucrose-diet-driven lipogenesis and body fat accumulation. *J. Funct. Foods* **2020**, *64*, 103646. [CrossRef]
206. Akiba, T.; Yaguchi, K.; Tsutsumi, K.; Nishioka, T.; Koyama, I.; Nomura, M.; Yokogawa, K.; Moritani, S.; Miyamoto, K.-I. Inhibitory mechanism of caffeine on insulin-stimulated glucose uptake in adipose cells. *Biochem. Pharmacol.* **2004**, *68*, 1929–1937. [CrossRef]
207. Kim, H.J.; Yoon, B.K.; Park, H.; Seok, J.W.; Choi, H.; Yu, J.H.; Choi, Y.; Song, S.J.; Kim, A.; Kim, J.-W. Caffeine inhibits adipogenesis through modulation of mitotic clonal expansion and the AKT/GSK3 pathway in 3T3-L1 adipocytes. *BMB Rep.* **2016**, *49*, 111–115. [CrossRef] [PubMed]
208. Velickovic, K.; Wayne, D.; Leija, H.A.L.; Bloor, I.; Morris, D.E.; Law, J.; Budge, H.; Sacks, H.; Symonds, M.E.; Sottile, V. Caffeine exposure induces browning features in adipose tissue In Vitro and In Vivo. *Sci. Rep.* **2019**, *9*, 9104. [CrossRef] [PubMed]

209. Mitani, T.; Nagano, T.; Harada, K.; Yamashita, Y.; Ashida, H. Caffeine-Stimulated Intestinal Epithelial Cells Suppress Lipid Accumulation in Adipocytes. *J. Nutr. Sci. Vitaminol.* **2017**, *63*, 331–338. [CrossRef] [PubMed]
210. Yamauchi, R.; Kobayashi, M.; Matsuda, Y.; Ojika, M.; Shigeoka, S.; Yamamoto, Y.; Tou, Y.; Inoue, T.; Katagiri, T.; Murai, A.; et al. Coffee and caffeine ameliorate hyperglycemia, fatty liver, and inflammatory adipocytokine expression in spontaneously diabetic KK-A^y mice. *J. Agric. Food Chem.* **2010**, *58*, 5597–5603. [CrossRef] [PubMed]
211. Pan, M.-H.; Tung, Y.-C.; Yang, G.; Li, S.; Ho, C.-T. Molecular mechanisms of the anti-obesity effect of bioactive compounds in tea and coffee. *Food Funct.* **2016**, *7*, 4481–4491. [CrossRef]
212. González, S.; Salazar, N.; Ruiz-Saavedra, S.; Gómez-Martín, M.; de los Reyes-Gavilán, C.G.; Gueimonde, M. Long-Term Coffee Consumption is Associated with Fecal Microbial Composition in Humans. *Nutrients* **2020**, *12*, 1287. [CrossRef]
213. Bhandarkar, N.S.; Mouatt, P.; Goncalves, P.; Thomas, T.; Brown, L.; Panchal, S.K. Modulation of gut microbiota by spent coffee grounds attenuates diet-induced metabolic syndrome in rats. *FASEB J.* **2020**, *34*, 4783–4797. [CrossRef]

Disclaimer/Publisher's Note: The statements, opinions and data contained in all publications are solely those of the individual author(s) and contributor(s) and not of MDPI and/or the editor(s). MDPI and/or the editor(s) disclaim responsibility for any injury to people or property resulting from any ideas, methods, instructions or products referred to in the content.

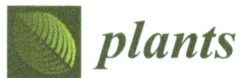 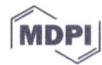

Article

Effects of *Spirulina maxima* on a Model of Sexual Dysfunction in Streptozotocin-Induced Diabetic Male Rats

Eduardo Osel Olvera-Roldán [1], José Melesio Cristóbal-Luna [1], Yuliana García-Martínez [1], María Angélica Mojica-Villegas [1], Ricardo Pérez-Pastén-Borja [1], Gabriela Gutiérrez-Salmeán [2], Salud Pérez-Gutiérrez [3], Rosa Virginia García-Rodríguez [4], Eduardo Madrigal-Santillán [5], José A. Morales-González [5] and Germán Chamorro-Cevallos [1,*]

[1] Laboratorio de Toxicología Preclínica, Departamento de Farmacia, Escuela Nacional de Ciencias Biológicas, Instituto Politécnico Nacional, Mexico City C.P. 07738, Mexico
[2] Facultad de Ciencias de la Salud/Centro de Investigaciones en Ciencias de la Salud (CICSA), Universidad Anáhuac, Mexico City C.P. 52786, Mexico
[3] Departamento de Sistemas Biológicos, Universidad Autónoma Metropolitana-Xochimilco, Mexico City C.P. 04960, Mexico
[4] Unidad de Servicios de Apoyo en Resolución Analítica, Universidad Veracruzana, Xalapa C.P. 91190, Mexico
[5] Laboratorio de Medicina de Conservación, Escuela Superior de Medicina, Instituto Politécnico Nacional, Mexico City C.P. 11340, Mexico
* Correspondence: gchamcev@yahoo.com.mx; Tel.: +52-55-4066-2631

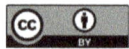

Abstract: *Arthrospira (Spirulina) maxima* (SM) is a cyanobacterium that has a long history of being used as human food. In recent years, several investigations have shown its beneficial biological effects, among which its antioxidant capacity has been highlighted. The purpose of this study was to evaluate the effects of SM on body weight, glycemia, sexual behavior, sperm quality, testosterone levels, sex organ weights, and the activity of antioxidant enzymes in diabetic male rats (a disease characterized by an increase in reactive oxygen species). The experiment consisted of six groups of sexually expert adult males (n = 6): (1) control (vehicle); (2) streptozotocin (STZ)-65 mg/kg; (3) SM-400 mg/kg; (4) STZ + SM-100 mg/kg; (5) STZ + SM-200 mg/kg; and (6) STZ + SM-400 mg/kg. Sexual behavior tests were performed during the first 3 h of the dark period under dim red illumination. Our results showed that SM significantly improved sexual behavior and sperm quality vs. diabetic animals. Likewise, while the enzymatic activities of SOD and GPx increased, TBARS lipoperoxidation decreased and testosterone levels increased. In view of the findings, it is suggested that SM may potentially be used as a nutraceutical for the treatment of diabetic male sexual dysfunction due to its antioxidant property.

Keywords: diabetes mellitus; sexual behavior; oxidative stress; *Spirulina maxima*

Citation: Olvera-Roldán, E.O.; Cristóbal-Luna, J.M.; García-Martínez, Y.; Mojica-Villegas, M.A.; Pérez-Pastén-Borja, R.; Gutiérrez-Salmeán, G.; Pérez-Gutiérrez, S.; García-Rodríguez, R.V.; Madrigal-Santillán, E.; Morales-González, J.A.; et al. Effects of *Spirulina maxima* on a Model of Sexual Dysfunction in Streptozotocin-Induced Diabetic Male Rats. *Plants* **2023**, *12*, 722. https://doi.org/10.3390/plants12040722

Academic Editor: Juei-Tang Cheng

Received: 15 December 2022
Revised: 19 January 2023
Accepted: 26 January 2023
Published: 6 February 2023

Copyright: © 2023 by the authors. Licensee MDPI, Basel, Switzerland. This article is an open access article distributed under the terms and conditions of the Creative Commons Attribution (CC BY) license (https://creativecommons.org/licenses/by/4.0/).

1. Introduction

Diabetes mellitus (DM) is characterized by an inability to regulate blood glucose in humans or animals due to either a deficiency of insulin or an erratic signaling pathway [1]. The dysfunction in blood glucose homeostasis affects the metabolism of all macronutrients, not only carbohydrates but lipids and proteins as well [2].

The scientific literature shows that diabetes is on the rise, irrespective of gender [3,4], to the extent that it has reached pandemic proportions [5,6]. DM is more frequent in developing countries due to poor dietary and exercise regimens [7], with 90% of patients presenting type 2 DM [8].

DM is also a risk factor for secondary disorders, such as coronary disease, stroke, chronic kidney disease, loss of vision, neuropathies, and sexual disorders [9]. Regarding sexual disorders, DM is closely associated with sexual dysfunction, leading to infertility due to alterations in spermatogenesis, structural changes in testicular tissue, the alteration of glucose metabolism in Sertoli cells, a decrease in testosterone concentrations, ejaculatory alteration, and a decrease in libido [7]. In fact, the incidence of erectile dysfunction in diabetic patients has been reported at between 35–75%, i.e., three times higher than that of non-diabetic men [10].

Although a sole isolated molecular pathway has not been identified as the cause of sexual dysfunction in DM, one of the suggested mechanisms is oxidative stress (OS) due to an overproduction of the reactive oxygen species (ROS) concomitant with a decrease in endogenous antioxidant activity [11].

There are certainly some synthetic drugs for improving sexual performance in men with DM; nevertheless, their high cost and the potential for adverse effects have engendered interest in natural products that are more economical and exhibit a safer profile while alleviating sexual dysfunction [12,13].

Arthrospira maxima (*Spirulina maxima*) (SM) is a filamentous cyanobacterium (previously considered blue-green algae) that has been cultivated and consumed in many parts of the world since ancestral times [14]. SM possesses a widely appreciated nutritional value and pharmacological effects, and attention has been drawn for some years both by in vivo and in vitro experiments [15–17] to its antioxidant activity, which is mainly due to its high content of antioxidant compounds, such as phycobiliproteins, beta-carotene, tocopherols, and phenolic acids [18]. In this sense, SM offers many functional bioactive ingredients with anti-inflammatory, antimetastatic, immunostimulatory, cardioprotective, and metalloprotective activity [19–22], and it has been effective in the treatment of neuropathies [23] and neurobehavioral and cognitive deficits [24,25]. Furthermore, it has been determined that the SM dose-dependently activates cellular antioxidant enzymes and inhibits peroxidation and DNA damage. In the same way, phycobiliproteins of SM, such as phycocyanin, have a broad capacity to capture free radicals, such as hydroxyl, alkoxyl, and peroxyl radicals, to inhibit liver microsome lipid peroxidation and increase the activity of the antioxidant enzymes superoxide dismutase (SOD) and catalase (CAT) during the process of oxidative stress [19,20]. However, to date, no study has, to our knowledge, been carried out to evaluate the benefits of the antioxidant effect of SM on the alterations generated in sexual behavior induced by the oxidative stress characteristic of diabetes.

Given the previously mentioned information, this study aimed to evaluate the potential effects of SM in restoring impaired sexual behavior, improving spermatic parameters, reducing oxidant effects in testicular tissue, increasing antioxidant enzyme activity, and restoring testosterone levels in streptozotocin/nicotinamide-induced diabetic male mice.

2. Results

2.1. Body Weight and Glycemia

Final body weights are presented in Figure 1. As observed, STZ, STZ + SM 100, and STZ + SM 200 were significantly lower compared with the control group, whereas this was not found for STZ + SM 400. Only SM 400 differed from STZ.

Glycemia is presented in Figure 2. Both the control and SM 400 groups demonstrated normal concentrations of ~90 mg/dL, whereas the remainder presented a significant increase in such values, reaching more than 300 mg/dL in STZ and STZ + SM 100. Hyperglycemia was, however, attenuated but significantly different compared with that of the control group when SM was administered at doses of 200 and 400 mg/kg.

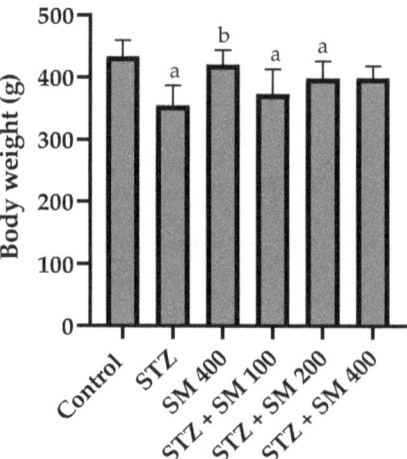

Figure 1. Effect of SM on body weight (g). STZ, streptozotocin; SM, *Spirulina maxima*. Each bar indicates the mean ± SEM (*n* = 6). Significant difference ($p < 0.05$) vs. [a] control; [b] STZ 65 mg/kg.

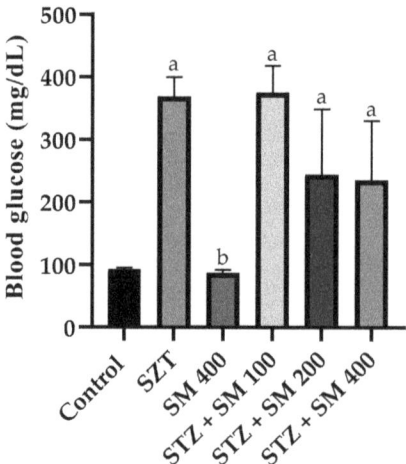

Figure 2. Effect of SM on blood glucose levels. STZ, streptozotocin; SM, *Spirulina maxima*. Each bar indicates the mean ± SEM (*n* = 6). Significant difference ($p < 0.05$) vs. [a] control; [b] STZ 65 mg/kg.

2.2. Copulatory Behavior

As depicted in Figure 3, mount latency (ML), intromission latency (IL), ejaculatory latency (EL), and ejaculatory series duration (ESD) were significantly longer in the STZ groups compared with the control group; contrariwise, mount frequency (MF) and intromission frequency (IF) were significantly lower, thus evidencing sexual dysfunction.

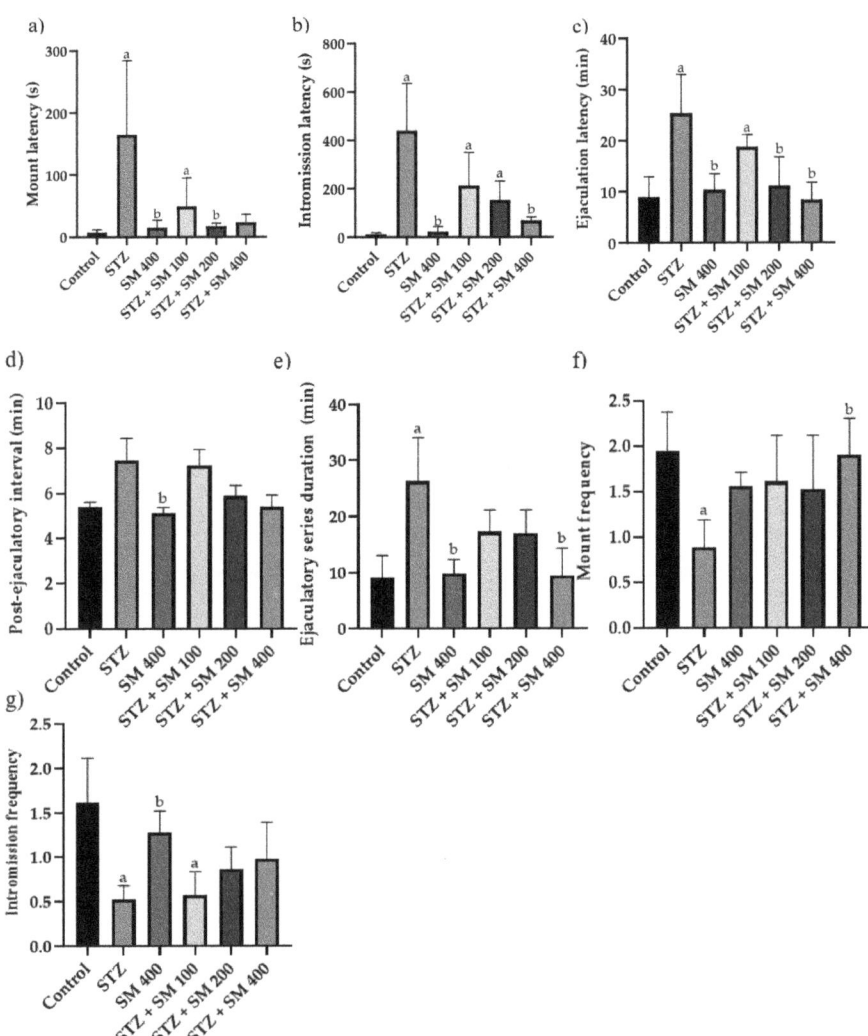

Figure 3. Effect of SM on copulatory behavior. (**a**) Mount latency; (**b**) intromission latency; (**c**) ejaculation latency; (**d**) post-ejaculatory interval; (**e**) ejaculatory series duration; (**f**) mount frequency; (**g**) intromission frequency. STZ, streptozotocin; SM, *Spirulina maxima* (SM). Each bar indicates the mean ± SEM (n= 6). Significant difference ($p < 0.05$) vs. [a] control; [b] STZ 65 mg/kg.

Compared with the STZ group, a significant difference ($p < 0.05$) was found for SM groups in mount latency (ML) for SM 400, STZ + SM 200, and STZ + 400, as well as in intromission latency (IL) for the SM 400 and STZ + SM 400 groups and ejaculatory latency (EL) with the treatments of SM 400, STZ + SM 200, and STZ + SM 400.

2.3. Sperm Quality

Table 1 presents the results of the spermatic quality analysis; it can be appreciated that sperm count, motility, and viability were significantly ($p < 0.05$) inhibited in diabetic rats. On the other hand, sperm abnormalities were markedly ($p < 0.05$) increased in this group.

Table 1. Effect of SM on count, motility, viability, and abnormality of the sperm of control and experimental groups.

Treatment (mg/kg)	Sperm Count (X10⁶/mL)	Sperm Motility	Sperm Viability	Sperm Abnormality (%)
Control	69.42 ± 2.72	29.77 ± 7.36	61.74 ± 1.20	3.93 ± 0.98
STZ	39.44 ± 6.05 [a]	9.48 ± 2.58 [a]	27.56 ± 2.94 [a]	6.08 ± 1.17 [a]
SM 400	75.29 ± 6.33 [b]	20.52 ± 2.99 [b]	61.49+ 2.20 [b]	4.3 ± 1.13 [b]
STZ + SM 100	64.04 ± 6.22 [b]	7.55 ± 1.89 [a]	33.45 ± 4.00	4.1 ± 1.24 [b]
STZ + SM 200	72.50 ± 2.81 [b]	16.38 ± 2.87 [b]	44.95 ± 2.68 [b]	3.9 ± 1.20 [b]
STZ + SM 400	74.20 ± 2.95 [b]	8.52 ± 1.52 [a]	43.82 ± 3.86 [b]	3.2 ± 1.12 [b]

The animals were given the corresponding treatment for 5 weeks. STZ, streptozotocin; SM, *Spirulina maxima*. Results are expressed as the mean ± SEM (n = 6). Significant difference ($p < 0.05$) vs. [a] control; [b] STZ 65 mg/kg.

All animals treated with SM exhibited a significantly ($p < 0.05$) higher total sperm count than those in the STZ group. Sperm motility was found to be diminished in the STZ + SM 100 and STZ + SM 400 groups compared with the control group, but it increased significantly ($p < 0.05$) in STZ + SM 200 compared with diabetic animals.

The viability analysis revealed a significant increase in all SM-treated groups, except for the STZ + SM 100 dose, which, notwithstanding this, exhibited a positive trend. Finally, the morphology of the sperm in SM-treated rats showed a significantly decreased percentage of abnormalities compared with that of diabetic animals.

2.4. Sex Organ Weight

No differences were found in the weight of seminal vesicles, testes, and epididymis among the groups (data not presented).

2.5. Biochemical Analyses

According to Table 2, a significant increase ($p < 0.05$) in lipoperoxidation was found in the diabetic groups, together with a decrease in SOD and GPX. However, treatment with SM significantly ($p < 0.05$) improved the activity of these antioxidant enzymes compared with that of the diabetic animals.

Table 2. Effect of SM on serum biochemical parameters in male diabetic rats.

Treatments (mg/kg)	TBARS (nmol/mg Protein)	SOD (U/mg Protein)	GPX (mU/mL)
Control	12.57 ± 0.42	4.11 ± 0.03	436.20 ± 24.63
STZ	17.65 ± 1.25 [a]	1.59 ± 0.04 [a]	209.83 ± 1.83 [a]
SM 400	13.91 ± 0.69 [b]	4.24 ± 0.02 [b]	430.10 ± 25.17 [b]
STZ + SM 100	13.79 ± 0.45 [b]	2.81 ± 0.06 [b]	332.65 ± 10.75
STZ + SM 200	11.86 ± 0.64 [b]	4.28 ± 0.03 [b]	451.55 ± 11.55 [b]
STZ + SM 400	12.38 ± 0.79 [b]	4.27 ± 0.02 [b]	447.42 ± 11.72 [b]

The animals were given the corresponding treatment for 5 weeks. STZ, streptozotocin; SM, *Spirulina maxima*. Results are expressed as the mean ± SEM (n = 6). Significant difference ($p < 0.05$) vs. [a] control; [b] STZ 65 mg/kg.

2.6. Testosterone Analysis

The results of the analysis of the serum testosterone concentration are presented in Figure 4. In the STZ group, a significant decrease ($p < 0.05$) in the concentration with regard to the control was manifested. However, in the group treated with SM and the diabetic groups treated with SM, the concentration of this hormone increased significantly ($p < 0.05$) in the diabetic group and was very similar to that in the control group.

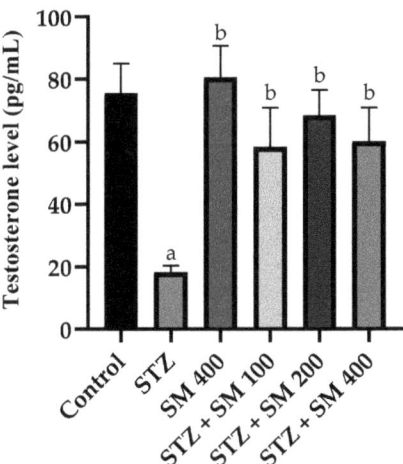

Figure 4. Effect of SM on testosterone levels. STZ, streptozotocin; SM, *Spirulina maxima*. Each bar indicates the mean ± SEM ($n = 6$). Significant difference ($p < 0.05$) vs. [a] control; [b] STZ 65 mg/kg.

3. Discussion

Sexual dysfunction is one of the most frequent complications in persons with diabetes for which, to our knowledge, there is no effective treatment to date [26], although some hypoglycemic agents may be useful in the treatment of diabetes [27]. Numerous authors have shown that male sexual dysfunction derived from diabetes is associated with oxidative stress and, consequently, a decrease in antioxidant concentrations in diabetic patients [28]. The said imbalance of prooxidant and antioxidant species gives rise to the production of free radicals [29], the increase in the destruction of nitric oxide (NO), and the increase in the peroxidation of polyunsaturated fatty acids (PUFA) [30]. For these reasons, we hypothesized that a natural product with great antioxidant activity, such as SM, when administered to diabetic male rats, would reduce or prevent damage to sexual behavior and other biochemical parameters related to it.

Almost all the components of SM, in addition to the pharmacological effects mentioned above and the absence of toxicity, have been effective in the treatment of neuropathies [23] and neurobehavioral and cognitive deficits [24,25]. In the present work, we tried to improve sexual behavior, blood and serum biochemical parameters and hormones, and antioxidant capacity by assessing the serum and testis MDA and Nrf2 pathway of reproductive organs of diabetic male rats by feeding the animals with SM [12]. No previous evidence, to our knowledge, has been reported on the effects of this algae in sexual dysfunction models, particularly assessing its antioxidant potential in diabetes models.

We found that, except for PEI, in which there was only an increasing trend in diabetic animals compared with controls, sexual behavior indicators significantly increased in ML, IL, and EL as well as in EDS, but these decreased in MF and IF, all of which is in agreement with the results of Al-Oanzi [29] and De [27], demonstrating deficiencies in the carrying out of copulation in diseased animals.

A significant amelioration in these disrupted parameters was observed in animals treated with SM. Thus, a decrease in ML, EL, and IL compared with the diabetic group indicates an increase in sexual motivation [31,32]. On the other hand, the significant increase in MF, as in the case of STZ + SM + 400, and the tendency of the increase in IF in the case of STZ + SM 200 and STZ + 400 reveal that diabetes did not interfere with the activity of cyanobacteria for sexual provocation in terms of the efficacy of raising penile posture and consequently sexual vigor, libido, and potency, characteristics demonstrating that the treated rats were aroused [33]. Likewise, because sexual dysfunction in diabetes is associated with inflammation [34], it is probable that the anti-inflammatory activity of

SM contributed to these results. The phycobiliproteins, β-carotene and other vitamins, chlorophyll, and phenols present in SM may have been responsible for sexual enhancement due to their antioxidant properties, which could be the subject of future studies.

Regarding the endocrine profile, the decrease in the serum testosterone level in male animals to which STZ was administered for the induction of diabetes was consistent with the results previously published by various authors [35,36], which showed that testosterone is necessary for normal development of male sexual behavior [28]. SM increased this level and reached values similar to those of the control group, which, similar to other agents, influenced erectile function, including sexual desire, until penile erection [30]. In this regard, it is noteworthy that in other studies, SM increased testosterone concentrations in the testes when it was administered to rats that had decreased concentrations of this hormone due to the administration of toxic agents, such as lead acetate [37], and when it was administered to mice via the administration of bifenthrin [38]. SM contains small concentrations of androgenic molecules, such as cholesterol and fatty acids, among other components that can influence testosterone production [33], as do quercetin, vitamin E, and vitamin C [39,40]. Moreover, it is thought that normality in the serum testosterone concentration may be more related to the cytoprotective effect of SM in the testicular tissue, specifically in Leydig cells. On the other hand, there are a few discrepancies in the influence of testosterone concentration on some parameters of sexual activity in rats [41].

In addition to the relationship between the improvement of sexual behavior and the concentration of testosterone, the reduction in oxidative stress caused by SM is probably a decisive factor in the pathophysiology of sexual dysfunction in that it is associated with an overproduction of free radicals [29]. In our work, which found a decrease in TBARS and an increase in the enzymatic activities of SOD and GPX in the testicular tissue of rats treated with SM, enzymes were considered to be the main antioxidants responsible for maintaining the optimal concentration of ROS [42]. Is important to note that, although SOD activity is typically assumed to be within cells, there is also an extracellular isoform—described in 1982—that differs from the cytoplasmatic SOD, as it is conformed as a tetramer (rather than a homodimer) and contains six Cys residues (vs. four in the intracellular). In this sense, both SODs catalyze the conversion of O_2^- into H_2O_2, which means that the changes in its activity have an impact not only on maintaining the balance between the prooxidant and antioxidant species but also decreasing blood glucose levels. Under hyperglycemic conditions, endothelial cells increase the levels of O_2^-; such an overproduction of O_2^- inhibits the activity of glyceraldehyde-3-phosphate dehydrogenase (GAPDH), a very important enzyme in the glycolytic pathway, and the inhibition of GAPDH leads to the accumulation of glucose and other intermediate metabolites of this pathway and shifts to other alternative pathways of glucose metabolism [43].

Regarding sperm parameters, diabetic rats exhibited lower sperm quality compared with the control group, presenting a lower sperm count, lower motility and viability, and an increase in the percentage of abnormalities; this again demonstrates the effects of oxidative stress and the production of free radicals, such as ROS, caused by hyperglycemia [35] due to the peroxidation of polyunsaturated fatty acids (PUFA) in sperm cell membrane spermatozoa [30]. Treatment with SM significantly increased the value of the previously mentioned parameters, which reveals its spermatic efficacy due to its antioxidant activity, although a dose–response relationship was not always observed. This antioxidant activity of SM has been the mechanism for explaining many of its pharmacological activities demonstrated in vivo and in vitro [44].

There were interesting results in this study, but prior to the extrapolation to humans mimicking the diabetic conditions of both species, it is necessary to better understand why SM improves sexual dysfunction parameters.

4. Materials and Methods

SM was kindly donated by Alimentos Esenciales para la Humanidad, S.A. de C.V. (Mexico City, Mexico) as a fine powder with a green-blue appearance. It was stored in trilaminate bags of metalized polyester to avoid light and air exposure and was maintained at room temperature until its use. In previous studies carried out in our laboratory, it was determined that the chemical and biochemical composition of this product for each 100 g was as follows: loss on drying (humidity) 4.65 g, lipids <0.50 g, saturated fats <0.10 g, crude fiber 0.96 g, proteins 60.08 g, ashes 6.71 g, total carbohydrates 27.60 g, sodium 114.99 mg, and energy supply 350 kcal. The microbiological analysis showed the following: fecal coliforms <3 NMP/100 mL, total coliforms <3 NMP/100 mL, *Escherichia coli* absent, mushrooms <1 CFU/g, yeasts <1 CFU/g, aerobic mesophilic 39,000 CFU/g, *Salmonella* absent, and *Staphylococcus aureus* absent. In addition, the metal analysis showed the following: As 0.054 mg/g, Al 0.352 mg/g, Cu <0.016 mg/g, Ca 1.1 mg/g, Fe 0.513 mg/g, Na 10.1 mg/g, K 12.6 mg/g, Cd <0.016 mg/g, Mn 0.030 mg/g, Ni <0.033 mg/g, Pb <0.033 mg/g, Mg 2.7 mg/g, Zn 0.016 mg/g, and Hg 0.0001 mg/g [14].

4.1. Animals

Thirty-six Wistar albino male rats of 350 ± 15 g ($n = 6$) and ten female Wistar albino rats 250 ± 15 g of eighty weeks old were obtained from the breeding colony of the Universidad Autónoma Metropolitana (UAM), Unidad Xochimilco, Mexico City, Mexico. They were housed in polypropylene cages with a sawdust floor and placed in an air-conditioned room (22–23 °C; 50–60 % humidity; and artificial illumination with an inverted light-dark cycle of 12h/12 h; lights on at 7:00 pm). The rats had access to standard rodent chow and purified water ad libitum, and they were adapted to the laboratory environment for 15 days prior to beginning the experimental protocols.

All procedures, including euthanasia, were performed in agreement with the Bioethics Committee of the National School of Biological Sciences of the National Polytechnic Institute, Mexico City ZOO-021-2019 and following the Mexican Official Regulation (NOM ZOO-062-200-199) entitled "Technical Specifications for Production, Care, and Use of Laboratory Animals".

4.2. Preparation of Females for Couplings, Animal Selection, and Preparation for Experiments

With the purpose of carrying out the definitive study of sexual behavior with sexually expert males, they were previously trained in mating with receptive females in circular acrylic cages 60 cm in diameter by 40 cm high on a bed of sawdust on alternate days to avoid sexual exhaustion. Only sexually apt healthy males were selected [45]. Only males who completed the copulatory sequence in <15 min from the entry of the female into the cages in three consecutive copulation sessions were considered sexually apt. Animals (males and females) that did not complete the copulatory sequence during training in the required time were removed from the study and replaced with other animals [45]. Receptive females were used for couplings, for which a bilateral ovariectomy was previously performed on female rats, as described by Khajuria [46]. Female rats were anesthetized with an i.p. dose of sodium pentobarbital, 60 mg/kg, and under the effect of anesthesia, both ovaries were excised, and the oviducts were ligated. The animals were maintained in recovery for 15 days after surgery. Finally, before initiating the sexual-behavior experiment, estrus was further induced in these ovariectomized rats by subcutaneous (s.c.) administration of estradiol benzoate (12 µg/kg) (Sigma Chemical Co., Ltd., St. Louis, MO, USA) 24 h before starting sexual behavior experiments and progesterone (3 mg/kg) (Sigma Chemical Co., Ltd.) 4 h before starting sexual experiments.

4.3. Induction of Diabetes Type II in Males

Once the sexually expert males were obtained, diabetes was induced (except for animals in the normal control group and SM 400 mg/kg group) with a single dose of STZ 65 mg/kg i.p. dissolved in citrate buffer at pH 4.6. One hour after STZ administration, 110 mg/kg of nicotinamide dissolved in saline solution was administered i.p., thus giving rise to the development of type II diabetes, according to the method described by Masiello [47]. After diabetes induction, blood glucose concentration was measured weekly from the dorsal tail vein by puncture under overnight fasting conditions using a glucometer (Accu-Chek Performa; Roche, Germany). Rats were considered diabetic when the blood glucose concentration was >200 mg/dL.

4.4. Mating Behavior Test

The sexually expert rat males (in whom diabetes was induced) were randomly distributed into six groups ($n = 6$), and the following treatments were administered for 5 weeks: 1. Control; 2. streptozotocin (STZ) 65 mg/kg; 3. SM 400 mg/kg; 4. STZ + SM 100 mg/kg; 5. STZ + SM 200 mg/kg, and 6. STZ + SM 400 mg/kg. The rats were then evaluated with sexual behavior tests. SM was suspended in water with 1% Tween-80 and administered orally (per os) in a constant volume per kg of weight. The doses of SM used in this study (100, 200, and 400 mg/kg) were selected on the basis of the results of pharmacological studies in rats carried out by our working group; such doses have shown good efficacy without producing mortality or altering body weights, tissues, and organs [14,48]. The evaluation in sexual behavior tests was performed during the first 3 h of the dark period under dim red illumination in a silent room, as previously described by Fumero [49]. Each male was introduced into a cage where it was first acclimatized for 10 min, then the female was introduced, and the registrations of the following parameters were videotaped with a digital camera (Sony HDR-CX405; China): mount latency (ML), counted as the time elapsed since the introduction of the female into the male box until the first mount; intromission latency (IL), calculated as time from introduction of the female to the first intromission by the male rat; mount frequency (MF), defined as the number of mounts before ejaculation; intromission frequency (IF), considered the number of intromissions before ejaculation; ejaculation latency (EL), recorded as the time elapsed from the first intromission to the first ejaculation; post-ejaculatory interval (PEI), calculated by the time from the first ejaculation to the next intromission by the male rat; and ejaculatory series duration (ESD), the time elapsed from the introduction of the female to the beginning of the second ejaculatory series (marked by the next intromission after the post-ejaculatory interval) [30,40].

Once tests were completed, the males were sacrificed by cervical decapitation. Blood was collected from the descending aorta vein, further incubated at room temperature for 10 min to allow coagulation, and subsequently centrifuged at 5000 rpm for 5 min to obtain the serum, which was frozen at $-70\ °C$ until analysis.

4.5. Sperm Collection and Analysis

Subsequently, the males' sacrificed testes, epididymis, and seminal vesicles were excised and weighed. A sperm sample was obtained from the vas deferens and the tail of the epididymis, which was suspended in 1 mL of Hanks' balanced salt solution preheated to 37 °C.

Staining was performed by incubating 10 μL of sperm sample with 10 μL of eosin–nigrosin vital dye at 36 °C for 5 min; this then was spread and dried on a slide to observe the viability of the cells under a microscope with a 100X objective. Viable (unstained) cells were distinguished from those that were not (stained), and the percentage of each was yielded from a count of at least 200 cells. Their morphology was also evaluated without characterization of the abnormality types found.

4.6. Biochemical Analysis

The determination of enzymatic activity in the testes was performed using commercial kits for superoxide dismutase (SOD) (Ransod; Randox Laboratories, Ltd., Crumlin, UK), which was based on the method described by Andersen [50], and glutathione peroxidase (GPX) (Ransel; Randox Laboratories, Ltd., Crumlin, UK) was determined according to the method of Paglia [51]. Lipoperoxidation was assessed by malondialdehyde (MDA), which was determined by the TBARS technique described by Matsuzawa [52].

Testosterone in the serum was determined with an ELISA kit (Cayman Chemical Company, Ann Arbor, MI, USA) following the manufacturer's instructions.

4.7. Statistical Analysis

The parametric data (body weight, blood glucose levels, mount latency, intromission latency, ejaculation latency, post-ejaculatory interval, and ejaculatory series duration; the count, motility, viability, and abnormality of the sperm; TBARS levels, SOD and GPX concentration; and testosterone levels) were expressed as the mean $\pm$ SEM ($n = 6$), while non-parametric data (mount and intromission frequencies) were expressed as frequencies. In the first case, after a normality test, analysis comparisons between multiple groups were performed with one-way ANOVA and post hoc Dunnett tests; in turn, for non-parametric data, Kruskal–Wallis with Dunnett post hoc tests were carried out [53]. In both cases, significant differences were considered when $p < 0.05$. All statistical analysis and the preparation of figures were made on GraphPad Prism v.8.

5. Conclusions

Oxidative stress in diabetic rats impairs sexual behavior in males, modifying mainly spermatic and biochemical parameters and testosterone levels. The antioxidant effect of SM, evidenced by the increase in the activity of SOD and GPX and the decrease in MDA in male diabetic rats, effectively counteracted the deterioration in parameters such as sexual conduct, sperm count, sperm motility, sperm viability, and sperm abnormalities and preserved sexual conduct together with higher sperm quality. These results show that antioxidant therapy, specifically with SM, could have a beneficial application in the treatment of diabetic sexual disorders in men.

Author Contributions: E.O.O.-R.: investigation, data curation; J.M.C.-L.: writing and review, Y.G.-M.: editing; M.A.M.-V.: procedures; R.P.-P.-B.: software analysis; G.G.-S.: visualization and revising content; S.P.-G.: resources; R.V.G.-R.: data analysis; E.M.-S.: conceptualization; J.A.M.-G.: validation; G.C.-C.: design and coordination of the study, supervision, project administration. All authors contributed to the study's conception and design. G.C.-C.: visualization, project administration; M.A.M.-V.: data curation; Y.G.-M.: methodology, data curation, investigation; S.P.-G.: supervision; E.M.-S.: software; J.A.M.-G.: writing—reviewing and editing; J.M.C.-L.: conceptualization, writing—original draft preparation, formal analysis. All authors have read and agreed to the published version of the manuscript.

Funding: This work was supported by the Secretaría de Investigación y Posgrado del Instituto Politécnico Nacional, grant number 20195923, Mexico City, Mexico.

Institutional Review Board Statement: The animal study protocol was approved by the Bioethics Committee of the National School of Biological Sciences of the National Polytechnic Institute, Mexico City (ZOO-021-2019, December 2019).

Informed Consent Statement: Not applicable.

Data Availability Statement: Not applicable.

Conflicts of Interest: The authors declare no conflict of interest.

References

1. Kong, Z.L.; Johnson, A.; Ko, F.C.; He, J.L.; Cheng, S.C. Effect of Cistanche Tubulosa Extracts on Male Reproductive Function in Streptozotocin–Nicotinamide-Induced Diabetic Rats. *Nutrients* **2018**, *10*, 1562. [CrossRef] [PubMed]
2. Ghaheri, M.; Miraghaee, S.; Babaei, A.; Mohammadi, B.; Kahrizi, D.; Saivosh Haghighi, Z.M.; Bahrami, G. Effect of Stevia rebaudiana Bertoni extract on sexual dysfunction in Streptozotocin-induced diabetic male rats. *Cell. Mol. Biol.* **2018**, *64*, 6–10. [CrossRef] [PubMed]
3. Kalka, D. Depression symptoms, sexual satisfaction and satisfaction with a relationship in individuals with type 2 diabetes and sexual dysfunctions. Objawy depresji i satysfakcja seksualna a zadowolenie ze związku u osób z cukrzycą typu 2 z dysfunkcjami seksualnymi. *Psychiatr. Pol.* **2018**, *52*, 1087–1099. [CrossRef] [PubMed]
4. Rai, A.; Das, S.; Chamallamudi, M.R.; Nandakumar, K.; Shetty, R.; Gill, M.; Sumalatha, S.; Devkar, R.; Gourishetti, K.; Kumar, N. Evaluation of the aphrodisiac potential of a chemically characterized aqueous extract of Tamarindus indica pulp. *J. Ethnopharmacol.* **2018**, *210*, 118–124. [CrossRef] [PubMed]
5. Maiorino, M.I.; Bellastella, G.; Esposito, K. Diabetes and sexual dysfunction: Current perspectives. *Diabetes. Metab. Syndr. Obes.* **2014**, *7*, 95–105. [CrossRef]
6. Wan, X.Z.; Li, T.T.; Zhong, R.T.; Chen, H.B.; Xia, X.; Gao, L.Y.; Gao, X.X.; Liu, B.; Zhang, H.Y.; Zhao, C. Anti-diabetic activity of PUFAs-rich extracts of Chlorella pyrenoidosa and Spirulina platensis in rats. *Food Chem. Toxicol.* **2019**, *128*, 233–239. [CrossRef]
7. Lert-Amornpat, T.; Maketon, C.; Fungfuang, W. Effect of Kaempferia parviflora on sexual performance in streptozotocin-induced diabetic male rats. *Andrologia* **2017**, *49*, e12770. [CrossRef]
8. Figueroa, M.C.; Pérez, I.; Mejía, R. Characterization of a type 2 diabetes model in female Wistar rats. *Rev. MVZ Córdoba* **2013**, *18*, 3699–3707. [CrossRef]
9. World Health Organization. *Informe Mundial Sobre la Diabetes*; WHO: Geneva, Switzerland, 2016; pp. 1–84. Available online: https://apps.who.int/iris/bitstream/handle/10665/254649/9789243565255-spa.pdf (accessed on 6 November 2022).
10. Yu, W.; Wan, Z.; Qiu, X.F.; Chen, Y.; Dai, Y.T. Resveratrol, an activator of SIRT1, restores erectile function in streptozotocin-induced diabetic rats. *Asian J. Androl.* **2013**, *15*, 646–651. [CrossRef]
11. Elbatreek, M.H.; Pachado, M.P.; Cuadrado, A.; Jandeleit-Dahm, K.; Schmidt, H. Reactive Oxygen Comes of Age: Mechanism-Based Therapy of Diabetic End-Organ Damage. *Trends Endocrinol. Metab.* **2019**, *30*, 312–327. [CrossRef]
12. Sahin, K.; Orhan, C.; Akdemir, F.; Tuzcu, M.; Gencoglu, H.; Sahin, N.; Turk, G.; Yilmaz, I.; Ozercan, I.H.; Juturu, V. Comparative evaluation of the sexual functions and NF-κB and Nrf2 pathways of some aphrodisiac herbal extracts in male rats. *BMC Complement. Altern. Med.* **2016**, *16*, 318. [CrossRef] [PubMed]
13. Duangnin, N.; Phitak, T.; Pothacharoen, P.; Kongtawelert, P. In vitro and in vivo investigation of natural compounds from seed extract of Mucuna pruriens lacking l-DOPA for the treatment of erectile dysfunction. *Asian Pac. J. Trop. Med.* **2017**, *10*, 238–252. [CrossRef] [PubMed]
14. Cristóbal-Luna, J.M.; Chamorro-Cevallos, G.; Monterubio-López, R.; Pérez-Ramos, J.; Pérez-González, C.; Pérez-Gutiérrez, S. Chapter 2: The effect of Arthrospira (Spirulina) maxima and its aqueous extract on fetal alcohol syndrome, induced in CD1 mice. In *Spirulina and Its Health Benefits*; Cochran, J., Ed.; NOVA: Hauppauge, NY, USA, 2021; pp. 45–92. [CrossRef]
15. Miranda, M.S.; Cintra, R.G.; Bsrros, S.B.M. Antioxidant activity of the microalga Spirulina maxima. *Braz. J. Med. Biol. Res.* **1998**, *31*, 1075–1079. [CrossRef] [PubMed]
16. Brito, A.F.; Silva, A.S.; de Souza, A.A.; Ferreira, P.B.; de Souza, I.L.L.; Araujo, L.C.D.C.; da Silva, B.A. Supplementation with Spirulina platensis Improves Tracheal Reactivity in Wistar Rats by Modulating Inflammation and Oxidative Stress. *Front. Pharmacol.* **2022**, *13*, 826649. [CrossRef]
17. Ferreira, P.B.; Diniz, A.F.A.; Lacerda Júnior, F.F.; Silva, M.D.C.C.; Cardoso, G.A.; Silva, A.S.; da Silva, B.A. Supplementation with Spirulina platensis Prevents Uterine Diseases Related to Muscle Reactivity and Oxidative Stress in Rats Undergoing Strength Training. *Nutrients* **2021**, *13*, 3763. [CrossRef]
18. Sadek, K.M.; Lebda, M.A.; Nasr, S.M.; Shoukry, M. Spirulina platensis prevents hyperglycemia in rats by modulating gluconeogenesis and apoptosis via modification of oxidative stress and MAPK-pathways. *Biomed. Pharmacother.* **2017**, *92*, 1085–1094. [CrossRef]
19. Deng, R.; Chow, T.J. Hypolipidemic, antioxidant, and antiinflammatory activities of microalgae Spirulina. *Cardiovasc. Ther.* **2010**, *28*, e33–e45. [CrossRef]
20. Shastri, D.; Kumar, M.; Kumar, A. Modulation of lead toxicity by Spirulina fusiformis. *Phytother. Res.* **1999**, *13*, 258–260. [CrossRef]
21. Al-Dhabi, N.A. Heavy metal analysis in commercial Spirulina products for human consumption. *Saudi J. Biol. Sci.* **2013**, *20*, 383–388. [CrossRef]
22. Gunes, S.; Tamburaci, S.; Dalay, M.C.; Deliloglu-Gurhan, I. In vitro evaluation of Spirulina platensis extract incorporated skin cream with its wound healing and antioxidant activities. *Pharm. Biol.* **2017**, *55*, 1824–1832. [CrossRef]
23. Abdel-Daim, M.M.; Shaaban-Ali, M.; Madkour, F.F.; Elgendy, H. Oral Spirulina Platensis Attenuates Hyperglycemia and Exhibits Antinociceptive Effect in Streptozotocin-Induced Diabetic Neuropathy Rat Model. *J. Pain Res.* **2020**, *13*, 2289–2296. [CrossRef]
24. Sinha, S.; Patro, N.; Patro, I.K. Amelioration of neurobehavioral and cognitive abilities of F1 progeny following dietary supplementation with Spirulina to protein malnourished mothers. *Brain Behav. Immun.* **2020**, *85*, 69–87. [CrossRef]
25. Sinha, S.; Patro, N.; Patro, I.K. Maternal Protein Malnutrition: Current and Future Perspectives of Spirulina Supplementation in Neuroprotection. *Front. Neurosci.* **2018**, *12*, 966. [CrossRef]

26. Shahzad, S.; Batool, Z.; Tabassum, S.; Ahmad, S.; Kamil, N.; Khaliq, S.; Nawaz, A.; Haider, S. Spirulina platensis (Blue-green algae): A miracle from sea combats the oxidative stress and improves behavioral deficits in an animal model of Schizophrenia. *Pak. J. Pharm. Sci.* **2020**, *33* (Suppl. 4), 1847–1853.
27. De, A.; Singh, M.F.; Singh, V.; Ram, V.; Bisht, S. Treatment effect of l-Norvaline on the sexual performance of male rats with streptozotocin induced diabetes. *Eur. J. Pharmacol.* **2016**, *771*, 247–254. [CrossRef] [PubMed]
28. Farzadi, L.; Khaki, A.; Ghasemzadeh, A.; Ouladsahebmadarek, E.; Ghadamkheir, E.; Shadfar, S.; Khaki, A.A. Effect of rosmarnic acid on sexual behavior in diabetic male rats. *Afr. J. Pharm. Pharmacol.* **2011**, *5*, 1906–1910. [CrossRef]
29. Al-Oanzi, Z.H. Erectile dysfunction attenuation by naringenin in streptozotocin-induced diabetic rats. *J. Food Biochem.* **2019**, *43*, e12885. [CrossRef] [PubMed]
30. Minaz, N.; Razdan, R.; Hammock, B.D.; Mujwar, S.; Goswami, S.K. Impact of diabetes on male sexual function in streptozotocin-induced diabetic rats: Protective role of soluble epoxide hydrolase inhibitor. *Biomed. Pharmacother.* **2019**, *115*, 108897. [CrossRef] [PubMed]
31. Chaturapanich, G.; Chaiyakul, S.; Verawatnapakul, V.; Pholpramool, C. Effects of Kaempferia parviflora extracts on reproductive parameters and spermatic blood flow in male rats. *Reproduction* **2008**, *136*, 515–522. [CrossRef] [PubMed]
32. Sing, R.; Ali, A.; Jeyabalan, G.; Semwal, A.; Jaikishan. An overview of the current methodologies used for evaluation of aphrodisiac agents. *J. Acute Dis.* **2013**, *2013*, 85–91. [CrossRef]
33. Erhabor, J.O.; Idu, M. Aphrodisiac potentials of the ethanol extract of Aloe barbadensis Mill. root in male Wistar rats. *BMC Complement. Altern. Med.* **2017**, *17*, 360. [CrossRef] [PubMed]
34. Arya, A.; Cheah, S.C.; Looi, C.Y.; Taha, H.; Mustafa, M.R.; Mohd, M.A. The methanolic fraction of Centratherum antihelminticam seed down regulates pro-inflammatory cytokines, oxidative stress, and hyperglycemia in STZ-nicotinamide-induced type 2 diabetic rats. *Food Chem. Toxicol.* **2012**, *50*, 4209–4220. [CrossRef]
35. Al-Roujeaie, A.S.; Abuohashish, H.M.; Ahmed, M.M.; Alkhamees, O.A. Effect of rutin on diabetic-induced erectile dysfunction: Possible involvement of testicular biomarkers in male rats. *Andrologia* **2017**, *49*, e12737. [CrossRef] [PubMed]
36. Pontes, D.A.; Fernandes, G.S.A.; Piffer, R.C.; Gerardin, D.C.C.; Pereira, O.C.M.; Kempinas, W.G. Ejaculatory dysfunction in streptozotocin-induced diabetic rats: The role of testosterone. *Pharmacol. Rep.* **2011**, *63*, 130–138. [CrossRef] [PubMed]
37. Abdrabou, M.I.; Elleithy, E.; Yasin, N.; Shaheen, Y.M.; Galal, M. Ameliorative effects of Spirulina maxima and Allium sativum on lead acetate-induced testicular injury in male albino rats with respect to caspase-3 gene expression. *Acta Histochem.* **2019**, *121*, 198–206. [CrossRef]
38. Barkallah, M.; Slima, A.B.; Elleuch, F.; Fendri, I.; Pichon, C.; Abdelkafi, S.; Baril, P. Protective Role of Spirulina platensis against Bifenthrin-Induced Reprotoxicity in Adult Male Mice by Reversing Expression of Altered Histological, Biochemical, and Molecular Markers Including MicroRNAs. *Biomolecules* **2020**, *10*, 753. [CrossRef] [PubMed]
39. Salama, A.F.; Kasem, S.M.; Tousson, E.; Elsisy, M.K. Protective role of L-carnitine and vitamin E on the testis of atherosclerotic rats. *Toxicol. Ind. Health* **2015**, *31*, 467–474. [CrossRef]
40. Allouh, M.Z.; Daradka, H.M.; Abu-Ghaida, J.H. Influence of Cyperus esculentus tubers (tiger nut) on male rat copulatory behavior. *BMC Complement. Altern. Med.* **2015**, *15*, 331. [CrossRef]
41. Cabrera, A.; Paredes, R.G. Effects of chronic estradiol or testosterone treatment upon sexual behavior in sexually sluggish male rats. *Pharmacol. Biochem. Behav.* **2012**, *101*, 336–341. [CrossRef]
42. Noberasco, G.; Odetti, P.; Boeri, D.; Maiello, M.; Adezati, L. Malondialdehyde (MDA) level in diabetic subjects. Relationship with blood glucose and glycosylated hemoglobin. *Biomed Pharmacother.* **1991**, *45*, 193–196. [CrossRef]
43. Younus, H. Therapeutic potentials of superoxide dismutase. *Int. J. Health Sci.* **2018**, *12*, 88–93.
44. Hernández-Lepe, M.A.; Wall-Medrano, A.; Juárez-Oropeza, M.A.; Ramos-Jiménez, A.; Hernández-Torres, R.P. Spirulina y su efecto hipolipemiante y antioxidante en humanos: Una revisión sistemática [Spirulina and its hypolipidemic and antioxidant effects in humans: A systematic review]. *Nutr. Hosp.* **2015**, *32*, 494–500. [CrossRef] [PubMed]
45. Lucio, R.A.; Tlachi, J.L.; López, A.A.; Zempoalteca, R.; Velázquez-Moctezuma, J. Análisis de los parámetros del eyaculado en la rata Wistar de laboratorio: Descripción de la técnica. *Vet. Mex.* **2008**, *40*, 405–415.
46. Khajuria, D.K.; Razdan, R.; Mahapatra, D.R. Description of a new method of ovariectomy in female rats. *Rev. Bras. Reumatol.* **2012**, *52*, 462–470.
47. Masiello, P.; Broca, C.; Gross, R.; Roye, M.; Manteghetti, M.; Hillaire-Buys, D.; Novelli, M.; Ribes, G. Experimental NIDDM: Development of a new model in adult rats administered streptozotocin and nicotinamide. *Diabetes* **1998**, *47*, 224–229. [CrossRef]
48. Garrido-Acosta, O.; Limón, I.D.; García, E.; Anguiano-Robledo, L.; Barrientos-Alvarado, C.; Chamorro-Cevallos, G. Efecto Protector de Spirulina maxima en un modelo experimental de enfermedad de Parkinson inducido con MPP+ Protective effect of Spirulina maxima in an experimental Parkinson´s disease model induced by MPP+. *Rev. Mex. Cienc. Farm.* **2017**, *48*, 56–64.
49. Fumero, B.; Fernandez-Vera, J.R.; Gonzalez-Mora, J.L.; Mas, M. Changes I, 5(6), n monoamine turnover in forebrain areas associated with masculine sexual behavior: A microdialysis study. *Brain Res.* **1994**, *662*, 233–239. [CrossRef]
50. Andersen, H.R.; Nielsen, J.B.; Nielsen, F.; Grandjean, P. Antioxidative enzyme activities in human erythrocytes. *Clin. Chem.* **1997**, *43*, 562–568. [CrossRef]
51. Paglia, D.E.; Valentine, W.N. Studies on the quantitative and qualitative characterization of erythrocyte glutathione peroxidase. *J. Lab. Clin. Med.* **1967**, *70*, 158–169.

52. Matsuzawa, T.; Saitoh, H.; Sano, M.; Tomita, I.; Ohkawa, M.; Ikekawa, T. Studies on Antioxidant Effects of Hypsizigus marmoreus. II. Effects of Hypsizigus marmoreus for Antioxidant Activities of Tumor-Bearing Mice. *Yakugaku Zasshi* **1998**, *118*, 476–481. [CrossRef]
53. Mitteer, D.R.; Greer, B.D. Using GraphPad Prism's Heat Maps for Efficient, Fine-Grained Analyses of Single-Case Data. *Behav. Anal. Pract.* **2022**, *15*, 505–514. [CrossRef] [PubMed]

Disclaimer/Publisher's Note: The statements, opinions and data contained in all publications are solely those of the individual author(s) and contributor(s) and not of MDPI and/or the editor(s). MDPI and/or the editor(s) disclaim responsibility for any injury to people or property resulting from any ideas, methods, instructions or products referred to in the content.

Review

Opuntia spp. in Human Health: A Comprehensive Summary on Its Pharmacological, Therapeutic and Preventive Properties. Part 2

Eduardo Madrigal-Santillán [1,*], Jacqueline Portillo-Reyes [1], Eduardo Madrigal-Bujaidar [2], Manuel Sánchez-Gutiérrez [3], Jeannett A. Izquierdo-Vega [3], Julieta Izquierdo-Vega [3], Luis Delgado-Olivares [3], Nancy Vargas-Mendoza [1], Isela Álvarez-González [2], Ángel Morales-González [4] and José A. Morales-González [1,*]

1 Escuela Superior de Medicina, Instituto Politécnico Nacional, "Unidad Casco de Santo Tomas", Ciudad de México 11340, Mexico
2 Escuela Nacional de Ciencias Biológicas, Instituto Politécnico Nacional, "Unidad Profesional A. López Mateos", Ciudad de México 07738, Mexico
3 Instituto de Ciencias de la Salud, Universidad Autónoma del Estado de Hidalgo, Ex-Hacienda de la Concepción, Tilcuautla, Pachuca de Soto 42080, Mexico
4 Escuela Superior de Cómputo, Instituto Politécnico Nacional, "Unidad Profesional A. López Mateos", Ciudad de México 07738, Mexico
* Correspondence: emadrigal@ipn.mx (E.M.-S.); jmorales101@yahoo.com.mx (J.A.M.-G.); Tel.: +52-55-5729-6300 (ext. 62733) (E.M.-S.)

Abstract: Plants of the genus *Opuntia* spp are widely distributed in Africa, Asia, Australia and America. Specifically, Mexico has the largest number of wild species; mainly *O. streptacantha, O. hyptiacantha, O. albicarpa, O. megacantha* and *O. ficus-indica*. The latter being the most cultivated and domesticated species. Its main bioactive compounds include pigments (carotenoids, betalains and betacyanins), vitamins, flavonoids (isorhamnetin, kaempferol, quercetin) and phenolic compounds. Together, they favor the different plant parts and are considered phytochemically important and associated with control, progression and prevention of some chronic and infectious diseases. Part 1 collected information on its preventive actions against atherosclerotic cardiovascular diseases, diabetes and obesity, hepatoprotection, effects on human infertility and chemopreventive capacity. Now, this second review (Part 2), compiles the data from published research (in vitro, in vivo, and clinical studies) on its neuroprotective, anti-inflammatory, antiulcerative, antimicrobial, antiviral potential and in the treatment of skin wounds. The aim of both reviews is to provide scientific evidences of its beneficial properties and to encourage health professionals and researchers to expand studies on the pharmacological and therapeutic effects of *Opuntia* spp.

Keywords: *Opuntia* spp.; neuroprotective; antiulcerative; antimicrobial; antiviral; skin wounds; anti-inflammatory effect

1. Introduction

The Traditional Medicine/Complementary and Alternative Medicine (TCAM) concept includes any practice, knowledge and belief in health that incorporates medicine based on plants, animals and/or minerals, spiritual therapies, manual techniques and exercises applied individually or in combination to improve human health. The World Health Organization (WHO) considers that TCAM have shown favorable factors that contribute to an increasing acceptance worldwide, such as easy access, diversity, relatively low cost and, most importantly, relatively low adverse toxic effects in comparison with allopathic medicine where these effects are frequently attributed to synthetic drugs. For this reason, TCAM continues to be used by different populations to treat and/or prevent the onset and progression of chronic and infectious diseases [1–3].

Throughout human history, plants and their phytochemicals have played an important role at improving human health care. *Opuntia* species have specifically shown many beneficial properties and high biotechnological capacity. These plants classified as angiosperm dicotyledonous are the most abundant of the Cactaceae family and are importantly distributed in America, Africa, Asia, Australia, and in the central Mediterranean area. Due to their capacity to store water in one or more of their organs, they are considered succulent plants whose cultivation is ideal in arid areas since they are very efficient to generate biomass in water scarcity conditions [4–7].

Most opuntioid cacti have flat and edible stems called cladodes (CLDs), paddles, nopales or stalks. Generally, young CLDs (also called nopalitos) are eaten as a vegetable in salads, while their fruits (called cactus pear fruits, tunas or prickly pear fruits (PPFs)) are widely eaten as fresh seasonal fruit. PPFs are oval berries with lots of seeds throughout all the pulp and a semi-hard bark that contains thorns. They are grouped in different colors (red, purple, orange/yellow, and white). Generally, the fruit with white flesh and green skin is the most consumed as food [4–7]. Some evidences indicate that *Opuntia* plants have been consumed by humans for more than 8000 years and due to their easy adaptation and spread in different types of soil, their domestication process has favored the constant collection of CLDs and PPFs by man [7–10].

2. Impact of the *Opuntia* Genus in Mexico and Other Countries

The Cactaceae family includes about 200 genera and 2000 species classified into three to six subfamilies. The Opuntioideae subfamily comprises between 15 and 18 genera, *Opuntia* being the most diverse and widely distributed genus in the American continent [10–12]. However, Mexico has the largest number of wild species. The most representaive are *O. streptacantha* (OS), *O. hyptiacantha* (OH), *O. albicarpa* (OA), *O. megacantha* (OM) and *O. ficus-indica* (Figure 1). The latter is highly cultivated and domesticated species due to its nutritional, medicinal, pharmaceutical, and economic impacts. It is believed to be a secondary crop with fewer thorns derived from OM, (a native species from central Mexico) [4,7,8,10–12]. Currently, *O. ficus-indica* (OFI) has become as important a vegetable crop as corn and agave-tequila; its economic relevance is significantly increasing in our country and in other parts of the world, especially for improving health when nopal and prickly pear are included in a diet. Therefore, the OFI domestication process has favored changes in the texture, flavor, size, color, quantity and quality of the cladodes and their fruits [4,7,8]. Mexico and Italy are the main producing and consuming countries of the approximately 590,000 ha cultivated around the world. The Annual Mexican production can reach 350,000 tons; for this reason, our country represents approximately 90% of the total production worldwide. In addition, Mexico is the main producer of prickly pear fruits, representing more than 45% of world production; however, only 1.5% of this production is exported, due to various factors such as a low level of technology in its production, climatic changes, the lack of a marketing plan (supply/demand) and that it is a seasonal product (it is obtained between the months of June to November) [4,7,12,13].

In relation to the impact of *Opuntia* species in other countries, there is evidence of positive and negative aspects. In the first case, due to their adaptability, which allows them to grow where no other crop can, their plants and fruits (specifically, PPFs) have become an essential and reliable crop for the diet of the inhabitants (As it happens in Ethiopia). Likewise, healers of the Kani tribes in the Tirunelveli hills of the Western Ghats of India, consider the opuntia species spiritual and esential for their first aid remedies; especially *O. dillenii* which is used to treat cough, headache, poisonous animal bites, cold and fever control [14,15].

Unfortunately, because they can survive in arid/semi-arid environments, high temperatures, little rainfall and limited nutrient supply, they are considered an invasive alien species in some South African and Kenyan communities that can threaten biodiversity and food security. For this reason, *Opuntia* (especially *O. stricta*) is included in the diet of animals (forage for livestock), as a measure to control its spread, mainly in dry seasons [16,17].

In general, in Mexico and other countries, *Opuntia* is a resource that has high agrotechnological potential, both as a food crop and as a base element to obtain derived products, which are used in the food industry (human and animal), medicine, agricultural industry and cosmetology (Table 1).

Table 1. Main products and by-products obtained from *Opuntia* (Nopal).

Products from Cladodes (CLDs)	Products from Prickly Pear Fruits (PPFs)	By-Products from CLDs and PPFs
Lacto-fermented pickles	Juices, nectars, pulps, purees	Fruit and seed oil
Candies, sweets	Jams, jellies	Peel pigments and/or fruit debris
jams	fruit leather and teas	Cladode extracts
flours	syrup, sweetener	Dietary fiber and cladode mucilage
Fresh and cooked vegetables	Bioethanol, wine	Pigments for cosmetics
Ethanol	Canned and frozen fruit	
Edible coating	Juice concentrates and spray dried juice powder	

Table modified from Feugang et al. (2006) [18].

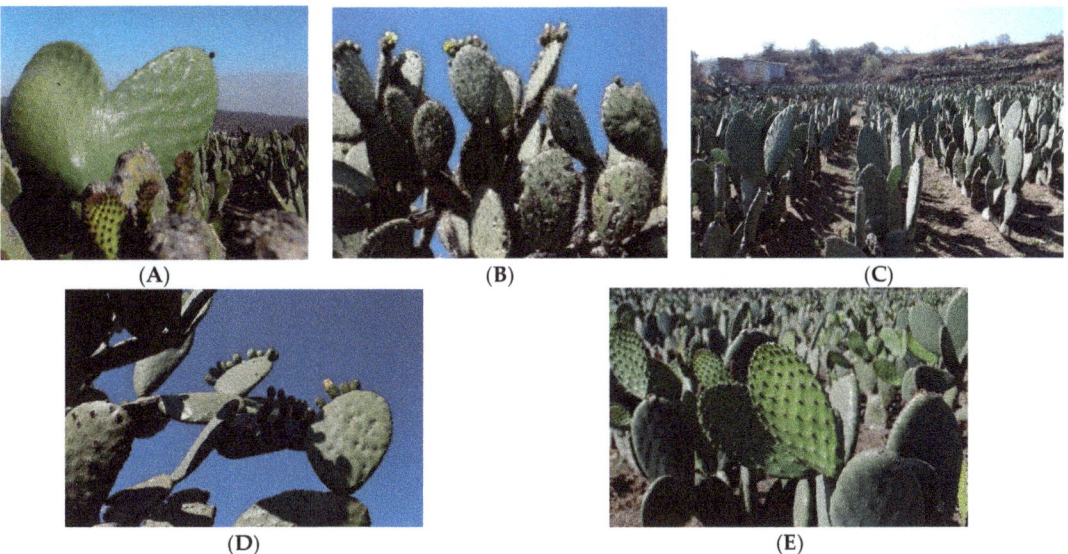

Figure 1. Mexican cultivars of *O. Streptacantha* (**A**), *O. megacantha* (**B**) and *O. ficus-indica* (**C**), *O. hyptiacantha* (**D**), and *O. albicarpa* (**E**).

3. Nutritionalcomposition and Mechanisms of Pharmacological Action of the *Opuntia* Genus

Different methods have documented the nutritional value of *Opuntia* spp. Most of these studies coincide in the differences among the phytochemical composition of their plant parts (fruits, roots, cladodes, flowers, seeds and stems) and the wild and domesticated species. These can be attributed to environmental conditions (climate, humidity), the type of soil that prevails in the cultivation sites, the age of maturity of the cladodes, and the harvest season [5–7]. The nutritional composition of the different parts of Opuntia ficus-indica (L.) Mill. is summarized in Table 2. In general, opuntioid cacti contain a large amount of water (80 and 95%), carbohydrates (3–7%), proteins (0.5–1%), soluble fiber (1–2%), fatty acids (palmitic, stearic, oleic, vaccenic and linoleic) and minerals (Potassium (K), calcium (Ca), phosphorus (P), magnesium (Mg), chrome (Cr) and sodium (Na)). They also have viscous and/or mucilaginous materials (made up of D-glucose, D-galactose, L-arabinose, D-xylose and polymers such as β-D-galacturonic acid linked to (1–4) and L-rhamnose residues linked with R (1–2)) whose function is to absorb and regulate the amount of cellular water in dry seasons [5–7,19]. Among the main bioactive compounds of prickly pear highlight the pigments (carotenoids, betalains, betaxanthins and betacyanins), vitamins (B1, B6, E, A, and C), flavonoids (isorhamnetin, kaempferol, quercetin, nicotiflorine, dihydroquercetin, penduletin, lutein), rutin, aromadendrine, myricetin vitexin, flavonones and flavanonols) and phenolic compounds (ferulic acid, feruloyl-sucrose and synapoyl-diglycoside) [5–7,19–22].

Table 2. Nutritional composition in different anatomical parts of Opuntia ficus-indica (L.) Mill.

Chemical Species	Main Component
Cladodes	
Minerals	K and Ca (mainly calcium oxalate crystals).
Vitamins	E, A, C, B1, B2, B3
Amino acids	Glutamine, arginine, leucine, isoleucine, lysine, valine and phenylalanine
Fatty acids	Palmitic acid, oleic acid, linoleic acid and linolenic acid
Carotenoids	Lutein, β-carotene and β-cryptoxanthin
Flavonoids	Quercetin, kaempferol, isoquercetin, isorhamnetin-3-O-glucoside, nicotiflorin, rutin
Phenolic compounds	Coumaric Gallic acid, 3,4-dihydroxybenzoic 4-hydroxybenzoic, and ferulic acid
Prickly pear fruits	
Minerals	K, Ca, and Mg
Vitamins	E, A, and C
Amino acids	Lysine, methionine, glutamine, and taurine
Organic acids	Maleic, malonic, succinic, tartaric, and oxalic
Pigments	Betaxanthins, betacyanins, and betalains
Fatty acids	Palmitic acid and linoleic acid
Flavonoids	Kaempferol, quercetin, and isorhamnetin
Seeds	
Minerals	K and P. Lower proportions of Mg, Na and Ca
Sterols	β-sitosterol and campesterol
Fatty acids	Palmitic acid, oleic acid, and linoleic acid
Phenolic compounds	Ferulic acid, sinapoyl-diglucoside, synapoyl-glucose, and feruloyl-sucrose
Pulp and peel	
Minerals	K, Ca and Mg
Sterols	β-sitosterol and campesterol
Fatty acids	Palmitic acid, oleic acid, linoleic acid, stearic acids and linolenic acid
Carotenoids	Lutein, β-carotene, violaxanthin, lycopene, and zeaxanthin
Flavonoids	Quercetin, isorhamnetin, kaempferol, luteolin, and isorhamnetin glycosides
Phenolic compounds	Ferulic acid, sinapoyl-diglucoside, and feruloyl-sucrose isomer
Flowers	
Flavonoids	Kaempferol, quercetin, and isorhamnetin glycosides
Organic acids	Mainly gallic acid

Table modified from Madrigal-Santillán et al. (2022) [23].

Specifically, the cladodes and prickly pears fruits of OFI have shown several kinds of bioactive compounds, among which flavonoids (such as quercetin, kaempferol, isorhamnetin), essential amino acids (Glutamine, arginine, leucine, isoleucine, lysine, valine and phenylalanine), vitamins (B1, B6, E, A, and C), minerals (mainly K and Ca), and betalains [such as betaxanthins (betanin and indicaxanthin) and betacyanins (betanidin, isobetanin, isobetanidine, and neobetanin) [5–7,19–22].

As mentioned in part 1 [23], various studies have shown the action of phytochemicals as substrates to activate different biochemical reactions that provide important health benefits. For that reason, they could be included in the definition of nutraceutical: "Any non-toxic food extract supplement that has been scientifically proven to be beneficial to health both intreating and preventing diseases" [5,23,24]. Different authors agree that the carotenoids are important compounds with great benefits for human health, related to the prevention and reduction of the development of some diseases, such as cardiovascular diseases, cancer and macular degeneration and that taurine (semi-essential amino acid) is involved in the modulation of the inflammatory response with potential antioxidant. As well as, that some plant sterols are incorporated into foods intended for human consumption to lower blood cholesterol levels [25,26]. On the other hand, the scientific evidence suggests that the phenolic acids (hydroxycinnamic acids and hydroxybenzoic acids), flavonoids, lignins and stilbenes have a high antioxidant potential that has been related in many health benefits such as prevention of inflammation, cardiovascular dysregulation, and neurodegenerative diseases [25,27]. In this same approach, it is known that the flavonoids are a group of bioactive compounds that exhibit many effects in the protection of the body, and their regular consumption is associated with reduced risk of several chronic diseases (especially, for its antioxidant, antiviral and antibacterial capacities). Finally, the Betalains are powerful radical eliminators in chemical systems and has act as efficient antioxidants in several biological models. Potential related as a possible strategy for intestinal inflammation [26–28]

In this context, opuntioid cacti reveal different mechanisms of action that can be interrelated and favor their biological effects. In general, they are organized in 7 groups: (I) Inhibition of the absorption of substances, favoring the absorption of protective agents and/or modification of the intestinal flora (action of soluble fiber and ascorbic acid), (II) Scavenging of reactive oxygen species and/or protection of DNA nucleophilic sites (antioxidant action), (III) Anti-inflammatory activity, (IV) Modification of transmembrane transport (effect of short-chain fatty acids and calcium in the diet), (V) Modulation of xenobiotic metabolising enzymes, inhibition of mutagen agents activation and induction of detoxification pathways (flavonoids, polyphenols and índoles), (VI) Enhancement of apoptosis (action of some flavonoids), and (VII) Maintenance of genomic stability (effect of some vitamins, minerals and polyphenols) [3,5–7,20–24].

Together, the bioactive compounds of *Opuntia* spp. favor its different plant parts to be considered phytochemically important and associated with the control, progression and prevention of some chronic and infectious diseases. This second review (Part 2) focuses on information from published research (in vitro, in vivo and clinical studies) on its anti-inflammatory, antiulcerative, neuroprotective, antimicrobial, antiviral properties and on the treatment of skin wounds; which will be discussed below.

4. Pharmacological, Therapeutic and Preventive Properties

4.1. Anti-Inflammator and Antiulcerative Effects

The inflammatory cascade includes a long chain of molecular reactions and cellular processes (highlighting phagocytosis, chemotaxis, mitosis, and cell differentiation) designed as a biological response to different noxious stimuli, including dust particles, chemical substances, physical injuries, bacteria, viruses, and parasites. This cascade is an important factor for the progression of various chronic disorders, such as obesity, arthritis, diabetes, cancer, cardiovascular diseases, eye disorders, autoimmune diseases and inflammatory bowel disorders; therefore, in recent decades it has become a highly studied field of research [29,30]. The stages of inflammation depend on the duration of the process and various immunological factors, classifying them into acute and chronic. The first is characterized by a rapid initial response that can last minutes and/or a few days. There is accumulation of plasma proteins and leukocytes, presenting increased blood flow, swelling, redness, pain and heat. When this response is prolonged, chronicity is established, which leads to an increase in the presence of lymphocytes, macrophages, and mast cells at the site of infection and/or damage. Simultaneously, repair mechanisms that can generate fibrosis and overproduction of connective tissue are activated. In general, inflammation is a vital response of the immune system; however, a chronic process can induce secondary consequences in the biological response associated with an increased risk of chronic diseases. This usually occurs through infections that are not cleared by endogenous protective mechanisms or by some type of genetic susceptibility [29,30].

Various investigations have confirmed that inflammation is related to the induction of oxidative stress (OXs) due to the increase in cells (lymphocytes, macrophages, and mast cells) that leads to greater oxygen uptake, increasing the production and release of reactive oxygen species (ROS) in the damaged area. In addition, the activation of signal transduction cascades and alteration in transcription factors (such as nuclear factor kappa B (NF-κB), signal transducer and activator of transcription 3, activator protein-1, factor 2 related to NF-E2, activated T-cell nuclear factor, and hypoxia-inducible factor-1α (HIF1-α)) [29,30]. Likewise, cyclooxygenase-2 (COX-2), nitric oxide synthase (iNOS), expression of inflammatory cytokines (such as tumor necrosis factor alpha (TNF-α)), interleukins (IL-1β, IL-6) and chemokines, are induced. Scientific findings of different anti-inflammatory agents have shown that bioactive extracts and their natural compounds exert their biological properties by blocking signaling pathways, such as NF-κB and mitogen-activated protein kinases (MAPK) [29,30].

On the other hand, Gastric Ulcers (GU) are open sores in the mucosa lining the stomach and/or duodenum. The most frequent symptomatology is pain and burning that can occur between meals or at night, with different durations (minutes and/or days). The worldwide incidence of GU varies depending on age, sex, and geographic location, but it remains a common condition and a major public health problem due to high healthcare costs and life-threatening complications (bleeding, perforation, and obstruction), that favor its high morbidity and mortality [31]. The pathophysiology of GU is multifactorial but is generally associated with the result of an imbalance between the protective and aggressive factors of the gastric mucosae; that is, when there is a significant increase in the acids that help digest food, damaging the walls of the stomach and/or duodenum. Among the harmful factors that favor its incidence are excessive gastric acid and pepsin secretion, increased ROS, *Helicobacter pylori* infection, constant alcohol consumption, and prolonged ingestion of nonsteroidal anti-inflammatory drugs (NSAIDs) [31–33]. While gastrointestinal defense mechanisms include mucus secretion, bicarbonate production, nitric oxide (NO), prostaglandin synthesis, normal gastric motility, and adequate tissue microcirculation. Currently, GU treatments are aimed at improving the defenses of the gastric mucosae or counteracting harmful factors. Among the most used are those that reduce gastric acid secretion (H2 receptor antagonists), those that inhibit the proton pump (omeprazole); and antibiotics that control *H. pylori*. However, its high costs and side effects of long-term treatments combined with recurrence of ulcers and some cases of rejection to conventional therapies have motivated the search for new antiulcer agents. In particular, those that improve the quality of ulcer healing to prevent abnormalities in mucosal regeneration and the persistence of chronic inflammation by reducing the infiltration of neutrophils and macrophages (i.e., prevent ulcer recurrence) [31–33].

Like anti-inflammatory agents extracted from natural compounds, herbal anti-ulcer medications have also become an excellent source to obtain them. In this sense, *Opuntia* spp. is no exception, and possibly, after the studies related to atherosclerotic cardiovascular diseases, diabetes, obesity and chemopreventive capacity (included in part 1) [23], the anti-inflammatory and antiulcerative evaluation field is of equal relevance to researchers.

Probably, the first study to break into this field of evaluation was aimed to confirm in rodents that a preparation of dried flowers of OFI reduced the discomfort of benign prostatic hypertrophy by suppressing the release of beta-glucuronidase (lysosomal enzyme of the neutrophils) [34]. Subsequently, two research groups, Park et al., (1998) [35] and Loro et al., (1998) [36], continued the studies. In the first, ethanolic extracts of fruits (EEOF) and stems (EEOS) of OFI were analyzed on the acetic acid writhing syndrome and paw edema induced by carrageenan (CRRG) in Sprague Dawley rats. Both extracts decreased writhing and edema; as well as the release of the same lysosomal enzyme. Their results suggested that EEOF and EEOS have analgesic and anti-inflammatory actions, and a possible protective effect against gastric injury [35]. Using similar techniques, the second group of scientists evaluated different lyophilisates (50–400 mg/kg, i.p.) from the fruits of *O. dillenii* Haw (OdHw); the result was similar when the chemical stimuli were dose-dependently inhibited (writhing test) and thermal (hot plate test) in Wistar rats; mainly in doses of 50 and 100 mg/kg [36]. The results of the previous studies motivated the fractionation of a methanolic extract of OFI stems and, together with a model of chronic inflammation induced by adjuvants in mice, β-sitosterol was isolated and identified as a possible anti-inflammatory active ingredient [37].

In relation to the first evidence of the anti-ulcer effect, Galati et al. [38–40] found that by previously administering lyophilized CLDs and/or OFI whole fruit juice on experimental ulcers induced by ethanol (EtOH) in rats, a cytoprotective action related to an increase in the production of gastric mucus was exerted. They attributed such effect to the mixture of mucilage and pectin present in OFI [38–40]. Table 3 shows the main studies that evidence the anti-inflammatory and antiulcerative effects of *Opuntia* spp. In summary, from 1993 to date, 16 of 39 have been in vitro studies; 20, using laboratory animals (mainly rodents) and 3, developed with patients (clinical studies). Mainly, different types of extracts (methanol (MeOH), hexane (Hx), chloroform (Chl), ethyl acetate (EtOAc), butanol and aqueous) obtained from CLDs and roots of OFI, OdHw and *O. humifusa* (OHF) have been analyzed. In addition, powders from the stems, juices, vinegars and oils of PPFs and/or their seeds extracted from *O. elatio* Mill, *O. macrorhiza* Engelm (OME), OFI and OdHw have been explored. Most studies confirm and agree that the main mechanism of action of both properties (anti-inflammatory and anti-ulcer) is related to its antioxidant capacity, which is attributed to a possible synergistic and/or combined effect between the different bioactive compounds (phenols, flavonoids (such as quercetin, kaempferol, isorhamnetin), betalains (betanin and indicaxanthin), betacyanins, α-pyrones (opuntiol and opuntioside glucoside), pectin and mucilage) present in the chemical composition of the *Opuntia* genus [41–75].

Table 3. Studies testing for anti-inflammatory and antiulcerative effects of *Opuntia* spp.

Type of Study	Objective and Characteristics	Results and Conclusion	Ref
Anti-Inflammatory Evidence			
In vitro	Considering that the inflammatory response depends on the redox state of an organism and the evidence of antioxidant properties of some OFI pigments, the protective effect of betalains on vascular endothelial cells as a direct target of OXs in inflammation was analyzed.	The result indicated that betalains protect the endothelium from oxidative alteration through the inhibition of some cytokines (such as ICAM-1).	[41]
In vivo	Using the rat paw edema model induced by CRRG, the anti-inflammatory effect of alcoholic extracts of flowers, fruits and stems from OdHw was evaluated. To analyze the analgesic potential of the same extracts, electric current was used as a noxious stimulus.	An important observation was that the flower extract (dose of 200 mg/kg) had the highest anti-inflammatory and analgesic capacity. Furthermore, by performing a bioassay-guided division by using VLC, Sephadex, and paper chromatography, three flavonoid glycosides (kaempferol 3-O-alpha-arabinoside, isorhamnetin-3-O-glucoside, and isorhamnetin-3-O-rutinoside) were obtained and related to its protective capacity.	[42]
In vitro	Hypochlorous acid (HOCl) is produced from H_2O_2 and chloride by the enzyme heme-myeloperoxidase (MPO). It is a powerful oxidant produced by Neut that contributes to the damage caused by these inflammatory cells. The objective of the study was to analyze the interaction of betanin and indicaxanthin (Ind) with HOCl and compounds I and II of MPO.	The conclusion was that both betalains were good substrates for MPO and function as one-electron reducing agents of their redox intermediates (compounds I and II). Moreover, the two pigments effectively removed HOCl at 25 °C with a pH between 5 and 7.	[43]

Table 3. Cont.

Type of Study	Objective and Characteristics	Results and Conclusion	Ref
	Anti-Inflammatory Evidence		
In vitro	The aim of the study was to determine the antioxidant potential and the anti-inflammatory effect in macrophages (RAW264.7 cells) producers of nitric oxide (NO) of different extracts (MeOH, Hx, Chl, EtOAc, butanol and water) prepared from the leaves of OHF	Using the 2,2-diphenyl-1-picrylhydrazyl (DPPH) scavenging assay, the presence of antioxidant activity in all the extracts was confirmed and the EtOAc fraction was the most significant. Regarding the anti-inflammatory effect, only Chl and EtOAc fractions suppressed the production of NO in RAW264.7 cells activated by lipopolysaccharide (LPS). A significant inhibition of the expression of inducible nitric oxide synthetase (iNOS) and interleukin-6 (IL-6) was also evidenced; hence, OHF can modulate the expression of inflammatory cytokines.	[44]
In vitro	Given that the conventional medications reduce symptoms of osteoarthritis (OA) but can cause significant side effects, the use of natural substances that reduce and/or delay the progression of that disease has begun to be explored. Therefore, the anti-inflammatory effect of some lyophilized extracts obtained from OFI cladodes on the production of NO, glycosaminoglycans (GAGs), prostaglandin G2 (PGE2), and ROS in cultured human chondrocytes stimulated by interleukin-1 beta (IL-1β) was analyzed.	The DPPH assay showed that the freeze-dried substances have a significant antioxidant effect. Besides, the results indicated that all extracts counteracted the deleterious effects of IL-1β by decreasing the production of key molecules released during the chronic inflammation. These data suggest that the extracts exert a chondroprotective capacity greater than that caused by hyaluronic acid commonly used as visco-supplementation in the treatment of OA.	[45]
In vitro	In order to increase the scientific information of OFI on its beneficial properties in the inflammatory response, the immunomodulatory activity of an aqueous extract supplemented to a mouse Macrop culture was studied.	The cells were cultured in RPMI-1640 to analyze the presence of NO, iNOS and NF-κB induced by LPS. The results of the immunosorbent assay and Western method showed that all inflammatory parameters were suppressed when adding the extract to the culture. This opens the possibility of considering the aqueous extract as a nutraceutical ingredient applicable to functional foods.	[46]
In vitro	Evidence from in vitro and in vivo studies with OHF suggests anti-cancer and anti-inflammatory activity on different cancer cells. Therefore, to confirm these biological properties, different OHF extracts were obtained and evaluated by the DPPH assay as well as analyzed their bioactive fractions to determine the cytotoxicity on human colon cancer (SW480) and breast cancer (MCF7) cells.	The EtOAc extract showed the highest cytotoxicity and regulated the expression of the proapoptotic protein Bax (bcl-2-associated X protein) in both cell lines. Likewise, the incubation of cells with this extract reduced the induction of inflammatory molecules (COX-2 and iNOS) mainly in SW480 cells. These results indicate that these cells are more susceptible to the bioactive compounds of the extract, which may be potentially preventive to cancer by modulating apoptotic markers and inhibiting inflammatory pathways.	[47]
In vitro	This study demonstrated the anti-inflammatory activity of Ind in an IBD model (i.e., intestinal Caco-2 cells stimulated by IL-1β; which induces ROS and iNOS to activate NF-κB and trigger the release of proinflammatory mediators).	Coincubation of cells with Ind (concentrations from 5 to 25 μM) prevented the release of proinflammatory cytokines (IL-6, IL-8, PGE2 and NO) in a dose-dependent manner. The expression of COX-2 and iNOS was also reduced. In conclusion, the findings indicate that betalain could modulate inflammatory processes in the intestine.	[48]

Table 3. Cont.

Type of Study	Objective and Characteristics	Results and Conclusion	Ref
Anti-Inflammatory Evidence			
In vivo	Using a rat model with acute inflammation, the protective activity of Ind from OFI was evaluated. Pleurisy was induced by injecting 0.2 mL of CRRG into the pleural cavity. Subsequently, the animals were sacrificed (4, 24 and 48 h) to collect exudates and analyze different inflammatory parameters.	Prior oral administration of Ind (0.5, 1, and 2 μmol/kg) decreased the volume of exudate and the number of leukocytes in the pleural cavity (95%). Likewise, the highest dose of Ind inhibited the expression of PGE2, NO, IL-1β, COX-2, iNOS and TNF-α. These results suggest that the pigment has the potential to improve health and prevent inflammatory disorders.	[49]
In vitro	In this research, natural flavonoid-rich concentrate (FRC) extracted from OFI juice was tested on intestinal inflammation induced in Caco-2 cells. Through an adsorption separation process, the FRC was obtained and its main components (isorhamnetin 3-O-rhamnose-rutinoside, isorhamnetin 3-O-rutinoside, and ferulic and piscidic acid) were identified. Subsequently, its effect (coincubation or preincubation) on the EOx induced by H_2O_2 in these human cells was evaluated.	Results showed that coincubation significantly attenuated ROS production; suggesting that bioactive compounds cannot freely cross the cell membrane. A similar phenomenon occurred in the inflammatory response, achieving a decrease in IL-8 secretion. FRC also reduced the expression of NO and TNF-α; however, there were no differences between pre and coincubation.	[50]
In vivo	Using the tail twisting and dipping test (Tail Flick) and the CRRG-induced paw edema test performed in albino Wistar rats, the antinociceptive and anti-inflammatory action of prickly pear juice extracted from O. elatio Mill was proved.	The results confirmed that the ED_{50} of the juice is between 0.919 and 9.282 mL/kg and that both pharmacological effects occur in a dose-dependent manner. Possibly, the betacyanins in the juice are responsible for exerting these potentials.	[51]
In vitro In vivo	Considering the biological properties of OFI attributed to different phytochemicals present in its composition, the effect of an extract and its main isorhamnetin glycosides on some inflammatory markers in vitro and in vivo was evaluated. Initially, the extract was obtained by alkaline hydrolysis, while the bioactive compounds were purified by preparative chromatography.	Using the croton oil-induced ear edema model, the expression of inflammatory markers was determined. The conclusion of the study is that the diglycoside isorhamnetin-glucosyl-rhamnoside (IGR) was the most significant bioactive compound. Both IGR and the extract suppressed the expression of NO, COX-2, TNF-α; IL-6; especially, NO production was decreased in LPS-stimulated RAW 264.7 cells.	[52]
In vitro	Filannino et al., (2016) studied the ability of lactic acid bacteria (Lactobacillus plantarum CIL6, POM1 and 1MR20, L. brevis POM2 and POM4, L. rossiae 2LC8 and Pediococcus pentosaceus CILSWE) to increase the antioxidant and anti-inflammatory potential of the pulp of OFI cladodes in intestinal Caco-2/TC7 cells. The pulp was fermented with the different strains of bacteria isolated from fruits and vegetables and the flavonoid profile was defined at the end of the study.	In conclusion, fermentation with L. plantarum and L. brevis favored the highest concentration of γ-amino butyric acid and had preservative effects on vitamin C and carotenoid levels. Using Caco-2/TC7 cells and after inducing oxidative EOx by IL-1β, an increase in antioxidant activity and an immunomodulatory effect was confirmed in the presence of the same bacteria. Kaempferol and isorhamnetin were identified as the main compounds responsible for the increase in radical scavenging activity.	[53]

Table 3. *Cont.*

Type of Study	Objective and Characteristics	Results and Conclusion	Ref
Anti-Inflammatory Evidence			
In vivo	*O. dillenii* (Nagphana) is a plant native to Central America traditionally used for its analgesic and anti-inflammatory effects. Unfortunately, there is little scientific evidence to support these properties. Therefore, in order to evaluate these properties, 12-O-tetradecanoyl-phorbol-13-acetate (TPA)-induced ear edema accompanied by histological studies of mice ear sections and phospholipase A2 (PLA2)-induced mice paw edema were used, parting from a MeOH extract. In parallel, levels of leukotriene B4 (LTB4) and ROS were also determined via HPLC and the levels of PGE2, TNF-α, IL-1β and -6 were measured by ELISA assay. Finally, its main α-pyrones [opuntiol (aglycone) and opuntioside glucoside (O-glucoside)] were isolated by vacuum liquid chromatography.	Both the extract and the α-pyrones reduced TPA-induced ear punch weight in a dose-dependent manner. IC_{50} values demonstrated a suppression of inflammatory features histologically observed. In addition, paw edema and peritonitis were also attenuated. In comparison to indomethacin and diclofenac sodium, opuntioside reduced PGE2 levels in the inflamed ear, which was 1.3 times better than opunthiol. However, opunthiol was more potent in reducing LTB4 levels in rat neutrophils and effectively suppressed ROS and cytokine (TNF-α, IL-1β and -6) levels. In general, the data justify the traditional use of *O. dillenii* and suggest that its CLDs possess anti-inflammatory properties through the inhibition of arachidonic acid metabolites and cytokines. Likewise, opunthiol can be considered a COX-2 inhibitor. However, opuntioside showed its selectivity towards PGE2 without affecting LTB4 levels.	[54] [55]
In vivo	The results obtained by Cho et al. [44] and Kim et al. [47] motivated to design this study to reveal the anti-nociceptive and anti-inflammatory effect of a MeOH extract of OHF stem. The first potential was evaluated by hot plate, acetic acid (AcOH)-induced writhing, and tail-flick assays in mice and rats. In contrast, the anti-inflammatory capacity was measured in tests of vascular permeability and paw edema induced by CRRG and serotonin. To confirm this effect, it was also measured using LPS-induced RAW 264.7 cells.	The extract inhibited writhing and delay reaction time of rodents to hot plate-induced thermal stimulation and tail-flick tests. Similarly, paw edema induced by CRRG and serotonin was attenuated. Evans blue concentration was significantly decreased in the vascular permeability test, confirming a strong anti-inflammatory effect. Finally, the n-butanol fraction reduced the expression of iNOS and NO in RAW 264.7 cells.	[56]
In vivo In vitro	The purpose of this study was to evaluate the antigenotoxic (using the Allium cepa test), analgesic and anti-inflammatory properties of *O. microdasys* in the post-flowering stage F3 (OMF3) by means of tests similar to previous studies.	The dose of the aqueous extract (100 mg/kg) decreased the writhing induced by AcOH and the edema produced by CRRG. Likewise, OMF3 had an antimutagenic potential against DNA damage mediated by H_2O_2.	[57]
In vivo	The fruit vinegars (FVs) available in Algeria are used in folk medicine for their hypolipidemic properties. The preventive effects of three types of FVs (PPFs from OFI, pomegranate and apple) against obesity-induced cardiomyopathy and their possible mechanisms of action were studied. Wistar rats on a high-fat diet (HFD) were treated with AcOH and different doses (3.5, 7.0 and 14.0 mL/kg) of the three types of FVs for 18 weeks. Subsequently, plasmatic biomarkers of inflammatory and cardiac enzymes were evaluated.	At the end of the treatment, the FVs decreased the increase in body weight induced by HFD, as well as the increase in plasma levels of fibrinogen and leptin. Furthermore, these treatments preserved the myocardial architecture and attenuated the cardiac fibrosis. These findings suggest that FVs (especially PPFs) can prevent obesity and its HFD-induced cardiac complications; This prevention is probably related to its anti-inflammatory and hypolipidemic properties.	[58]

Table 3. Cont.

Type of Study	Objective and Characteristics	Results and Conclusion	Ref
Anti-Inflammatory Evidence			
In vivo	In this study, we did a research on the effects of polyphenol-rich infusions of OFI cladodes on obesity-associated inflammation and ulcerative colitis induced by dextran sulfate sodium (DSS) in Swiss HFD mice. For 4 weeks, the animals received an infusion of 1.0% CLDs and were subjected to the administration of DSS for the following 7 days. At the end, the rodents were sacrificed to determine the levels of proinflammatory cytokines.	The infusion decreased the severity of inflammation associated with obesity and acute colitis exerted by DSS. The expression of TNF-α, and IL-6 in the colon and spleen was significantly reduced. Therefore, the anti-inflammatory potential of the infusion could be attributed to the polyphenols present in its chemical composition.	[59]
In vivo In vitro	The food industry maintains a continuous search for ingredients that provide beneficial properties to its products, whether considering their nutritional value, bioactivity, flavoring and/or technological aspects. The crude oil from the seed of *O. macrorhiza* Engelm (OMESO) is an ideal candidate for this type of ingredient, so it was chemically characterized and its in vitro and in vivo bioactivities were determined.	OMESO presented a low acidity index and oxidation stability; properties that favored its antioxidant and α-glucosidase inhibitory activity. In addition, it presented anti-inflammatory, analgesic and antibacterial potential (mainly against Gram-positive bacteria) and did not show any signs of acute toxicity in animals. This highlights its possible use in different food applications.	[60]
In vitro	The purpose of the study was to analyze the antioxidant and anti-inflammatory properties of OFI cladode extracts in BV-2 microglia cells. The inflammation associated with the activation of microglia in neuronal injury was achieved by exposing it to LPS and revealing its action on fatty acid β-oxidation and antioxidant enzymes in peroxisomes.	The different extracts showed an antioxidant effect through microglial catalase and an anti-inflammatory effect by reducing the production of NO LPS-dependent. These results suggest that the extracts have a neuroprotective activity through the induction of peroxisomal antioxidant activity.	[61]
Clinical study	Various scientific evidences have shown that products containing extracts of fruits and/or OFI cladodes have been favorably used to control obesity, lipid profile and glycemia. Therefore, the beneficial potential of a paste added with 3% of CLDs extract to human health was analyzed. A study was developed with 42 healthy volunteers who were administered 500 g/week of this paste for 30 days.	The paste demonstrated hypoglycemic, antioxidant and anti-inflammatory properties with a supposed effect on the aging process. Although the results were preliminary, there is a strong possibility that the paste would be considered an effective food for the prevention of some metabolic diseases.	[62]
Clinical study	As has been shown, dietary ingredients and food components are important factors in stimulating the immune system and preventing chronic inflammation responsible for some age-related diseases. In this randomized 2-period (2-week/period), controlled-feeding study involving 28 healthy patients, a diet supplemented with PPFs pulp (200 g/twice daily) on inflammatory plasmatic markers was explored.	At the end of the period, there was a reduction in proinflammatory markers (TNF-α, IL-8, IL-6, IL-1β, interferon-γ, and C-reactive protein (CRP)). Likewise, an increase in dermal carotenoids ("skin carotenoid score", a biomarker of the antioxidant status of the human body) was established. The observed modulation of both inflammatory markers and antioxidant balance suggests that prickly pear may be a beneficial food for human health.	[63]
In vivo	The purpose of the study was to characterize the phytochemical composition of a hydroalcoholic extract from PPFs seeds by High-Performance Liquid with Diode-Array Detection (HPLC-DAD) analysis and to evaluate its anti-inflammatory and/or analgesic activity in rodents using again the edema assay of legs induced by CRRG, the resistance exerted by AcOH and the tail dip test.	The extract dose (500 mg/kg) showed a significant increase in the mean latency of the TAIL FLICK test and a decrease in the mean number of twisting movements in the KOSTER test. As well as an important anti-inflammatory activity in the pattern of paw edema. Which suggests that OFI seeds may be a possible natural source of new active ingredients with therapeutic action.	[64]

Table 3. *Cont.*

Type of Study	Objective and Characteristics	Results and Conclusion	Ref
Anti-Inflammatory Evidence			
In vivo	Because different plants have been used as a source of effective and safe alternative of therapeutic agents for various ailments, the topical anti-inflammatory and antioxidant potential of pumpkin seed oil (*Cucurbita pepo*), flaxseed (*Linum usitatissimum*) and OFI were compared using the CRRG plantar edema test, hematological and biochemical analysis, EOx test and histological study.	All oils proved to be effective against acute inflammation. Animals treated, especially with OFI, revealed a significant decrease in hematological parameters (white blood cells and platelets) and concentrations of CRP and fibrinogen. Another observation was an increase in the activity of glutathione peroxidase (GPx), catalase (CAT) and superoxide dismutase (SOD) in the skin by reducing lipid peroxidation. The suggestion is that the anti-inflammatory effect of oils is related to the antioxidant properties of their bioactive compounds (polyunsaturated fatty acids, vitamin E and phytosterols).	[65]
In vitro	The study investigated betalain-rich extracts as a promising strategy for intestinal inflammation management. After obtaining the prickly pear betalain-rich extracts by means of a QuEChERS method and characterizing it by LC-DAD-ESI-MS/MS analysis, mainly betanin and indicaxanthin were found.	The extracts showed potent antioxidant and anti-inflammatory activities. Significant inhibition of ROS and inflammatory markers (IL-6, IL-8 and NO), even greater than dexamethasone, was observed in an in vitro model of IL-1β-induced intestinal inflammation.	[39]
In vivo	Due to the fact that exposure to Particulate matter (PM) can cause respiratory disorders. It was evaluated the protective effect of various extracts (water, ethanolic 30 and 50%) from OFI on airway inflammation associated with exposure to PM10D (diameter aerodynamic less than 10 µm). BALB/c mice were exposed to PM10D via intranasal tracheal injection three times over a period of 12 days and the extracts were administered orally for the same time.	All extracts suppressed neutrophil infiltration and the number of immune cells ($CD3^+/CD4^+$, $CD3^+/CD8^+$, and $Gr-1^+/CD11b$) in bronchoalveolar lavage fluid and lungs. They also decreased the expression of cytokines, TNF-α, COX-2 and different interleukins (IL-17, IL-1α, IL-1β, IL-5, IL-6). These results suggest that OFI extracts may be used to prevent and treat respiratory diseases.	[66]
Antiulcer evidence			
In vivo	The effects of dry stem powder of OFI var. Saboten (OFIS) were studied in models of gastric ulcers and injuries induced by ethanol (EtOH) and acetylsalicylic acid (ASA), respectively.	OFIS showed a significant inhibition at doses of 200 and 600 mg/kg for gastric lesions produced by both chemical compounds (EtOH and ASA). In the same sense, it was determined that OFIS do not affect gastric juice secretion, acid production and pH. Which indicates that they only have an inhibitory action on gastric injury without anti-ulcer activity.	[67]
Clinical study	Some evidence suggest that the severity of alcoholic hangovers is related to inflammation induced by impurities in the beverage and byproducts of EtOH metabolism. Therefore, to try to reduce it, natural agents have been used. In this double-blind, crossover trial, 64 volunteers consumed an OFI extract (1600 IU) 5 h before ingesting 1.75 g/EtOH/Kg for 4 h. At the end of the period, symptoms of alcoholic hangover were evaluated and blood and urine samples were obtained.	In general, the symptom index was reduced; especially, the presence of nausea, dry mouth and anorexia. It was also observed that CRP levels were associated with the hangover severity; which decreased with the previous intake of OFI. These data confirm that hangover symptoms are mainly due to the activation of inflammation and that OFI has a moderate effect in reducing hangover symptoms.	[68]

Table 3. Cont.

Type of Study	Objective and Characteristics	Results and Conclusion	Ref
	Antiulcer evidence		
In vivo	Considering the previous studies of Wiese et al. [68] as well as that OFI mucilage can slow down the rate of digestion and/or intestinal absorption, its effect (5 mg/kg per day) on the healing of gastritis induced by EtOH was evaluated in rats. Consequently, the lipid composition, expression of 5′-nucleotidase (membrane-associated ectoenzyme), cytosolic activity of alcohol dehydrogenase (ADH) in the gastric mucosal plasma membrane were determined. In addition, a histological analysis was included.	Results showed that EtOH induced loss of surface epithelium and infiltration of polymorphonuclear leukocytes. The activity of ADH and phosphatidylcholine (PC) diminished and the content of cholesterol in plasma membranes increased. In contrast, the administration of mucilage rapidly corrected these enzymatic changes and restored histological alterations and also reduced the damage to the plasmatic membranes of the gastric mucosa; showing an anti-inflammatory effect. Therefore, the beneficial action of the mucilage seems to be correlated with the stabilization of the plasmatic membranes of the damaged gastric mucosa. Molecular interactions between its monosaccharides and membrane phospholipids favor the healing process.	[69]
In vivo In vitro	Some phytochemical analyzes of the MeOH extract from the root of O. ficus-indica f. inermis (MEROfi) agree that it is rich in flavonoids and phenols, which is why its antioxidant activity was quantified in vitro (DPPH assay) and its gastroprotective capacity against EtOH-induced ulcer was evaluated in vivo.	The antiradical activity showed an EC_{50} of 119 µg/mL. Whereas the pretreatment of three doses of MEROfi (200, 400 and 800 mg/kg) reduced the ulcerative lesion at a rate of 82, 83 and 93% respectively. It also prevented the depletion of antioxidant enzymes, SOD, CAT and GPx.	[70]
In vivo In vitro	Since MEROfi demonstrated a positive effect on the ulcerative lesion [70], now we studied the same antiulcer action, antioxidant activity and reducing power of a 50% MeOH extract of the flowers obtained from the same species of Opuntia (MEFOfi).	Animals pretreated with MEFOfi (250, 500 and 1000 mg/kg) evidenced a dose-dependent protection against gastric damage caused by EtOH, avoiding deep epithelial necrotic lesions. The reduction of the ulcerative lesion was accompanied by an inhibition of lipid peroxidation, protein oxidation and restitution of the enzymatic activity of SOD and CAT. Possibly, the antiulcerogenic activity is attributed to a synergistic effect of antioxidant and antihistamine type.	[71]
In vivo	In this third approach, the research group of Alimi et al., (2010, 2011) explored the efficacy of administering two doses (2 and 4 mL/100g p.v.) of a fruit juice of O. ficus indica f. inermis (FJOfi) for 90 days on the reversal of oxidative damage induced by chronic EtOH intake in Wistar rat erythrocytes and with the use of HPLC, they determined the content of phenols and flavonoids.	HPLC analysis revealed high concentrations of phenolic acids and flavonoids. On the other hand, EtOH markedly decreased the activity of SOD and CAT. These changes in the antioxidant capacity of erythrocytes were accompanied by a greater oxidative modification of lipids and proteins (increase in carbonyl groups). In contrast, both doses of FJOfi significantly reversed decreases in enzymatic and non-enzymatic antioxidant parameters in erythrocytes. The protective effect of FJOfi highlights the inhibition of free radical chain reactions induced by EtOH.	[72]

Table 3. *Cont.*

Type of Study	Objective and Characteristics	Results and Conclusion	Ref
Antiulcer evidence			
In vivo	In order to develop this study, pectin was isolated from peel (WNPE) and pulp (WNPU) of *O. microdasys* var. rufida's (OMR) and its main polysaccharides were characterized by gas chromatography coupled to mass spectrometer (GC-MS), nuclear magnetic resonance (1H NMR) and Fourier transform infrared spectroscopy (FTIR). Subsequently, the biopolymers were administered intraperitoneally (50-100 mg/kg) to mice to determine their gastroprotective, analgesic and anti-inflammatory effects.	The results showed that WNPE and WNPU are mainly composed of uronic acids and neutral sugars (such as arabinose, galactose, rhamnose, and mannose). A significant gastroprotective effect was observed with both biopolymers, reducing the presence of gastric ulcer at a dose of 100 mg/kg (between 67 and 82%). Regarding the analgesic and anti-inflammatory action, tests with chemical stimuli (writhing test) and thermal stimuli (hot plate test) determined a dose-dependent effect (especially between 50 and 100 mg/kg)	[73]
In vivo	The objective was to evaluate the protective effect of *O. dillenii* Haw fruit juice. (FJOdHw) on AcOH-induced ulcerative colitis in rats. FJOdHw was administered orally for 7 consecutive days before inducing colitis on the eighth day. Subsequently, biochemical tests and histopathological examinations of the colon were performed to assess the damage.	Pretreatment with FJOdHw (2.5 and 5 mL/kg) attenuated macroscopic damage and showed significantly reduced levels of myeloperoxidase, malondialdehyde, and serum lactate dehydrogenase. The results suggest that the antiulcer effect may be due phenols, flavonoids and betalains present in FJOdHw.	[74]
In vivo	As shown in the evidence included in this table, the different OFI extracts have been used in traditional folk medicine for various purposes, including action on inflammatory processes. This last experiment explored the prophylactic effect of an OFI fruit peel petroleum ether extract (FPPEE) against irradiation-induced colitis in rats.	A previous analysis with gas chromatography and mass spectrometry (GC/MS) identified 33 compounds in the unsaponifiable fraction and 15 fatty acid methyl esters in the saponifiable part. Of these, 13 terpenes and sterols were isolated; and 10 of their compounds had not been isolated before from any part of this species. On the other hand, FPPEE pretreatment decreased elevated levels of MPO, NO, COX-2, TNF-α, NF-κB, IL-10, and SOD. The conclusion was that FPPEE can limit the colonic complications generated by irradiation, possibly due to its antioxidant and anti-inflammatory properties.	[75]

4.2. Neuroprotective Effect

Neurodegenerative disease (ND) is a progressive dysfunction and/or loss of neuronal structure and function, generally irreversible, that alters intellectual and cognitive faculties. This disorder occurs in various diseases that affect the central nervous system (CNS) and may be acute or chronic [76–79]. The first case refers to a condition where neurons are rapidly damaged and can die in response to a sudden insult or traumatic event (such as head injury, stroke, traumatic brain injury, brain hemorrhage, or ischemic brain damage). On the other hand, chronic neurodegeneration is a state where a degenerative process that begins slowly and worsens over time due to multifactorial causes, is experienced; resulting in the progressive and irreversible destruction of specific neuronal populations. Among the most significant chronic neurodegenerative disorders are Alzheimer's disease (AD), Huntington's disease, Parkinson's disease (PD), and amyotrophic lateral sclerosis. As mentioned, the causes of ND are multifactorial and are associated with different types of biological mechanisms, which in general can be summarized as: (a) oxidative stress (EOx), (b) neuroinflammation, (c) excitotoxicity, (d) mitochondrial dysfunction, (e) induction of apoptosis and (f) abnormal protein folding and aggregation [76–79].

Specifically, imbalanced ROS production and poor antioxidant defense (endogenous and/or exogenous) cause EOx resulting in cell damage, impaired DNA repair system, and mitochondrial dysfunction; accelerating the neurodegenerative process. On the other hand, neuroinflammation involves both the innate and adaptive CNS immune systems, playing an important role in the pathophysiology of DN. Since microglia are the main components of the innate immune defense, and if there are pathological changes within the CNS, they secrete inflammatory mediators (cytokines, chemokines, COX-2), which activate astrocytes to induce a secondary inflammatory response in a population of neurons that respond to a survival process [76–79].

Excitotoxicity [neuronal death caused by excessive or prolonged activation of glutamate (Glu) receptors by excitatory amino acids or CNS excitotoxins] is also involved in degenerative pathogenesis. Excitotoxins that bind to Glu receptors, as well as pathologically high levels of their release, are known to cause toxicity by allowing a rapid entry of calcium ions (Ca^{2+}) into the cell, activating various Ca^{2+}-dependent enzymes (iNOS, phospholipases, lipase endonucleases, xanthine oxidase, protein phosphatases, proteases, and protein kinase). These enzymes continue to damage cellular structures (such as components of the cytoskeleton, membrane, and DNA) and/or generate ROS, mitochondrial dysfunction, and other inflammatory responses, which together lead to neuronal death [76–79].

Finally, combining apoptosis (a highly regulated form of cell death that is triggered by intrinsic and extrinsic signals) and the mitochondria (site of oxidative phosphorylation and cellular respiration), a significant role is played in maintaining a low concentration of Ca^{2+} cytosolic [76–79]. Excessive uptake of this ion and generation of ROS cause the opening of mitochondrial permeability transition pores, inducing matrix inflammation, mitochondrial uncoupling, and membrane rupture that releases cytochrome-c (Cyt-c) and apoptosis inducing factor. Cyt-c, a caspase-dependent pathway, binds to apoptotic protease-activating factor 1 and procaspase-9 to form an apoptosome complex and activate the caspase-3 pathway, producing apoptotic neuronal death. While the apoptosis-inducing factor, a caspase-independent mechanism, moves to the nucleus and induces the DNA fragmentation, chromatin condensation and subsequently cell collapse [76–79].

Progressive degeneration and/or neuronal death causes characteristic symptoms such as problems with movement (ataxia) or alterations in cognitive functioning (dementia), and since, unfortunately, most NDs have no cure, conventional treatments focuson improving symptoms and relieving pain. For example, in individuals with PD there are low concentrations of dopamine (DA) in the brain, so the main drugs (Carbidopa-levodopa, Dopamine agonists, Inhibitors of the enzyme monoamine oxidase type B or Inhibitors of catechol -O-methyltransferase), mimic, increase or replace this neurotransmitter (NT) [76–79]. In the case of AD, cholinesterase inhibitors are prescribed to patients with mild and/or moderate symptoms to prevent the breakdown of Acetylcholine (Ach), a brain neurotransmitter that is related to memory and thought. Unfortunately, these medications often lose their therapeutic effect over time. Another example is the so-called "disease-modifying agent", "aducanumab", a human antibody that targets β-amyloid protein (Aβ) to reduce brain lesions (amyloid plaques) associated with AD [76–79].

Various studies have tried to elucidate mechanisms and possible therapeutic objectives to combat NDs, in order to avoid neuronal damage and preserve the integrity and functionality of these cells; all resultingin a concept known as Neuroprotection. A strategy that includes three approaches: (1) before the onset of the disease to avoid any risk factors might affect the neurons. (2) during the progression of the disease to avoid the spread of the lesion from one neuron to another; and (3) to try to delay and /or stop progressive neurodegeneration [76–79].

Again, natural products and their bioactive compounds are an excellent source of neuroprotective agents for the treatment of ND. The early agents studied limited their mechanism of action to intervene in NT receptors through agonists and antagonists; the best known example was caffeine, adenosine A2 receptor antagonist, which has been shown to protect dopaminergic neurons in an experimental model of PD induced by 1-methyl-4-phenyl-1,2,3,6-tetrahydropyridine. It is now known that microglial cells also express the A2 receptor, and A2 receptor antagonist or caffeine can reduce the activation of these cells. Therefore, drinking coffee, maintaining a healthy lifestyle and having moderate physical activity has been considered a neuroprotective strategy, and added to the fact that A2 antagonists can protect neurons and minimize the activation of microglial cells, the field of research of phytotherapy continues to be active in the search for new and innovative neuroprotective agents [76–79].

Since multifactorial pathological mechanisms (EOx, neuroinflammation, excitotoxicity, mitochondrial dysfunction, and apoptosis) are associated with neurodegeneration, current research look for multiplemechanisms of action that intervene in the complexity of the disease with natural neuroprotective agents instead of looking for a single biological objective.

Table 4 shows the main evidence of the neuroprotective effect of *Opuntia* spp. Since the year 2000, when the exploration of this scientific field began, most of the studies have been carried out in vitro (mouse cortical cells, primary cultured rat cortical cells, PC12 cells) where extracts of CLDs and prickly pear fruits have been evaluated. Some phytochemicals (Quercetin, quercetin 3-methyl ether, indicaxanthin, polysaccharides) from 6 species of *Opuntia*; where the most studied are OFI and OFI var. Saboten (OFIS). Basically, neuronal damage and toxicity have been induced by different agents and/or substances; such as xanthine/xanthine oxidase (X/XO), FeCl2/ascorbicFeCl2/ascorbic acid, N-methyl-d-aspartate (NMDA), kainate (KA), oxygen-glucose deprivation (OGD, LPS, AlCl3 and Aβ. Although, probably, the neuroprotective effect of *Opuntia* spp. can be carried out through multiple mechanisms, most authors agree that the antioxidant capacity is the most significant and/or representative [80–93].

Table 4. Scientific evidence of the neuroprotective effect of *Opuntia* spp.

Type of Study	Objective and Characteristics	Results and Conclusion	Ref
In vitro	The author examined the inhibitory action of two concentrations of OFI methanolic extracts (10 µg/mL and 1 mg/mL) on xanthine/xanthine oxidase (X/XO)-, FeCl2/ascorbicFeCl2/ascorbic acid- and arachidonic acid (AA)- induced neurotoxicity in mouse cortical cell cultures.	The highest concentration showed a reduction of 89 and 100% of the toxic effect exerted by X/XO and FeCl2/ascorbicFeCl2/ascorbic acid, respectively. While the neuronal injury induced by AA decreased by 22%. Presumably, OFI exerts protection against certain neuronal injuries caused by the excessive presence of free radicals.	[80]
In vitro	Quercetin, (+)-dihydroquercetin, and quercetin 3-methyl ether were isolated from EtOAc fractions originating from OFIS fruits and stems to determine their protective effect against H_2O_2 and X/XO induced neuronal injury in primary cultured rat cortical cells.	Results indicate that all flavonoids decreased neuronal injury and significantly inhibited lipid peroxidation. However, quercetin had the best effect, with an IC_{50} between 4 and 5 µg/mL. It is suggested that these active ingredients have a neuroprotective action related to their antioxidant capacity.	[81]
In vitro In vivo	In the first study, a methanolic extract of OFI (MEOFI) was tested against neuronal injury induced by NMDA, KA and oxygen-glucose deprivation (OGD) in cortical cell culture from mouse. Subsequently, it was evaluated its protective effect in the CA1 region of the hippocampus against neuronal damage caused by global ischemia in gerbils.	The treatment of the extract (30, 300 and 1000 µg/mL) inhibited the neurotoxicity induced by NMDA, KA and OGD in a dose-dependent manner in cortical cells. Likewise, in animals previously treated with MEOFI (0.1, 1.0 and 4.0 g/kg, p.o.) every 24 h for 3 days and 4 weeks, the neuronal damage in the hippocampus was reduced by approximately 35%;suggesting that preventive administration of MEOFI can alleviate excitotoxic damage induced by global ischemia.	[82]
In vitro	Considering that high concentrations of ROS, especially superoxide anion (O_2^-) and peroxynitrite ($ONOO^-$), product of the NO reaction, contribute to the oxidative toxicity generated in NDs. The neuroprotective activity of two butanolic fractions prepared from the 50% ethanolic extract of OFIS stems was evaluated.	Both the stem fraction (SK OFB901) and its hydrolysis product (SK OFB901H) inhibited the NO production in microglia activated by LPS in a dose-dependent manner. In addition, they suppressed iNOS mRNA expression in microglia cells observed by western blot analysis and RT-PCR. These results demonstrate that the neuroprotective property of OFI is through the reduction of NO by activated microglial cells and the uptake of $ONOO^-$	[83]

Table 4. Cont.

Type of Study	Objective and Characteristics	Results and Conclusion	Ref
In vitro	The results obtained by Lee et al., (2006) [83] motivated another experiment with the SK OFB901 fraction to determine its action on neuronal lesions induced by EOx, excitotoxins and Aβ in primary cultured rat cortical cells. In addition, through cell-free bioassays, its antioxidant potential was determined.	SK OFB901 inhibited H_2O_2- and X/XO-induced neuronal damage and Glu-, NMDA- and KA-induced excitotoxicity. Likewise, the neurotoxicity exerted by Aβ and the lipid peroxidation initiated by Fe^{2+} and L-ascorbic acid in rat brain homogenates were attenuated. All these data indicate that the butanolic fraction has antioxidant and neuroprotective capacities through multiple mechanisms, which imply the possible application to prevent and treat NDs.	[84]
In vitro In vivo	Huang et al., (2008, 2009) carried out two experiments in order to determine the neuroprotective effects of Cactus polysaccharides (CP) extracted from OdHw. In the first, this capacity was evaluated on the damage induced by OGD and reoxygenation (REO) in the cortical and hippocampal slices of rat brain. Cell viability and quantification of cell survival were quantified using the 2, 3, 5-triphenyl tetrazolium chloride (TTC) method and The fluorescence of propidium iodide (PI) staining, respectively. Subsequently, they analyzed the mechanisms of ischemia-reperfusion injury of the middle cerebral artery in Sprague-Dawley rats and the damage induced by EOx in PC12 cells.	Both studies demonstrated that: (a) The ischemic condition decreased cell viability and increased lactate dehydrogenase (LDH) release, (b) CP protected brain slices from the OGD injury, decreased PI intensity and LDH release. Likewise, it prevented the increase in iNOS activity, (c) With a dose of 200 mg/kg of CP, the volume of the infarction and the neuronal loss in the cerebral cortex of rats were reduced, and d) Finally, the in vitro conditions confirmed that the CP pretreatment significantly increases cell viability, protects PC12 cells from H_2O_2 damage, and reduces apoptosis and ROS production. The results suggest that the protective mechanism of CP may be partially mediated by the NO/iNOS system and induced by the OGD aggression. In addition, it can be considered a candidate compound for the treatment of ischemia and DN induced by EOx	[85] [86]
In vitro	The objective was to determine the chemical constituent of O. Milpa Alta polysaccharides (MAP) and its neuroprotective potential in an in vitro model of cerebral ischemic injury. By using the gas chromatograph and GC-MS it was observed that MAP mainly contained galactose, arabinose, rhamnose and glucose.	On the other hand, the three concentrations of MAP (0.5, 5, and 50 µg/mL) increased the cell viability [methylthiazolyltetrazolium (MTT) assay], inhibited LDH-induced cellular cytotoxicity, suppressed ROS production and decreased intracellular Ca^{2+} concentrations; significantly preventing neuronal cell death.	[87]
In vitro	Inflammation associated with microglia activation in neuronal injury can be achieved by exposure to LPS. Thus, using 4 different serotypes of LPS, a differential effect related to β-oxidation of fatty acids and antioxidant enzymes in peroxisomes was identified.	Using various OFI cladode extracts, an antioxidant effect was demonstrated through microglial catalase and an anti-inflammatory effect by reducing the production of NO LPS-dependent; suggesting that these extracts have a neuroprotective activity through the induction of peroxisomal antioxidant activity.	[61]
In vitro	A hallmark of age-related neurodegenerative proteinopathies is the misfolding and aggregation of proteins, usually Aβ in AD and α-synuclein (α-syn) in PD, which in soluble oligomeric structures are often highly neurotoxic. Using two different experimental models, we investigated whether prickly pear extracts from OFI (PPEOFI) alleviated the neurodegenerative effects of AD and PD in yeast (Saccharomyces cerevisiae) and fly (Drosophila melanogaster).	Pretreatment with PPEOFI in the culture medium increased the viability of yeast expressing the Arctic mutant Aβ42 (E22G). Likewise, dietary supplementation of PPEOFI dramatically improved the lifespan and behavioral signs of flies with brain-specific expression of wild-type Aβ42 (late-onset AD model) or the Arctic variant of Aβ42 (early-onset AD model). Increased fly survival was observed in a PD model where the human α-syn A53T mutant is expressed. These findings indicate that PPEOFI interferes with the neurodegenerative mechanisms of AD and PD. Probably they inhibit both Aβ42 and α-syn fibrillogenesis by accumulating remodeled oligomeric aggregates that are less toxic to the lipid membrane.	[88]

Table 4. Cont.

Type of Study	Objective and Characteristics	Results and Conclusion	Ref
In vitro	The purpose of the study was to detect the specific areas of the brain where Ind, derived from OFI, can be localized in significant quantities after an oral administration and to highlight its possible local effects on the excitability of individual neuronal units.	HPLC analysis of brain tissue after ingestion of 2 μmol/kgInd indicates that it accumulates primarily in the cortex, hippocampus, diencephalon, brainstem, and cerebellum. Using electrophysiological recordings and microiontophoretic technique, its influence on neuronal firing rate was evaluated, confirming that neuronal bioelectrical activity is modulated after the local injection of Ind. These findings constitute the justification to explore the biological mechanisms through which bioactive compounds could modulate the neuronal function with a relapse in the cognitive brain process and neurodegenerative conditions.	[89]
In vitro	Different studies agree that Ind has anti-inflammatory and neuromodulatory effects. Therefore, discovering new physiological targets plays an important role in understanding its biochemical mechanism. In this regard, combined reverse pharmacophore mapping, reverse docking, and a search of some databases identified Inositol Trisphosphate 3-Kinase, Glutamate carboxypeptidase II, Leukotriene-A4 hydrolase, Phosphoserine phosphatase, Phosphodiesterase 4D, and Kainate receptor (GluK1 isoform) as potential targets for indicaxanthin.	The results suggest that these targets are involved in neuromodulation and inflammatory regulation, normally expressed in the CNS and in cancerous tissues (especially breast, thyroid and prostate). Furthermore, this study provides insights into the dynamic interactions of Ind at the binding site of target proteins, through molecular dynamics simulations and MM-GBSA.	[90]
In vitro	Although several studies have reported that OFIS has antidiabetic, antiasthmatic and analgesic properties; its action mode is not clearly described. Therefore, the anti-inflammatory and neuroprotective capacity of an ethanolic extract (EEOFIS) was analyzed individually or in combination with Vitamin C (Vit C). NO, iNOS and COX-2 levels were evaluated in macrophage cells. In addition, a cell viability assay was performed to confirm its protection against Aβ-induced neurotoxicity.	At the conclusion of the study, elevated levels of cAMP response element-binding protein were found and brain-derived neurotrophic factor expression upon evaluation of the regulation of synaptic plasticity by EEOFIS in SH-SY5Y neuroblastoma cells. A synergistic effect was also confirmed in the combined treatment with Vit C. These results suggest that EEOFIS can improve the cognitive function through an anti-inflammatory response, cell protection and regulation of synaptic plasticity.	[91]
In vivo	In this work, 37 OFI metabolites were characterized using HPLC-MS/MS and the main polysaccharides of its fruit pulp and CLDs were identified, as well as their neuroprotective activity under in vitro conditions of AD induced by AlCl3.	All the tested extracts presented antioxidant activity; however, the most representative effects were for those from CDLs (possibly due to their high phenolic content). A significant decrease in learning and memory impairment induced by AlCl3 was observed (Passive avoidance test). In addition, elevated brain levels of proinflammatory cytokines (NF-κB and TNF-α) were reduced.	[92]

Table 4. Cont.

Type of Study	Objective and Characteristics	Results and Conclusion	Ref
In vitro	Organic extracts of spines, flowers, roots and fruits of *O. microdasys* var. rufida (OMR) and *O. leptocaulis* (OL) were studied for their phytochemical composition and their anticholinesterase, cytotoxic and neuroprotective activity. The catalase test result was that the extracts have a potent antioxidant activity. The anticholinesterase activity was determined by butyrylcholinesterase (BChE) and revealed that all extracts were endowed with excellent inhibitory efficacy against BChE; however, the EtOAc extract of OMR flowers was the most significant.	On the other hand, the neuroprotective effect of the extracts was evaluated against the toxicity induced by Aβ in PC12 cell lines; confirming that the MeOH extract of OMR spines was the one that increased cell viability the most (approximately 80%). The MTT assay showed that the extracts presented an evident cytotoxic activity on HeLa cells. Finally, the column chromatography of the EtOAc extract of OMR flowers identified 5 flavonol glycosides (isorhamnetin-3-O-α-rhamnopyranosyl-(1 → 2)[α-rhamnopyranosyl-(1 → 6)]-β galactopyranoside, quercetin-3-O-β-pyranogalactoside (hyperoside, isorhamnetin-3-O-β-galacto (1 → 6)-α-rhamnoside, isorhamnetin-3-O-β-glucoside and kaempferol-3-O-β-arabinoside.	[93]

4.3. Antiviral and Antimicrobial Effects

Despite the incredible progress in human medicine, Viral Infections (VI) continue to be responsible for various chronic and acute diseases. Diseases such as Acquired Immunodeficiency Syndrome (AIDS), hepatitis, and respiratory syndromes, especially the one caused by the severe acute respiratory syndrome virus type-2 (SARS-CoV-2) are associated with high rates of morbidity and mortality [94,95]. Again, natural products are a rich source of bioactive compounds with possible antiviral effects; thus, identifying them is of critical importance. A wide variety of phytochemicals, including coumarins, flavonoids, terpenoids, organosulfur compounds, lignans, polyphenols, saponins, proteins, and peptides, have been found to influence cell functions, membrane permeability, and viral replication. Therefore, natural-based pharmacotherapy may be a good alternative for VI treatment. Antiviral agents can be classified according to their chemical nature or their activity against viral proteins and/or host cellular proteins. Particularly, the antiviral activity can be exerted based on its ability to inhibit any viral entry, viral DNA and RNA synthesis, as well as viral replication/reproduction. Differences in viral structure and replication cycle are crucial to the design of any antiviral medication [94,95].

The antiviral activity of phytochemicals can be established by different biological assays, commonly used to assess cytotoxicity, cytopathic effect, and the ability to block viral cell-to-cell propagation. Purified natural products are considered a rich resource for the development of new antiviral drugs. However, their extraction and isolation can be a difficult process, since many bioactive compounds are present in low concentration in the natural source and due to their complex chemical structures they are not easy to synthesize. In addition, the majority of the natural compounds are used as unpurified crude extracts, which makes it very important to isolate each biomolecule individually and to establish their pharmacokinetics (absorption, distribution, metabolism, excretion), therapeutic effects, dose and possible toxicity events [94,95].

Among the isolated bioactive compounds with recognized antiviral action is rutin (known as quercetin-3-rutinoside), a flavonoid glycoside effective against avian influenza virus, herpes simplex virus 1 and 2 (HSV-1, HSV-2) and parainfluenza -3 virus [94,95]. Quercetin, an aglycone of rutin, has demonstrated its therapeutic potential against influenza A virus (IFV-A), rhinovirus, dengue virus type 2 (DENV-2), HSV-1, poliovirus type 1 (PV- 1), adenovirus, Epstein-Barr virus, Mayaro virus, Japanese encephalitis virus, Respiratory Syncytial Virus (RSV), and Hepatitis C virus (HCV) [94,95]. Among the mechanisms of action of quercetin are limiting the activity of some thermal shock proteins involved in viral translation (Internal Ribosome Entry Site or IRES) mediated by the non-structural protein 5A (NS5A), inhibiting NS3 protease and viral replication of HCV, reducing endocytosis, blocking viral genome transcription and rhinovirus protein synthesis, and decreasing DENV-2 replication [94,95]. Other flavonoids, such as myricetin (3,3′,4′,5,5′,7-hexahydroxyflavone), quercetagetin (3,3′,4′,5,6,7-hexahydroxyflavone), and Baicalein (5,6,7-trihydroxyflavone) block the reverse transcriptase of the Rauscher murine leukemia virus and the human immunodeficiency virus (HIV). Finally, Baicalin (the glucuronide of baicalein) inhibits the synthesis of DNA and viral proteins of the hepatitis B virus (HBV); it is also active against HIV, DENV, RSV, enterovirus, and Newcastle disease virus [94,95].

Thus far, only three investigations have evaluated the antiviral effect of *Opuntia* spp. In the first, administration of an OS stem extract to mice, horses, and humans inhibited the intracellular replication of several DNA and RNA viruses, such as HSV-2, RSV, HIV, IFV-A, equine herpes and pseudorabies virus. Although a viral inactivation at the extracellular level was also observed, there were no answers about the possible inhibitory components of the extract [96]. On the other hand, Bouslama et al., (2011) analyzed the inhibitory effect of two extracts (aqueous and/or EtOH) from OFI stems on the replication of two enveloped viruses (HSV-2 and IFV-A) and a non-enveloped virus (PV-1). Given that only the EtOH extract showed significant antiviral activity in vitro, two stem chlorophyll derivatives (pheophorbide a and pyropheophorbide a) were isolated; which demonstrated a virucidal effect only on both enveloped viruses. These findings suggest that both phytochemicals could recognize specific glycoproteins of enveloped viruses, preventing their binding to the host cell receptors and inhibiting VI [97]. In the latest study, an antiviral protein (named Opuntin B) from OFI was purified; which shows the total degradation of genomic RNA of the plant and causes a displacement of the electrophoretic mobility of the RNAs of the cucumber mosaic virus (CMV). Using CMV as prey protein and Opuntin B as bait protein, far western dot blot analysis showed no interaction between antiviral protein and viral coat protein [98].

On the other hand, microbial pathogens (MP) can enter a host using different transmission mechanisms, which are generally classified as: (a) direct contact (cutaneous lesions, urogenital tract and/or sexual transmission), (b) indirect contact (contaminated hands and/or inanimate instruments), and (c) airway (inhalation of droplets of different diameters through the respiratory tract and/or ingestion of contaminated food or drink). Regardless of the route of transmission, MPs are responsible for producing various diseases that generate public health problems and cause excessive economic costs [99,100]. Unfortunately, antimicrobial resistance has also become an increasingly important and pressing global problem, as of the millions of people who acquire bacterial infections, approximately 70% of cases involve strains that are resistant at least to one drug [99–101]. Therefore, in response to this problem, pharmaceutical companies are focusing their efforts on improving antimicrobial agents; however, the researchers acknowledge that they are reaching the end game in terms of alterations to their chemical structures. For this reason, natural products can be a rich source of anti-infective agents that work at different target sites and can replace synthetic compounds [99–101].

Obtaining natural antimicrobial agents also has an impact on food preservation to prevent disease transmission after ingestion of contaminated food and/or beverages. These bioconservatives must keep and preserve nutritional values and/or guarantee food safety; all these aspects are not usually met with synthetic conservation methods (nitrates, benzoates, sulfites, sorbates, formaldehyde) that despite being approved by government agencies continue to threaten health, by frequently inducing allergic reactions.

Some studies suggest that natural antimicrobials may be safer than synthetic ones; therefore, obtaining anti-infective agents from plants and algae can be an alternative strategy to develop new drugs that are safer, more effective and avoid bacterial resistance [99,100].

In general, the mechanisms of action of natural antimicrobials include disruption of the cytoplasmic membrane, inhibition of nucleic acid synthesis, decrease in proton motive force, and inhibition of energy metabolism (ATP depletion) [99,100]. Most antimicrobials derived from plants have been found in herbs and spices. These agents have different structural configurations that provide their antimicrobial action; the presence of hydroxyl groups (-OH) is believed to be the main cause of this property. Possibly due to the interaction of the -OH groups with the bacterial cell membrane that alters its structures and causes the leakage of its components. The antioxidant capacity is usually linked to the antimicrobial effect, which together (antioxidant/-OH groups) makes the compound more effective [99,100].

Currently, more than 1300 plants have shown antimicrobial activity, from which more than 30,000 compounds with this characteristic have been extracted. Plants and herbs (such as oregano, garlic, parsley, sage, coriander, rosemary, lemongrass, ginger, and chili), spices (cinnamon, cloves, curry, and pepper), and some essential oils (such as citral) have been shown to be effective against *Escherichia coli*, *Listeria monocytogenes*, *Campylobacter* spp., *Staphylococcus aureus*, *Salmonella* spp., *Pseudomonas aeruginosa*, *Vibrio cholerae* and *Bacillus cereus* [99–103]. Among the most relevant antimicrobial phytochemicals are thiosulfinates, glucosinolates, phenols, organic acids, flavonoids and saponins. However, those with the highest activity are phenols (terpenes, aliphatic alcohols, aldehydes, ketones, acids and isoflavonoids [99–103].

Although Ginestra et al., (2009) indicated that cladodes of *O. ficus indica* contain glucose, kaempherol and isorhamnetin, and apparently do not have antimicrobial activity, even after an enzymatic treatment; it was not a reason to rule out the development of further investigations [104]. In this sense, Sánchez et al., (2010) measured the synthesis of ATP, minimal bactericidal concentrations (MBCs), and changes in the integrity and potential of the *Vibrio cholerae* membrane after exposing it to methanolic, ethanolic and aqueous extracts of OFI var. Villanueva L. The three types of extracts were active against the bacteria (MBCs ranged between 0.5 and 3.0 mg/mL), were able to break cell membranes and cause an increase in their permeability [105].

These results opened the studies to the control of bacterial contamination in food and subsequently, the antimicrobial activity of non-polar extracts (petroleum ether and Chl) and polar extracts (MeOH and water) from the dried stems of OdHw and rhizome of *Zingiber officinale* were compared with *Bacillus subtilis*, *Staphylococcus aureus* and *Salmonella typhi*. The results also confirmed that this last bacterium is resistant to all extracts of both plants. Unlike *E. coli* and *B. subtilis* that were inhibited with the ether and chloroform extracts of OdHw, as well as with the MeOH and aqueous extracts of *Z. officinale*. These data suggest that the beneficial property of both plants is affected by the polarity of the extraction solvent [106].

In general, the studies developed to date (Table 5) suggest that different extracts (Hx, MeOH, EtOH, Chl, EtOAc, acetone (Ace), aqueous, dichloromethane (DCM) and mucilage) and/or oils from PPFs, CLDs (ripe and nopalitos), flowers, seeds and fruit peel especially obtained from OFI, OdHw, *O. xoconostle* (OX), *O. albicarpa* (OA), *O. stricta*, *O. microdasys* (OMs) and *O. macrorhiza* Engelm (OME) have shown antimicrobial action against Gram-positive bacteria (such as *Staphylococcus aureus*, *Staphylococcus haemolyticus*, *Listeria Monocytogenes*, *Bacillus cereus*, *Bacillus subtilis*, *Bacillus thuringiensis*, *Enterococcus faecalis*, *Streptococcus pneumoniae* and *Micrococcus flavus*) and Gram-negative bacteria (*Escherichia coli*, *Vibrio parahaemolyticus*, *Klebsiella pneumoniae*, *Pseudomonasaeruginosa*, *Pseudomonas fluorescens*, *Salmonella typhimurium*, *Acinetobacter lwoffii*, *Acinetobacter baumannii*, *Campylobacter coli*, *Campylobacter jejuni*, *Porphyromonas gingivalis*, *Prevotella intermedia*, *Enterobacter cloacae*, *Stenotrophomonas maltophilia*, and *Neisseria gonorrhoeae*) [107–129].

Table 5. Scientific evidence of the antimicrobial effects of *Opuntia* spp.

Type of Study	Objective and Characteristics	Results and Conclusion	Ref
In vitro In vivo	The food industry is continually looking for ingredients that provide advantageous properties to food products, especially protecting their nutritional value. Because crude oils are examples of this type of ingredient, the in vitro and in vivo bioactivities of *O. macrorhiza* Engelm (OMESO) seed oil were chemically characterized and evaluated.	OMESO presented a low acidity index, oxidation stability and a high content of unsaturated fatty acids. It also showed antioxidant activity, cytotoxicity against human tumor cell lines and antibacterial capacity, especially against Gram (+) species such as *S. aureus*, *E. faecalis*, *B. cereus* and *L. monocytogenes*. The latter was the one with the greatest diameter of inhibition. These properties and its low toxicity in animals favor the use of OMESO compared to synthetic bioactive agents (ampicillin, amphotericin B) that induce greater adverse effects.	[60]
In vitro	The aim of the study was to determine the antimicrobial effects of Mexican medicinal plant extracts, including OX, against some pathogenic bacteria [both Gram (+) and Gram (−) species] using the disk diffusion assay. The cytotoxicity of the extracts on human breast cancer cells (MCF-7) was also evaluated with the MTT assay.	Most of the extracts evidenced this beneficial effect. However, OX presented the best antimicrobial capacity against *Acinetobacter lwoffii* and more resistant strains such as *A. baumannii*, *S. aureus* and *S. haemolyticus*. Although, unfortunately, it did not show any cytotoxic action on MCF-7 cells; unlike the extract of *Justicia spicigera* and *Phoradendron serotinum*.	[107]
In vitro	Adherence and cytotoxicity of *Campylobacter* spp to host mucosa are critical steps in inducing bacterial gastroenteritis. The proposal is to use natural food products to reduce its pathogenesis. With that purpose, the bactericidal potential of 28 plant species (including OFI) on the growth of *C. jejuni* and *C. coli* was analyzed.	The OFI extract was one of the most effective against both microorganisms at MBCs of 0.3, 0.5, 0.4 and 2.0 mg/mL. This same extract also diminished the adherence and cytotoxicity of bacteria on Vero cells. Thus, OFI may be a candidate for the control of food contamination by Campylobacter and/or as a feed supplement to reduce the prevalence of this bacterium on farms.	[108]
In vitro	In this investigation, the antimicrobial activity of an extract of PPFs from OX against four strains of *Escherichia coli* O157: H7 was determined, by means of brain-heart infusion (BHI) medium to analyze bacterial growth over time and in agar well diffusion.	The results showed that the extract had a significant inhibitory effect at concentrations of 4.0, 6.0, 8.0 and 10% at 8 h of incubation at 37 °C which confirmed that such potential was concentration dependent. Therefore, prickly pear fruits of OX could be considered a natural means to control the pathogenic contamination in food and reduce its risks.	[109]
In vitro	The chemical composition of hexane extracts from flowers belonging to two species of *Opuntia* (OFI and OdHw) were studied by gas chromatography–mass spectrometry in four developmental stages of flower (vegetative, initial flowering, full flowering, and post-flowering stages).	The differences observed in the composition of the two species of flowers were mainly carboxylic acid, terpenes, esters and alcohols. Furthermore, both *Opuntia* species showed inhibitory activity against *P. aeruginosa*, *S. aureus* and *E. coli*. Therefore, OFI and OdHw could be used as food preservative agents.	[110]
In vitro	Because there are few reports on the chemical composition and biological activity of OFI in its flowering development, the percentage of nutrients and antibacterial activity of a hexane extract of its flowers were studied in different 4 stages of flowering.	The results showed that during flowering there were no significant variations in its chemical composition; finding you mainly fiber, proteins and minerals. Also observed a high efficacy against *E. coli* and *S. aureus*, making it a botanical source with possible additive food control potential.	[111]
In vitro	Some evidence suggest that OdHw endophytic fungi may help the host to overcome biotic and abiotic stress by producing biologically active metabolites. To confirm this, we evaluated the antimicrobial activities of endophytes isolated from their CLDs and flowers against 5 bacteria [3 Gram (+) and 2 Gram (−)].	Of the 8 fungi isolated, *Fusarium* spp was the most bioactive and presented equisetin (derived from tetramic acid) as an antibacterial compound. Their MBCs ranged from 8 to 16 µg/mL for *S. aureus* and Methicillin Resistant *S. aureus* (MRSA). The conclusion is that these fungi can help the host to resist the stressful environmental conditions and produce biologically active secondary metabolites.	[112]

Table 5. *Cont.*

Type of Study	Objective and Characteristics	Results and Conclusion	Ref
In vivo In vitro	Ammar et al., (2015) investigated the healing (excision wound model in rats), antioxidant (Trolox equivalent antioxidant capacity and DPPH assay) and antibacterial (agar-well diffusion assay) activity of mucilaginous and methanolic extracts from OFI flowers.	The conclusión was that both extracts showed significant results and the mucilage extract was the most effective. In practically all the microorganisms tested (*L. monocytogenes, E. coli, P. aeruginosa, S. aureus,* and *B. subtilis*) inhibition halos were observed. However, *L. monocytogenes* was the most sensitive.	[113]
In vitro	Initially, the synthesis of HAP nanoparticles was made using pectin (extracted from the shell of prickly pear fruits from OFI) as a base template. Subsequently, the evaluation focused on its efficiency and antimicrobial activity against *S. aureus* and *E. coli* in the absence and presence of pectin at a concentration of 0.15%.	The results showed that the HAP nanoparticles synthesized with pectin had better antimicrobial activity against both bacteria compared to those without pectin. On average, the inhibition halos ranged from 6 to 8 mm in diameter. Therefore, these little crystalline and granular nanoparticles can be useful in the field of biomedicine.	[114]
In vitro	Biofilm is a complex microbial community that is highly resistant to antimicrobial agents, and its formation is associated with high rates of morbidity and mortality in hospitalized patients. Considering that the use of medicinal plants is a new proposal for the control of hospital infections, the antimicrobial and antibiofilm activities of 8 methanolic plant extracts were evaluated, (including OFI) against 5 nosocomial pathogens (*K. pneumoniae, E. faecalis, E. coli, S. maltophilia* and *S. aureus*).	Preliminary antimicrobial tests performed by the well diffusion method showed that OFI induces zones of inhibition ranging from 0.7 to 1.3 cm and the MBCs were between 1.0 and 15 mg/mL. Besides, most pathogens were inhibited and the most sensitive were *E. coli* and *S. aureus*. The specific biofilm formation index (SBF) was evaluated before and after the addition of plant extracts and again OFI caused the greatest reduction in SBF.	[115]
In vitro	The presence of multiresistant pathogenic bacteria in food is known to be a major public health problem, especially Diarrheagenic *Escherichia coli* pathotypes (DEPs). In the case of nopalitos (raw whole and chopped) and in nopalitos salad samples, generic *E. coli* and multiresistant DEPs were found. The generic *E. coli* was determined using the most probable number procedures and for DEPs two multiplex polymerase chain reaction procedures were used and their susceptibility to 16 antibiotics was evaluated for the DEPs strains.	Of the 300 samples of nopalitos (100 for each type evaluated), both generic *E. coli* and DEPs between 10 and 80% per type were identified in them. The DEPs that were identified, include Shiga toxin-producing *E. coli*, enteropathogenic *E. coli*, and enterotoxigenic *E. coli*. Finally, all the isolated strains exhibited resistance to at least six antibiotics.	[116]
In vitro	The objective of the study was to characterize the phytochemical profile and determine the cytotoxic and antimicrobial properties in flowers of *O. microdasys* (OMs) at different stages of maturity. An initial observation was that OMs stand out for their high content of dietary fiber, potassium and camphor.	The vegetative stage showed the highest cytotoxic and antifungal (*A. versicolor* and *P. funiculosum*) activities, while the full bloom stage was particularly active against bacterial species (*S. aureus, B. cereus, M. flavus, L. monocytogenes, E. coli, P. aeruginosa, S. typhimurium,* and *E. cloacae*). Of these, *S. aureus* was the most susceptible species, while *L. monocytogenes* and *E. cloacae* stood out as the most resistant.	[117]
In vitro	Seed oils extracted with different solvents (Hx, EtOH and EtOAc) and from two Mexican varieties of PPFs [red: OFI and green: *O. albicarpa* (OA)] were evaluated to determine their antioxidant and antimicrobial activity. The fatty acid profile of the oils was also quantified by gas chromatography-mass spectrometry (GC-MS), which confirmed that both varieties of PPFs were similar and exhibited a high content of linoleic acid.	Because OA oil obtained with EtOH and EtOAc showed the highest antioxidant activity (323 and 316 µmol TE/20 mg, respectively), it was used to analyze the antimicrobial potential; which showed inhibition halos in most of the microorganisms evaluated (*E. coli* O58:H21 and O157:H7, *S. aureus, L. monocytogenes, P. aeruginosa,* and *S. Typhi*). *S. typhi* and *E. coli* O157:H7 were the most resistant species.	[118]

Table 5. Cont.

Type of Study	Objective and Characteristics	Results and Conclusion	Ref
In vitro	Various evidences have confirmed that the oils from the seeds of *Opuntia* species have a significant content of unsaturated fatty acids and antioxidant compounds. Therefore, the focus of the study was to compare the effectiveness of conventional extraction methods (extraction with hexane) and new ones (supercritical (SC)-CO$_2$) for oil recovery, obtaining phenolic compounds and action of the antimicrobial effect of the *O. stricta* seeds.	Using liquid chromatography-high-resolution mass spectrometry, the conclusion is that similar yields of oil are obtained in both extraction methods; although when using the SC-CO2 method, it is more enriched in polyphenols, which favors an increase in antioxidant potential and its percentage of antibacterial inhibition (especially against *B. thuringiensis* and *B. subtilis*). This extraction method favors the beneficial properties of *O. stricta* to suggest its oil as high quality.	[119]
In vitro	Aqueous extracts of OFI, *Artemisia herba-alba*, *Camellia sinensis* and *Phlomis crinita* were evaluated by the disc method against two Gram-negative bacterial strains (*Porphyromonas gingivalis* and *Prevotella intermedia*) commonly involved in periodontal diseases.	All extracts showed a powerful activity against these strains, especially OFI whose inhibitory concentration varied between 0.03 and 590 mg/mL. In summary, the statistical analysis showed that the most significant antimicrobial effect was on *P. intermedia*	[120]
In vitro	Considering the previous results of Gómez-Aldapa et al. (2016) [105], in this study the presence of Salmonella strains resistant to antibiotics in nopalitos (raw whole and cut) and in samples of nopalitos salad was found. The analysis also covered the behavior of multiresistant Salmonella isolates.	Bacterial strains were found between 10 and 30% of the samples. From all the samples, 70 multiresistant Salmonella strains were isolated, which survived longer in whole raw nopales at 25 °C; unlike the strains found in the other nopalitos samples where their growth was inhibited at 3 °C. Possibly, this is an important factor that contributes to alimentary gastroenteritis.	[121]
In vitro	Antimicrobial resistance is a serious health problem of the 21st century, which is intended to be solved by searching for new agents with this therapeutic property in plants. Consequently, fresh OFI fruits were collected to extract their bioactive compounds using solvents such as EtOH, MeOH, Chl. Afterwards, the antimicrobial potential of these extracts against *E. coli*, *S. pneumoniae*, *S. typhi* and *B. subtilis* was determined by the diffusion method in agar wells.	All the extracts demonstrated antibacterial activity against the 4 bacteria, showing an inhibition diameter between 9.0 and 23.0 mm. The highest activity was against *S. typhi*, *B. subtilis* and *S. pneumoniae*, whch was significantly higher when compared to synthetic antimicrobials (tetracycline and vancomycin). These results suggest that OFI extracts could be used for prevention and treatment of different bacterial diseases.	[122]
In vitro	With the purpose of expanding the knowledge about natural bioactive compounds for food preservation, an aqueous extract of purple-red prickly pears obtained from the first flowering of OFI and the total content of polyphenols, betacyanins, and betaxanthins was evaluated; as well as the antimicrobial against food spoilage induced by different pathogenic bacteria (*E. coli*, *S. enterica*, *P. fluorescens*, *L. innocua*, *S. aureus*, *B. subtilis*, *B. cereus*). The extract was applied through the immersion technique to sliced beef meat in order to determine its physical and chemical parameters, and maintenance of color and texture.	The addition of the extract preserved the color, texture and extended the shelf life of the meat during the storage period. Likewise, the agar well diffusion test showed that the extract has a broad-spectrum activity by inhibiting the growth of all bacterial strains; especially against *B. cereus*, *P. fluorescens* and *E. coli*. These results support the possibility that the betacyanins and betaxanthins of the extract favor the general quality of the meat under refrigeration conditions.	[123]

Table 5. Cont.

Type of Study	Objective and Characteristics	Results and Conclusion	Ref
In vitro	Considering the previous results of Ammar et al., (2015) [102], the antimicrobial, antifungal activity and skin wound healing effect of the oil extracted from the seeds of PPFs from OFI were evaluated. For the first properties, minimal inhibitory concentrations (MICs) and minimal bactericidal concentrations (MBCs) were calculated against 4 bacterial strains (E. coli, S. aureus, S. agalactiae, and E. cloacae), and 3 fungi (A. niger, P. digitatum, and F. oxysporum).	The oil was able to mainly inhibit E. cloacae, A. niger, P. digitatum and F. oxysporum. (On average, the inhibition halos were 16 mm compared to the 23 mm obtained by the positive control of Ceftazidime). In addition, a good wound healing effect was observed, preventing skin infections and reducing the re-epithelialization phase. These data suggest that OFI oil exerts both bacteriostatic and bactericidal effects on E. cloacae and appears to be effective for the treatment of skin infections.	[124]
In vitro	Sexually transmitted infections (STIs) continue being a major health problem and unfortunately, antimicrobial drugs are becoming ineffective due to the increasing resistance of bacteria and viruses; thus, the use of medicinal plants has become a good alternative. Using the disk diffusion model and the microdilution technique to determine the zone of inhibition and MICs, some plant extracts (including OFI) were tested against N. gonorrhoeae and some fungal strains (C. albicans, C. krusei, C. parapsilosis, C. tropicalis and C. neoformans)	The extracts (MeOH, Hx, Ace and DCM) presented different levels of phytoconstituents such as alkaloids, steroids, terpenes, flavonoids, tannins and saponins. Especially the Ace and MeOH extracts of OFI showed potency against N. gonorrhoeae and fungal strains. These results open the field of new studies to consider plants as an alternative method for STIs control.	[125]
In vitro	The shell of the PPFs is usually an agroindustrial waste that has been little studied in the nutraceutical area. Consequently, the main components of the shell were isolated and characterized in order to subsequently quantify their antibacterial capacity. Initially, a MeOH extract was fractionated using Hx, Chl and EtOAc. The GC-MS analysis confirmed that the Hx fraction had 60% linolenic acid; while the study of the EtOAc fraction by ultra-performance liquid chromatography electrospray tandem mass spectrometry (UPLC-ESI-MS/MS), revealed caffeic acid and quercetin.	This EtOAc fraction was also subjected to column chromatography, resulting in the isolation of four flavanols (astragalin, quercetin 5,4′-dimethyl ether, isorhamnetin-3-O-glucoside, and isorhamnetin). The antibacterial evaluation revealed that the EtOAc fraction (specifically, quercetin 5,4′-dimethyl ether) was more potent against pneumonia pathogens. These findings indicate that OFI fruit debris containinvaluable components against some pathogens.	[126]
Systematic review	Of all the studies carried out to date, this is the only one where a bibliographic search has been carried out on fruit extracts and agro-industrial residues with antimicrobial activity that can be applied to meat products.	The data obtained confirm that: a) Opuntia extracts have antimicrobial effects against L. monocytogenes, B. cereus, S. aureus and E. coli, b) Other important extracts and/or by-products were those of the grape that show inhibition of S aureus, L. monocytogenes, P. aeruginosa, E. coli. These data reinforce the possibility of substituting synthetic preservatives by natural versions. For this reason, it is necessary to investigate in detail the effective concentrations that maintain the sensory properties of foods.	[127]
In vitro	By comparing two fractionation processes (semi-preparative high-performance countercurrent chromatography (HPCCC) and HPLC) of O. stricta extracts to obtain secondary metabolites, it was confirmed that HPCCC has a better separation capacity; obtaining two 14-ring cyclopeptide alkaloids (Opuntisine A and B)	In determining its antimicrobial potentials, we found that opuntisin A had moderate activity against E. coli. Therefore, a strong suggestion is to extend the studies in these new natural products of the Cactaceae family.	[128]

Table 5. *Cont.*

Type of Study	Objective and Characteristics	Results and Conclusion	Ref
In vitro	Urinary tract infections (UTI) are caused by different microorganisms, highlighting *E. coli* in 90% of female cases. Considering all previous OFI studies, the antimicrobial efficacy of ethanolic and ethyl acetate extracts of the OFI cactus on this Gram (−) bacterium isolated from UTI patient samples was assesed. The results were compared against reference antibiotics (gentamicin and ampicillin).	An important observation was that the EtOH extract had a higher activity against *E. coli* compared to EtOAc and the reference antibiotics. In the same way, it was established that the EtOAc extract may have activity on bacteria from food (*B. subtilis*, *S. aureus*, *S. typhimurium* and *P. fluorescens*). In conclusion, the inhibitory effect of both extracts against Gram (+) and (−) bacteria can be attributed to the presence of the different bioactive ingredients.	[129]

4.4. Action in the Treatment of Skin Wounds

The skin is the largest organ of the human body that acts as a protective barrier against harmful agents from the external environment. It controls thermal regulation and homeostasis of water and electrolytes. When this barrier is damaged, the body promotes the healing and/or scarring process to regenerate the injured area, involving molecular, cellular, and biochemical mechanisms that are divided into four phases (hemostasis, inflammatory, proliferative, and remodeling) (Figure 2). Any disruption in the balance of these processes causes problems and delays in wound healing; deteriorations related to aging, pathological situations (such as diabetes, obesity and/or arterial diseases) and multiple local and systemic factors (hypoxia, OXs, diminished immune response, poor nutrition, medications and infectious agents) [130].

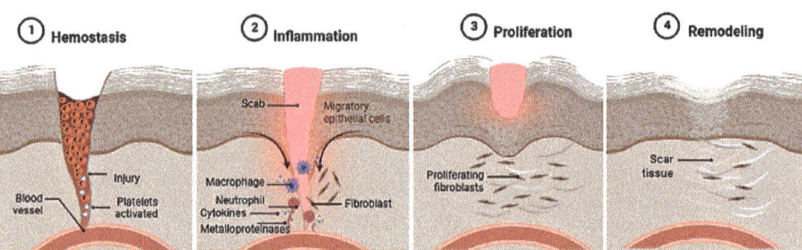

Figure 2. Stages of skin healing.

Cicatrization is a physiological process that involves perfect interactions of numerous cells and molecules, so the imbalance of these interactions generates alterations during the process that are expressed as excessive yellow discharge, pain, swelling, redness and fever. Among the most relevant is the chronic inflammatory state, where pro- and anti-inflammatory mediators produce an exacerbated recruitment of neutrophils and macrophages with overexpression of inflammatory cytokines and excessive release of ROS, which together interfere with the proliferation/differentiation of keratinocytes and fibroblasts in the injured area and leads to cell apoptosis [130]. In addition, the increase in proinflammatory cytokines affects subsequent wound healing mechanisms, increasing matrix metalloproteinases (MMPs) and other proteases that alter cell proliferation/migration and reduce the accumulation of extracellular matrix components. Normally, there must be a balance between proliferation/activation and maturation/apoptosis of blood vessels; and if this is not done correctly, neovascularization and blood flow in the area are reduced, delaying the subsequent mechanisms of the proliferative and remodeling phase. Another mistake is the involvement of wound keratinocytes, which acquire a hyperproliferative state due to overexpression of the β-catenin/c-myc pathway, and express low levels of keratins 1, 2, and 10. This alters the migratory potential of these cells, which is related to the proteolytic degradation of growth factors and extracellular matrix proteins necessary for migration. Impaired remodeling is another major failure, as injured cells synthesize excessive amounts of MMPs and other proteases, degrading not only extracellular matrix components, but also cell surface receptors, growth factors, and the cytokines. In addition, inhibitors of metalloproteinases (TIMP) are reduced, contributing to the deregulation of proteases in these lesions, and consequently, the degradation of important molecules of the extracellular matrix such as collagen, elastin, fibronectin and chondroitin sulfate [130].

Over the years, adequate therapies have been sought to improve or promote the wound healing process. Currently, there are several treatments that can be classified into surgical procedures (autografts, allografts and xenografts), non-surgical therapies (topical formulations, dressings and skin substitutes) and pharmacological agents. However, depending on the size, type of wound, and factors that caused the damage, existing therapies are not completely effective [131]. Once again, phytomedicine, being popular among the general population in different regions of the world, opens new avenues of pharmacological intervention for the healing of skin wounds. Among the known phytotherapeutic agents are Aloe vera, mimosa (*Mimosa sensitive*), grape vine (*Vitis vinifera*), chamomile (*Matricaria chamomilla*), ginseng (*Panax ginseng*), jojoba (*Simmondsia chinensis*), rosemary (*Salvia rosmarinus*), lemon (*Citrus limon*), comfrey (*Symphytum officinale*), papaya (*Carica papaya*), oats (*Avena sativa*), garlic (*Allium sativum*), ginkgo (*Ginkgo biloba*), ocimum (*Ocimum basilicum*), tree oil, and olive oil [131].

In the case of *Opuntia* spp. and its extracts, there is various evidence of its use in traditional medicine for the treatment of burns, skin disorders and wound healing. The first study in this field of research compared the healing activity of a base cream containing lyophilized cladodes of OFI at 15% against a commercial ointment on wounds produced on the back of rats. After 5 days of treatment, the epithelialization process was evident and complete, suggesting that cladodes accelerate the proliferation and migration of keratinocytes in the cicatrization process [132]. The previous result was confirmed when two lyophilized polysaccharide extracts obtained from OFI were applied topically for 6 days and observed that they induce a beneficial effect (accelerate the re-epithelialization-remodeling phases and favor cell-matrix interactions) in the skin wounds of rats [133].

Using benzopyrene- or TNF-α-stimulated keratinocytes, Nakahara et al., (2015) demonstrated that CLD extracts protect the epidermal barrier and keratinocyte function by increasing the expression of filaggrin and loricrin, two proteins present in keratinocytes and corneocytes differentiated. In addition, they attribute the protective effect to an inhibition of ROS production caused by inflammatory agents. This property is probably related to the activation of nuclear erythroid factor (Nrf2) and NAD(P)H:quinone oxidoreductase 1 [134]. It is considered that the cicatrizant properties of OFI cladodes may involve high molecular weight polysaccharide components (such as linear galactan polymer and highly branched xyloarabinan) as well as low molecular weight components [lactic acid, D-mannitol, piscidic, eucomic, and 2-hydroxy-4-(4′-hydroxyphenyl)-butanoic acid]. These extracts could accelerate cell regeneration in a keratinocyte monolayer, which suggest that OFI components exhibit high anti-inflammatory and wound-healing properties [135].

Likewise, polysaccharides extracted from OFI stimulate the proliferation of fibroblasts and keratinocytes [136]. Among the protective agents present in *Opuntia* extracts, isorhamnetin glucoside components [such as isorhamnetin-glucosyl-rhamnoside diglucoside (IGR)], could inhibit COX-2, TNF-α and IL-6 production and induction of NO evoked by LPS [52].Not only OFI has shown beneficial effects, *O. humifusa* (OHF) extracts regulate the production of hyaluronic acid (HA) by increasing the expression of HA synthase in keratinocytes exposed to UV-B treatment. Treatment with these extracts could decrease the increased expression of hyaluronidase UV-B. The same protective effect on HA has been observed in SKH-1 hairless mice exposed to UV-B, which indicates that OHF extracts have a great capacity for skin care [137]. Table 6 presents all the studies of *Opuntia* spp. that justify its efficacy at the molecular and cellular level for the healing of skin wounds, as well as its use in dermatological preparations.

Table 6. Scientific evidence of *Opuntia* spp. on the healing of skin wounds.

Type of Study	Objective and Characteristics	Results and Conclusion	Ref
In vitro	As mentioned, OFI flowers are used for various medicinal purposes. Therefore, the healing activity (excision wound model in rats) and antioxidant activity (Trolox equivalent antioxidant capacity and DPPH assay) of mucilaginous and methanolic extracts of its flowers were studied.	After 13 days of treatment with both extracts, a beneficial effect on skin repair was observed, evaluated by the acceleration of the phases of contraction and remodeling of the wound. Histopathological studies of the granulation tissue indicated that the dermis was properly corrected and that the mucilage extract was more effective. In addition, it was confirmed that the extracts showed a significant antioxidant capacity.	[113]
In vivo	After isolating, washing, drying and cold pressing PPFs seeds from OFI, their oil was obtained to determine the effect of cicatrization of skin wounds and its antimicrobial potential against 4 bacterial strains and 3 fungi. The skin wounds of three experimental groups of rats were topically treated once a day with the oil, observing the healing process and calculating the percentage of wound contraction. At the same time, a histological study was performed on skin biopsies.	At the end of the study, it was shown that the oil exerted a good wound-cicatrization effect, preventing skin infections (especially against *E. cloacae*, and *A. niger*) and reducing the re-epithelialization phase. It is suggested to increase the studies to confirm the capacity of the oil in the promotion of the cicatrization process.	[124]
In vivo	The purpose of this study was to investigate the effect of spraying an extract of *O. stricta* on wounds on the ventral surface of rabbit ears. After the wounds healed, hypertrophic scar tissue was obtained and histological analysis was performed. Using immunohistochemistry and real-time quantitative polymerase chain reaction, the expression of type I and III collagen and matrix metalloproteinase-1 (MMP-1) was evaluated.	The results indicated: a) the expression of type I collagen in the animals treated with the extract was lower than in the control group, unlike type III collagen that gradually increased, b) the scar that was less prominent and expression of MMP-1 decreased with the application of the extract. In conclusion, the extract decreased the formation of hypertrophic scars by inhibiting type I collagen, and increasing type III collagen and MMP-1.	[138]
In vivo	Despite advances in modern medicine, to date there is no effective natural treatment for second-degree burns. Therefore, the healing efficacy of oil extracted from PPFs on partial-thickness burns induced by fractional CO_2 laser in rats was evaluated. All the burns were measured and treated topically for 7 days. The response to treatment was determined by macroscopic, histological and biochemical parameters.	The oil showed improvements in the general appearance of the wound and in the formation of scabs; besides, it significantly decreased the healing time. The histological evaluation confirmed that the oil has comparatively good healing properties and favors collagen content. This is scientific evidence of the efficacy of PPF oils on partial thickness burns.	[139]
In vitro	The purpose of the research was to compare the effects of OFI and Milk Thistle (MT) (*Silybum marianum* L.) on adult keratinocytes (HaCaT) functioning in basal conditions or in the presence of mechanical damage (wounded cells). Natural compounds were tested on HaCaT in monoculture and triculture configurations. In three-culture models, HaCaTs were treated with conditioned media obtained by co-cultures of normal human dermal fibroblasts and human dermal microvascular endothelial cells.	After determining cell viability, mechanisms of EOx (cytokine release and lipid peroxidation), cell remodeling (modulation of metalloproteinases), and migratory potential of HaCaT (in vitro wound healing assay); OFI and MT were found to favor migratory properties of HaCaT under both physiological conditions and mechanical damage. In addition, the response to EOx was modulated. The conclusion was that OFI and MT are good alternatives in skin repair.	[140]

Table 6. *Cont.*

Type of Study	Objective and Characteristics	Results and Conclusion	Ref
In vivo	This last study investigated the potential of opuntiol, isolated from OFI, against UVA radiation-mediated inflammation and skin photoaging in mice. The animals were shaved and exposed to UVA rays (dose of 10 J/cm^2/day) for ten days. One hour before each exposure, opuntiol (50 mg/kg) was applied topically.	Opuntiol pretreatment prevented UVA-linked clinical macroscopic skin lesions and histological changes in the mouse skin. In addition, opuntiol prevented dermal collagen fiber loss and collagen I and III breakdown in animal skin. Opuntiol was found to inhibit UVA-induced activation of iNOS, TNF-α, COX-2 MMP-2, and MMP-9. In conclusion, opuntiol exerted skin protection to the photoaging response associated with UVA radiation by reducing inflammatory responses and activating MAPK.	[141]
In vitro	*O. humifusa* (OHF) is considered a possible candidate to design cosmetic formulations that prevent the harmful effects of Particulate Matter (PM). Unfortunately, its high viscosity does not allow its adequate use in these formulations. Therefore, the effect of a high-power microwave treatment on an *O. humifusa* extract (MA-OHF) was investigated.	The results indicated that MA-OHE showed reasonable viscosity and outstanding anti-inflammatory activity to suppress PM-induced ROS production. In addition, COX-2 and MMP-9 expression was decreased in HaCaT keratinocytes. It is suggested that MA-OHE may be a suitable natural cosmetic ingredient to prevent PM-induced skin oxidative stress and inflammation.	[142]
In vivo	Considering that delayed wound healing represents a common health hazard, we compared the wound cicatrization activity of OFI seed oil and an auto-nanoemulsifying drug delivery system (OFI-SNEDDS) formulation in a full-thickness skin excision rat model. The OFI-SNEDDS formulation was prepared using a droplet size of 50.02 nm and applied directly to the animals.	The results showed that the formula exhibited healing activities superior to the oil, which was confirmed by histopathological examinations. In addition, OFI-SNEDDS presented greater antioxidant and anti-inflammatory capacity and improved angiogenesis (a phenomenon that was demonstrated by increasing the expression of vascular endothelial growth factor). The conclusion was that OFI has wound healing properties that are enhanced by the self-emulsion of the oil in nanodroplets. This is probably attributed to its anti-inflammatory, procollagenous and angiogenic properties.	[143]
In vitro	In this study, chitosan-based wound dressings loaded with an OFI extract were prepared. Chitosan (Ch) was crosslinked with a low molecular weight diepoxy-poly(ethylene glycol) (PEG), and hydrogel films with different Ch/PEG composition and OFI content were prepared. Using FTIR spectroscopy (Fourier transform infrared spectroscopy) the appearance of the crosslinking reaction was determined.	The analyses suggested that ionic interactions between Ch and OFI occur. The swelling characteristics, the water vapor transmission rate and the release kinetics showed that these films are suitable for their application. Finally, a scratch test on a keratinocyte monolayer showed that the rate of cell migration in the presence of OFI-loaded samples is approximately 3 times higher compared to unloaded films, confirming its restorative activity.	[144]

5. Toxic Evidence of the Genus *Opuntia*

The cacti family contains approximately 200 genera and 2000 species, which favors a wide genetic diversity that, together with environmental conditions (climate, humidity), type of soil, age of maturity of the cladodes and the harvest season, generates differences in the phytochemical composition of its vegetable parts (PPFs, CLDs, roots, flowers, seeds and stems) between wild and domesticated species, inducing changes in its nutritional values and undoubtedly in its functional and therapeutic properties. In this sense, although the public and some health professionals consider herbal medicines to be relatively safe because they are "natural", there is very little data to support this assumption. Therefore, *Opuntia* spp. species are not exempt from possible adverse and toxic effects.

Saleem et al., (2005) evaluated for the first time its toxicological safety by determining the hypotensive activity of a methanolic extract of OdHw and its alpha-pyrone glycoside (opuntioside-I) in normotensive rats. At the end of their study, they observed no mortality with the extract and/or opuntioside-I orally administered, even at high doses of 1000 mg/kg/day. However, histopathological analysis revealed slight changes in the liver and spleen of the animals [145]. Subsequently, in 2012, the physicochemical characteristics (acidity, percentage of free fatty acids, saponification value, refractive index and density), lethal dose 50 (LD_{50}) and toxicity of an OFI seed oil in mice were determined. Finding that the LD_{50} values ranged between 40.7 and 45.4 mL/kg body wt for oral administration and 2.52–2.92 mL/kg body wt for intraperitoneal administration [146].

These results and variations in doses called the attention to analyze other species of *Opuntia*, e.g., Osorio-Esquivel et al., (2012) who determined the acute toxicity of a MeOH extract of *O. xoconostle* (OX) seeds in mice fed with a hypercholesterolemic diet; finding that it was greater than 5000 mg/kg of body weight without the presence of apparent toxic manifestations [147]. Similar data on the absence of any sign of acute toxicity were observed in two other studies; the first, when orally administering up to 5 mL/kg of cactus pear seed oil (CPSO) to Wistar rats to determine its hypoglycemic effect [148] and/or by evaluating the in vitro and in vivo bioactivities of *O. macrorhiza* Engelm seed oil (OMESO) [60].

Considering that OFI is an important dietary source, a toxicological evaluation of aqueous extracts from different parts of the plant was performed and compared using three types of assays (MTT, Comet and the γH2AX In-Cell Western). The conclusion was that the fruit pulp extracts showed the best antigenotoxic effect against H_2O_2 and that no extract induced genotoxicity and/or cytotoxicity in the cell lines used [149].

To confirm the above findings, Han et al. (2019) investigated the genotoxicity of three doses of an OFIS extract (500, 1000 and 2000 mg/kg/day) orally administered for one week in rodents using the Ames test (*S. typhimurium* strains TA100, TA1535, TA98 and TA153 and *E. coli* strain WP2 urvA), chromosomal aberration assay in Chinese hamster lung cells and micronucleus test in bone marrow cells. In summary, it was observed that: (a) OFIS did not alter normal animal behavior or body weight gain, (b) mutagenicity was not present in both bacterial strains with or without S9 activation and (c) the number of micronucleated polychromatic erythrocytes (MPE) was not increased [150].

Recently, two groups of researchers addressed the safety of OdHw, considering that it is a cactaceae traditionally used in several countries to treat ailments such as inflammation, gastric ulcers, diabetes, hepatitis, asthma, and intestinal spasms. In the first study, the acute toxicity of the oil obtained from its seeds was evaluated in albino mice and Wistar rats. After a single administration of the established doses (1.0, 2.0, 3.0, 5.0 and 7.0 mL/kg), adverse signs and/or mortality were observed for four weeks. The conclusion was that the oil produced no variations in the body weight of the animals and no mortality or signs of toxicity during the entire monitoring period. In addition, cell viability was not affected when human hepatoma HepG2 culture was analyzed [151,152].

Finally, when evaluating a MeOH extract of cladodes by MTT assay in human embryonic kidney cell line, genomic DNA fragmentation using agarose gel electrophoresis and bone marrow micronuclei frequency, it was proved that a 7-day treatment of 5 g/kg of the extract orally had no effect on DNA integrity, neither did it induce cytotoxicity or stimulate MPE formation [153]. Unfortunately, although *Opuntia* spp. could be considered a reliable and safe plant, some authors have identified and reported the presence of certain side effects during oral consumption of OFI, such as mild diarrhea, increased stool volume and frequency, nausea, headache and lower colonic obstruction [6,20,103,149].

Despite these secondary effects, plants of the *Opuntia* genus are traditional foods frequently consumed and their cladodes and fruits are still considered with high agrotechnological potential. Besides, studies suggesting an LD_{50}, above 5000 mg/kg are safe levels. To date, there is no established dose and/or concentration for its consumption and there are different intervals that depend on the route of administration, the species (humans/animals) in which they are used; the approach to use it whether it is food (fresh, juices or extracts) or for experimental evaluation.

Some authors recommend an intake between 10 to 17 g/person/day of *Opuntia* and/or prickly pear fruits (PPFs) to have a healthy life. Others suggest between 100 and 500 g/day of roasted CLDs to significantly reduce the complications of diabetes mellitus. There are products, such as PPFs, in commercial presentations of capsules, tablets, powders, and juices whose oral dosage regimens are established at 250 mg/3 times a day/every 8 h [18,154,155].

In general, summarizing the information from both documents (part 1 and 2) it can be seen that the doses range from 50 mg/kg to 7 g/kg [23].

6. Conclusions and Perspectives

Although modern medicine is available in most countries for the control and treatment of many diseases, phytomedicine and/or TCAM continue being popularly used in different populations for historical, cultural reasons, easy access, low cost, diversity, and especially, a relative lower quantity of adverse effects. The set of studies presented in both reviews (Part 1 and 2) demonstrate the beneficial properties of the different vegetative parts of *Opuntia* spp. (wild and domesticated). For this reason, scientific research on this genus of plants (known as succulents, due to their ability to generate biomass by storing water in one or more of their organs) has deepened and may continue to increase, in order to better understand their nutritional and therapeutic properties.

In general, most of the evidence confirms that CLDs, PPFs, oils and/or extracts (MeOH, Hx, EtOAc, Chl and aqueous) coming mainly from OFI, OS, OdHw, OHF, OX and *O. macrorhiza* Engelm have presented relevant therapeutic and/or pharmacological potentials; whose mechanisms of action are mainly related to the inhibition of the absorption of substances, modification of the intestinal flora, elimination of reactive oxygen species and/or protection of nucleophilic DNA sites, anti-inflammatory activity, induction of detoxification pathways, and activation of apoptosis. However, it is convenient to extend the investigations to other species in order to analyze and confirm their pharmacological capacities.

Likewise, the results of the investigations confirm and coincide that these beneficial properties are possible attributed to a synergistic and/or combined effect among the different bioactive compounds (vitamins, flavonoids (isorhamnetin, kaempferol, quercetin), phenolic compounds, pigments (carotenoids, betalains and betacyanins), α-pyrones (opunthiol and opuntioside glucoside), pectin and mucilage). Nonetheless, it is convenient to increase the individual studies of each phytochemical, to determine its protective action; given that as substrates they can activate different biochemical reactions to provide important health benefits and be recognized as significant nutraceutical agents. All of the above, added to the fact that several *Opuntia* plants have been consumed by humans for more than 8000 years, which are easily adapted and/or propagated in different types of soil. In addition to their relatively low presence of adverse and toxic effects, they favor their domestication process, the increase in economic interest and new advances in the field of biotechnology.

It is convenient to remember that the process to discover drugs and/or medications is complex and costly. In that process different types of studies converge (such as those presented in this document; in vitro, in vivo and clinical). In recent years, computational methods (also called in-silico) have been integrated into this multidisciplinary effort, contributing to efficient data analysis, filtering and/or selecting individual bioactive molecules for their subsequent experimental evaluation, and also to generate hypotheses that favor the understanding of its mechanism of action and the design of new chemical structures. Again, *Opuntia* species are not exempt from participating in this area of research. Among the most significant studies, those carried out by Elkady et al., (2020), who isolated and characterized constituents of the prickly pear peel to determine their antibacterial activity stand out. This latter assay revealed that quercetin 5,4'-dimethyl ether found in EtOAc fraction exerted an inhibitory effect against pneumonia pathogens. Virtual docking of the isolated compounds showed promise in silico anti-quorum sensing efficacy, suggesting that unused waste from fruits contains bioactive components with possible beneficial potential [126]. On the other hand, an In Silico Investigation on the Interaction of Chiral Phytochemicals from *O. ficus-indica* with SARS-CoV-2 Mpro (main viral protease) was developed. Using two web-based molecular docking programs (1-Click Mcule and COVID-19 Docking Server) several flavonols and flavonol glycosides were identified; highlighting the chiral compound astragalin with high binding affinity for Mpro and a low toxicity profile. Emerging the possibility of a protease inhibitor agent as an anti-COVID-19 strategy [156]. In the most recent study, the possible targets in the PI3K/Akt/mTOR pathway acted upon by an *O. xoconostle* extract were modeled and simulated in silico using the Big Data-Cellulat platform, as well as the concentration range of LD_{50} to be used in breast cancer cells. The in silico results showed that the activation of I3K and Akt is related to angiogenesis and inhibition of apoptosis, and that the extract has an antiproliferative effect on cancer cells, causing the cells to interrupt in the G2/M phase of the cell cycle [157]. Taken together, these three studies demonstrate that the use of in silico tools is a valuable method for conducting virtual experiments and discovering new therapeutic agents.

In conclusion, there is still a long way to go on scientific research to understand in more detail the significant beneficial properties of all species of *Opuntia* spp.

Author Contributions: E.M.-S., E.M.-B., J.A.M.-G. and J.P.-R. designed the concept, wrote the majority of the paper and managed the authors; N.V.-M., J.A.I.-V., M.S.-G. and L.D.-O. conducted the literature search, wrote key sections of the paper; I.Á.-G., Á.M.-G. and J.I.-V. wrote sections of the paper and managed the reference list. All authors have read and agreed to the published version of the manuscript.

Funding: This research received no external funding.

Institutional Review Board Statement: Not applicable.

Informed Consent Statement: Not applicable.

Data Availability Statement: Not applicable.

Acknowledgments: The authors thank Florencia Ana María Talavera Silva for all her academic support. Her comments and observations in reviewing articles are always valuable and we give her immense recognition for her efforts.

Conflicts of Interest: The authors declare no conflict of interest.

References

1. Mendoza-Pérez, J.; Fregoso-Aguilar, T. Chemistry of Natural Antioxidants and Studies Performed with Different Plants Collected in Mexico. In *Oxidative Stress and Chronic Degenerative Diseases—A Role for Antioxidants*; Morales-González, J.A., Ed.; IntechOpen: Rijeka, Croatia, 2013; pp. 59–85; ISBN 978-953-51-1123-8.
2. Peltzer, K.; Pengpid, S. Utilization and Practice of Traditional/Complementary/Alternative Medicine (T/CAM) in Southeast Asian Nations (ASEAN) Member States. *Stud. Ethno-Med.* **2015**, *9*, 209–218. [CrossRef]
3. López-Romero, D.; Izquierdo-Vega, J.A.; Morales-González, J.A.; Madrigal-Bujaidar, E.; Chamorro-Cevallos, G.; Sánchez-Gutiérrez, M.; Betanzos-Cabrera, G.; Alvarez-Gonzalez, I.; Morales-González, Á.; Madrigal-Santillán, E. Evidence of Some Natural Products with Antigenotoxic Effects. Part 2: Plants, Vegetables, and Natural Resin. *Nutrients* **2018**, *10*, 1954. [CrossRef]
4. Madrigal-Santillán, E.; García-Melo, F.; Morales-González, J.A.; Vázquez-Alvarado, P.; Muñoz-Juárez, S.; Zuñiga-Pérez, C.; Sumaya-Martínez, M.T.; Madrigal-Bujaidar, E.; Hernández-Ceruelos, A. Antioxidant and Anticlastogenic Capacity of Prickly Pear Juice. *Nutrients* **2013**, *5*, 4145–4158. [CrossRef]
5. Angulo-Bejarano, P.I.; Martínez-Cruz, O.; Paredes-López, O. Phytochemical Content, Nutraceutical Potential and Biotechnological Applications of an Ancient Mexican Plant: Nopal (*Opuntia ficus-indica*). *Curr. Nutr. Food. Sci.* **2014**, *10*, 196–217. [CrossRef]
6. El-Mostafa, K.; El Kharrassi, Y.; Badreddine, A.; Andreoletti, P.; Vamecq, J.; El Kebbaj, M.S.; Latruffe, N.; Lizard, G.; Nasser, B.; Cherkaoui-Malki, M. Nopal Cactus (*Opuntia ficus-indica*) as a Source of Bioactive Compounds for Nutrition, Health and Disease. *Molecules* **2014**, *19*, 14879–14901. [CrossRef]
7. Del Socorro Santos Díaz, M.; Barba de la Rosa, A.-P.; Héliès-Toussaint, C.; Guéraud, F.; Nègre-Salvayre, A. *Opuntia* spp.: Characterization and Benefits in Chronic Diseases. *Oxid. Med. Cell Longev.* **2017**, *2017*, 8634249. [CrossRef]
8. Griffith, M.P. The Origins of an Important Cactus Crop, *Opuntia ficus-indica* (Cactaceae): New Molecular Evidence. *Am. J. Bot.* **2004**, *91*, 1915–1921. [CrossRef]

9. Ochoa, M.; Giuseppe Barbera, G. History and Economic and Agro-Ecological Importance. In *Crop Ecology, Cultivation and Uses of Cactus Pear*; Inglese, P., Mondragon, C., Eds.; Food and Agriculture Organization of the United: Rome, Italy, 2017; pp. 1–11; ISBN 978-92-5-109860-8.
10. Kiesling, R.; Metzing, D. Origin and Taxonomy of *Opuntia ficus-indica*. In *Crop Ecology, Cultivation and Uses of Cactus Pear*; Inglese, P., Mondragon, C., Eds.; Food and Agriculture Organization of the United: Rome, Italy, 2017; pp. 13–16; ISBN 978-92-5-109860-8.
11. Griffith, P.; Porter, M. Phylogeny of Opuntioideae (Cactaceae). *Int. J. Plant Sci.* **2009**, *170*, 107–116. [CrossRef]
12. Reyes-Aguero, J.A.; Rivera, J.R.A. Agrobiodiversity of Cactus Pear (*Opuntia*, Cactaceae) in the Meridional Highlands Plateau of Mexico. *J. Nat. Resour. Dev.* **2011**, *1*, 1–9. [CrossRef]
13. Madrigal-Santillán, E.; Madrigal-Bujaidar, E.; Álvarez-González, I.; Sumaya-Martínez, M.T.; Gutiérrez-Salinas, J.; Bautista, M.; Morales-González, Á.; García-Luna y González-Rubio, M.; Aguilar-Faisal, J.L.; Morales-González, J.A. Review of Natural Products with Hepatoprotective Effects. *World J. Gastroenterol.* **2014**, *20*, 14787–14804. [CrossRef]
14. Silva, M.A.; Gonçalves-Albuquerque, T.; Pereira, P.; Ramalho, R.; Vicente, F.; Oliveira, M.B.P.P.; Costa, H.S. *Opuntia ficus-indica* (L.) Mill.: A Multi-Benefit Potential to Be Exploited. *Molecules* **2021**, *26*, 951. [CrossRef] [PubMed]
15. Ayyanar, M.; Ignacimuthu, S. Ethnobotanical survey of medicinal plants commonly used by Kani tribals in Tirunelveli hills of Western Ghats, India. *J. Ethnopharmacol.* **2011**, *134*, 851–864. [CrossRef]
16. Githae, E.W. Status of Opuntia invasions in the arid and semi-arid lands of Kenya. *CAB Reviews.* **2018**, *13*, 1–9. [CrossRef]
17. Chakale, M.V.; Asong, J.A.; Struwig, M.; Mwanza, M.; Aremu, A.O. Ethnoveterinary Practices and Ethnobotanical Knowledge on Plants Used against Cattle Diseases among Two Communities in South Africa. *Plants* **2022**, *11*, 1784. [CrossRef]
18. Feugang, J.M.; Konarski, P.; Zou, D.; Stintzing, F.C.; Zou, C. Nutritional and medicinal use of Cactus pear (*Opuntia* spp.) cladodes and fruits. *Front. Biosci.* **2006**, *11*, 2574–2589. [CrossRef]
19. El-Samahy, S.; El-Hady, E.A.; Habiba, R.; Moussa, T. Chemical and Rheological Characteristics of Orange-Yellow Cactus-Pear Pulp from Egypt. *J. Prof. Assoc. Cact. Dev.* **2006**, *8*, 39–51.
20. Osuna-Martínez, U.; Reyes-Esparza, J.; Rodríguez-Fragoso, L. Cactus (*Opuntia ficus-indica*): A Review on Its Antioxidants Properties and Potential Pharmacological Use in Chronic Diseases. *Nat. Prod. Chem. Res.* **2014**, *2*, 153–159. [CrossRef]
21. Kaur, M. Pharmacological Actions of *Opuntia ficus indica*: A Review. *J. App. Pharm. Sci.* **2012**, *2*, 15–18. [CrossRef]
22. Aragona, M.; Lauriano, E.R.; Pergolizzi, S.; Faggio, C. *Opuntia ficus-indica* (L.) Miller as a Source of Bioactivity Compounds for Health and Nutrition. *Nat. Prod. Res.* **2018**, *32*, 2037–2049. [CrossRef]
23. Madrigal-Santillán, E.; Portillo-Reyes, J.; Madrigal-Bujaidar, E.; Sánchez-Gutiérrez, M.; Mercado-Gonzalez, P.E.; Izquierdo Vega, J.; Vargas-Mendoza, N.; Álvarez-González, I.; Fregoso-Aguilar, T.; Delgado-Olivares, L.; et al. Opuntia Genus in Human Health: A Comprehensive Summary on Its Pharmacological, Therapeutic and Preventive Properties. Part 1. *Horticulturae.* **2022**, *8*, 88. [CrossRef]
24. Dillard, C.J.; German, J.B. Phytochemicals: Nutraceuticals and Human Health. *J. Sci. Food Agric.* **2000**, *80*, 1744–1756. [CrossRef]
25. Lichtenstein, A.H.; Deckelbaum, R.J. Stanol/Sterol ester-containing foods and blood cholesterol levels a statement for healthcare professionals from the Nutrition Committee of the Council on Nutrition, Physical Activity, and Metabolism of the American Heart Association. *Am. Heart J.* **2001**, *103*, 1177–1179.
26. Zeghbib, W.; Boudjouan, F.; Vasconcelos, V.; Lopes, G. Phenolic Compounds' Occurrence in *Opuntia* Species and Their Role in the Inflammatory Process: A Review. *Molecules* **2022**, *27*, 4763. [CrossRef] [PubMed]
27. Kozłowska, A.; Szostak-Wegierek, D. Flavonoids-Food sources and health benefits. *Rocz. Pa'nstw. Zakł. Hig.* **2014**, *65*, 79–85.
28. Smeriglio, A.; De Francesco, C.; Denaro, M.; Trombetta, D. Prickly Pear Betalain-Rich Extracts as New Promising Strategy for Intestinal Inflammation: Plant Complex vs. Main Isolated Bioactive Compounds. *Front. Pharmacol.* **2021**, *12*, 722398. [CrossRef] [PubMed]
29. Fernández-Sánchez, A.; Madrigal-Santillán, E.; Bautista, M.; Esquivel-Soto, J.; Morales-González, A.; Esquivel-Chirino, C.; Durante-Montiel, I.; Sánchez-Rivera, G.; Valadez-Vega, C.; Morales-González, J.A. Inflammation, Oxidative Stress, and Obesity. *Int. J. Mol. Sci.* **2011**, *12*, 3117–3132. [CrossRef]
30. Arulselvan, P.; Fard, M.T.; Tan, W.S.; Gothai, S.; Fakurazi, S.; Norhaizan, M.E.; Kumar, S.S. Role of Antioxidants and Natural Products in Inflammation. *Oxid. Med. Cell Longev.* **2016**, *2016*, 5276130. [CrossRef]
31. Escobedo-Hinojosa, W.I.; Gomez-Chang, E.; García-Martínez, K.; Guerrero Alquicira, R.; Cardoso-Taketa, A.; Romero, I. Gastroprotective Mechanism and Ulcer Resolution Effect of Cyrtocarpa Procera Methanolic Extract on Ethanol-Induced Gastric Injury. *Evid. Based Complement. Alternat. Med.* **2018**, *2018*, 2862706. [CrossRef]
32. Bi, W.-P.; Man, H.-B.; Man, M.-Q. Efficacy and Safety of Herbal Medicines in Treating Gastric Ulcer: A Review. *World J. Gastroenterol.* **2014**, *20*, 17020–17028. [CrossRef]
33. Kangwan, N.; Park, J.-M.; Kim, E.-H.; Hahm, K.B. Quality of Healing of Gastric Ulcers: Natural Products beyond Acid Suppression. *World J. Gastrointest. Pathophysiol.* **2014**, *5*, 40–47. [CrossRef]
34. Palevitch, D.; Earon, G.; Levin, I. Treatment of Benign Prostatic Hypertrophy with *Opuntia ficus-indica* (L.) Miller. *J. Herbs Spices Med. Plants.* **1993**, *2*, 45–49. [CrossRef]
35. Park, E.H.; Kahng, J.H.; Paek, E.A. Studies on the Pharmacological Action of Cactus: Identification of Its Anti-Inflammatory Effect. *Arch. Pharm. Res.* **1998**, *21*, 30–34. [CrossRef]
36. Loro, J.F.; del Rio, I.; Pérez-Santana, L. Preliminary Studies of Analgesic and Anti-Inflammatory Properties of Opuntia Dillenii Aqueous Extract. *J. Ethnopharmacol.* **1999**, *67*, 213–218. [CrossRef]
37. Park, E.H.; Kahng, J.H.; Lee, S.H.; Shin, K.H. An Anti-Inflammatory Principle from Cactus. *Fitoterapia* **2001**, *72*, 288–290. [CrossRef]

38. Galati, E.M.; Monforte, M.T.; Tripodo, M.M.; d'Aquino, A.; Mondello, M.R. Antiulcer Activity of *Opuntia ficus indica* (L.) Mill. (Cactaceae): Ultrastructural Study. *J. Ethnopharmacol.* **2001**, *76*, 1–9. [CrossRef]
39. Galati, E.M.; Pergolizzi, S.; Miceli, N.; Monforte, M.T.; Tripodo, M.M. Study on the Increment of the Production of Gastric Mucus in Rats Treated with *Opuntia ficus indica* (L.) Mill. Cladodes. *J. Ethnopharmacol.* **2002**, *83*, 229–233. [CrossRef]
40. Galati, E.M.; Mondello, M.R.; Giuffrida, D.; Dugo, G.; Miceli, N.; Pergolizzi, S.; Taviano, M.F. Chemical Characterization and Biological Effects of Sicilian *Opuntia ficus indica* (L.) Mill. Fruit Juice: Antioxidant and Antiulcerogenic Activity. *J. Agric. Food Chem.* **2003**, *51*, 4903–4908. [CrossRef]
41. Gentile, C.; Tesoriere, L.; Allegra, M.; Livrea, M.A.; D'Alessio, P. Antioxidant Betalains from Cactus Pear (*Opuntia ficus-indica*) Inhibit Endothelial ICAM-1 Expression. *Ann. N. Y. Acad. Sci.* **2004**, *1028*, 481–486. [CrossRef]
42. Ahmed, M.S.; El Tanbouly, N.D.; Islam, W.T.; Sleem, A.A.; El Senousy, A.S. Antiinflammatory Flavonoids from *Opuntia dillenii* (Ker-Gawl) Haw. Flowers Growing in Egypt. *Phytother. Res.* **2005**, *19*, 807–809. [CrossRef]
43. Allegra, M.; Furtmüller, P.G.; Jantschko, W.; Zederbauer, M.; Tesoriere, L.; Livrea, M.A.; Obinger, C. Mechanism of Interaction of Betanin and Indicaxanthin with Human Myeloperoxidase and Hypochlorous Acid. *Biochem. Biophys. Res. Commun.* **2005**, *332*, 837–844. [CrossRef]
44. Cho, J.Y.; Park, S.-C.; Kim, T.-W.; Kim, K.-S.; Song, J.-C.; Kim, S.-K.; Lee, H.-M.; Sung, H.-J.; Park, H.-J.; Song, Y.-B.; et al. Radical Scavenging and Anti-Inflammatory Activity of Extracts from *Opuntia humifusa* Raf. *J. Pharm. Pharmacol.* **2006**, *58*, 113–119. [CrossRef]
45. Panico, A.M.; Cardile, V.; Garufi, F.; Puglia, C.; Bonina, F.; Ronsisvalle, S. Effect of Hyaluronic Acid and Polysaccharides from *Opuntia ficus indica* (L.) Cladodes on the Metabolism of Human Chondrocyte Cultures. *J. Ethnopharmacol.* **2007**, *111*, 315–321. [CrossRef]
46. Jung, J.; Shin, J.H. Effect of *Opuntia ficus-indica* Extract on Anti-Inflammatory in Murine Macrophages. *FASEB J.* **2010**, *24*, 929.5. [CrossRef]
47. Kim, J.; Jho, K.H.; Choi, Y.H.; Nam, S.-Y. Chemopreventive Effect of Cactus (*Opuntia humifusa*) Extracts: Radical Scavenging Activity, pro-Apoptosis, and Anti-Inflammatory Effect in Human Colon (SW480) and Breast Cancer (MCF7) Cells. *Food Funct.* **2013**, *4*, 681–688. [CrossRef]
48. Tesoriere, L.; Attanzio, A.; Allegra, M.; Gentile, C.; Livrea, M.A. Indicaxanthin Inhibits NADPH Oxidase (NOX)-1 Activation and NF-KB-Dependent Release of Inflammatory Mediators and Prevents the Increase of Epithelial Permeability in IL-1β-Exposed Caco-2 Cells. *Br. J. Nutr.* **2014**, *111*, 415–423. [CrossRef]
49. Allegra, M.; Ianaro, A.; Tersigni, M.; Panza, E.; Tesoriere, L.; Livrea, M.A. Indicaxanthin from Cactus Pear Fruit Exerts Anti-Inflammatory Effects in Carrageenin-Induced Rat Pleurisy. *J. Nutr.* **2014**, *144*, 185–192. [CrossRef]
50. Matias, A.; Nunes, S.L.; Poejo, J.; Mecha, E.; Serra, A.T.; Madeira, P.J.A.; Bronze, M.R.; Duarte, C.M.M. Antioxidant and Anti-Inflammatory Activity of a Flavonoid-Rich Concentrate Recovered from *Opuntia ficus-indica* Juice. *Food Funct.* **2014**, *5*, 3269–3280. [CrossRef]
51. Chauhan, S.P.; Sheth, N.R.; Suhagia, B.N. Analgesic and Anti-Inflammatory Action of *Opuntia elatior* Mill Fruits. *J. Ayurveda Integr. Med.* **2015**, *6*, 75–81. [CrossRef]
52. Antunes-Ricardo, M.; Gutiérrez-Uribe, J.A.; Martínez-Vitela, C.; Serna-Saldívar, S.O. Topical Anti-Inflammatory Effects of Isorhamnetin Glycosides Isolated from *Opuntia ficus-indica*. *Biomed. Res. Int.* **2015**, *2015*, 847320. [CrossRef]
53. Filannino, P.; Cavoski, I.; Thlien, N.; Vincentini, O.; De Angelis, M.; Silano, M.; Gobbetti, M.; Di Cagno, R. Lactic Acid Fermentation of Cactus Cladodes (*Opuntia ficusindica* L.) Generates Flavonoid Derivatives with Antioxidant and Anti-Inflammatory Properties. *PLoS ONE* **2016**, *11*, e0152575. [CrossRef]
54. Siddiqui, F.; Abidi, L.; Poh, C.F.; Faizi, S.; Farooq, A.D. Analgesic Potential of Opuntia Dillenii and Its Compounds Opuntiol and Opuntioside against Pain Models in Mice. *Rec. Nat. Prod.* **2016**, *10*, 721.
55. Siddiqui, F.; Naqvi, S.; Abidi, L.; Faizi, S.; Avesi, L.; Mirza, T.; Farooq, A.D. Opuntia Dillenii Cladode: Opuntiol and Opuntioside Attenuated Cytokines and Eicosanoids Mediated Inflammation. *J. Ethnopharmacol.* **2016**, *182*, 221–234. [CrossRef]
56. Sharma, B.R.; Park, C.M.; Choi, J.W.; Rhyu, D.Y. Anti-Nociceptive and Anti-Inflammatory Effects of the Methanolic Extract of *Opuntia humifusa* Stem. *Avicenna J. Phytomed.* **2017**, *7*, 366–375.
57. Chahdoura, H.; El Bok, S.; Refifa, T.; Adouni, K.; Khemiss, F.; Mosbah, H.; Ben-Attia, M.; Flamini, G.; Achour, L. Activity of Anti-Inflammatory, Analgesic and Antigenotoxic of the Aqueous Flower Extracts of *Opuntia microdasys* Lem.Pfeiff. *J. Pharm. Pharmacol.* **2017**, *69*, 1056–1063. [CrossRef]
58. Bounihi, A.; Bitam, A.; Bouazza, A.; Yargui, L.; Koceir, E.A. Fruit Vinegars Attenuate Cardiac Injury via Anti-Inflammatory and Anti-Adiposity Actions in High-Fat Diet-Induced Obese Rats. *Pharm. Biol.* **2017**, *55*, 43–52. [CrossRef]
59. Aboura, I.; Nani, A.; Belarbi, M.; Murtaza, B.; Fluckiger, A.; Dumont, A.; Benammar, C.; Tounsi, M.S.; Ghiringhelli, F.; Rialland, M.; et al. Protective Effects of Polyphenol-Rich Infusions from Carob (*Ceratonia siliqua*) Leaves and Cladodes of Opuntia ficus-indica against Inflammation Associated with Diet-Induced Obesity and DSS-Induced Colitis in Swiss Mice. *Biomed. Pharmacother.* **2017**, *96*, 1022–1035. [CrossRef]
60. Chahdoura, H.; Barreira, J.C.M.; Adouni, K.; Mhadhebi, L.; Calhelha, R.C.; Snoussi, M.; Majdoub, H.; Flamini, G.; Ferreira, I.C.F.R.; Achour, L. Bioactivity and Chemical Characterization of *Opuntia macrorhiza* Engelm. Seed Oil: Potential Food and Pharmaceutical Applications. *Food Funct.* **2017**, *8*, 2739–2747. [CrossRef]
61. Saih, F.-E.; Andreoletti, P.; Mandard, S.; Latruffe, N.; El Kebbaj, M.S.; Lizard, G.; Nasser, B.; Cherkaoui-Malki, M. Protective Effect of Cactus Cladode Extracts on Peroxisomal Functions in Microglial BV-2 Cells Activated by Different Lipopolysaccharides. *Molecules* **2017**, *22*, 102. [CrossRef]

62. Aiello, A.; Di Bona, D.; Candore, G.; Carru, C.; Zinellu, A.; Di Miceli, G.; Nicosia, A.; Gambino, C.M.; Ruisi, P.; Caruso, C.; et al. Targeting Aging with Functional Food: Pasta with Opuntia Single-Arm Pilot Study. *Rejuvenation Res.* **2018**, *21*, 249–256. [CrossRef]
63. Attanzio, A.; Tesoriere, L.; Vasto, S.; Pintaudi, A.M.; Livrea, M.A.; Allegra, M. Short-Term Cactus Pear [*Opuntia ficus-indica* (L.) Mill] Fruit Supplementation Ameliorates the Inflammatory Profile and Is Associated with Improved Antioxidant Status among Healthy Humans. *Food Nutr. Res.* **2018**, *62*, 1262. [CrossRef]
64. Benattia, F.K.; Arrar, Z.; Dergal, F.; Khabbal, Y. Pharmaco-Analytical Study and Phytochemical Profile of Hydroethanolic Extract of Algerian Prickly Pear (*Opuntia ficus-indica* L.). *Curr. Pharm. Biotechnol.* **2019**, *20*, 696–706. [CrossRef] [PubMed]
65. Bardaa, S.; Turki, M.; Ben Khedir, S.; Mzid, M.; Rebai, T.; Ayadi, F.; Sahnoun, Z. The Effect of Prickly Pear, Pumpkin, and Linseed Oils on Biological Mediators of Acute Inflammation and Oxidative Stress Markers. *Biomed. Res. Int.* **2020**, *2020*, 5643465. [CrossRef] [PubMed]
66. Lee, Y.S.; Yang, W.K.; Park, Y.R.; Park, Y.C.; Park, I.J.; Lee, G.J.; Kang, H.S.; Kim, B.K.; Kim, S.H. Opuntia ficus-indica Alleviates Particulate Matter 10 Plus Diesel Exhaust Particles (PM10D)-Induced Airway Inflammation by Suppressing the Expression of Inflammatory Cytokines and Chemokines. *Plants* **2022**, *11*, 520. [CrossRef] [PubMed]
67. Lee, E.B.; Hyun, J.E.; Li, D.W.; Moon, Y.I. Effects of *Opuntia ficus-indica* Var. Saboten Stem on Gastric Damages in Rats. *Arch. Pharm. Res.* **2002**, *25*, 67–70. [CrossRef]
68. Wiese, J.; McPherson, S.; Odden, M.C.; Shlipak, M.G. Effect of *Opuntia ficus indica* on Symptoms of the Alcohol Hangover. *Arch. Intern. Med.* **2004**, *164*, 1334–1340. [CrossRef]
69. Vázquez-Ramírez, R.; Olguín-Martínez, M.; Kubli-Garfias, C.; Hernández-Muñoz, R. Reversing Gastric Mucosal Alterations during Ethanol-Induced Chronic Gastritis in Rats by Oral Administration of *Opuntia ficus-indica* Mucilage. *World J. Gastroenterol.* **2006**, *12*, 4318–4324. [CrossRef]
70. Alimi, H.; Hfaiedh, N.; Bouoni, Z.; Hfaiedh, M.; Sakly, M.; Zourgui, L.; Rhouma, K.B. Antioxidant and Antiulcerogenic Activities of *Opuntia ficus indica* f. Inermis Root Extract in Rats. *Phytomedicine* **2010**, *17*, 1120–1126. [CrossRef]
71. Alimi, H.; Hfaiedh, N.; Bouoni, Z.; Sakly, M.; Ben Rhouma, K. Evaluation of Antioxidant and Antiulcerogenic Activities of *Opuntia ficus indica* f. Inermis Flowers Extract in Rats. *Environ. Toxicol. Pharmacol.* **2011**, *32*, 406–416. [CrossRef]
72. Alimi, H.; Hfaiedh, N.; Bouoni, Z.; Sakly, M.; Rhouma, K.B. Ameliorative Effect of *Opuntia ficus indica* Juice on Ethanol-Induced Oxidative Stress in Rat Erythrocytes. *Exp. Toxicol. Pathol.* **2013**, *65*, 391–396. [CrossRef]
73. Jouini, M.; Abdelhamid, A.; Chaouch, M.A.; le Cerf, D.; Bouraoui, A.; Majdoub, H.; Ben Jannet, H. Physico-Chemical Characterization and Pharmacological Activities of Polysaccharides from *Opuntia microdasys* Var. Rufida Cladodes. *Int. J. Biol. Macromol.* **2018**, *107*, 1330–1338. [CrossRef]
74. Babitha, S.; Bindu, K.; Nageena, T.; Veerapur, V.P. Fresh Fruit Juice of Opuntia Dillenii Haw. Attenuates Acetic Acid-Induced Ulcerative Colitis in Rats. *J. Diet. Suppl.* **2019**, *16*, 431–442. [CrossRef] [PubMed]
75. Elsawi, S.A.; Radwan, R.R.; Elbatanony, M.M.; El-Feky, A.M.; Sherif, N.H. Prophylactic Effect of *Opuntia ficus indica* Fruit Peel Extract against Irradiation-Induced Colon Injury in Rats. *Planta Med.* **2020**, *86*, 61–69. [CrossRef] [PubMed]
76. Iriti, M.; Vitalini, S.; Fico, G.; Faoro, F. Neuroprotective Herbs and Foods from Different Traditional Medicines and Diets. *Molecules* **2010**, *15*, 3517–3555. [CrossRef]
77. Khazdair, M.R.; Anaeigoudari, A.; Hashemzehi, M.; Mohebbati, R. Neuroprotective Potency of Some Spice Herbs, a Literature Review. *J. Tradit. Complement. Med.* **2019**, *9*, 98–105. [CrossRef]
78. Chang, R.; Ho, Y. Introductory Chapter: Concept of Neuroprotection—A New Perspective. In *Neuroprotection*; Chang, R.C., Ho, Y., Eds.; IntechOpen: Rijeka, Croatia, 2019; pp. 1–19.
79. Mohd Sairazi, N.S.; Sirajudeen, K.N.S. Natural Products and Their Bioactive Compounds: Neuroprotective Potentials against Neurodegenerative Diseases. *Evid. Based Complement. Alternat. Med.* **2020**, *2020*, 6565396. [CrossRef] [PubMed]
80. Wie, M.-B. Protective Effects of *Opuntia ficus-indica* and Saururus Chinensis on Free Radical-Induced Neuronal Injury in Mouse Cortical Cell Cultures. *Yakhak. Hoeji.* **2000**, *44*, 613–619.
81. Dok-Go, H.; Lee, K.H.; Kim, H.J.; Lee, E.H.; Lee, J.; Song, Y.S.; Lee, Y.-H.; Jin, C.; Lee, Y.S.; Cho, J. Neuroprotective Effects of Antioxidative Flavonoids, Quercetin, (+)-Dihydroquercetin and Quercetin 3-Methyl Ether, Isolated from *Opuntia ficus-indica* Var. Saboten. *Brain Res.* **2003**, *965*, 130–136. [CrossRef]
82. Kim, J.-H.; Park, S.-M.; Ha, H.-J.; Moon, C.-J.; Shin, T.-K.; Kim, J.-M.; Lee, N.-H.; Kim, H.-C.; Jang, K.-J.; Wie, M.-B. *Opuntia ficus-indica* Attenuates Neuronal Injury in in Vitro and in Vivo Models of Cerebral Ischemia. *J. Ethnopharmacol.* **2006**, *104*, 257–262. [CrossRef]
83. Lee, M.H.; Kim, J.Y.; Yoon, J.H.; Lim, H.J.; Kim, T.H.; Jin, C.; Kwak, W.-J.; Han, C.-K.; Ryu, J.-H. Inhibition of Nitric Oxide Synthase Expression in Activated Microglia and Peroxynitrite Scavenging Activity by *Opuntia ficus indica* Var. Saboten. *Phytother Res.* **2006**, *20*, 742–747. [CrossRef]
84. Cho, J.-S.; Han, C.-K.; Lee, Y.-S.; Jin, C.-B. Neuroprotective and Antioxidant Effects of the Butanol Fraction Prepared from *Opuntia ficus-indica* Var. Saboten. *Biomol Ther.* **2007**, *15*, 205–211. [CrossRef]
85. Huang, X.; Li, Q.; Zhang, Y.; Lü, Q.; Guo, L.; Huang, L.; He, Z. Neuroprotective Effects of Cactus Polysaccharide on Oxygen and Glucose Deprivation Induced Damage in Rat Brain Slices. *Cell Mol. Neurobiol.* **2008**, *28*, 559–568. [CrossRef]
86. Huang, X.; Li, Q.; Li, H.; Guo, L. Neuroprotective and Antioxidative Effect of Cactus Polysaccharides in Vivo and in Vitro. *Cell Mol. Neurobiol.* **2009**, *29*, 1211–1221. [CrossRef]

87. Chen, Y.; Zhao, B.; Huang, X.; Zhan, J.; Zhao, Y.; Zhou, M.; Guo, L. Purification and Neuroprotective Effects of Polysaccharides from Opuntia Milpa Alta in Cultured Cortical Neurons. *Int. J. Biol. Macromol.* **2011**, *49*, 681–687. [CrossRef]
88. Briffa, M.; Ghio, S.; Neuner, J.; Gauci, A.J.; Cacciottolo, R.; Marchal, C.; Caruana, M.; Cullin, C.; Vassallo, N.; Cauchi, R.J. Extracts from Two Ubiquitous Mediterranean Plants Ameliorate Cellular and Animal Models of Neurodegenerative Proteinopathies. *Neurosci. Lett.* **2017**, *638*, 12–20. [CrossRef]
89. Gambino, G.; Allegra, M.; Sardo, P.; Attanzio, A.; Tesoriere, L.; Livrea, M.A.; Ferraro, G.; Carletti, F. Brain Distribution and Modulation of Neuronal Excitability by Indicaxanthin from *Opuntia ficus indica* Administered at Nutritionally-Relevant Amounts. *Front. Aging Neurosci.* **2018**, *10*, 133. [CrossRef]
90. Tutone, M.; Virzì, A.; Almerico, A.M. Reverse Screening on Indicaxanthin from *Opuntia ficus-indica* as Natural Chemoactive and Chemopreventive Agent. *J. Theor. Biol.* **2018**, *455*, 147–160. [CrossRef]
91. Kim, J.K.; Lim, M.L. Anti-Inflammatory and Neuroprotective Effects of *Opuntia ficus-indica* Var. Saboten Alone or Combined with Vitamin C. *J. Korean Soc. Food Sci. Nutr.* **2019**, *48*, 613–621. [CrossRef]
92. El-Hawary, S.S.; Sobeh, M.; Badr, W.K.; Abdelfattah, M.A.O.; Ali, Z.Y.; El-Tantawy, M.E.; Rabeh, M.A.; Wink, M. HPLC-PDA-MS/MS Profiling of Secondary Metabolites from *Opuntia ficus-indica* Cladode, Peel and Fruit Pulp Extracts and Their Antioxidant, Neuroprotective Effect in Rats with Aluminum Chloride Induced Neurotoxicity. *Saudi J. Biol. Sci.* **2020**, *27*, 2829–2838. [CrossRef]
93. Jouini, M.; Horchani, M.; Zardi-Bergaoui, A.; Znati, M.; Romdhane, A.; Krisa, S.; Waffo-Téguo, P.; Ben, J. Phytochemical Analysis, Neuroprotective, Anticholinesterase, Cytotoxic and Catalase Potentials of *Opuntia microdasys* Var. *Rufida* and *Opuntia leptocaulis*. *Chem. Africa.* **2021**, *4*, 285–298. [CrossRef]
94. Musarra-Pizzo, M.; Pennisi, R.; Ben-Amor, I.; Mandalari, G.; Sciortino, M.T. Antiviral Activity Exerted by Natural Products against Human Viruses. *Viruses* **2021**, *13*, 828. [CrossRef]
95. Ben-Shabat, S.; Yarmolinsky, L.; Porat, D.; Dahan, A. Antiviral Effect of Phytochemicals from Medicinal Plants: Applications and Drug Delivery Strategies. *Drug Deliv. Transl. Res.* **2020**, *10*, 354–367. [CrossRef] [PubMed]
96. Ahmad, A.; Davies, J.; Randall, S.; Skinner, G.R. Antiviral Properties of Extract of Opuntia Streptacantha. *Antivir. Res.* **1996**, *30*, 75–85. [CrossRef]
97. Bouslama, L.; Hayashi, K.; Lee, J.-B.; Ghorbel, A.; Hayashi, T. Potent Virucidal Effect of Pheophorbide a and Pyropheophorbide a on Enveloped Viruses. *J. Nat. Med.* **2011**, *65*, 229–233. [CrossRef] [PubMed]
98. Rasoulpour, R.; Izadpanah, K.; Afsharifar, A. Opuntin B, the Antiviral Protein Isolated from Prickly Pear (*Opuntia ficus-indica* (L.) Miller) Cladode Exhibits Ribonuclease Activity. *Microb. Pathog.* **2020**, *140*, 103929. [CrossRef] [PubMed]
99. Quinto, E.J.; Caro, I.; Villalobos-Delgado, L.H.; Mateo, J.; De-Mateo-Silleras, B.; Redondo-Del-Río, M.P. Food Safety through Natural Antimicrobials. *Antibiotics* **2019**, *8*, 208. [CrossRef]
100. Karunaratne, D.N.; Pamunuwa, G. Natural Antimicrobials, Their Sources and Food Safety. In *Food Additives*; IntechOpen: Rijeka, Croatia, 2017; pp. 87–102. ISBN 978-953-51-3489-3.
101. Nascimento, G.; Locatelli, J.; Freitas, C.; Silva, G. Antibacterial Activity of Plant Extracts and Phytochemicals on Antibiotic-Resistant Bacteria Antibacterial Activity of Plant Extracts and Phytochemicals on Antibiotic-Resistant Bacteria. *Braz. J. Microbiol.* **2000**, *31*, 247–256. [CrossRef]
102. Cushnie, T.P.T.; Lamb, A.J. Antimicrobial Activity of Flavonoids. *Int. J. Antimicrob. Agents.* **2005**, *26*, 343–356. [CrossRef]
103. Aruwa, C.E.; Amoo, S.O.; Kudanga, T. *Opuntia* (Cactaceae) Plant Compounds, Biological Activities and Prospects—A Comprehensive Review. *Food Res. Int.* **2018**, *112*, 328–344. [CrossRef]
104. Ginestra, G.; Parker, M.L.; Bennett, R.N.; Robertson, J.; Mandalari, G.; Narbad, A.; Lo Curto, R.B.; Bisignano, G.; Faulds, C.B.; Waldron, K.W. Anatomical, Chemical, and Biochemical Characterization of Cladodes from Prickly Pear [*Opuntia ficus-indica* (L.) Mill.]. *J. Agric. Food Chem.* **2009**, *57*, 10323–10330. [CrossRef]
105. Sánchez, E.; García, S.; Heredia, N. Extracts of Edible and Medicinal Plants Damage Membranes of Vibrio Cholerae. *Appl. Environ. Microbiol.* **2010**, *76*, 6888–6894. [CrossRef] [PubMed]
106. Umar, M.; Javeed, A.; Ashraf, M.; Riaz, A.; Mukhtar, M.; Afzal, S.; Altaf, R. Polarity-Based Solvents Extraction of *Opuntia dillenii* and *Zingiber officinale* for In Vitro Antimicrobial Activities. *Int. J. Food Prop.* **2010**, *16*, 114–124. [CrossRef]
107. Jacobo-Salcedo, M.D.R.; Alonso-Castro, A.J.; Salazar-Olivo, L.A.; Carranza-Alvarez, C.; González-Espíndola, L.A.; Domínguez, F.; Maciel-Torres, S.P.; García-Lujan, C.; González-Martínez, M.D.R.; Gómez-Sánchez, M.; et al. Antimicrobial and Cytotoxic Effects of Mexican Medicinal Plants. *Nat. Prod. Commun.* **2011**, *6*, 1925–1928. [CrossRef]
108. Castillo, S.L.; Heredia, N.; Contreras, J.F.; García, S. Extracts of Edible and Medicinal Plants in Inhibition of Growth, Adherence, and Cytotoxin Production of *Campylobacter jejuni* and *Campylobacter coli*. *J. Food Sci.* **2011**, *76*, M421–M426. [CrossRef] [PubMed]
109. Hayek, S.A.; Ibrahim, S.A. Antimicrobial Activity of Xoconostle Pears (*Opuntia matudae*) against *Escherichia coli* O157:H7 in Laboratory Medium. *Int. J. Microbiol.* **2012**, *2012*, 368472. [CrossRef]
110. Ammar, I.; Ennouri, M.; Khemakhem, B.; Yangui, T.; Attia, H. Variation in Chemical Composition and Biological Activities of Two Species of Opuntia Flowers at Four Stages of Flowering. *Ind. Crop. Prod.* **2012**, *37*, 34–40. [CrossRef]
111. Ennouri, M.; Ammar, I.; Khemakhem, B.; Attia, H. Chemical Composition and Antibacterial Activity of *Opuntia ficus-indica* f. *inermis* (Cactus Pear) Flowers. *J. Med. Food.* **2014**, *17*, 908–914. [CrossRef]
112. Ratnaweera, P.B.; de Silva, E.D.; Williams, D.E.; Andersen, R.J. Antimicrobial Activities of Endophytic Fungi Obtained from the Arid Zone Invasive Plant *Opuntia dillenii* and the Isolation of Equisetin, from Endophytic *Fusarium* sp. *BMC Complement. Altern. Med.* **2015**, *15*, 220. [CrossRef]

113. Ammar, I.; Bardaa, S.; Mzid, M.; Sahnoun, Z.; Rebaii, T.; Attia, H.; Ennouri, M. Antioxidant, Antibacterial and in Vivo Dermal Wound Healing Effects of Opuntia Flower Extracts. *Int. J. Biol. Macromol.* **2015**, *81*, 483–490. [CrossRef]
114. Gopi, D.; Kanimozhi, K.; Kavitha, L. *Opuntia ficus indica* Peel Derived Pectin Mediated Hydroxyapatite Nanoparticles: Synthesis, Spectral Characterization, Biological and Antimicrobial Activities. *Spectrochim. Acta A Mol. Biomol. Spectrosc.* **2015**, *141*, 135–143. [CrossRef]
115. Sánchez, E.; Rivas Morales, C.; Castillo, S.; Leos-Rivas, C.; García-Becerra, L.; Ortiz Martínez, D.M. Antibacterial and Antibiofilm Activity of Methanolic Plant Extracts against Nosocomial Microorganisms. *Evid. Based Complement. Alternat. Med.* **2016**, *2016*, 1572697. [CrossRef]
116. Gómez-Aldapa, C.A.; Cerna-Cortes, J.F.; Rangel-Vargas, E.; Torres-Vitela, M.R.; Villarruel-López, A.; Gutiérrez-Alcántara, E.J.; Castro-Rosas, J. Presence of Multidrug-Resistant Shiga Toxin-Producing Escherichia Coli, Enteropathogenic *E. coli* and Enterotoxigenic *E. coli*, on Raw Nopalitos (*Opuntia ficus-indica* L.) and in Nopalitos Salads from Local Retail Markets in Mexico. *Foodborne Pathog. Dis.* **2016**, *13*, 269–274. [CrossRef] [PubMed]
117. Chahdoura, H.; Barreira, J.C.M.; Fernández-Ruiz, V.; Morales, P.; Calhelha, R.C.; Flamini, G.; Soković, M.; Ferreira, I.C.F.R.; Achour, L. Bioactivity, Proximate, Mineral and Volatile Profiles along the Flowering Stages of *Opuntia microdasys* (Lehm.): Defining Potential Applications. *Food Funct.* **2016**, *7*, 1458–1467. [CrossRef] [PubMed]
118. Ramírez-Moreno, E.; Cariño-Cortés, R.; Cruz-Cansino, N.D.S.; Delgado-Olivares, L.; Ariza-Ortega, J.A.; Montañez-Izquierdo, V.Y.; Hernández-Herrero, M.M.; Filardo-Kerstupp, T. Antioxidant and Antimicrobial Properties of Cactus Pear (*Opuntia*) Seed Oils. *J. Food Qual.* **2017**, *2017*, e3075907. [CrossRef]
119. Koubaa, M.; Mhemdi, H.; Barba, F.J.; Angelotti, A.; Bouaziz, F.; Chaabouni, S.E.; Vorobiev, E. Seed Oil Extraction from Red Prickly Pear Using Hexane and Supercritical CO_2: Assessment of Phenolic Compound Composition, Antioxidant and Antibacterial Activities. *J. Sci. Food Agric.* **2017**, *97*, 613–620. [CrossRef] [PubMed]
120. Arbia, L.; Chikhi-Chorfi, N.; Betatache, I.; Pham-Huy, C.; Zenia, S.; Mameri, N.; Drouiche, N.; Lounici, H. Antimicrobial Activity of Aqueous Extracts from Four Plants on Bacterial Isolates from Periodontitis Patients. *Environ. Sci. Pollut. Res. Int.* **2017**, *24*, 13394–13404. [CrossRef] [PubMed]
121. Gómez-Aldapa, C.A.; Gutiérrez-Alcántara, E.J.; Torres-Vitela, M.R.; Rangel-Vargas, E.; Villarruel-López, A.; Castro-Rosas, J. Prevalence and Behavior of Multidrug-Resistant Salmonella Strains on Raw Whole and Cut Nopalitos (*Opuntia ficus-indica* L.) and on Nopalitos Salads. *J. Sci. Food Agric.* **2017**, *97*, 4117–4123. [CrossRef]
122. Welegerima, G.; Zemene, A.; Tilahun, Y. Phytochemical composition and antibacterial activity of *Opuntia ficus-indica* cladodes extracts. *J. Med. Plants Stud.* **2018**, *6*, 243–246.
123. Palmeri, R.; Parafati, L.; Restuccia, C.; Fallico, B. Application of Prickly Pear Fruit Extract to Improve Domestic Shelf Life, Quality and Microbial Safety of Sliced Beef. *Food Chem. Toxicol.* **2018**, *118*, 355–360. [CrossRef]
124. Khémiri, I.; Essghaier Hédi, B.; Sadfi Zouaoui, N.; Ben Gdara, N.; Bitri, L. The Antimicrobial and Wound Healing Potential of *Opuntia ficus indica* L. Inermis Extracted Oil from Tunisia. *Evid. Based Complement. Alternat. Med.* **2019**, *2019*, 9148782. [CrossRef]
125. Maema, L.P.; Potgieter, M.; Masevhe, N.A.; Samie, A. Antimicrobial Activity of Selected Plants against Fungal Species Isolated from South African AIDS Patients and Their Antigonococcal Activity. *J. Complement. Integr. Med.* **2020**, *17*, 20190087. [CrossRef]
126. Elkady, W.M.; Bishr, M.M.; Abdel-Aziz, M.M.; Salama, O.M. Identification and Isolation of Anti-Pneumonia Bioactive Compounds from *Opuntia ficus-indica* Fruit Waste Peels. *Food Funct.* **2020**, *11*, 5275–5283. [CrossRef] [PubMed]
127. Gonçalves, L.A.; Lorenzo, J.M.; Trindade, M.A. Fruit and Agro-Industrial Waste Extracts as Potential Antimicrobials in Meat Products: A Brief Review. *Foods* **2021**, *10*, 1469. [CrossRef] [PubMed]
128. Surup, F.; Minh Thi Tran, T.; Pfütze, S.; Budde, J.; Moussa-Ayoub, T.E.; Rohn, S.; Jerz, G. Opuntisines, 14-Membered Cyclopeptide Alkaloids from Fruits of *Opuntia stricta* Var. *Dillenii* Isolated by High-Performance Countercurrent Chromatography. *Food Chem.* **2021**, *334*, 127552. [CrossRef] [PubMed]
129. Pourmajed, R.; Jabbari Amiri, M.; Karami, P.; Khaledi, A. Antimicrobial Effect of *Opuntia ficus-indica* Extract on *Escherichia coli* Isolated from Patients with Urinary Tract Infection. *Iran J. Public Health* **2021**, *50*, 634–636. [CrossRef]
130. Gushiken, L.F.S.; Beserra, F.P.; Bastos, J.K.; Jackson, C.J.; Pellizzon, C.H. Cutaneous Wound Healing: An Update from Physiopathology to Current Therapies. *Life* **2021**, *11*, 665. [CrossRef]
131. Pazyar, N.; Yaghoobi, R.; Rafiee, E.; Mehrabian, A.; Feily, A. Skin Wound Healing and Phytomedicine: A Review. *Skin Pharmacol. Physiol.* **2014**, *27*, 303–310. [CrossRef]
132. Galati, E.M.; Mondello, M.R.; Monforte, M.T.; Galluzzo, M.; Miceli, N.; Tripodo, M.M. Effect of *Opuntia ficus-indica* (L.) Mill. Cladodes in the Wound-Healing Process. *J. Prof. Assoc. Cact. Dev.* **2003**, *5*, 1–16.
133. Trombetta, D.; Puglia, C.; Perri, D.; Licata, A.; Pergolizzi, S.; Lauriano, E.R.; De Pasquale, A.; Saija, A.; Bonina, F.P. Effect of Polysaccharides from *Opuntia ficus-indica* (L.) Cladodes on the Healing of Dermal Wounds in the Rat. *Phytomedicine* **2006**, *13*, 352–358. [CrossRef]
134. Nakahara, T.; Mitoma, C.; Hashimoto-Hachiya, A.; Takahara, M.; Tsuji, G.; Uchi, H.; Yan, X.; Hachisuka, J.; Chiba, T.; Esaki, H.; et al. Antioxidant *Opuntia ficus-indica* Extract Activates AHR-NRF2 Signaling and Upregulates Filaggrin and Loricrin Expression in Human Keratinocytes. *J. Med. Food* **2015**, *18*, 1143–1149. [CrossRef]
135. Deters, A.M.; Meyer, U.; Stintzing, F.C. Time-Dependent Bioactivity of Preparations from Cactus Pear (*Opuntia ficus indica*) and Ice Plant (*Mesembryanthemum crystallinum*) on Human Skin Fibroblasts and Keratinocytes. *J. Ethnopharmacol.* **2012**, *142*, 438–444. [CrossRef]

136. Di Lorenzo, F.; Silipo, A.; Molinaro, A.; Parrilli, M.; Schiraldi, C.; D'Agostino, A.; Izzo, E.; Rizza, L.; Bonina, A.; Bonina, F.; et al. The Polysaccharide and Low Molecular Weight Components of *Opuntia ficus indica* Cladodes: Structure and Skin Repairing Properties. *Carbohydr. Polym.* **2017**, *157*, 128–136. [CrossRef] [PubMed]
137. Park, K.; Choi, H.-S.; Hong, Y.H.; Jung, E.Y.; Suh, H.J. Cactus Cladodes (*Opuntia humifusa*) Extract Minimizes the Effects of UV Irradiation on Keratinocytes and Hairless Mice. *Pharm. Biol.* **2017**, *55*, 1032–1040. [CrossRef]
138. Fang, Q.; Huang, C.; You, C.; Ma, S. Opuntia Extract Reduces Scar Formation in Rabbit Ear Model: A Randomized Controlled Study. *Int. J. Low Extrem. Wounds.* **2015**, *14*, 343–352. [CrossRef] [PubMed]
139. Bardaa, S.; Chabchoub, N.; Jridi, M.; Moalla, D.; Mseddi, M.; Rebai, T.; Sahnoun, Z. The Effect of Natural Extracts on Laser Burn Wound Healing. *J. Surg. Res.* **2016**, *201*, 464–472. [CrossRef]
140. Bassino, E.; Gasparri, F.; Munaron, L. Natural Dietary Antioxidants Containing Flavonoids Modulate Keratinocytes Physiology: In Vitro Tri-Culture Models. *J. Ethnopharmacol.* **2019**, *238*, 111844. [CrossRef] [PubMed]
141. Kandan, P.V.; Balupillai, A.; Kanimozhi, G.; Khan, H.A.; Alhomida, A.S.; Prasad, N.R. Opuntiol Prevents Photoaging of Mouse Skin via Blocking Inflammatory Responses and Collagen Degradation. *Oxid. Med. Cell Longev.* **2020**, *2020*, 5275178. [CrossRef]
142. Moon, J.Y.; Ngoc, L.T.N.; Chae, M.; Tran, V.V.; Lee, Y.C. Effects of Microwave-Assisted *Opuntia humifusa* Extract in Inhibiting the Impacts of Particulate Matter on Human Keratinocyte Skin Cell. *Antioxidants* **2020**, *9*, 271. [CrossRef] [PubMed]
143. Koshak, A.E.; Algandaby, M.M.; Mujallid, M.I.; Abdel-Naim, A.B.; Alhakamy, N.A.; Fahmy, U.A.; Alfarsi, A.; Badr-Eldin, S.M.; Neamatallah, T.; Nasrullah, M.Z.; et al. Wound Healing Activity of *Opuntia ficus-indica* Fixed Oil Formulated in a Self-Nanoemulsifying Formulation. *Int. J. Nanomedicine.* **2021**, *16*, 3889–3905. [CrossRef]
144. Catanzano, O.; Gomez d'Ayala, G.; D'Agostino, A.; Di Lorenzo, F.; Schiraldi, C.; Malinconico, M.; Lanzetta, R.; Bonina, F.; Laurienzo, P. PEG-Crosslinked-Chitosan Hydrogel Films for in Situ Delivery of *Opuntia ficus-indica* Extract. *Carbohydr. Polym.* **2021**, *264*, 117987. [CrossRef]
145. Saleem, R.; Ahmad, M.; Azmat, A.; Ahmad, S.I.; Faizi, Z.; Abidi, L.; Faizi, S. Hypotensive Activity, Toxicology and Histopathology of Opuntioside-I and Methanolic Extract of *Opuntia dillenii*. *Biol. Pharm. Bull.* **2005**, *28*, 1844–1851. [CrossRef]
146. Boukeloua, A.; Belkhiri, A.; Djerrou, Z.; Bahri, L.; Boulebda, N.; Hamdi Pacha, Y. Acute Toxicity of *Opuntia ficus indica* and *Pistacia lentiscus* Seed Oils in Mice. *Afr. J. Tradit. Complement. Altern. Med.* **2012**, *9*, 607–611. [CrossRef] [PubMed]
147. Osorio-Esquivel, O.; Ortiz-Moreno, A.; Garduño-Siciliano, L.; Alvarez, V.B.; Hernández-Navarro, M.D. Antihyperlipidemic Effect of Methanolic Extract from *Opuntia joconostle* Seeds in Mice Fed a Hypercholesterolemic Diet. *Plant Foods Hum. Nutr.* **2012**, *67*, 365–370. [CrossRef] [PubMed]
148. Berraaouan, A.; Ziyyat, A.; Mekhfi, H.; Legssyer, A.; Sindic, M.; Aziz, M.; Bnouham, M. Evaluation of Antidiabetic Properties of Cactus Pear Seed Oil in Rats. *Pharm. Biol.* **2014**, *52*, 1286–1290. [CrossRef] [PubMed]
149. Tsafantakis, N.; Katsanou, E.S.; Kyriakopoulou, K.; Psarou, E.-C.; Raptaki, I.; Skaltsounis, A.L.; Audebert, M.; Machera, K.A.; Fokialakis, N. Comparative UHPLC-HRMS Profiling, Toxicological Assessment, and Protection Against H_2O_2-Induced Genotoxicity of Different Parts of *Opuntia ficus indica*. *J. Med. Food.* **2019**, *22*, 1280–1293. [CrossRef] [PubMed]
150. Han, E.H.; Lim, M.K.; Lee, S.H.; Rahman, M.M.; Lim, Y.-H. An Oral Toxicity Test in Rats and a Genotoxicity Study of Extracts from the Stems of *Opuntia ficus-indica* Var. Saboten. *BMC Complement. Altern. Med.* **2019**, *19*, 31. [CrossRef]
151. Bouhrim, M.; Ouassou, H.; Boutahiri, S.; Daoudi, N.E.; Mechchate, H.; Gressier, B.; Eto, B.; Imtara, H.; A Alotaibi, A.; Al-Zharani, M.; et al. *Opuntia dillenii* (Ker Gawl.) Haw., Seeds Oil Antidiabetic Potential Using In Vivo, In Vitro, In Situ, and Ex Vivo Approaches to Reveal Its Underlying Mechanism of Action. *Molecules* **2021**, *26*, 1677. [CrossRef]
152. Bouhrim, M.; Boutahiri, S.; Kharchoufa, L.; Mechchate, H.; Mohamed Al Kamaly, O.; Berraaouan, A.; Eto, B.; Ziyyat, A.; Mekhfi, H.; Legssyer, A.; et al. Acute and Subacute Toxicity and Cytotoxicity of *Opuntia dillenii* (Ker-Gawl) Haw. Seed Oil and Its Impact on the Isolated Rat Diaphragm Glucose Absorption. *Molecules* **2021**, *26*, 2172. [CrossRef]
153. Siddiqui, F.; Farooq, A.D.; Kabir, N.; Fatima, L.; Abidi, L.; Faizi, S. Toxicological Assessment of *Opuntia dillenii* (Ker Gawl.) Haw. Cladode Methanol Extract, Fractions and Its Alpha Pyrones: Opuntiol and Opuntioside. *J. Ethnopharmacol.* **2021**, *280*, 114409. [CrossRef]
154. Torres-Ponce, R.L.; Morales-Corral, D.; Ballinas-Casarrubias, M.L.; Nevárez-Moorillón, G.V. Nopal: Semi-desert plant with applications in pharmaceuticals, food and animal nutrition. *Rev. Mex. Cienc. Agr.* **2015**, *6*, 1129–1142.
155. Stintzing, F.C.; Carl, R. Cactus stems (*Opuntia* spp.): A review on their chemistry, technology, and uses. *Mol. Nutr. Food Res.* **2005**, *49*, 175–194. [CrossRef]
156. Vicidomini, C.; Roviello, V.; Roviello, G.N. In Silico Investigation on the Interaction of Chiral Phytochemicals from *Opuntia ficus-indica* with SARS-CoV-2 Mpro. *Symmetry* **2021**, *13*, 1041. [CrossRef]
157. Ortiz-González, A.; González-Pérez, P.P.; Cárdenas-García, M.; Hernández-Linares, M.G. In silico Prediction on the PI3K/AKT/mTOR Pathway of the Antiproliferative Effect of *O. joconostle* in Breast Cancer Models. *Cancer Inform.* **2022**, *21*, 1–17. [CrossRef]

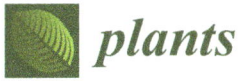

Review

A Complete Review of Mexican Plants with Teratogenic Effects

Germán Chamorro-Cevallos [1], María Angélica Mojica-Villegas [1], Yuliana García-Martínez [2], Salud Pérez-Gutiérrez [3], Eduardo Madrigal-Santillán [4], Nancy Vargas-Mendoza [4], José A. Morales-González [4] and José Melesio Cristóbal-Luna [1,*]

1. Laboratorio de Toxicología Preclínica, Departamento de Farmacia, Escuela Nacional de Ciencias Biológicas, Instituto Politécnico Nacional, Av. Wilfrido Massieu 399, Col. Nueva Industrial Vallejo, Del. Gustavo A. Madero, Ciudad de México 07738, Mexico; gchamcev@yahoo.com.mx (G.C.-C.); moviangel13@yahoo.com.mx (M.A.M.-V.)
2. Laboratorio de Neurofisiología, Departamento de Fisiología "Mauricio Russek", Instituto Politécnico Nacional, Escuela Nacional de Ciencias Biológicas, Av. Wilfrido Massieu 399, Col. Nueva Industrial Vallejo, Del. Gustavo A. Madero, Ciudad de México 07738, Mexico; ygarciamart@hotmail.com
3. Departamento de Sistemas Biológicos, Universidad Autónoma Metropolitana-Xochimilco, Calzada del Hueso 1100, Del. Coyoacán, Ciudad de México 04960, Mexico; msperez@correo.xoc.uam.mx
4. Laboratorio de Medicina de Conservación, Escuela Superior de Medicina, Instituto Politécnico Nacional, Plan de San Luis y Díaz Mirón, Col. Casco de Santo Tomás, Del. Miguel Hidalgo, Ciudad de México 11340, Mexico; eomsmx@yahoo.com.mx (E.M.-S.); nvargasmendoza@gmail.com (N.V.-M.); jmorales101@yahoo.com.mx (J.A.M.-G.)
* Correspondence: josmcl@hotmail.com; Tel.: +52-5520670441

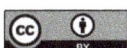

Citation: Chamorro-Cevallos, G.; Mojica-Villegas, M.A.; García-Martínez, Y.; Pérez-Gutiérrez, S.; Madrigal-Santillán, E.; Vargas-Mendoza, N.; Morales-González, J.A.; Cristóbal-Luna, J.M. A Complete Review of Mexican Plants with Teratogenic Effects. *Plants* 2022, 11, 1675. https://doi.org/10.3390/plants11131675

Academic Editor: Jose M. Soriano

Received: 3 June 2022
Accepted: 21 June 2022
Published: 24 June 2022

Publisher's Note: MDPI stays neutral with regard to jurisdictional claims in published maps and institutional affiliations.

Copyright: © 2022 by the authors. Licensee MDPI, Basel, Switzerland. This article is an open access article distributed under the terms and conditions of the Creative Commons Attribution (CC BY) license (https://creativecommons.org/licenses/by/4.0/).

Abstract: In Mexico, the use of medicinal plants is the first alternative to treat the diseases of the most economically vulnerable population. Therefore, this review offers a list of Mexican plants (native and introduced) with teratogenic effects and describes their main alterations, teratogenic compounds, and the models and doses used. Our results identified 63 species with teratogenic effects (19 native) and the main alterations that were found in the nervous system and axial skeleton, induced by compounds such as alkaloids, terpenes, and flavonoids. Additionally, a group of hallucinogenic plants rich in alkaloids employed by indigenous groups without teratogenic studies were identified. Our conclusion shows that several of the identified species are employed in Mexican traditional medicine and that the teratogenic species most distributed in Mexico are *Astragalus mollissimus*, *Astragalus lentiginosus*, and *Lupinus formosus*. Considering the total number of plants in Mexico (≈29,000 total vascular plants), to date, existing research in the area shows that Mexican plants with teratogenic effects represent ≈0.22% of the total species of these in the country. This indicates a clear need to intensify the evaluation of the teratogenic effect of Mexican plants.

Keywords: traditional medicine; Mexican plants; alkaloids; pregnancy exposure; teratogenic effects

1. Introduction

Since ancient times, humans have used the elements in their environment to satisfy their basic needs. Such is the case of plants, which for millennia have been utilized by humans to produce food, shelter, clothing, footwear, dyes and stains, means of transport, fertilizers, fragrances, cosmetics, as fuel and, of course, to alleviate their diseases [1,2]. There is solid evidence that plants have been cultivated for their biological effects for over 60,000 years [3], with the earliest written records on the preparation of herbal remedies and their biological effects being found in Sumerian tablets [4] and in Egyptian, Indian, and Chinese inscriptions aged approximately 5000 years, such as Ebers papyrus [5], Rigveda texts [6], and the book Pen T'Sao [7], respectively.

In places such as Greece and Central Asia, these first records have been found in more recent times, that is, approximately 2500 years ago [8], while in Mexico it is possible to find records of the use of plants with medicinal purposes (by the Olmec, Mayan, Mixtec, and Aztec), such as the *Códice De la Cruz Badiano* or the *Libellus de Medicinalibus Indorum*

Herbis [9]. It is difficult to establish a concise period for the first records of their medicinal use, because the majority of Mesoamerican literature, in the form of *códices*, were burned in the years after the Conquest by Spanish missionaries [10]. In this regard, according to archaeological records, the process of domestication and the use of plants in Mesoamerica began about 7000 and 5000 years ago, respectively [11]. The latter can provide us with an idea of the important role that plants have played as a means of health in the native societies of the current territory of México.

1.1. From Plants to Drugs

According to the significance that Greece, the cradle of philosophical thought and Western civilization, has held in the sciences and arts, it should not come as a surprise to us that the Greeks were the fathers of Medicine, Botany, and Pharmacology (Hippocrates, Theophrastus, and Pedanius Dioscorides, respectively), who laid the foundations of the therapeutic value of medicinal plants through detailed compilations of the knowledge of medicinal plants during their respective times and in their respective regions [12–14], as well as that herbal medicine is denominated phytotherapy, a compound word formed by the Latin prefix *phyto* "plant", and the Latin word *therapia*, "to treat medically", in the study of the use of extracts of natural origin as medicines [15].

With the fall of the Western Roman Empire (476 AD), there began a period of time that stretched from the V to the XV century, called the "Middle Ages" or the "Dark Ages", which involved a notable lag in the development of the sciences [16], despite that knowledge on the use of medicinal plants (and many others) survived during being confined for several centuries inside the walls of monasteries in countries such as England, Ireland, France, and Germany [17], among others. The Arab people were responsible for the preservation of a great part of Greco–Roman knowledge (along with that of the Chinese and the Indians, mainly in terms of plants), and later with the establishment of the first private pharmacies in Baghdad, Irak, at the end of the 8th century [18,19]. Later, the Persian pharmacist and poet Avicena (980–1037 AD) contributed to the dissemination of the knowledge of therapeutic plants with his work *"Canon Medicinae"*, considered the latest translation of all Greco–Roman Medicine [1] and the starting point for the development of medicinal-plant texts throughout Europe, such as *"The Corpus of Simples"* by Ibn al-Baitar, or the Florentine *"Nuovo Receptario Composito"*, which, alongside other manuscripts in England (1518), laid out the concept of "pure compounds" and promoted their development; a century later, these manuscripts would comprise the basis of the emergence of the first pharmacopoeia (First London Pharmacopoeia) [20]. Deriving from this idea, the first natural product to be marketed as isolated and pure was morphine, by Merck in 1826; while the first semi-synthetic medicine based on a natural product was aspirin by Bayer in 1899 [21].

The health needs of our increasing population have intensified the interest in developing more effective chemically synthesized compounds. In this context, since 1910, there was the "magic bullet" (Salvarsan or compound 606) by the German bacteriologist Paul Ehrlich [22], continuing all the way to modern times with the development of drugs used for chronic obstructive pulmonary disease, such as umeclidinium bromide [23]. Despite the good results obtained with chemical synthesis, the therapeutic potential of medicinal plants was not lost from sight. From plants such as meadowsweet (*Spiraea ulmaria*), poppy (*Papaver somniferum*), foxglove (*Digitalis purpurea*), and *barbasco* (*Lonchocarpus utilis*), drugs as remarkable as acetylsalicylic acid [24], morphine [25], digoxin [26], and diosgenin [27], respectively, have been obtained. Currently, this approach has become diversified thanks to the boom in novel processes for the extraction and identification of organic compounds, but mainly due to the increasing use of traditional medicine, which has been the starting point for information obtained throughout scientific research for the development of molecules that, under different conditions, would have been difficult or virtually impossible to conceive. In this regard, nature arises and is constituted, with chemical synthesis [28] and with biotechnology [29], one of the three main ways to obtain biologically active molecules today [30]. This said fact can be observed as reflected in the growing number of studies during the last decades that have provided valuable information to this scientific field, confirming the molecules present in the structures of numerous plants that possess a biological effect against diseases. However, in addition to the development of the knowledge of plant curative properties, the misconception of the safety of natural products has become a health problem that can be confirmed in several epidemiological and experimental assays.

1.2. Mexican Plants

Worldwide, Mexico has one of the richest diversities of plants composed of native and introduced species from various parts of the planet [31] that, together with their cultural wealth, constitute Mexican Traditional Medicine. In general terms, the concept of traditional medicine refers to a conventional denomination adopted by researchers to refer to empirical medical systems that are organized and based on various cultures of the world [32]. Thus, traditional medicine is made up of three main types according to the source of the remedy: that obtained from animal products; that of processed minerals, and Botany [33]. With regard to the latter, it is difficult to accurately determine the number of families, genera, or species of existing Mexican plants. Some reports estimate that Mexico has approximately 22,351 species of vascular plants (native and introduced) and calculate that at least 6500 species must be added to this calculation [34,35]. Of this total number ($\approx$29,000 total vascular plants), it is suggested that between 3000 and 5000 plants are currently utilized with medicinal purposes in the country [36].

The Teratogenic Effects of Mexican Plants

During pregnancy, the organogenesis phase is the most critical period for generating birth defects, because it is at this time that the differentiation and specialization of tissues, structures, organs, and systems in the *conceptus* begin, with the grouping of cells in early patterns directed by gene expression toward specific sites in an organ [37]. Thus, during this period, it is most likely (but not exclusively so) that there occurs a multifactorial process known as teratogenesis. The latter, as a result of multiple interactions between environmental (physical, chemical, biological, and maternal diseases, clinical states, etc.) and endogenous (genetic background of the mother and the embryo/fetus) factors, can produce a wide range of congenital deformities in the developing fetus or in the newborn [38]. Although the mechanisms by which this process occurs are varied, the main ones include oxidative stress, folate antagonism, vascular disruption, neural crest cell disruption, endocrine disruption, and specific receptor- or enzyme-mediated actions, among others [39]. Therefore, the severity and type of alterations will depend, among other things, on the time of the interaction of the teratogenic agent with the embryo/fetus, as well as on the mechanism(s) involved in the disruptive process.

The wide diversity of plants in Mexico allows some of these to be used by humans to alleviate their diseases or as food [40,41], even for livestock. In Mexico, as in other developing countries, the use of medicinal plants remains the first health care available in many rural areas to alleviate the diseases of the most economically vulnerable population, without social security [42,43], as a substantially less expensive and affordable alternative to conventional therapies. Unfortunately, in this practice, quality is generally unproven and is solely based on the population's beliefs. In contrast, insufficient attention is paid to their possible toxicity (unlike what happens with drugs), with the belief espoused for generations, e.g., "the natural remedy" is totally safe, without taking into consideration that plants could contain toxic compounds. Thus, although plants are undeniably an important source of health for vulnerable persons, it is important to make it known to the general population that "natural is not always safe".

The data provided by several investigations demonstrate than an important number of herbs and herbal products have been implicated in poisoning [44], health problems [45], and alterations in embryonic/fetal development in humans [46] and animals [47]. This latter toxic effect of plants comprises an important problem worldwide, not only for public health, where birth defects are one of the main preventable causes of morbidity, mortality, and childhood disability [48], but also in the economic sector, since in different parts of the world, the consumption of teratogenic plants by pregnant females produces a wide variety of congenital anomalies in livestock, generating, in this manner, considerable losses of capital for companies and local ranchers [49].

This work provides an updated catalog of native and introduced vascular plants in Mexico with a teratogenic effect, in order to describe the main birth defects produced by these in different models, as well as their implications during pregnancy. In addition, we underscore those plants that should be avoided during the critical period of pregnancy because of their harmful effects on the developing embryo/fetus (abortifacient and/or teratogenic potential). Additionally, this review seeks to serve as the basis for generating novel research projects, new questions, a better understanding of the Mexican flora, and as a promoter of the responsible and safe use of medicinal plants. For example, in Mexico, there are a considerable number of plants termed "sacred" that are employed with religious purposes due to their hallucinogenic effects, plants that are rich in alkaloids (these will be discussed later), plants without (to our knowledge) studies that support their safety or that warn of their toxicity during pregnancy and that are currently used without any type of regulation by ethnic populations.

2. Methodology

A scoping review of Mexican plants with a teratogenic effect was conducted in the principal academic research databases (DOAJ, PubMed, ScienceDirect, Scopus, Web of Sciences and Springer) and academic search engines (Google Scholar, Science.gov, and Microsoft Academic). The search was carried out in the first instance by faceting the main ideas that make up our research, which were later condensed into keywords and which in turn were utilized in different combinations to feed the academic search engines and databases in order to identify potentially relevant studies for their inclusion in our review as follows: "teratogenesis, teratogen, teratogenic effect, teratogenic plants, plant extracts, sacred plants, Mexican plants, herbal, herbal medicine, medicinal plants, traditional Mexican medicine, natural products, phytotherapy, pregnancy, birth defects, and congenital malformations".

To achieve this goal, we adopted as inclusion criteria, articles, papers, books, book chapters, reports, patents, and theses on plants native to or introduced into Mexico with proven teratogenic effects, published during the last 72 years (1950–2022) and, as exclusion criteria, studies that address another type of toxicity not related to our main objective, information on compounds or molecules other than those obtained from plants, information from unreliable sources, information from years prior to 1950, information that does not refer to the keywords raised, repeated teratogenic plants previously found, and works on teratogenic plants that are not present in Mexico. To perform this selection, we compared the plants in the studies found with the checklist of the native vascular plants of Mexico [34] and with the databases of the Invasive Species Compendium [50], the Herbario Virtual of the Comisión Nacional para el Conocimiento y Uso de la Biodiversidad [51], the platform iNaturalist (citizen science social network) [52], and the Red de Herbarios del Noroeste de México [53], to differentiate between native plants, plants introduced from other countries, and plants that do not present in Mexico.

Please note that this review was focused only on the variety of plants with teratogenic effects. Therefore, no information is included on the number of investigations conducted on the same plant by different authors, with different animal species, doses, or any other different variable.

3. Results

3.1. Teratogenic Plants from Mexico

In this review, 63 species of Mexican plants with teratogenic effects distributed in 56 genera were identified (Table 1). Compared to the enormous number of plant species in Mexico, this figure scarcely represents ≈0.21% of the total number of species in the country. In the studies consulted, the main plant parts employed were leaves, followed by seeds, fruits, roots, flowers, and bark. Evidently, this fact depended on the amount and type of the compound suspected as the teratogenic agent in the studied species. For example, alkaloids are mainly found in leaves, barks and, to a lesser extent, in roots [54], and cyanides are often found in rhizomes and, at lesser amounts, in fruits and seeds [55]. However, essential oils (a complex mixture of fatty acids, aldehydes, esters, phenols, ketones, alcohols, nitrogen, and Sulphur) are isolated from various plant structures, such as peel, stem, leaves, flowers, roots, and woods [56]. Although the majority of the studies were conducted on livestock, complete plants were administered to pregnant animals through their diet, mixed with food; in laboratory animals such as rats, mice, fish, frogs, and chickens, the majority of the investigations opted to extract the representative compounds of the plant-in-question, utilizing different types of solvents according to the compound that the plants were suspected to obtain; for example, aqueous extracts for flavonoids, alkaloids, steroids, terpenoids, phenols, and terpenes; methanolic extracts for sterols, flavonoids, some alkaloids, and lectins; ethanolic extracts for diterpenes, aldehydes, and polyketides, and organic extracts for lycopene, fatty acids, some alkaloids, sterols, and terpenes. As can be observed, the relative polarity of the solvents employed ranges from the lowest with hexane (0.009) and continues in increasing order with benzene (0.111), methylene chloride (0.309), ethanol (0.654), and methanol (0.762), to the compound with the highest relative polarity: water (1.0). That is, the authors played with the intensity of the interactions of solvents with their molecules-of-interest to extract apolar compounds by applying non-polar solvents, and vice versa [57].

The case of the alkaloids is very interesting because, as bases, they are scarcely soluble in water, but are very soluble in polar (alcohols) and apolar (ether, chloroform, hexane) organic solvents [58] Nevertheless, in the various studies in which they were identified, alkaloids were obtained through aqueous extracts and, in very few cases, by hydroalcoholic or organic extracts. This is most likely because the experiments involved attempted to imitate the way in which the plant is ingested by humans, in the form of teas (aqueous extracts).

The main compounds identified as the cause of the developmental alteration observed in different studies, in descending order, were as follows; alkaloids (22); unknown (20); terpenes (5); flavonoids (3); steroids (3); carbohydrates (2); cyanide (2) M lycopene (2); polyphenols (2); acids (1); aldehydes (1); amino acids (1); β-carotenes (1); fatty acids (1); lactones (1); gingerols (1); lectins (1); peroxides (1); polyketides (1), and sterols (1). It is not surprising that the majority of these investigations found alkaloids to be responsible for the teratogenic effect, as for decades there has been full knowledge that these compounds generate a wide variety of developmental defects in humans and animals [59]. However, due to the large number of studies in which the compound responsible for the teratogenic effect is not mentioned, leads us to think that this is because determining this data was not a priority for the study. It is curious that a wide variety of natural compounds with a low incidence of teratogenic effects was identified as teratogenic compounds. Thus, it is essential to consider these for future studies, as for several of these there are insufficient reports or citations in the literature specifying their teratogenic properties.

Table 1. List of Mexican plants screened for their teratogenicity.

Plant	Teratogen					Animal/Model			Origin	Citation
	Used Part	Doses	Route of Administration	Compound	Mechanism	Species	Status	Malformations		
Acanthospermum hispidum	Leaves, stalk, and seeds; AqEx	AqEx 10%, 0–600 mg/kg/day	IG, during organogenic period	Sesquiterpenoids (terpenoids) and phenolic compounds	-	Wistar rats	Normal	Anomalies in urinary system, palatosquisis, acampsia, ear heterotopic, cranial alterations, micrognathia, gastroschisis, extra ribs.	Introduced from Brazil	[60]
Acanthus montanus	Leaves; Met:MCEx (1:1)	1000 mg/kg	IG, GD6–15	β-sitosterol (sterol)	-	Wistar rats	Normal	Embryotoxicity, reduction in fetal body weight, crown-rump, tail lengths; reduced ossification of extremities bones.	Introduced from Africa	[61]
Ageratum conyzoides	Leaves; HAEx (80:20)	1000 mg/kg	Oral, GD17–20	Pyrrolizidine alkaloids	Oxidative stress	Wistar rats	Normal	Decrease fetal weight.	Native of Mexico	[62]
Aloe barbadensis miller	Leaf; juice	3 mL/rat	IG, GD4–15	-	-	Wistar rats	Normal	Reduction in fetal body weight, crown rump length, tail length; renal alterations as shrunken tubules, mild degeneration of glomeruli, narrowing of capsular spaces.	Introduced from Africa	[63]
Alstonia macrophylla	Leaves; EtEx	10 mg/mice	IG, GD8–15	Acetogenins (polyketides), styryl-lactones and alkaloids	-	ICR mice	Normal	Head shape angular, reduced elongation in the snout, abnormalities in digits of forelimbs and hindlimbs (separate fully or lack of some digits), altered body shape morphology, dead implants.	Introduced from Indonesia	[64]
Alstonia scholaris	Stem bark; HAEx (85:15)	480 mg/kg	IP, GD11	-	-	Swiss albino mice	Normal	Mortality, growth retardation, body length reduction, bent tails, syndactyly, delay in fur development, eye opening, pinna detachment, and vaginal opening, testes descent, ear unfolding.	Introduced from India	[65]

Table 1. Cont.

Plant	Teratogen						Animal/Model			Origin	Citation
	Used Part	Doses	Route of Administration	Compound	Mechanism		Species	Status	Malformations		
Artemisia annua L.	Leaves; OEx	70 mg/kg	IG, GD14-20	Artemisinin (sesquiterpene)	-		Wistar rats	Normal	Post-implantation losses.	Introduced from Asia	[66]
Astragalus lentiginosus (locoweed)	Leaves	25%	Oral, mixed with food during pregnancy	-	-		Columbia sheeps	Normal	Abortion, skeletal malformations (flexure of carpal joint, lateral rotation front legs, hypermobility hock and stifle joint), fetal edema, ascites, fetal hemorrhage, less gross effect on fetal cotyledons.	Native of Mexico	[67]
Astragalus mollissimus Torr	Leaves and stems	-	Oral, during pregnancy	Swainsonine alkaloids	-		Horses, lambs,	Normal	Skeletal defects, limb contractures.	Native of Mexico	[68]
Astragalus pubentissimus	Leaves and stems	-	Oral, mixed with food during pregnancy	Swainsonine alkaloids	-		Sheep and cattle	Normal	Abortions, lateral rotation of forelimbs, contracted tendons, anterior flexure, looseness of hock joints, flexure of the carpus, decreased length.	Introduced from North America	[69]
Azadirachta indica	Seeds oil	1.2 mL	IG, during whole pregnancy	-	Oxidative stress		Sprague Dawley rats	Normal	Anophthalmia, enlarged trachea, abnormally shaped sternebrae, macroglossia, exencephaly.	Introduced from India	[70]
Cajanus cajan	Leaves; AqEx	0-600 mg/kg/day	IG, during organogenic period	-	-		Wistar rats	Normal	Anomalies in urinary system, palatosquisis, acampsia, ear heterotopic, cranial alterations, micrognathia, gastroschisis, extra ribs.	Introduced from Brazil	[71]
Cannabis sativa L. (ganga)	Resin	4.2 mg/kg	IP, GD1-6	Cannabinoid alkaloids	-		Wistar rats; mice	Normal	Higher rate of resorptions and syndactyly, encephalocele, phocomelia; decrease in fetal weight and size; dental asymmetry.	Introduced from Asia	[72,73]

Table 1. Cont.

Plant	Used Part	Teratogen Doses	Route of Administration	Compound	Mechanism	Animal/Model Species	Status	Malformations	Origin	Citation
Carthamus tinctorius	Flowers; AqEx	1.2 mg/kg	IG, GD0-8	-	Cytotoxicity	Albino mice	Normal	Changes in external, internal and longitudinal diameters, open neuropore, changes in cellular orientation and cellular degeneration, disconnected lateral folds.	Introduced from Mediterranean	[74]
Caryocar brasiliense	Fruits (dried pulp); Oex	1000 mg/kg	IG, GD6-15	Oleic acid (fatty acid), β-carotene and lycopene	High antioxidant capacity, probably	Wistar rats	Normal	Bruises, developmental delay, distended abdomen, incomplete ossification, vertebra in dumbbell, sternebra misaligned or bipartite, ribs wavy or supernumerary, change in shape of bones, absent sternebra or ribs, shortening of forelimbs and hindlimbs.	Introduced from Brazil	[75]
Cinnamomum zeylanicum	Leaves; AqEx, Cex	70 mg/kg	IP, throughout pregnancy	-	-	Wistar rats	Normal	Fetal resorption.	Introduced from South Asia	[71]
Conium maculatum	Leaves, fruits	2 and 1 mL/day	IG; GD25-35 sheep and GD55-75 cows	Piperidine alkaloids (coniine, N-methyl-coniine, conhydrine, pseudoconhydrine, γ-coniceine)	Restricted fetal movement (sedative or anesthetic effect of alkaloids)	Columbia sheep, cows	Normal	Cleft palate, under-extension of carpals and pastern joints, limb and spinal deformities.	Introduced from Europe	[76,77]
Cortex cinnamom L. (Lauraceae)	Cortex; EtEx	0.5 mmol/embryo	In ovo	Cinnamaldehyde (aldehyde)		Chick	Whole embryo culture	Malformations and lethality.	Introduced from India	[78]
Croton megalocarpus	Leaves; MetEx	1000 mg/kg	IG, GD6-16	-	Interference with the mechanisms involved in the production or removal of amniotic fluid	Swiss albino mice	Normal	Fetal resorption, microcephaly, polyhydramnios.	Introduced from Africa	[79]

Table 1. Cont.

Plant	Teratogen						Animal/Model			Origin	Citation
	Used Part	Doses	Route of Administration	Compound	Mechanism		Species	Status	Malformations		
Curcuma longa	Rhizome; MetEx	125.0 µg/mL	In medium, 6 hpf	Catechin, epicatechin, and naringenin (flavonoids)	Weakened or damaged embryo protective layer (chorion)		Zebra fish	Whole embryo culture	Body deformities of larvae, kink tail, bend trunk, enlarged yolk sac edema.	Introduced from Southeast Asia	[80]
Datura stramonium	-	-	-	Unknown, possibly alkaloids	-		Pigs	Normal	Cleft palate, contracture-type skeletal defects.	Native of Mexico	[81]
Derris elliptica	Leaves; AqEx	0.50%	Culture medium	-	-		Zebra fish	Whole embryo culture	Reduced hatchability, lower heartbeat, delayed formation, undeveloped head and tail region, coagulation and death of embryos.	Introduced from India	[82]
Descurainia sophia	Leaves	10%	Oral, mixed with food during first 2 months of pregnancy	3-butenyl glucosinolate (glycosides)	-		Goats	Normal	Hypothyroidism, absence of hair, goiter, abnormally large birth weights.	Introduced from Eurasia	[83]
Garcinia kola	Seeds; AqEx	200 mg/kg	IG, GD1–5	Flavonoids	-		Sprague Dawley rats	Normal	Decrease in fetal weight, malformed left upper limb.	Introduced from Africa	[84]
Ginseng (Spp)	Root	780–1560 mg/kg	IG, throughout pregnancy	Ginsenoside (steroid glycosides and triterpene saponins)	Activation of ginseng saponins		Albino mice	Whole embryo culture	Malformation of sternum, defects in the lumbar vertebrae, bad union of transverse processes with vertebral body.	Introduced from China and Korea	[85]
Indigofera spicata	Seeds; ion-exchange extraction	1 mL/100 g (1 mL of extract equals to 10 g seeds)	IG, GD13	Canavanine (amino acid)	Amino acid antagonism		Sprague Dawley rats	Normal	Cleft secondary-palate, somatic dwarfism, hepatic toxic change.	Introduced from Africa	[86]
Ipomoea carnea	Leaves; AqEx	15.0 mg/kg	IG, GD5–21	Swainsonine (alkaloid) and caligestines	Inhibition of acidic/lysosomal amannosidase and Golgi mannosidase II; and glicosydases		Wistar rats	Normal	Reduction in ossification centers, kidney symmetry, dilated renal pelvis, hemorrhagic kidney, dilated cerebral ventricle, hemorrhagic cerebrum, hemorrhagic thyroid gland, spongy lung, and embryotoxicity.	Native of Mexico	[87]

Table 1. Cont.

Plant	Teratogen					Animal/Model			Origin	Citation
	Used Part	Doses	Route of Administration	Compound	Mechanism	Species	Status	Malformations		
Krameria cytisoides Cav	Leaves; MetEx	1000 mg/kg	IG, GD6–15	Kramecyne (hexamer of cyclic peroxide monomers)	Inhibition of cyclooxygenase 2 and consequent inhibition of prostaglandin synthesis; and ROS imbalance due to an increase in antioxidant enzymes (most likely)	Wistar rats	Normal	Decrease of fetal length and weight, live fetuses; increase of post-implantation loss; incomplete ossification in cranial vault, pelvis, sternum; asymmetric sternebrae; rudimentary and undulate ribs.	Native of Mexico	[88]
Lantana camara	Leaves; HAEx (70:30)	7 g/kg	IG, 14 days prior to mating and over the pregnancy (GD21)	-	-	Wistar rats	Normal	Increase of resorption rate and post-implantation loss index, forelimbs poorly ossification, sternebra with incomplete ossification.	Native of Mexico	[89]
Lavandula angustifolia	Leaves; AqEx	15 mg/kg	IP, GD3–6	Linalool (terpene)	-	BALB/c mice	Normal	Limb displacement from symmetry axis, encephalocele, no brain development, scoliosis, hemorrhage, spinal cord protrusion, eye protrusion, lack of limb, ear, eye and exohepatic development.	Introduced from Mediterranean	[90]
Lawsonia inermis	Leaves; AqEx	10 mg/kg	IP, GD1–7	-	Decreased levels of progesterone and increased levels of estrogen	BALB/c mice	Normal	Abortion (fetal death).	Introduced from Africa	[91]
Leucaena leucocephala	Leaves	50%	Oral, mixed with food during pregnancy	Mimosine (alkaloid)	-	Goats	Normal	Abortions at different stages of pregnancy, congenital goiter.	Native of Mexico	[92]

Table 1. Cont.

Plant	Teratogen					Animal/Model			Origin	Citation
	Used Part	Doses	Route of Administration	Compound	Mechanism	Species	Status	Malformations		
Luffa operculata	Fruits; AqEx	4 mL/kg	IG, GD1–9	-	-	CD1 mice	Normal	Cleft palate, anencephaly, exophthalmia, delayed bone development; and decrease in implantation sites, live fetuses, and birth rate.	Native of Mexico	[93]
Lupinus caudatus	Leaves and stems	-	Oral, mixed with food GD40–70	Anagyrine (alkaloid)	-	Cows	Normal	Multiple congenital contractures, torticollis, arthrogryposis, kyphosis, rib cage deformities, scoliosis.	Introduced from North America	[94]
Lupinus formosus	Whole plant	2.25–3.16 g/kg	IG, twice daily GD40–70	Ammodendrine, piperidine and quinolizidine alkaloids	Restricted fetal movement (sedative or anesthetic effect of alkaloids)	Cows	Normal	Cleft palate, spinal curvature, rib cage depression, and multiple congenital contractures involving limbs, spinal column, and neck.	Native of Mexico	[95]
Lycopersicon esculentum	Leaves	-	Oral, mixed with food	Solanidanes, spirosolanes alkaloids, glycoalkaloids, and lycopenes	-	Columbia sheep, cows	Normal	Brain defects and cleft palate.	Native of Mexico	[96]
Manihot esculenta	Rhizome	50 and 80%	Oral, mixed with food during GD0–15	Cyanide and cyanogenic compounds (linamarin)	-	Albino rats	Normal	Growth retardation, limb defects, microcephaly, open eyes, low fetal body weight, embryonic death.	Native of Mexico	[97]
Mimosa tenuiflora	Seeds	10%	Oral, mixed with food during GD6–21	Alkaloids	-	Wistar rats	Normal	Cleft palate, scoliosis, bifid sternum, aplasia of sternebraes, hypoplastic sternebrae, hypoplasia of ischium, femur, nasal bone, deformed occipital bone, microphthalmia, lordosis, a shorter head, and weight increased.	Native of Mexico	[98]

Table 1. Cont.

Plant	Teratogen					Animal/Model			Origin	Citation
	Used Part	Doses	Route of Administration	Compound	Mechanism	Species	Status	Malformations		
Momordica charantia	Fruits and seeds; AqEx	2 mL/rat	IG, GD7, 11 or 13	-	-	Sprague Dawley rats	Normal	Cryptorchidism, splenomegaly; bilateral testicular, hepatic atrophy; renal hypertrophy; splenomegaly; anencephaly and spinabifida.	Introduced from Africa	[99]
Montanoa tomentosa	Leaves; HAEx (70:30)	25 mg/kg	IG, GD14-21	-	Ischemia and oxytocic effect	Wistar rats	Normal	Fetal mortality, increased fetal body weight, and maternal bleeding.	Native of Mexico	[100]
Morinda citrifolia	Fruit; AqEx	300 mg/kg	IG, GD7-15	-	-	Wistar rats	Normal	Delayed ossification and variations in skull, vertebral column, ribs, forelimbs, hindlimbs, and sternum.	Introduced from Asia	[101]
Moringa oleifera	Leaves; AqEx	3000 ppm	In medium, at segmentation phase during 48 h	-	-	Zebra fish	Whole embryo culture	Absence or low heartbeat rate, growth retardation, yolk deformity, stunted tail, and embryotoxicity.	Introduced from India	[102]
Nicotiana glauca	Leaves, stems, flowers, and woody (contained 0.175–0.23% anabasine)	5–8 mg/kg	IG, twice a day GD32-41	Anabasine (alkaloid)	Reduction in fetal movement during by fetal pharmacologic neuromuscular blockade	Spanish-goats	Normal	Bilateral cleft palate, embryonic/fetal death, resorptions, maxillary hypoplasia, midfacial retrusion, contracture in spine, neck, and legs.	Introduced from Argentina and Bolivia	[103]
Nicotiana humilis (plumbaginifolia)	Leaves; MetEx	0.5 mg/kg	IG, throughout gestational period	Nicotinic alkaloids	-	Sprague Dawley rats	Normal	Increased the body weight, length; decreased tail length; dysplastic tail, curved tail; behavioral disturbance; delayed opening eyes, incisor eruption and hair appearance.	Native of Mexico	[104]

Table 1. Cont.

Plant	Teratogen					Animal/Model			Origin	Citation
	Used Part	Doses	Route of Administration	Compound	Mechanism	Species	Status	Malformations		
Nicotiana tabacum	Leaves and stalks; juice	-	IG, GD4–53	Nicotinic alkaloids	-	Duroc pig	Normal	Congenital limb deformities and contractures; arthrogryposis.	Introduced from Peru	[105]
Oxytropis sericea	Leaves and stems	-	Oral, mixed with food during pregnancy	Swainsonine alkaloids	-	Sheep and cattle	Normal	Abortions, lateral rotation of forelimbs, contracted tendons, anterior flexure, looseness of hock joints, flexure of the carpus, decreased length.	Introduced from North America	[69]
Perovskia abrotanoides	Flowers; EtEx (95%)	0.25 g/kg	IP, GD8–11	Tanshinones (abietane diterpene)	Cytotoxicity and apoptosis induction	CD1 mice	Normal	Resorption, stillborn, polydactyly, spina bifida, aglossia, exencephaly, hydrocephaly, tarsal extensor, gastroschisis, skeletal abnormalities, cranium anomaly, variation in vertebrae, ribs, sternum, pelvis and hind limbs.	Introduced from Asia	[106]
Peumus boldus	Leaves; HAEx	800 mg/kg	IG, GD7–12	Boldine (alkaloid)	-	Wistar rats	Normal	Absence of paw inferior, external ear, and tail; increase of resorptions; weight decrease.	Introduced from Chile	[107]
Pinus ponderosa	Pine needles; isolated acids	152 mg/kg	IG, twice daily GD250–252	Isocupressic acid	-	Cows	Normal	Abortion.	Native of Mexico	[108]
Podophyllum peltatum	Roots; AEx	Five times	Topic, 4 h at the end of 23rd, 24th, 25th, 28th, and 29th weeks of pregnancy	Podophyllotoxin (β-D-glucoside)	Probably by interference with cellular mitosis	Humans	Normal	Simian crease on the left hand and a preauricular skin tag; polyneuritis, limb malformations, septal heart defects, and intrauterine death.	Introduced from North America	[109, 110]
Prunus serotina	Fruits and leaves	-	Oral, ad libitum	Cyanide	-	Yorkshire pig	Normal	No tail, no anus, very small external sex organs, hind legs plantarflexed below the hock (most were female).	Native of Mexico	[111]

Table 1. Cont.

Plant	Teratogen						Animal/Model		Malformations	Origin	Citation
	Used Part	Doses	Route of Administration	Compound	Mechanism		Species	Status			
Rauwolfia vomitoria	Leaves and roots; EtEx	250 mg/kg	IG, GD7-11	-	-		Wistar rats	Normal	Distortion of cardiac muscle nicleiand myocaridial fibers.	Introduced from Africa	[112]
Ricinus communis-linn	Seeds; MetEx	600 mg/kg	IG, GD1-12	Ricin and lectin	-		Wistar rats	Normal	Prevention of implantation, abortion, and significant reduction of fetal parameters; crown-rump length, tail length, and weigh.	Introduced from Africa	[113]
Ruta chalepensis L.	Leaves; AqEx	10 mg/kg	IP, GD9-17	-	-		Swiss Rockefeller mice	Normal	Increased frequency of fetal resorption, lower fetal weight, hemivertebra, mesocephaly, spina bifida and skeletal malformations.	Introduced from Mediterranean	[114]
Ruta graveolens	Leaves; AqEx	20%	Oral, mixed with water GD0-4	-	-		Swiss albino mice	Normal	Abnormal compacted and uncompacted morula, extruded blastomere, embryo transport slightly delayed, retarded embryonic development.	Introduced from southern Europe	[115]
Senna alata	Leaves; HEx	1000 mg/kg	IG, GD10-18	Alkaloids	-		Wistar rats	Normal	Fetal death, decrease of implantation sites and corpora lutea; increase of resorption index, pre- and post-implantation losses.	Introduced from South America	[116]
Silybum marianum	Seeds (probably); AqEx	200 mg/kg	IP, GD6-15	Silibinin (flavonolignans)	Inhibition of cyclooxygenase and apoptosis		BALB/c mice	Normal	Reduction of fetal body weight, and crown-rump length; growth retardation; limb malformations, mandibular hypoplasia, vertebral deviations in normal curvatures, kyphotic body, increased fetal resorption.	Introduced from Mediterranean	[117]

Table 1. Cont.

Plant	Teratogen					Animal/Model			Origin	Citation
	Used Part	Doses	Route of Administration	Compound	Mechanism	Species	Status	Malformations		
Solanum tuberosum	Isolated from root; α-chaconine and α-solanine	4.6 and 10.9 mg/L, respectively	In medium, during 96 h	Steroidal glycosides and alkaloids	Carbohydrate side chain attached to the 3-OH group of solanidine, appears to be an important factor in teratogenicity	Xenopus	Whole embryo culture	Growth inhibition, loose gut coiling (miscoiling), misshapen eyes, muscular kinking, microencephaly, lacking in facial and brain structures, mortality.	Introduced from Bolivia	[118]
Treculia africana	Outer coat fruit; HAEX (50%)	2.5 mg/kg	SC, GD6	Polyphenol	-	Wistar rats	Normal	Reduction of fetal body weight, hydrocephaly, anophthalmia, omphalocele, shift in position, bipartite vertebral, rudimentary ribs, fused ribs, extra ribs.	Introduced from Africa	[119]
Trigonella foenum graecum	Seeds; AqEx	1000 mg/kg	IG, during entire period of pregnancy	Diosgenin (steroid) and alkaloids	-	Swiss albino mice	Normal	Decrease in litter size and in fetal body weight, aplasia of external ear, bump on the head, median cleft of lower lip, fetotoxicity.	Introduced from Asia	[120]
Urtica dioica	Leaves; MetEx	1000 mg/kg	Oral, GD6-16	-	-	Swiss albino mice	Normal	Fetal resorption.	Native of Mexico	[101]
Veratrum californicum	Root and top structures; Oex	200 g	Oral, twice on GD14	Alkaloids	-	Sheep	Normal	Cyclopia, fetal death.	Native of Mexico	[121]
Zingiber officinale	Rhizome; AqEx	50 g/L	Oral, mixed with water GD6-15	Gingerols and shaogoals	-	Sprague Dawley rats	Normal	Embryonic loss, advanced skeletal development, increased fetal weight.	Introduced from Asia	[122]

Information on the teratogenic effect of Mexican plants, details of the part used, type of extract, mechanism, animal model, and congenital anomalies found is presented. Alcoholic extract, AEx; aqueous extract, AqEx; chloroform extract, CEx; ethanolic extract, EtEx; hours post-fertization, hpf; hexane extract, Hex; hydroalcoholic extract, HAEx; intragastric, IG; intravaginal, IVG; methanol/methylene chloride, Met; MCEx; methanolic extract, MetEx; oily extract, OEx; organic extract, Oex.

According to what was found in this review, the animal species employed for carrying out these investigations were very varied; according to their incidence in the publications, the preferred species was rat (Wistar 20, Sprague Dawley 6, albino 1), followed by mouse (Swiss albino 5, BALB/c 3, CD1 2, albino 2, ICR 1, Swiss Rockefeller 1, not specified 1), and in a few species such as sheep 6 (Columbia 3, not specified 3), cows (5 not specified), goats 3 (Spanish 1, not specified 2), pigs (Duroc 1, Yorkshire 1, not specified 1), fish (zebra 3) cattle (not specified 2), chicken (not specified 1), frog (Xenopus 1), horses (not specified 1), human (Homo sapiens 1), and lambs (not specified 1). The latter demonstrates one of our main premises for conducting this review: livestock is seriously affected by teratogenic plants. Similarly, the preferred route of treatment administration was intragastric by gavage (31), followed by orally mixed with food or water (16), intraperitoneally (8), in culture medium (5), subcutaneously (1), and topically (1). All were administered during the critical period of gestation (organogenesis) or during the most susceptible stages of pregnancy in order to obtain suspected alterations.

The majority of species used in the teratogenicity studies in this review are rat and mouse, which is not uncommon, because, for a long time, they have been utilized as the preferred species for scientific research due to being readily available, small in size, easy to handle, easy to maintain, they have a short life cycle, etc. This is not to mention that there is much accessible information on their very similar physiological, anatomical, and genetic characteristics to those of humans [123], a similarity that would be more difficult to obtain in other models, such as fish, birds, or amphibians. In this context, the remarkable anatomical and physiological similarities between animals (particularly mammals) and humans have made possible the development of studies in different areas to investigate the physiological processes, mechanisms of action, efficacy, and the toxicity of drugs in developmental animal models before applying these models to humans [124].

While in preclinical toxicology the use of animals is a highly appreciated resource due to their resemblance to humans, it is evident that not all of the results obtained in animals can be directly translated into a very complex organism. In organisms such as humans, the organs perform distinct highly integrated and regulated physiological functions that involve a complex network of hormones, circulating factors, and cross communication between cells in other compartments, to say the least. Therefore, before thinking about extrapolating to humans the results obtained in animal models, it is necessary to investigate these at all required levels in order to obtain a complete description and an understanding of the involved mechanisms. In this latter aspect, many authors consider that a predominant reason for the poor rate of translation in some studies between animals and humans lies not in the lack of similarity between the species, but in problems of internal validity in preclinical animal studies (poor study design, lack of measures to control bias, etc.) [125].

Since in toxicity tests it is possible to reproduce the toxic effects in different species, for several years investigators have sought an animal species that responds in the same manner as humans to intoxications, to establish a practical model that aids in efficiently extrapolating the toxic effects observed in animals toward humans. However, the conclusion reached was that no animal, not even the higher primates, responds precisely in the same way that humans do against toxic substances [126]. Variability among species is so significant that even within a species such as that of the human, we can find individuals of the same race who respond differently to the same substance/molecule [127]. However, as Litchfield [128] demonstrated, more than one half century ago by comparing 89 effects of 6 toxic substances on rat, dog, and human, the problem is not qualitative, but quantitative. The author concluded that when a toxic effect does not appear in any of the former two species (dog or rat), it will not appear in humans either. However, if the substance affects only one of these, it will also affect humans. Thus, these toxicity tests are not designed to prove that a compound is safe, but instead to characterize the effects that it can produce in animals to produce a series of considerations such as metabolic rate, size, anatomical compartments, pathological state, physiological barriers, among others, which allow for an estimation of the intensity of the expected effects on humans.

Herein we find the importance of the data collected in this review, in which we can observe that the majority of the studies were carried out in species that share physiological similarities with human, rat, and mouse (and only one of these in human). Therefore, according to what has already been stated, it is to be expected that the plants analyzed in this review (or their extracts), when ingested or exposed to developing humans, produce similar alterations (qualitative) to those generated in rat or mouse murine models, varying only in the intensity of said alteration (quantitative).

Although in our review only a sole case of teratogenicity in humans by plants was found, this does not imply that plants do not generate alterations in the development of humans. Simply, at the time of birth, various alterations can go unnoticed if the medical staff does not have adequate preparation, not to mention that the population that uses plants to relieve their ailments and illnesses are mostly low-income persons who do not usually present at medical care centers. In this way, the lack of evidence of teratogenicity in humans (clinical cases) in this bibliographic review due to the consumption of medicinal plants does not comprise evidence of their absence. However, it is evidence of the need to intensify research in this area.

Second, the developmental alterations found in both livestock and laboratory animals were varied to such a degree that their specific description would be unsuccessful. Therefore, we will only mention the most significant alterations produced by the main compounds. The main alterations produced by plants with alkaloids were a decrease in fetal weight and length, altered body-shape morphology, and contracted tendons; encephalocele, phocomelia, and cleft palate, abnormalities in digits, forelimbs, hindlimbs, skull, spinal deformities, a reduction in ossification centers, and a higher rate of resorption, embryotoxicity, and fetal death. For plants with terpenes, we find palatosquisis, acampsia, ear heterotopic, micrognathia, gastroschisis, encephalocele, polydactyly, scoliosis, hemorrhage, spinal cord protrusion, eye protrusion, exencephaly, hydrocephaly and anomalies in the urinary system, variation in vertebrae, ribs, sternum, pelvis, hind limbs and skull post-implantation losses, and resorption. For plants with flavonoids, these are as follows: body deformities; kink tail; bent trunk; limb malformations; mandibular hypoplasia; decrease in fetal weight and crown–rump length; malformed limbs; vertebral deviations, and increased and fetal resorption. For plants with cyanide, these are the following: growth retardation; limb defects; microcephaly; open eyes; low fetal body weight; no tail; no anus; very small external sex organs, and embryonic death. The exact mechanisms by which these alterations occurred have not been fully clarified. However, the consulted authors point out or suspect that the main causing mechanisms in the observed teratogenic effect include oxidative stress [62], ischemia [100], enzymatic inhibition [88,117], alteration in levels of estrogens [91], cytotoxicity [106], apoptosis [117], interference with cellular mitosis [109,110], and restricted fetal movement [76,77,95], among others. Obviously, such alterations can be produced by each one of these or by combinations of these mechanisms (Figure 1).

The last important data obtained from our review are the number of native and introduced teratogenic plants in Mexico. According to our results, of the 63 teratogenic species of Mexican plants found, 19 are native to the country while the 44 remaining plants were introduced during the last 5 centuries from Africa (10), Asia (10), South America (8), India (5), the Mediterranean region (4), North America (4), and Europe (3) (Figure 2). These data, in addition to exhibiting the botanical wealth of Mexico, also reveal to us an important part of the notable cultural influences that Mexico has received from the world. Note that, with respect to these 44 introduced species, many of their genera are present natively (with different species) in Mexico, including *Solanum* (143), *Croton* (127), *Astragalus* (92), *Lupinus* (80), *Senna* (62), *Indigofera* (33), *Cinnamomum* (23), *Artemisia* (11), *Nicotiana* (10), *Descurainia* (8), *Morinda* (3), *Garcinia* (2), and *Alstonia* (1) [34]. It is logical to suppose that many of these "not studied species", by sharing the genus with species that have shown teratogenic effects in the laboratory, must share the same or similar families of metabolites with the ability to modify fetal/embryonic development.

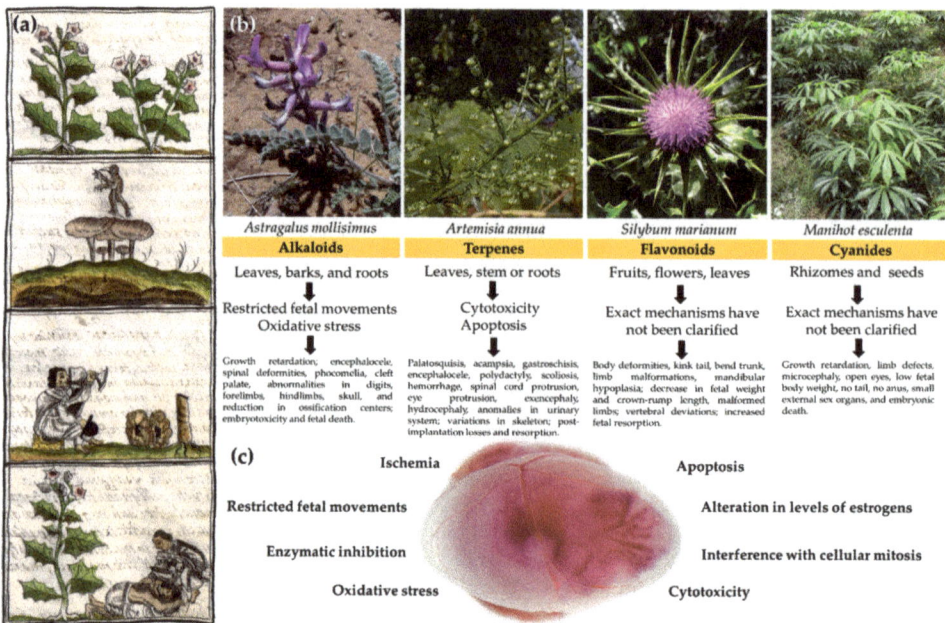

Figure 1. Developmental defects and the mechanisms of teratogenicity of the main compounds identified in Mexican plants. (**a**) In the upper part, this fragment of the Florentino codex shows the importance of the role that plants played in the pre-Hispanic Mexican culture (a reflection of the current one). Hallucinogenic plants, from top: *tlapatl, nanacatl, peyotl,* and *tolo* (bottom) used by the ancient indigenous people to stimulate the nervous system, for ritual or medicinal purposes as in love sickness [129]. (**b**) Four of the following teratogenic plants most used by the Mexican population as medicine or food are depicted: *Astragalus mollissimus* [130]; *Artemisia annua* [131]; *Silybum marianum* [132], and *Manihot esculenta* [133]. At the bottom of the fragment, we find the responsible compound, the part of the plant in which the compound predominates, the proposed mechanisms of teratogenicity, and the observed teratogenic effects. (**c**) A 12.5 GD mouse embryo is shown inside its amniotic sac to represent the teratogenic mechanisms identified in Mexican plants that can affect its development. Although the exact mechanisms have not been fully clarified, the authors suspect that the main mechanisms in the observed teratogenic effect are as follows: oxidative stress; ischemia; enzymatic inhibition; alteration in levels of estrogens; cytotoxicity; apoptosis; interference with cellular mitosis; restricted fetal movements, among others. It is noteworthy that such alterations can be produced not only by a single mechanism, but also by the interaction of several of these.

In this regard, *Astragalus* and *Lupinus* are the more interesting genera due to their high number of species distributed in Mexico and the severe malformations that they generate in livestock. Additionally, although *Solanum* and *Croton* are two of the most important genera in Mexico due to their high variety of species, in our review no reports were found indicating that they have affected livestock (the teratogenic effect of these two genera were proven only in mouse and frog). This does not mean that these genera do not affect livestock, but simply that these effects have not yet been documented or studied, rendering novel opportunities.

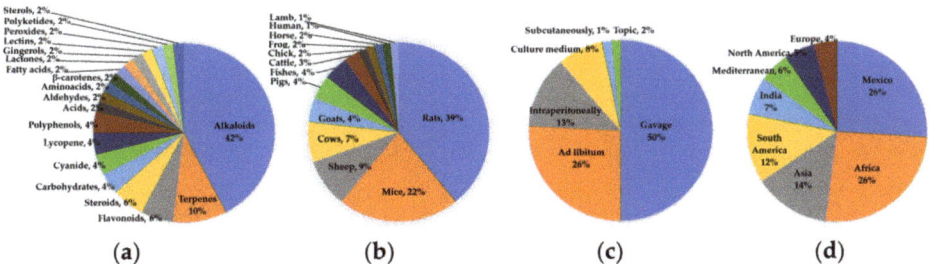

Figure 2. Graphic summary of the most relevant data obtained in the documentary research. (**a**) Abundance of the families of compounds identified in the teratogenic plants analyzed; (**b**) percentages of the main animal species (models) used to evaluate the teratogenicity of plants in the collected studies; (**c**) main routes of administration utilized in the evaluation of teratogenicity in the studies consulted, and; (**d**) distribution of identified teratogenic plants, native to or introduced from other countries.

3.2. Sacred Plants from Mexico

Additionally, it is important to consider that there are some species of Mexican plants that contain considerable amounts of the most common teratogenic compounds in nature, that is, alkaloids, but their teratogenic effect, to our knowledge, has not been investigated. Such is the case of *Borago officinalis* [134], the genus *Senecio* [135], and, of course, an important group of Mexican plants termed "sacred" (Table 2). In ancient Mexico (before the Spanish Conquest), plants with toxic properties were usually considered sacred, because their consumption induces mystical outbursts, fear, and alteration of the human mind in order to experience an elevation in consciousness; for this reason, they were bestowed with the personality of deities based on their effects [136]. In this manner, even today, the act of consuming *peyote* (*Lophophora williamsii*, America's most famous sacred hallucinogen) is called by an indigenous group, the *Huicholes*, as receiving "*hikuri*," which means receiving the "heart of the Deer God," who in turn is known as *Tatewari* and represents the grandfather god (God of Fire). This deity, the original shaman, collects *peyote* every year and guides his followers on a mystical pilgrimage to a sacred place where their ancestors rest: *Wirikuta* [137].

The Mexican sacred plants mentioned in Table 2 possess an important role in rituals and in their medicinal use due to the presence of psychoactive alkaloids, such as psilocybin, mescaline, and ergotamine, among others [138]. However, an important case that we must specify here is that of *Salvia devious* or *hierba de la virgen*, which contains a powerful hallucinogenic substance called "salvinorin A," with a structure similar to that of alkaloids. Nonetheless, it does not contain any nitrogen atom, and, thus, it is not considered as one of these, but rather the first documented diterpene nonalkaloid hallucinogen [139–141]. Despite the fact that *Salvia divinorum* is a sacred plant of great relevance in Mexico, it is addressed outside of Table 2 because, in said table, we find grouped only the Mexican sacred plants whose main hallucinogen components are alkaloids (molecules with great teratogenic capacity), while salvinorin A is a nonalkaloid hallucinogen whose teratogenic potential has not yet been evaluated or related to its particular structure.

The use of plants with ornamental, nutritional, aromatic, medicinal, and religious purposes is widely extended in Mexico [142]. In this respect, sacred plants with biological effects comprise an important element in indigenous medical and religious practices [143]. According to the lack of studies found in this review to evaluate the risks of these sacred plants for embryonic and fetal development, which are commonly used in Mexico, it is necessary to emphasize the danger of their use in the indigenous medical and religious systems. The fact is more alarming if we consider that about 80% of persons worldwide depend on traditional medicine to treat their ailments [144], and that, as stated by the Cámara de Diputados del Congreso de la Unión, the use of sacred plants in Mexico still continues not to be evaluated. Although it is true that Mexico, in subscribing to international treaties, is obliged to prohibit any substance decreed by the World Health Organization (WHO), there is no law in Mexico that punishes the use of these substances. In other words, Mexican legislation sanctions the possession, but not the consumption, of illegal substances, including sacred plants. Therefore, the consumption of hallucinogenic plants such as *peyote* is legal with only certain restrictions (trafficking) that do not apply to indigenous groups because "ot is an issue of rights regarding the culture and native communities of our country" [145].

Table 2. List of Mexican sacred plants without studies of teratogenicity.

Scientific Name	Common Name	Compound	Type	Cite
Ariocarpus retusus	Peyote cimarron	Alkaloids	Cactaceae	[146]
Argemone mexicana	Chicalote	Alkaloids	Plat	[147]
Conocybe	Teonanácatl	Alkaloids	Mushroom	[148]
Coryphantha compacta	Biznaga Partida Compacta	Alkaloids	Cactaceae	[149]
Datura ceratocaula Ortega	Torna loco	Alkaloids	Plant	[150]
Datura inoxia Mill	Toloache	Alkaloids	Plant	[151]
Echinocereus triglochidiatus	Alicoche Copa de Vino	Alkaloids	Cactaceae	[152]
Epithelantha micromeris	Ikuli mulato	Alkaloids	Cactaceae	[153]
Erytrhina americana Mill	Zumpantle	Alkaloids	Plant	[154]
Heimia salicifolia	Sinicuichi	Alkaloids	Plant	[155]
Ipomoea violacea	Quiebra platos	Alkaloids	Plant	[156]
Lophophora williamsii	Peyote	Alkaloids	Cactaceae	[157]
Lycoperdon mixtecorum	Hongo de primera clase	Alkaloids	Mushroom	[158]
Mammillaria senilis	Biznaga cabeza de viejitos	Alkaloids	Cactaceae	[149]
Pachycereus pecten-aboriginum	Cardón Barbón	Alkaloids	Cactaceae	[159]
Panaeolus sphinctrinus	Toshka	Alkaloids	Mushroom	[160]
Psilocybe caerulescens	Quélet	Alkaloids	Mushroom	[160]
Rhynchosia phaseoloides	Ojo de cangrejo	Alkaloids	Plant	[136]
Solandra brevicalyx	Tecomaxóchitl	Alkaloids	Plant	[161]
Sophora secundiflora	Mezcal frijol	Alkaloids	Plant	[162]
Stropharia cubensis	San Isidro	Alkaloids	Mushroom	[163]
Tagetes lucida	Yauhtli	Alkaloids	Plant	[164]
Turbina corymbose	Ololiuhqui	Alkaloids	Plant	[156]
Turnera Diffusa	Damiana	Alkaloids	Plant	[165]
Ungnadia speciosa	Monilla	Alkaloids	Plant	[166]

Information is shown on the alkaloid-rich main Mexican sacred plants that do not, to our knowledge, have scientific studies that evaluate their toxicity on embryo–fetal development.

Finally, we would like to mention that it is advisable to develop a database on non-teratogenic plants, as it is difficult to determine which plants lack a teratogenic effect because, to our knowledge, there are no published studies reporting this. In other words, the corresponding studies may have been carried out, but due to the lack of a teratogenic effect, these resulted as being unattractive for their publication. This catalog of non-teratogenic plants would be very useful in various investigations, both experimental and theoretical.

4. Conclusions

The information compiled in this bibliographic review reveals that there are a considerable number of Mexican plants used in traditional medicine with proven teratogenic effects in laboratory animals and in livestock. The main substances responsible for the teratogenic effects of the plants studied were those of alkaloids, terpenes, and flavonoids. Among the most notable teratogenic effects, alterations to the nervous system, the axial skeleton, and specific systems/structures are highlighted, for which the alkaloids are those mostly responsible.

Many of these plant species share the genus and, most likely, the teratogenic effects with other Mexican plant species on which, to our knowledge, teratogenic studies have not been conducted. Of the 63 species of Mexican plants with a teratogenic effect, 30.15%

are native to Mexico, while 69.84% derive from other regions such as Africa, Asia, and South America.

It was determined that there is a group of sacred Mexican plants, attractive due to the presence of alkaloids in their chemical composition and because of the use that they are afforded in traditional medicine and religious practices because of their hallucinogenic effects, which have, to our knowledge, no studies ascribed to them that describe their effects on development.

The biodiversity of plants in Mexico is very extensive: the 63 species with teratogenic effects found in this review barely refer to ≈0.21% of the total species in the country. Therefore, the need to continue exploring the teratogenic potential of Mexican plants is evident, at least beginning with the genera of other species that have already demonstrated their teratogenic effect in the laboratory.

Author Contributions: All authors contributed to the study conception and design. G.C.-C.: Visualization, project administration; M.A.M.-V.: data curation; Y.G.-M.: methodology, data curation, investigation; S.P.-G.: supervision; E.M.-S.: software; N.V.-M.: validation; J.A.M.-G.: writing—reviewing and editing; J.M.C.-L.: conceptualization, writing—original draft preparation, formal analysis. All authors have read and agreed to the published version of the manuscript.

Funding: This research received no external funding.

Institutional Review Board Statement: Not applicable.

Informed Consent Statement: Not applicable.

Data Availability Statement: Not applicable.

Acknowledgments: Melesio Cristóbal wants to express his very great appreciation to Yuliana García-Martínez for her valuable and constructive suggestions during the planning and development of this research work. Likewise, he wishes to reciprocate her love, support and patience throughout the last years: Yuli, do you want to conduct research with me for the rest of our lives? I mean, will you marry me?

"Est osculo gratum speculari semper amatum"
Medieval Aphorism

Conflicts of Interest: The authors declare no conflict of interest.

References

1. Newman, D.J.; Cragg, G.M.; Snader, K.M. The influence of natural products upon drug discovery. *Nat. Prod. Rep.* **2000**, *17*, 215–234. [CrossRef] [PubMed]
2. Jamshidi-Kia, F.; Lorigooini, Z.; Amini-Khoei, H. Medicinal plants: Past history and future perspective. *J. Herbmed. Pharmacol.* **2018**, *7*, 1–7. [CrossRef]
3. Solecki, R. Shanidar IV a Neanderthal flower burial in Northern Iraq. *Science* **1975**, *190*, 880–881. [CrossRef]
4. Qiu, J. Traditional medicine: A culture in the balance. *Nature* **2007**, *448*, 126–128. [CrossRef]
5. Hartmann, A. Back to the roots-dermatology in ancient Egyptian medicine. *J. Dtsch. Dermatol. Ges.* **2016**, *14*, 389–396. [CrossRef]
6. Balkrishna, A.; Mishra, R.K.; Srivastava, A.; Joshi, B.; Marde, R.; Prajapati, U.B. Ancient Indian rishi's (Sages) knowledge of botany and medicinal plants since Vedic period was much older than the period of Theophrastus, A case study—Who was the actual father of botany? *Int. J. Unani Integr. Med.* **2019**, *3*, 40–44.
7. Petrovska, B.B. Historical review of medicinal plants' usage. *Pharmacogn. Rev.* **2012**, *6*, 1–5. [CrossRef]
8. Ang-Lee, M.K.; Moss, J.; Yuan, C.S. Herbal medicines and perioperative care. *JAMA* **2001**, *286*, 208–216. [CrossRef]
9. Palencia, J.S. Presentación. El códice de la cruz Badiano libellus de medicinalibus indorum herbis. *Salud Pub. Mex.* **1990**, *32*, 603–617.
10. Casas, A.; Blancas, J.; Lira, R. Mexican Ethnobotany: Interactions of people and plants in Mesoamerica. In *Ethnobotany of Mexico*; Springer: New York, NY, USA, 2016; Chapter 1; pp. 1–20.
11. Pickersgill, B. Domestication of plants in the Americas: Insights from Mendelian and molecular genetics. *Ann Bot.* **2007**, *100*, 925–940. [CrossRef]
12. Ríos, J.L.; Recio, M.C. Medicinal plants and antimicrobial activity. *J. Ethnopharmacol.* **2005**, *100*, 80–84. [CrossRef]
13. Madsen, H.L.; Bertelsen, G. Spices as antioxidants. *Trends Food Sci. Technol.* **1995**, *6*, 271–277. [CrossRef]
14. Staub, P.O.; Casu, L.; Leonti, M. Back to the roots: A quantitative survey of herbal drugs in Dioscorides' De Materia Medica (ex Matthioli, 1568). *Phytomedicine* **2016**, *23*, 1043–1052. [CrossRef]

15. Singh, N.; Savita, S.; Rithesh, K.; Shivanand, S. Phytotherapy: A novel approach for treating periodontal disease. *J. Pharm. Biomed. Sci.* **2016**, *6*, 205–210. [CrossRef]
16. McIntyre, L. *Dark Ages: The Case for a Science of Human Behavior*; The MIT Press: Cambridge, MA, USA, 2006; p. 15.
17. Guthrie, L.S. Monastic cataloging and classification and the beginnings of "class b" at the library of congress. *Cat. Classif Q.* **2003**, *35*, 447–465. [CrossRef]
18. Cragg, G.; Newman, D.J. Natural product drug discovery in the next millennium. *Pharm. Biol.* **2001**, *39*, 8–17. [CrossRef]
19. Hamarneh, S. The rise of professional pharmacy in Islam. *Med. Hist.* **1962**, *6*, 59–66. [CrossRef]
20. Dunlop, D.M.; Denston, T.C. The history and development of the British Pharmacopoeia. *Br. Med. J.* **1958**, *2*, 1250–1252. [CrossRef]
21. Grabley, S.; Thiericke, R. Bioactive agents from natural sources: Trends in discovery and application. *Adv. Biochem. Eng. Biotechnol.* **1999**, *64*, 101–154. [CrossRef]
22. Thorburn, A.L. Paul Ehrlich: Pioneer of chemotherapy and cure by arsenic (1854–1915). *Br. J. Vener. Dis.* **1983**, *59*, 404–405. [CrossRef]
23. Gu, J.; Zhang, J.; Wang, X.; Wang, G. Convenient new synthesis of umeclidinium bromide. *Synth. Commun.* **2018**, *48*, 995–1000. [CrossRef]
24. Tsoucalas, G.; Karamanou, M.; Androutsos, G. Travelling through time with aspirin, a healing companion. *Eur. J. Inflamm.* **2011**, *9*, 13–16. [CrossRef]
25. Bulduk, I.; Gezer, B.; Cengiz, M. Optimization of ultrasound-assisted extraction of morphine from capsules of *Papaver somniferum* by response surface methodology. *Int. J. Anal. Chem.* **2015**, *2015*, 796349. [CrossRef]
26. Whayne, T.F., Jr. Clinical use of digitalis: A state of the art review. *Am. J. Cardiovasc. Drugs* **2018**, *18*, 427–440. [CrossRef]
27. Colorado, I.R. Obtaining diosgenin from the barbasco. *Rev. Inst. Salubr. Enferm. Trop.* **1962**, *22*, 71–73.
28. Blakemore, D.C.; Castro, L.; Churcher, I.; Rees, D.C.; Thomas, A.W.; Wilson, D.M.; Wood, A. Organic synthesis provides opportunities to transform drug discovery. *Nat. Chem.* **2018**, *10*, 383–394. [CrossRef]
29. Tandon, S.; Sharma, S.; Rajput, R.; Semwal, B.; Yadav, P.K.; Singh, K. Biotech drugs: The next boom in pharmaceutical market. *JPRP* **2011**, *1*, 76–79.
30. Shen, B. A new golden age of natural products drug discovery. *Cell* **2015**, *163*, 1297–1300. [CrossRef] [PubMed]
31. Juárez, A.; Carranza, C.; Alonso, A.; González, V.; Bravo, E.; Chamarro, F.; Solano, E. Ethnobotany of medicinal plants used in Xalpatlahuac, Guerrero, México. *J. Ethnopharmacol.* **2013**, *148*, 521–527. [CrossRef] [PubMed]
32. Consejo Estatal Para el Desarrollo Integral de los Pueblos Indígenas del Estado de México (CEDIPIEM). (S.F.). La Medicina Tradicional. Available online: http://portal2.edomex.gob.mx/cedipiem/pueblosindigenas/cultura/medicinatradicional/index.html (accessed on 6 May 2015).
33. Lee, J.W.; Lee, W.B.; Kim, W.; Min, B.I.; Lee, H.; Cho, S.H. Traditional herbal medicine for cancer pain: A systematic review and meta-analysis. *Complement. Ther. Med.* **2015**, *23*, 265–274. [CrossRef] [PubMed]
34. Villaseñor, J.L. Checklist of the native vascular plants of Mexico. *Rev. Mex. Biodivers.* **2016**, *87*, 559–902. [CrossRef]
35. Villaseñor, J.L. Diversidad y distribución de las magnoliophyta de México. *Interciencia* **2003**, *28*, 160–167.
36. Palma-Tenango, M.; Miguel-Chávez, R.S.; Soto-Hernández, R.M. Aromatic and Medicinal Plants in Mexico. Chapter 7: Aromatic and medicinal plants in Mexico. In *Aromatic and Medicinal Plants*; InTech: London, UK, 2017. [CrossRef]
37. McAleer, I. Renal Development. In *Avery's Diseases of the Newborn*, 10th ed.; Elsevier Inc.: Amsterdam, The Netherlands, 2018; pp. 1238–1249. [CrossRef]
38. Vargesson, N.; Fraga, L. Teratogenesis. *eLS* **2017**, *a0026056*, 1–7. [CrossRef]
39. Cassina, M.; Cagnoli, G.A.; Zuccarello, D.; Di Gianantonio, E.; Clementi, M. Human teratogens and genetic phenocopies. Understanding pathogenesis through human genes mutation. *Eur. J. Med. Genet.* **2017**, *60*, 22–31. [CrossRef]
40. Jacobo-Herrera, N.J.; Jacobo-Herrera, F.E.; Zentella-Dehesa, A.; Andrade-Cetto, A.; Heinrich, M.; Pérez-Plasencia, C. Medicinal plants used in Mexican traditional medicine for the treatment of colorectal cancer. *J. Ethnopharmacol.* **2016**, *179*, 391–402. [CrossRef]
41. Bautista-Cruz, A.; Arnaud-Viñas, M.R.; Martínez-Gutiérrez, G.A.; Sánchez-Medina, P.S.; Pacheco, R.P. The traditional medicinal and food uses of four plants in Oaxaca, Mexico. *J. Med. Plants Res.* **2011**, *5*, 3404–3411.
42. Laveaga, G.S. Mexico's Historical Models for Providing Rural Healthcare. In *Health for All: The Journey of Universal Health Coverage*; Medcalf, A., Bhattacharya, S., Momen, H., Saavedra, M., Jones, M., Eds.; Orient Blackswan: Hyderabad, Indian, 2015; Chapter 4. Available online: https://www.ncbi.nlm.nih.gov/books/NBK316259/ (accessed on 12 November 2021).
43. van Gameren, E. Health insurance and use of alternative medicine in Mexico. *Health Policy* **2010**, *98*, 50–57. [CrossRef]
44. Govea-Salas, M.; Morlett-Chávez, J.; Rodriguez-Herrera, R.; Ascacio-Valdés, J. Some Mexican Plants Used in Traditional Medicine. In *Aromatic and Medicinal Plants—Back to Nature*; InTech: London, UK, 2017; Chapter 10. [CrossRef]
45. Valdivia-Correa, B.; Gómez-Gutiérrez, C.; Uribe, M.; Méndez-Sánchez, N. Herbal Medicine in Mexico: A Cause of Hepatotoxicity. A Critical Review. *Int. J. Mol. Sci.* **2016**, *17*, 235. [CrossRef]
46. Alonso-Castro, A.J.; Ruiz-Padilla, A.J.; Ruiz-Noa, Y.; Alba-Betancourt, C.; Domínguez, F.; Ibarra-Reynoso, L.; Maldonado-Miranda, J.J.; Carranza-Álvarez, C.; Blanco-Sandate, C.; Ramírez-Morales, M.A.; et al. Self-medication practice in pregnant women from central Mexico. *Saudi Pharm. J.* **2018**, *26*, 886–890. [CrossRef]
47. Cortinovis, C.; Caloni, F. Alkaloid-Containing Plants Poisonous to Cattle and Horses in Europe. *Toxins* **2015**, *7*, 5301–5307. [CrossRef]

48. Almli, L.M.; Ely, D.M.; Ailes, E.C.; Abouk, R.; Grosse, S.D.; Isenburg, J.L.; Waldron, D.B.; Reefhuis, J. Infant Mortality Attributable to Birth Defects—United States, 2003–2017. *Morb. Mortal. Wkly. Rep.* **2020**, *69*, 25–29. [CrossRef]
49. Soares, M.C.; Pupin, R.C.; Guizelini, C.C.; Gaspar, A.O.; Gomes, D.C.; Brumatti, R.C.; Lemos, R.A.A. Economic losses due to Vernonia rubricaulis poisoning in cattle. *Pesq. Vet. Bras.* **2018**, *38*, 2217–2223. [CrossRef]
50. Invasive Species Compendium (ISC). CAB International: Wallingford, UK. Available online: www.cabi.org/isc (accessed on 30 August 2021).
51. Herbario Virtual Conabio (HVC). Available online: http://www.conabio.gob.mx/otros/cgi-bin/herbario.cgi (accessed on 5 August 2021).
52. Naturalista. CONABIO. Available online: http://www.naturalista.mx (accessed on 15 August 2021).
53. Flora del Noroeste de México. 2021. Available online: http://www.herbanwmex.net/portal/index.php (accessed on 4 September 2021).
54. Jing, H.; Liu, J.; Liu, H.; Xin, H. Histochemical investigation and kinds of alkaloids in leaves of different developmental stages in Thymus quinquecostatus. *Sci. World J.* **2014**, *2014*, 839548. [CrossRef]
55. Jaszczak, E.; Polkowska, Ż.; Narkowicz, S.; Namieśnik, J. Cyanides in the environment-analysis-problems and challenges. *Environ. Sci. Pollut. Res. Int.* **2017**, *24*, 15929–15948. [CrossRef]
56. Butnariu, M.; Sarac, I. Essential oils from plants. *J. Biotechnol. Biomed. Sci.* **2018**, *1*, 35–43. [CrossRef]
57. Dey, P.; Kundu, A.; Kumar, A.; Gupta, M.; Lee, B.M.; Bhakta, T.; Dash, S.; Kim, H.S. Analysis of alkaloids (indole alkaloids, isoquinoline alkaloids, tropane alkaloids). In *Recent Advances in Natural Products Analysis*; Elsevier: Amsterdam, The Netherlands, 2020; pp. 505–567. [CrossRef]
58. Funayama, A.S.; Cordell, G.A. *Alkaloids: A Treasury of Poisons and Medicines*; Elsevier: Amsterdam, The Netherlands, 2015; pp. 1–10.
59. Green, B.T.; Lee, S.T.; Welch, K.D.; Panter, K.E. Plant alkaloids that cause developmental defects through the disruption of cholinergic neurotransmission. *Birth Defects Res. C Embryo Today* **2013**, *99*, 235–246. [CrossRef]
60. Lemonica, I.P.; Alvarenga, C.M. Abortive and teratogenic effect of Acanthospermum hispidum DC. and *Cajanus cajan* (L.) Millps. in pregnant rats. *J. Ethnopharmacol.* **1994**, *43*, 39–44. [CrossRef]
61. Nana, P.; Asongalem, E.A.; Foyet, H.S.; Folefoc, G.N.; Dimo, T.; Kamtchouing, P. Maternal and developmental toxicity evaluation of *Acanthus montanus* leaves extract administered orally to Wistar pregnant rats during organogenesis. *J. Ethnopharmacol.* **2008**, *116*, 228–233. [CrossRef]
62. Diallo, A.; Batomayena, B.; Povic, L.; Eklu-Gadegbeku, K.; Aklikokou, K.; Creppy, E.; Gbeassor, M. Fetal toxicity of hydroalcoholic extract of *Ageratum conyzoides* L. leaves (asteraceae) in rats. *Int. J. Pharm. Pharm. Sci.* **2015**, *7*, 264–266.
63. Eluwa, M.A.; Otung, G.; Udo-Affah, G.; Ekanem, T.B.; Mesembe, O.; Au, A. Teratogenic effect of maternal administration of aloe vera extract on foetal morphology and the histology of the foetal kidney. *Glob. J. Med. Sci.* **2006**, *5*, 41–44. [CrossRef]
64. Herrera, A.A.; Dee, A.M.O.; Ipulan, L.A. Detection of congenital anomalies in Mus musculus induced by crude leaf extracts of *Goniothalamus amuyon* (Blanco) Merr. and *Alstonia macrophylla* Wall. Ex G. Don. *J. Med. Plant Res.* **2010**, *4*, 327–334. [CrossRef]
65. Jagetia, G.C.; Baliga, M.S. Induction of developmental toxicity in mice treated with *Alstonia scholaris* (Sapthaparna) In utero. *Birth Defects Res. B Dev. Reprod. Toxicol.* **2003**, *68*, 472–478. [CrossRef] [PubMed]
66. Boareto, A.C.; Muller, J.C.; Bufalo, A.C.; Botelho, G.G.K.; De Araujo, S.L.; Foglio, M.A.; Dalsenter, P.R. Toxicity of artemisinin [*Artemisia annua* L.] in two different periods of pregnancy in Wistar rats. *Reprod. Toxicol.* **2008**, *25*, 239–246. [CrossRef] [PubMed]
67. James, L.F. Effect of locoweed (*Astragalus lentiginosus*) feeding of fetal lamb development. *Can. J. Comp. Med.* **1976**, *40*, 380–384. [PubMed]
68. Hanson, G. The Toxicity of Plants in Equines, a Modern Three-Point Approach to Disseminating Information. Master's Thesis, University of Idaho, Moscow, ID, USA, 2008; pp. 83–89.
69. James, L.F.; Shupe, J.L.; Binns, W.; Keeler, R.F. Abortive and teratogenic effects of locoweed on sheep and cattle. *Am. J. Vet. Res.* **1967**, *28*, 379–1388.
70. Dallaqua, B.; Saito, F.H.; Rodrigues, T.; Calderon, I.M.; Rudge, M.V.; Volpato, G.T.; Damasceno, D.C. Azadirachta indica treatment on the congenital malformations of fetuses from rats. *J. Ethnopharmacol.* **2013**, *150*, 1109–1113. [CrossRef]
71. Lemonica, I.P.; Macedo, A.M.R.B. Borro Macedo. Abortive and/or embryofetotoxic effect of *Cinnamomum zeylanicum* leaf extracts in pregnant rats. *Fitoter* **1994**, *65*, 431–434.
72. Abel, E.L.; Rockwood, G.A.; Riley, E.P. The Effects of Early Marijuana Exposure. In *Handbook of Behavioral Teratology*; Riley, E.P., Vorhees, C.V., Eds.; Springer: Boston, MA, USA, 1986. [CrossRef]
73. Persaud, T.V.; Ellington, A.C. The effects of *Cannabis sativa* L. (Ganja) on developing rat embryos–preliminary observations. *West Indian Med. J.* **1968**, *17*, 232–234.
74. Nobakht, M.; Fattahi, M.; Hoormand, M.; Milanian, I.; Rahbar, N.; Mahmoudian, M. A study on the teratogenic and cytotoxic effects of safflower extract. *J. Ethnopharmacol.* **2000**, *73*, 453–459. [CrossRef]
75. Traesel, G.K.; De Lima, F.F.; Dos Santos, A.C.; Souza, R.I.C.; Cantadori, D.T.; Kretschmer, C.R.; Navarini, V.J.; Oesterreich, S.A. Evaluation of embryotoxic and teratogenic effects of the oil extracted from *Caryocar brasiliense Cambess* pulp in rats. *Food Chem. Toxicol.* **2017**, *110*, 74–82. [CrossRef]
76. Green, B.T.; Lee, S.T.; Panter, K.E.; Brown, D.R. Piperidine alkaloids: Human and food animal teratogens. *Food Chem. Toxicol.* **2012**, *50*, 2049–2055. [CrossRef]

77. Keeler, R.F. Coniine, a teratogenic principle from *Conium maculatum* producing congenital malformations in calves. *Clin. Toxicol.* **1974**, *7*, 195–206. [CrossRef]
78. Keller, K. Cinnamomum Species. In *Adverse Reactions of Herbal Drugs*; De Smet, P.A.G.M., Keller, K., Hänsel, R., Chandler, R.F., Eds.; Springer: Berlin/Heidelberg, Germany, 1992; pp. 105–114.
79. Wabai, Y.W.; Maina, M.K.J.; Mwaniki, N.E. Teratogenic potential of *Urtica massaica* (Mildbr.) and *Croton megalocarpus* (Hutch) in mice. *J. Phytopharmacol.* **2018**, *7*, 460–463. [CrossRef]
80. Alafiatayo, A.A.; Lai, K.S.; Syahida, A.; Mahmood, M.; Shaharuddin, N.A. Phytochemical Evaluation, Embryotoxicity, and Teratogenic Effects of *Curcuma longa* Extract on Zebrafish (*Danio rerio*). *Evid. Based Complement. Altern. Med.* **2019**, *2019*, 3807207. [CrossRef]
81. Ramesh, C.G. *Reproductive and Developmental Toxicology*; Chapter 51: Toxic Plants; Academic Press: San Diego, CA, USA, 2011; p. 690.
82. Tolentino, J.J.V.; Undan, J.R. Embryo-Toxicity and Teratogenicity of *Derris elliptica* Leaf Extract on Zebra Fish (*Danio rerio*) Embryos. *Int. J. Pure App. Biosci.* **2016**, *4*, 16–20. [CrossRef]
83. Kuete, V. *Toxicological Survey of African Medicinal Plants*; Elsevier: New York, NY, USA, 2014; p. 266.
84. Akpantah, A.O.; Oremosu, A.A.; Noronha, C.C.; Ekanem, T.B.; Okanlawon, A.O. Effects of garcinia kola seed extract on ovulation, oestrous cycle and foetal development in cyclic female sprague-dawley rats. *Niger. J. Physiol. Sci.* **2005**, *20*, 58–62.
85. Khalid, M.; Tahir, M.; Shoro, A. Ginseng induced fetal skeletal malformations. *Biomedica* **2008**, *24*, 96–98.
86. Pearn, J.H. Studies on a site-specific cleft palate teratogen. The toxic extract from Indigofera spicata Forssk. *Br. J. Exp. Pathol.* **1967**, *48*, 620–626.
87. Zoriki-Hosomi, R.; Spinosa, H.; Lima-Górniak, S.; Ferreira-Habr, S.; Witaker-Penteado, S.; Fantinato-Varoli, F.M.; Bernardi, M.M. Embryotoxic effects of prenatal treatment with *Ipomoea carnea* aqueous fraction in rats. *Braz. J. Vet. Res. Anim. Sci.* **2008**, *45*, 67–75. [CrossRef]
88. Cristóbal-Luna, J.M.; Paniagua-Castro, N.; Escalona-Cardoso, G.N.; Pérez-Gutiérrez, M.S.; Álvarez-González, I.; Madrigal-Bujaidar, E.; Chamorro-Cevallos, G. Evaluation of teratogenicity and genotoxicity induced by kramecyne (KACY). *Saudi Pharm. J.* **2018**, *26*, 829–838. [CrossRef]
89. Mello, F.B.; Jacobus, D.; Carvalho, K.; Mello, J.R.B. Effects of *Lantana camara* (Verbenaceae) on general reproductive performance and teratology in rats. *Toxicon* **2005**, *45*, 459–466. [CrossRef]
90. Sarhadi, Z.; Torabzadeh, P.; Ramezani, M. Assessment of the Teratogenic Effects of Aqueous Extract of *Lavandula angustifolia* on BALB/c Female Mouse's Embryos in the 3rd, 4th, 5th and 6th Days of Gestation. *J. Anim. Biol.* **2019**, *11*, 35–45.
91. Esteki, E.; Miraj, S. The Abortificient Effects of Hydroalcoholic Extract of Lawsonia Inermis on BALB/c Mice. *Electron. Physician* **2016**, *8*, 2568–2575. [CrossRef]
92. Sastry, M.S.; Singh, R. Toxic effects of subabul (*Leucaena leucocephala*) on the thyroid and reproduction of female goats. *Indian J. Anim. Sci.* **2008**, *78*, 251–253.
93. Barilli, S.L.S.; Dos Santos, S.T.; Montanari, T. Efeito do Decocto dos Frutos de Buchinha-do-Norte (*Luffa operculata* Cogn.) Sobre a Reprodução Feminina e o Desenvolvimento Embrionário e fetal, 10 a 12 de maio. Semana da Enfermagem: A enfermagem e o Desafio da Integralidade em Saúde. 2006. Available online: www.tinyurl.com/ybd3h4ye (accessed on 14 August 2021).
94. Panter, K.E.; James, L.F.; Keeler, R.F.; Bunch, T.D. Radio-ultrasound observations of poisonous plant–induced fetotoxicity in livestock. In *Poisonous Plants: Proceedings of the Third International Symposium*; James, L.F., Keeler, R.F., Bailey, E.M., Panter, K.E., Bunch, T.D., Eds.; Iowa State University Press: Ames, IA, USA, 1992; pp. 481–488.
95. Keeler, R.F.; Panter, K.E. Piperidine alkaloid composition and relation to crooked calf disease–inducing potential of *Lupinus formosus*. *Teratology* **1989**, *40*, 423–432. [CrossRef]
96. James, L.F.; Keeler, R.F.; Binns, W. Sequence in the abortive and teratogenic effects of locoweed fed to sheep. *Am. J. Vet. Res.* **1969**, *30*, 377–380.
97. Singh, J.D. The teratogenic effects of dietary cassava on the pregnant albino rat: A preliminary report. *Teratology* **1981**, *24*, 289–291. [CrossRef]
98. Medeiros, R.M.T.; De Figueiredo, A.P.M.; Benício, T.M.A.; Dantas, F.P.M.; Riet-Correa, F. Teratogenicity of *Mimosa tenuiflora* seeds to pregnant rats. *Toxicon* **2008**, *51*, 316–319. [CrossRef]
99. Uche-Nwachi, E.O.; McEwen, C. Teratogenic effect of the water extract of bitter gourd (*Momordica charantia*) on the Sprague Dawley rats. *Afr. J. Tradit. Complement. Altern. Med.* **2009**, *7*, 24–33. [CrossRef]
100. Moy, N.A. *Efectos Farmacológicos y Toxicológicos de Extractos Hidroalcohólicos de Zoapatle (Montanoa tomentosa) en Rata Biodisponibilidad Después de Administración Intravaginal*; Universidad de Colima: Colima, México, 1998; pp. 3–4.
101. Marques, N.F.; Marques, A.P.; Iwano, A.L.; Golin, M.; De-Carvalho, R.R.; Paumgartten, F.J.; Dalsenter, P.R. Delayed ossification in Wistar rats induced by *Morinda citrifolia* L. exposure during pregnancy. *J. Ethnopharmacol.* **2010**, *128*, 85–91. [CrossRef]
102. David, C.R.S.; Angeles, A.; Angoluan, R.C.; Santos, J.P.E.; David, E.S.; Dulay, R.M.R. *Moringa oleifera* (Malunggay) Water Extracts Exhibit Embryo-toxic and Teratogenic Activity in Zebrafish (*Danio rerio*) Embryo Model. *Der Pharm. Lett.* **2016**, *8*, 163–168. [CrossRef]
103. Panter, K.E.; Weinzweig, J.; Gardner, D.R.; Stegelmeier, B.L.; James, L.F. Comparison of cleft palate induction by *Nicotiana glauca* in goats and sheep. *Teratology* **2000**, *61*, 203–210. [CrossRef]

104. Khalki, H.; Khalki, L.; Aboufatima, R.; Ouachrif, A.; Mountassir, M.; Benharref, A.; Chait, A. Prenatal exposure to tobacco extract containing nicotinic alkaloids produces morphological and behavioral changes in newborn rats. *Pharmacol. Biochem. Behav.* **2012**, *101*, 342–347. [CrossRef] [PubMed]
105. Crowe, M.W.; Swerczek, T.W. Congenital arthrogryposis in offspring of sows fed tobacco (*Nicotiana tabacum*). *Am. J. Vet. Res.* **1974**, *35*, 1071–1073.
106. Moallem, S.A.; Niapour, M. Study of embryotoxicity of *Perovskia abrotanoides*, an adulterant in folk-medicine, during organogenesis in mice. *J. Ethnopharmacol.* **2008**, *117*, 108–114. [CrossRef]
107. Almeida, E.R.; Melo, A.M.; Xavier, H. Toxicological evaluation of the hydro-alcohol extract of the dry leaves of *Peumus boldus* and boldine in rats. *Phytother. Res. PTR* **2000**, *14*, 99–102. [CrossRef]
108. Gardner, D.R.; Molyneux, R.J.; James, L.F.; Panter, K.E.; Stegelmeier, B.L. Ponderosa Pine Needle-Induced abortion in beef cattle: Identification of isocupressic acid as the principal active compound. *J. Agric. Food Chem.* **1994**, *42*, 756–761. [CrossRef]
109. Karol, M.D.; Conner, C.S.; Watanabe, A.S.; Murphrey, K.J. Podophyllum: Suspected teratogenicity from topical application. *Clin. Toxicol.* **1980**, *16*, 283–286. [CrossRef]
110. Chamberlain, M.J.; Reynolds, A.L.; Yeoman, W.B. Medical memoranda. Toxic effect of podophyllum application in pregnancy. *Br. Med. J.* **1972**, *3*, 391–392. [CrossRef]
111. Selby, L.A.; Menges, R.W.; Houser, E.C.; Flatt, R.E.; Case, A.A. Outbreak of swine malformations associated with the wild black cherry, *Prunus serotina*. *Arch. Environ. Health* **1971**, *22*, 496–501. [CrossRef]
112. Eluwa, M.A.; Udoaffah, M.T.; Vulley, M.B.; Ekanem, T.B.; Akpantah, A.O.; Asuquo, O.A.; Ekong, M.B. Comparative study of teratogenic potentials of crude ethanolic root bark and leaf extract of *Rauwolfia vomitoria* (apocynaceae) on the fetal heart. *N. Am. J. Med. Sci.* **2010**, *2*, 592–595. [CrossRef]
113. Ucheya, R.E.; Biose, I.J. Teratogenic effects of methanolic extract of *Ricinus communis* seed oil on the morphology of foetal wistar rats. *Biosci. Biotechnol. Res. Asia* **2010**, *7*, 719–723.
114. Gonzales, J.; Benavides, V.; Rojas, R.; Pino, J. Embryotoxic and teratogenic effect of *Ruta chalepensis* L. «rue», in mouse (*Mus musculus*). *Rev. Peru. Biol.* **2007**, *13*, 223–226.
115. Gutiérrez-Pajares, J.L.; Zúñiga, L.; Pino, J. Ruta graveolens aqueous extract retards mouse preimplantation embryo development. *Reprod. Toxicol.* **2003**, *17*, 667–672. [CrossRef]
116. Yakubu, M.T.; Musa, I.F. Effects of Post-coital Administration of Alkaloids from *Senna alata* (Linn. Roxb) Leaves on some Fetal and Maternal Outcomes of Pregnant Rats. *J. Reprod. Infertil.* **2012**, *13*, 211–217.
117. Gholami, M.; Moallem, S.A.; Afshar, M.; Amoueian, S.; Etemad, L.; Karimi, G. Teratogenic effects of silymarin on mouse fetuses. *Avicenna J. Phytomed.* **2016**, *6*, 542–549.
118. Friedman, M.; Rayburn, J.R.; Bantle, J.A. Developmental toxicology of potato alkaloids in the frog embryo teratogenesis assay–Xenopus (FETAX). *Food Chem. Toxicol.* **1991**, *29*, 537–547. [CrossRef]
119. Lawal, R.O. Effects of dietary protein on teratogenicity of polyphenols obtained from the outer coat of the fruit of *Treculia africana*. *Food Chem.* **1997**, *60*, 495–499. [CrossRef]
120. Khalki, L.; M'hamed, S.B.; Bennis, M.; Chait, A.; Sokar, Z. Evaluation of the developmental toxicity of the aqueous extract from *Trigonella foenum-graecum* (L.) in mice. *J. Ethnopharmacol.* **2010**, *131*, 321–325. [CrossRef]
121. Keeler, R.F.; Binns, W. Teratogenic compounds of *Veratrum californicum* (Durand). II. Production of ovine fetal cyclobia by fractions and alkaloid preparations. *Can. J. Biochem.* **1966**, *44*, 829–838. [CrossRef]
122. Wilkinson, J.M. Effect of ginger tea on the fetal development of Sprague-Dawley rats. *Reprod. Toxicol.* **2000**, *14*, 507–512. [CrossRef]
123. Bryda, E.C. The Mighty Mouse: The impact of rodents on advances in biomedical research. *Mo. Med.* **2013**, *110*, 207–211.
124. Barré-Sinoussi, F.; Montagutelli, X. Animal models are essential to biological research: Issues and perspectives. *Future Sci. OA* **2015**, *1*, FSO63. [CrossRef]
125. Pound, P.; Ritskes-Hoitinga, M. Is it possible to overcome issues of external validity in preclinical animal research? Why most animal models are bound to fail. Pound and Ritskes? *Hoitinga J. Transl. Med.* **2018**, *16*, 304. [CrossRef]
126. Van Norman, G.A. Limitations of Animal Studies for Predicting Toxicity in Clinical Trials: Is it Time to Rethink Our Current Approach? *JACC Basic Transl. Sci.* **2019**, *4*, 845–854. [CrossRef]
127. Templeton, A.R. Biological races in humans. *Stud. Hist. Philos. Biol. Biomed. Sci.* **2013**, *44*, 262–271. [CrossRef]
128. Litchfield, J.T. Symposium on clinical drug evaluation and human pharmacology. XVI. Evaluation of the safety of new drugs by means of tests in animals. *Clin. Pharmacol. Ther.* **1962**, *3*, 665–672. [CrossRef]
129. Library of Congress. Image 286 of General History of the Things of New Spain by Fray Bernardino de Sahagún: The Florentine Codex. Book XI: Natural Things. Available online: https://www.loc.gov/resource/gdcwdl.wdl_10622/?sp=286 (accessed on 13 June 2022).
130. Red de Herbarios del Noroeste de México. *Astragalus mollissimus* Torr. Available online: https://herbanwmex.net/portal/taxa/index.php?tid=4122 (accessed on 13 June 2022).
131. Red de Herbarios del Noroeste de México. *Artemisia annua* L. Available online: https://herbanwmex.net/portal/taxa/index.php?taxon=Artemisia+annua+&formsubmit=Search+Terms (accessed on 13 June 2022).
132. Red de Herbarios del Noroeste de México. *Silybum marianum* (L.) Gaertn. Available online: https://herbanwmex.net/portal/taxa/index.php?taxon=Silybum+marianum&formsubmit=Search+Terms (accessed on 13 June 2022).

133. TRAMILE Programa de Investigación Aplicada a la Medicina Popular del Caribe. Available online: https://www.tramil.net/es/plant/manihot-esculenta#:~:text=Descripci%C3%B3n%20bot%C3%A1nica,con%20c%C3%A1liz%20campanulado%2C%205%20lobado (accessed on 13 June 2022).
134. Vacillotto, G.; Favretto, D.; Seraglia, R.; Pagiotti, R.; Traldi, P.; Mattoli, L. A rapid and highly specific method to evaluate the presence of pyrrolizidine alkaloids in *Borago officinalis* seed oil. *J. Mass Spectrom.* **2013**, *48*, 1078–1082. [CrossRef]
135. Langel, D.; Ober, D.; Pelser, P.B. The evolution of pyrrolizidine alkaloid biosynthesis and diversity in the Senecioneae. *Phytochem. Rev.* **2001**, *10*, 3–74. [CrossRef]
136. Barba, B. Las plantas sagradas mexicanas. *Ciencia* **2015**, *66*, 48–59.
137. Schultes, R.E.; Hofmann, A. *Plants of the Gods: Their Sacred, Healing, and Hallucinogenic Powers*, 2nd ed.; Healing Arts Press: Rochester, VT, USA, 2001; p. 148.
138. Díaz, J.L. Ethnopharmacology of sacred psychoactive plants used by the Indians of Mexico. *Annu. Rev. Pharmacol. Toxicol.* **1977**, *17*, 647–675. [CrossRef] [PubMed]
139. Rossi, A.; Pace, S.; Tedesco, F.; Pagano, E.; Guerra, G.; Troisi, F.; Werner, M.; Roviezzo, F.; Zjawiony, J.K.; Werz, O.; et al. The hallucinogenic diterpene salvinorin A inhibits leukotriene synthesis in experimental models of inflammation. *Pharmacol. Res.* **2016**, *106*, 64–71. [CrossRef] [PubMed]
140. Roth, B.L.; Baner, K.; Westkaemper, R.; Siebert, D.; Rice, K.C.; Steinberg, S.; Ernsberger, P.; Rothman, R.B.; Salvinorin, A. A potent naturally occurring nonnitrogenous kappa opioid selective agonist. *Proc. Natl. Acad. Sci. USA* **2002**, *99*, 11934–11939. [CrossRef] [PubMed]
141. Valdés, L.J., 3rd. Salvia divinorum and the unique diterpene hallucinogen, Salvinorin (divinorin) A. *J. Psychoact. Drugs* **1994**, *26*, 277–283. [CrossRef]
142. Reimers, E.A.L.; Fernández, E.C.; Reimers, D.J.L.; Chaloupkova, P.; Del Valle, J.M.Z.; Milella, L.; Russo, D. An Ethnobotanical Survey of Medicinal Plants Used in Papantla, Veracruz, Mexico. *Plants* **2019**, *8*, 246. [CrossRef]
143. Heinrich, M.; Ankli, A.; Frei, B.; Weimann, C.; Sticher, O. Medicinal plants in Mexico: Healers' consensus and cultural importance. *Soc. Sci. Med.* **1998**, *47*, 1859–1871. [CrossRef]
144. Yabesh, J.E.M.; Prabhu, S.; Vijayakumar, S. An ethnobotanical study of medicinal plants used by traditional healers in silent valley of Kerala, India. *J. Ethnopharmacol.* **2014**, *154*, 774–789. [CrossRef]
145. Cámara de Diputados del Congreso de la Unión, LXIV Legislatura. *Necesario Legislar Sobre Plantas Sagradas*; Boletín 3979; son Patrimonio Nacional: Nava Palacios. México, 2017. Available online: http://www5.diputados.gob.mx/index.php/esl/Comunicacion/Boletines/2017/Agosto/29/3979-Necesario-legislar-sobre-plantas-sagradas-son-patrimonio-nacional-Nava-Palacios (accessed on 24 August 2020).
146. Rodríguez, R.G.; Morales, M.E.; Verde, M.J.; Oranday, A.; Rivas, C.; Núñez, M.A.; González, G.M.; Treviño, J.F. Actividad antibacteriana y antifúngica de las especies *Ariocarpus kotschoubeyanus* (Lemaire) y *Ariocarpus retusus* (Scheidweiler) (Cactaceae). *Rev. Mex. Cienc. Farm.* **2010**, *41*, 55–59.
147. Singh, S.; Verma, M.; Malhotra, M.; Prakash, S.; Singh, T.D. Cytotoxicity of alkaloids isolated from *Argemone mexicana* on SW480 human colon cancer cell line. *Pharm. Biol.* **2016**, *54*, 740–745. [CrossRef]
148. Reingardiene, D.; Vilcinskaite, J.; Lazauskas, R. Haliucinogeniniai grybai [Hallucinogenic mushrooms]. *Medicina* **2005**, *41*, 1067–1070.
149. Mandujano, M.C.; Gulovob, J.; Reyes, J. Lo que usted siempre quiso saber sobre las cactaceas y nunca se atrevio a preguntar. CONABIO. *Biodiversitas* **2002**, *40*, 4–7.
150. Berkov, S. Alkaloids of *Datura ceratocaula*. *Z. Naturforsch. C. J. Biosci.* **2003**, *58*, 455–458. [CrossRef]
151. Malinowska, I.; Studziński, M.; Niezabitowska, K.; Gadzikowska, M. Comparison of TLC and Different Micro TLC Techniques in Analysis of Tropane Alkaloids and Their Derivatives Mixture from *Datura inoxia* Mill. Extract. *Chromatographia* **2013**, *76*, 1327–1332. [CrossRef]
152. Ferrigni, N.R.; Nichols, D.E.; McLaughlin, J.L.; Bye, R.A. Cactus alkaloids. XLVII. N alpha-dimethylhistamine, a hypotensive component of *Echinocereus triglochidiatus*. *J. Ethnopharmacol.* **1982**, *5*, 359–364. [CrossRef]
153. Štarha, R. Alkaloids of *Epithelantha micromeris*. *Fitoterapia* **1995**, *66*, 375.
154. Garín-Aguilar, M.E.; Luna, J.E.; Soto-Hernández, M.; Valencia del Toro, G.; Vázquez, M.M. Effect of crude extracts of *Erythrina americana* Mill. on aggressive behavior in rats. *J. Ethnopharmacol.* **2000**, *69*, 189–196. [CrossRef]
155. Rumalla, C.S.; Jadhav, A.N.; Smillie, T.; Fronczek, F.R.; Khan, I.A. Alkaloids from *Heimia salicifolia*. *Phytochemistry* **2008**, *69*, 1756–1762. [CrossRef]
156. Steiner, U.; Leistner, E. Ergot Alkaloids and their Hallucinogenic Potential in Morning Glories. *Planta Med.* **2018**, *84*, 751–758. [CrossRef]
157. Cassels, B.K.; Sáez-Briones, P. Dark Classics in Chemical Neuroscience: Mescaline. *ACS Chem. Neurosci.* **2018**, *9*, 2448–2458. [CrossRef]
158. Schultes, R.; Farnsworth, N. Ethnomedical, botanical and phytochemical aspects of natural hallucinogens. In *Botanical Museum Leaflets*; Harvard University: Cambridge, MA, USA, 1980; Volume 28, pp. 123–214.
159. Strömbom, J.; Bruhn, J.G. Alkaloids of *Pachycereus pecten*-aboriginum, a Mexican cactus of ethnopharmacologic interest. *Acta Pharm. Suec.* **1978**, *15*, 127–132.
160. Mahmood, Z.A. Bioactive Alkaloids from Fungi: Psilocybin. In *Natural Products*; Ramawat, K., Mérillon, J.M., Eds.; Springer: Berlin/Heidelberg, Germany, 2013. [CrossRef]

161. Qu, J.; Hu, Y.C.; Li, J.B.; Wang, Y.H.; Zhang, J.L.; Abliz, Z.; Yu, S.S.; Liu, Y.B. Structural characterization of constituents with molecular diversity in fractions from *Lysidice brevicalyx* by liquid chromatography/diode-array detection/electrospray ionization tandem mass spectrometry and liquid chromatography/nuclear magnetic resonance. *Rapid Commun. Mass Spectrom.* **2008**, *22*, 755–765. [CrossRef]
162. Izaddoost, M.; Harris, B.G.; Gracy, R.W. Structure and toxicity of alkaloids and amino acids of *Sophora secundiflora*. *J. Pharm. Sci.* **1976**, *65*, 352–354. [CrossRef]
163. Bogusz, M.J.; Maier, R.D.; Schäfer, A.T.; Erkens, M. Honey with *Psilocybe mushrooms*: A revival of a very old preparation on the drug market? *Int. J. Legal Med.* **1998**, *111*, 147–150. [CrossRef]
164. Salvaña, F.R. Morphological and Histochemical Characterization of Callus from Leaf Explant of *Tagetes lucida* Cav. (Asteraceae). *JNBR* **2019**, *8*, 172–178.
165. Esquivel-Gutiérrez, E.R.; Alcaraz-Meléndez, L.; Hernández-Herrera, R.; Torres, A.; Rodríguez-Jaramillo, C. Effects of damiana (*Turnera diffusa*; var. diffusa and var. aphrodisiaca) on diabetic rats. *Acta Univ.* **2018**, *28*, 84–92. [CrossRef]
166. Dayton, W.A. *Important Western Browse Plants*; Miscellaneous Publication, 101; U.S. Department of Agriculture: Washington, DC, USA, 1931; Volume 214, p. 768.

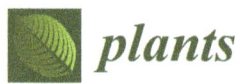 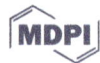

Article

Bauhinia forficata Link, Antioxidant, Genoprotective, and Hypoglycemic Activity in a Murine Model

Erika Anayetzi Chávez-Bustos [1], Angel Morales-González [2], Liliana Anguiano-Robledo [3], Eduardo Osiris Madrigal-Santillán [4], Cármen Valadez-Vega [5], Olivia Lugo-Magaña [6], Jorge Alberto Mendoza-Pérez [7] and Tomás Alejandro Fregoso-Aguilar [1,*]

[1] Escuela Nacional de Ciencias Biológicas, Instituto Politécnico Nacional, Department de Fisiología. Av., Wilfrido Massieu S/N, Col. Nueva Industrial Vallejo, Alcaldía Gustavo A. Madero, Ciudad de México C.P. 07700, Mexico
[2] Escuela Superior de Cómputo, Instituto Politécnico Nacional, Av. Juan de Dios Bátiz S/N Esquina Miguel Othón de Mendizabal, Unidad Profesional Adolfo López Mateos, Ciudad de México C.P. 07738, Mexico
[3] Escuela Superior de Medicina, Laboratorio de Farmacología Molecular, Instituto Politécnico Nacional, Alcaldía Miguel Hidalgo, Ciudad de México C.P. 11340, Mexico
[4] Laboratorio de Medicina de Conservación, Escuela Superior de Medicina, Instituto Politécnico Nacional, México, Plan de San Luis y Díaz Mirón, Col. Casco de Santo Tomás, Alcaldía. Miguel Hidalgo, Ciudad de México C.P. 11340, Mexico
[5] Área Académica de Medicina, Instituto de Ciencias de la Salud, Universidad Autónoma del Estado de Hidalgo, Ex-Hacienda de la Concepción, Tilcuautla, San Agustín Tlaxiaca C.P. 42080, Mexico
[6] Preparatoria Número 1, Universidad Autónoma del Estado de Hidalgo, Av. Benito Juárez S/N, Constitución, Pachuca de Soto C.P. 42060, Mexico
[7] Escuela Nacional de Ciencias Biológicas, Instituto Politécnico Nacional, Department de Ingeniería en Sistemas Ambientales. Av., Wilfrido Massieu S/N, Col. Nueva Industrial Vallejo, Alcaldía Gustavo A. Madero, Ciudad de México C.P. 07700, Mexico
* Correspondence: tfregoso@ipn.mx

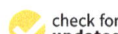

Abstract: *Bauhinia forficata* L. is a tree used in alternative medicine as an anti-diabetic agent, with little scientific information about its pharmacological properties. The hypoglycemic, antioxidant, and genoprotective activities of a methanolic extract of *B. forficata* leaves and stems combined were investigated in mice treated with streptozotocin (STZ). Secondary metabolites were determined by qualitative phytochemistry. In vitro antioxidant activity was determined by the DPPH method at four concentrations of the extract. The genoprotective activity was evaluated in 3 groups of mice: control, anthracene (10 mg/kg), and anthracene + *B. forficata* (500 mg/kg) and the presence of micronuclei in peripheral blood was measured for 2 weeks. To determine the hypoglycemic activity, the crude extract was prepared in a suspension and administered (500 mg/kg, i.g.) in previously diabetic mice with STZ (120 mg/kg, i.p.), measuring blood glucose levels every week as well as the animals' body weight for six weeks. The extract showed good antioxidant activity and caused a decrease in the number of micronuclei. The diabetic mice + *B. forficata* presented hypoglycemic effects in the third week of treatment, perhaps due to its secondary metabolites. Therefore, *B. forficata* is a candidate for continued use at the ethnomedical level as an adjuvant to allopathic therapy.

Keywords: *Bahuinia forficata*; diabetes; antioxidant; hypoglycemic activity; mice

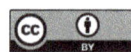

1. Introduction

According to the International Diabetes Federation, currently 537 million persons suffer from diabetes, which corresponds to 10.5% of the world's population, and it is expected that by the year 2030, there will be 643 million, and by 2045, there will be 783 million patients with diabetes [1]. On the other hand, in Mexico in 2021, 14.1 million patients were diagnosed, ranking 7th worldwide. It is expected that by 2045, this amount will increase to 21.1 million [1]. Likewise, in the National Survey of Health and Nutrition in Mexico (ENSANUT) it was

Citation: Chávez-Bustos, E.A.; Morales-González, A.; Anguiano-Robledo, L.; Madrigal-Santillán, E.O.; Valadez-Vega, C.; Lugo-Magaña, O.; Mendoza-Pérez, J.A.; Fregoso-Aguilar, T.A. *Bauhinia forficata* Link, Antioxidant, Genoprotective, and Hypoglycemic Activity in a Murine Model. *Plants* 2022, 11, 3052. https://doi.org/10.3390/plants11223052

Academic Editor: Corina Danciu

Received: 4 October 2022
Accepted: 8 November 2022
Published: 11 November 2022

Publisher's Note: MDPI stays neutral with regard to jurisdictional claims in published maps and institutional affiliations.

Copyright: © 2022 by the authors. Licensee MDPI, Basel, Switzerland. This article is an open access article distributed under the terms and conditions of the Creative Commons Attribution (CC BY) license (https://creativecommons.org/licenses/by/4.0/).

found that in 2018, the population with diabetes was 16.8%, while by 2020 it had increased to 15.7% [2,3]. For these reasons, it is clear that this chronic-degenerative disease (CDD) is a global health problem that has worsened with the arrival of the COVID-19 pandemic, as it was found that patients with COVID-19 who were hospitalized and had a diabetic comorbidity accounted for between 17 and 30% of all admissions to health centers around the world during 2020–2021 [4]. As an example of the latter, in a study conducted with patients hospitalized for COVID-19 in 2020 in Mexico, from a sample of 89, 756 patients, 17.5% also suffered from diabetes [5]. If we add to all of the latter the fact that Mexico is among the developing countries, with a high percentage of the population living in poverty, it is clearly understood that many of these low-income persons make use of alternative treatments for diabetes [6].

In México, herbalism has been employed since pre-colonial times to treat all types of diseases, including chronic degenerative diseases (CDD) such as diabetes [7,8]. In this regard, species such as nopal (*Opuntia* spp.) are widely utilized to lower blood glucose levels [9,10]. It has been found that, among the secondary metabolites contained in this plant, we find ascorbic acid, flavonoids, and phenolic acids [9] such as catechol, cinnamic acid, and 3-phenylpropionic acid, among others [11]. Another example is represented by the leaves of the Neem tree, which contain quercetin-3-O-glucoside, quercetin-3-O-rutinoside, and rutin derivatives, azadirachtin, and nimbidiol, among others [12,13]. Thus, there are many examples of plants that are used in México to treat diabetes [14], many of these originating in this country and others brought from other countries. In this regard, in some regions of Mexico, such as the state of Nuevo León and the capital Mexico City, the leaves of the plant *Bahuinia forficata* Link (Cow's paw) are used to treat diabetes [15]. This species is thought to be an evergreen tree native to Asia or South America; it is a tree in the Fabaceae family and the tribe Cercideae, whose leaves are petiolate in the shape of a heart at their base and resemble the hoofprints left by cattle [15,16]. In various communities, therapeutic properties are attributed to it, such as diuretic, healing, antiseptic, astringent, and hypoglycemic [15]. However, although there are some publications on its different pharmacological and foraging properties [17], there are few recent studies, to our knowledge, on the therapeutic properties of this tree in Mexico. Studies have reported its anti-cancer properties [18] and its use for the treatment of infections, pain, inflammation, microbial diseases, malaria, etc., all of which are likely due to its content of secondary metabolites such as flavonoids [19]. It has also been found effective for treating cardiovascular disorders (CVD) [20] and CDD such as diabetes [21,22]. In this regard, we consider that by testing the hypoglycemic properties of this species, this could be added to the therapeutic properties mentioned above and could make this plant a multifunctional tool in the field of traditional and allopathic medicine.

Considering all of the above and the knowledge that one of the main signs of diabetes is hyperglycemia [1], this work aimed to conduct a series of experiments to determine whether *Bahuinia forficata* Link possesses antioxidant, genoprotective, and hypoglycemic properties in a murine model of chemical diabetes. For this, albino Swiss mice were chosen because of their size, which is suitable for experimental manipulation compared to other larger models (e.g., non-human primates), their short life cycle, and their adaptability to laboratory conditions.

2. Results
2.1. Qualitative Phytochemical Analysis

Thirty-one chemical reactions were carried out to identify the main secondary metabolites of the methanolic extract of the leaves of *B. forficata* Link. Table 1 summarizes the chemical reactions in which a positive result was observed for the presence of secondary metabolites in the extract.

Table 1. Secondary metabolites detected by qualitative phytochemistry in the dry extract of the combination of leaves and stems of *Bahuinia forficata*.

Secondary Metabolite	Test
Alkaloids	Dragendorff
	Sonnenschain
	Wagner
Flavonoids	Shinoda (Flavones)
	10% sodium hydroxide (Flavonols)
Saponins	Liebermann Buchard (triterpenoids)
	Rosenthaler (triterpenoids)
Quinones	Ammonium hydroxide (Anthraquinones)
	Börntraguer (Anthraquinones)
Reducing sugars	Fehling
	Benedict
Tannins	1% ferric chloride (Phenolic compounds)

2.2. Spectroscopic Analysis

Figure 1 depicts the spectrum obtained by means of a Fourier-transform infrared spectroscopy (FTIR) analysis. At the wavelength 630–735 cm^{-1}, a vibration of C-H CIS bonds was located, and at the wavelength close to 1638 cm^{-1}, the carbonyl functional group was located. Between 2800 and 2900 cm^{-1}, C-C-H bonds were detected, and in 3295 cm^{-1}, evidence of the functional carboxyl group or perhaps that of the bridged hydroxyl was found.

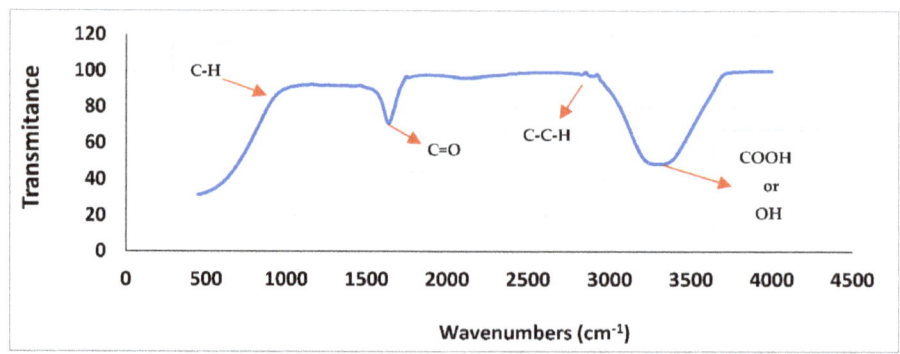

Figure 1. The spectrum obtained through Fourier-transform infrared (FTIR) analysis of the methanolic extract of *Bahuinia forficata* leaves and stems.

Several aliquots of *B. forficata* extract were taken where there was greater detection of functional groups to be subjected to other spectroscopic tests. Figure 2 presents the spectrum obtained with HPLC coupled to mass spectroscopy, where the main peak with a higher area (retention time of 3.805 min) is associated with a higher concentration of glycoside-type compounds (red circle) detected. Different reference evidence from previously published works confirms this result [23].

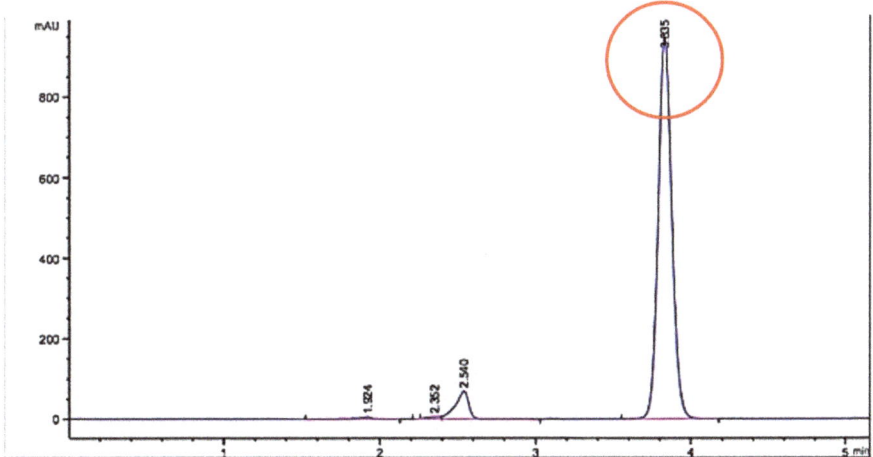

Figure 2. Spectrum obtained with coupled HPLC-mass spectroscopy from some aliquots of the *Bahuinia forficata* extract. Red circle denotes the retention time of 3.805 min corresponding to glycoside-type compounds.

In several of these aliquots, when subjected to the additional HPLC-MS technique, mass peaks detected have a corresponding peak in 95% of the samples, with a flavonoid similar to kaempferol bonded with one or two glucose or arabinoside units, so the mass fragments observed of 286 m/z, 466 m/z, and 576 m/z are closely related to kaempferol derivatives such as kaempferol-3-O-arabinoside, astragalin, and kaempferitrin (Figure 3).

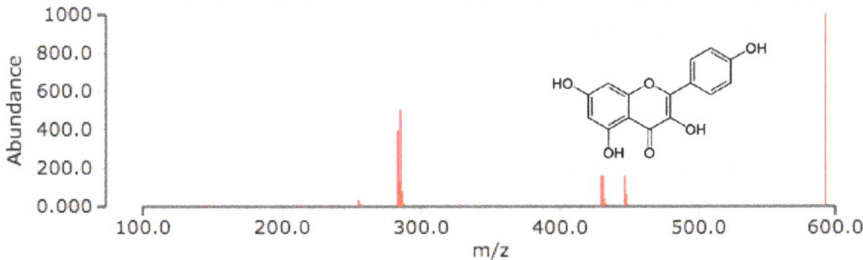

Figure 3. The spectrum obtained with HPLC showing the zone of the functional groups that may correspond to secondary metabolites derivatives of kaempferol.

2.3. Evaluation of In-Vitro Antioxidant Activity

Figure 4 summarizes the antioxidant activity of the four concentrations of *B. forficata* tested by the in vitro DPPH method, where the percentage of inhibition of the presence of DPPH by the extract was evaluated. Ascorbic acid (2%) was employed as the reference standard, and it reached its maximal inhibition in the presence of DPPH (90.84%) when 15 min of the reaction had elapsed. The first three concentrations (50, 25, and 12.5 mg/mL) presented about 80% inhibition in the presence of DPPH in the first 5 min of the reaction and remained stable, with slight decreases at the end of the reaction (78.78%). Paradoxically, the lowest concentration (6.25 mg/mL) exhibited an inhibition in the presence of DPPH of less than 50% during the first 5 min of the reaction. Notwithstanding this, it achieved the highest percentage of inhibition (88%) within 10 min of the reaction, remaining at that level throughout the rest of the measurement time.

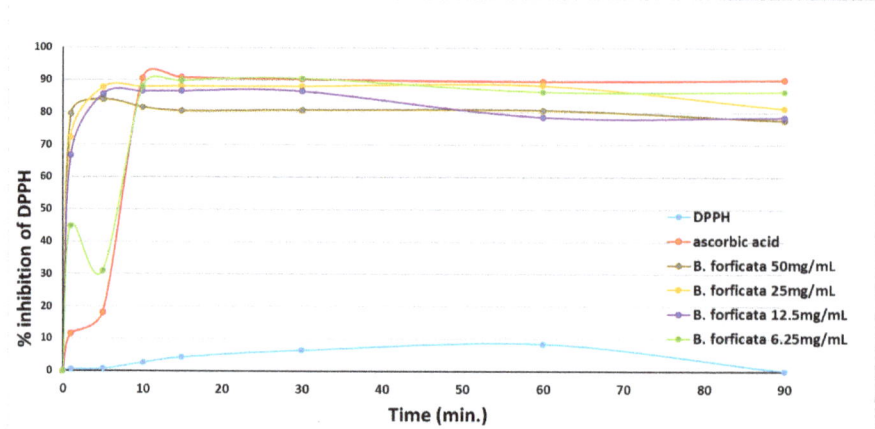

Figure 4. Percentage of inhibition in the presence of DPPH of four concentrations of *B. forficata* during 90 min of the reaction. Each point represents the average of two absorbance measurements (517 nm) substituted in Equation (1), as described in the methodology.

2.4. Assessment of Genoprotective Activity

Figure 5 presents the number of micronuclei in mouse peripheral blood over a period of 2 weeks, the first with the administration of anthracene and/or *B. forficata* extract (500 mg/kg), and the second without the administration of treatment. Anthracene was used because it is a mutagenic agent with a low mortality risk when used in low doses and for a short period of time. The group of mice administered anthracene (10 mg/kg) had the highest number of micronuclei on day 3 of administration, and that number decreased slightly when the mutagenic agent was no longer administered. On the other hand, animals administered with anthracene plus *B. forficata* extract had a significantly lower number of micronuclei on days 2 and 3 of the administration (19 micronuclei; $p < 0.05$; two-way repeated measures ANOVA), and when the treatment was no longer administered in week 2, that number continued to decrease significantly (two micronuclei).

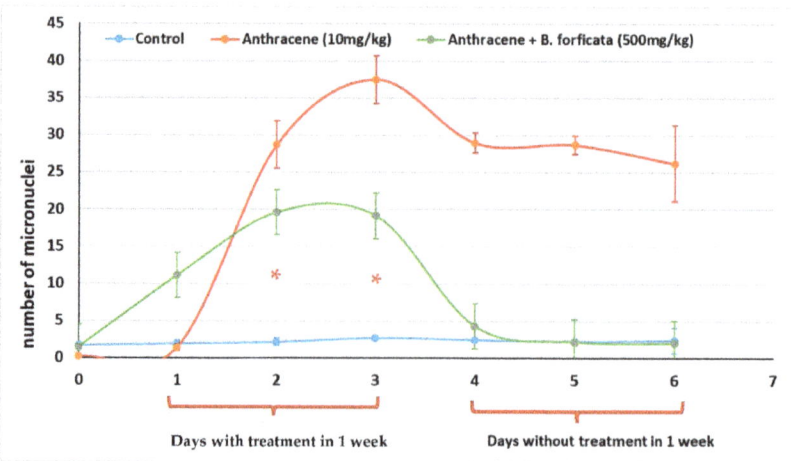

Figure 5. Genoprotective activity measured as the number of micronuclei in peripheral mouse blood. Data is expressed as mean ± standard error of the mean (SEM). * denotes a $p < 0.05$; comparison of anthracene + *B. forficata* vs. anthracene as determined by a two-way repeated measures ANOVA.

2.5. Assessment of Hypoglycemic Activity

Because during diabetic states a loss in body weight can also occur, in this experiment, the body weight of the mice was also measured weekly during the 36-day treatment. Figure 6 shows changes in the body weight of the mice under different treatments. Diabetic mice administered with *B. forficata* prevented weight loss caused by Streptozocin administration in weeks 5 and 6 of treatment ($p < 0.05$ with a two-way repeated measures ANOVA) and, although the animals in that group had a lower weight than the controls, this was not significant ($p > 0.05$).

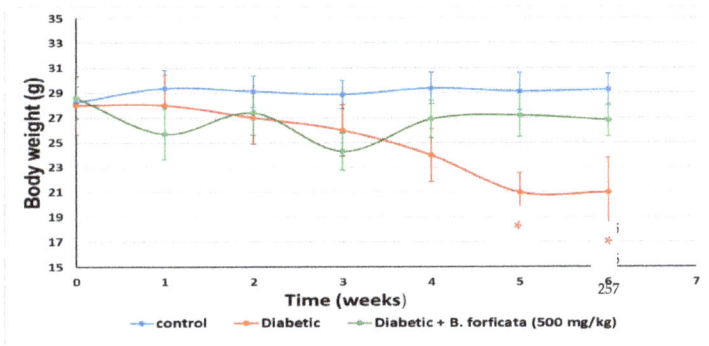

Figure 6. Changes in the body weight of mice under different treatments for 36 days (6 weeks). Data is expressed as mean ± SEM. * denotes a $p < 0.05$; comparison of diabetic + *B. forficata* vs. diabetic and control groups as determined by a two-way repeated measures ANOVA.

Figure 7 shows changes in the blood glucose values of mice under different treatments. Statistical analysis found significant differences among treatments ($p < 0.001$; two-way repeated measures ANOVA), between weeks and measurements ($p < 0.001$), as well as a significant interaction between the treatment factor and the weeks of measurement ($p < 0.001$). Overall, the administration of *B. forficata* extract to diabetic mice significantly decreased blood glucose levels from week 2 of treatment ($p < 0.05$, the post-hoc multiple comparisons test of Student–Newman–Keuls). It is noteworthy that in week 3 of treatment, the animals' glucose levels were equal to those of the control group, and although they rose again later, this increase was significantly lower ($p < 0.05$) than that observed in the diabetic group.

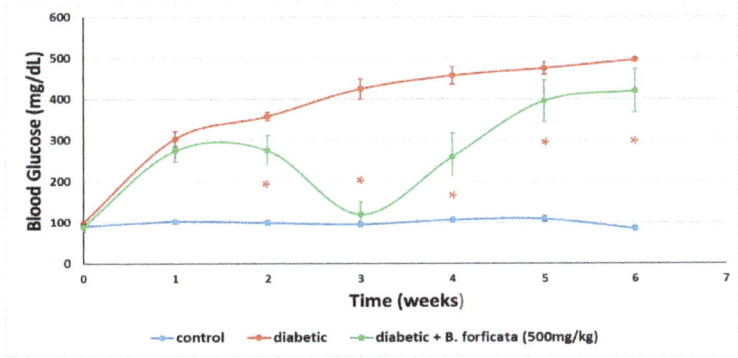

Figure 7. Glucose levels recorded in mice under different treatments for 36 days (6 weeks). Data is expressed as mean ± SEM. * denotes a $p < 0.05$; comparison of diabetic + *B. forficata* vs. diabetic as determined by a two-way repeated measures ANOVA.

3. Discussion

The presence of flavonoids, saponins, and tannins, among other secondary metabolites, in the methanolic extract of *Bahuinia forficata* Link leaves could aid in explaining the effects found in this work, considering that these polar compounds possess many pharmacological properties that may be in opposition to the mechanism of action of the diabetogenic agent used, streptozotocin (STZ). Several mechanisms of action for streptozotocin have been described, including DNA methylation, the activation of poly ADP-ribosylation that causes NAD^+ and ATP depletion, the formation of free radicals, and the release of nitric oxide, all of which contribute to the death of pancreatic beta cells [24,25]. In addition, STZ has been found to inhibit the enzyme O-GlcNAcase (N-acetyl-β-D-glucosaminidase), increasing the O-glycosylation of the B-cells and their death. This in turn decreases insulin concentrations and causes hyperglycemia [26].

In this work, qualitative phytochemistry was employed as a primary tool that, although it does not establish the amount of secondary metabolites present in an extract, can provide an indication of which of those metabolites are present [27].

In this regard, the information obtained with qualitative phytochemistry was complemented with three spectroscopic analyses, including infrared with Fourier transform, GC-MS, and HPLC, finding that the most abundant secondary metabolite in the methanolic extract of *B. forficata* was a flavonoid very similar to kaempferol; however, perhaps the other metabolites detected qualitatively also contributed to the effects found in this work. Several of the secondary metabolites detected qualitatively in this work have been studied separately by different authors and share different mechanisms of action that could oppose the mechanism of action of STZ and therefore the onset and development of diabetes. For example, Ajebli et al. conducted a review of natural alkaloids and mentioned that these have a therapeutic effect on the treatment of diabetes through actions such as the blockade of protein tyrosine phosfatase 1B and the deactivation of dipeptydil peptidase-IV, increasing insulin sensitivity, modulating oxidative stress, and the inhibition of the enzyme α-glucosidase [28–31]. As for triterpenoids, it has been reported that these can be intermediates in phytosteroid synthesis and, in addition, it has been proposed that several of their biological effects, such as the inhibition of feeding, are due to the presence of hydroxyl groups [32]. Quinones (anthraquinones) have been linked to anticancer properties [33], inhibiting the activity of the enzyme P450 [34], with anti-inflammatory and antioxidant properties, among others, being the entire structure of the molecule plus the alizarin-type substituents responsible for this latter property [35]. Moreover, phenolic compounds and flavonoids have been reported to possess antioxidant properties and the ability to inhibit acetylcholinesterase and alpha-glucosidases [36], which are important features for explaining the results of this work. Prior studies had already mentioned that *B. forficata* has hypoglycemic, antioxidant, and diuretic effects, among others [19,37], and several of these studies also reported that a secondary metabolite of the flavonoid type, such as kaempferol, is abundant in the leaves of this species [38]. The latter was confirmed in this work when the HPLC analysis of our extract was performed. Several studies have found that kaempferol is also involved in the anticancer, anti-inflammatory, and anti-diabetic properties of many plants [39,40]. All of this serves as a basis for affirming that metabolites detected in the methanolic extract of *B. forficata* leaves oppose the mechanisms of action of streptozotocin, which was the agent used in our chemical model of diabetes. The four concentrations employed for the evaluation of antioxidant activity in vitro presented a high percentage in their inhibitory effect in terms of the presence of the DPPH radical during the 90 min that the reaction lasted, including the lowest concentration of the extract (6.25 mg/mL), which presented this effect after 5 min of starting the reaction. In all cases, this percentage was higher than that presented by the reference standard (ascorbic acid); thus, the extract was able to donate electrons (or donate hydrogen ions) to stabilize the last electron-deficient orbit in the DPPH, thus transforming it into its reduced form (DPPH-H). This experiment was performed in vitro, but the results can be scaled to what occurs in the chemical model of diabetes, where the STZ gave rise to the generation of free radicals such as the hydroxyl radical and peroxinitrites that, in excess, cause oxidative stress [22], which in turn causes damage to the DNA of the pancreatic beta cells of mice and therefore the death of those cells. It should be noted that in this work, the antioxidant activity of all concentrations utilized exceeded 80%, something similar to that found in another study, where the extract reached 75% of antioxidant activity with the same in vitro test [41]. It is important to note that this plant possesses great antioxidant activity that, as already mentioned, may be mediated by the presence of metabolites such as tannins, quinones, and flavonoids like kaempferol, since this property would oppose the oxidative stress that would be caused during the course of diabetes. In fact, one study found that *B. forficata* decreased hepatic oxidative stress in rats treated with bisphenol, decreasing malondialdehyde levels and increasing catalase activity [42]. For the evaluation of the genoprotective activity by the micronucleus technique in mouse peripheral blood, anthracene was used instead of streptozotocin because several studies employed this type of mutagenic agent in genotoxicity tests [43–45]. Anthracene is a mutagenic agent with low carcinogenic capacity [44], and its application in this work attempted to resemble the action of STZ on the DNA of pancreatic beta cells by methylating the DNA of these cells and causing their death. In the case of anthracene, alterations in the mitotic process would be caused, and consequently, the mature erythrocytes would preserve the remains of the genetic material in the form of micronuclei. In this experiment, it was found that the extract of *B. forficata* significantly decreased the number of micronuclei in the peripheral blood erythrocytes of mice compared to animals treated only with the mutagenic agent, an indication that the secondary metabolites of the extract of this species avoided the alterations of the genetic material caused by anthracene and perhaps also counteracted the methylization action of the STZ pancreatic-beta cells in the chemical model of diabetes. In other words, the extract of *B. forficata* did indeed exhibit genoprotective activity. This would agree with works in which anthracene has been used to evaluate genotoxicity [46] and with other studies in which variants of this technique have also been utilized to explore the genoprotective activity of *B. forficata*. For example, in 2013, a study was conducted in rats to determine chromosomal aberrations, and it was found that *B. forficata* did not present cytotoxic effects (mutagenicity) on the chromosomes of the bone marrow cells at a concentration of 4.65 g/L and even presented a significant antioxidant effect, all attributable to the presence of secondary metabolites such as kaempferol [47]. In another study, 7,12-dimethylbenz[a]anthracene (30 mg/kg) was utilized as a mutagenic agent, and the authors also found an elevation in the number of micronuclei in golden Syrian hamster erythrocytes [48]. It is important to note that, in the present work, the methanolic extract of *B. forficata* was employed in all experiments, and that there are studies that used the ethanolic extract and also reported antioxidant and antimutagenic effects, but it was also found that the ethereal extract does indeed possess genotoxic activity [49], leading us to consider that more and further studies still need to be conducted to clearly determine the genoprotective activity of this species. It is proposed herein that the methanolic extract had genoprotective activity of long duration in that it decreased the number of micronuclei in the erythrocytes of mice treated with anthracene both during the week of treatment as well as during the week in which the mutagenic agent was no longer administered.

In this work, two of the main signs of diabetes were reproduced: weight loss and hyperglycemia. Both in our chemical model of STZ and in diabetes, weight loss is due to the fact that when beta-pancreatic cells die, there is insufficient production of insulin to capture glucose in the different tissues and maintain homeostasis. This gives rise to the fact that the tissues use other sources of energy, such as fats and proteins, resulting in a loss of body mass and thereby the weight loss that is observed in this CDD [50–52]. In this respect, the *B. forficata* extract gave rise to oscillations in the body weight of diabetic mice, but such levels were maintained and were similar to those of the control group; they also had a protective effect against weight loss caused by the administration of STZ. The latter was also observed in another study, where the *Bauhinia variegata* extract was employed at doses ranging from 100–1000 mg/kg in type 1 and type 2 STZ-induced models of diabetes in rats [53]. The dose of *B. forficata* extract used in this work was 500 mg/kg, and it caused a maximal hypoglycemic effect during week 3 of treatment. Although this latter effect apparently began to fade from week 4, the glucose levels of the animals administered with the extract were always below those of the diabetic animals. This leads us to think that if a higher dose (e.g., 1000 mg/kg) had been used, the hypoglycemic effect would have lasted longer. Considering everything that has been commented on so far, we propose that the extract of *B. forficata* prevented the development of the mechanisms of action of the STZ. That is, the presence of secondary metabolites such as tannins and saponins, and especially those of the flavonoid type such as kaempferol, prevented the formation of free radicals (antioxidant activity), prevented DNA damage (genoprotective effect), and exerted a hypoglycemic and antihyperglycemic effect. In this regard, the hypoglycemic effect could also be due to the ability of the metabolites described to optimize the use and uptake of glucose by tissues other than hepatic and muscle cells, optimizing the activity of some enzymes involved in the metabolic pathways of glucose management. In this respect, there are relatively recent studies that propose mechanisms of action of *B. forficata* extract to explain the effects found in our study [22,54–56]. For example, a 2012 review conducted in Brazil with several species including *B. forficata* notes that tannins and flavonoids are responsible for antioxidant effects and that this justifies their use in the treatment of diabetes [57].

It is possible that the effects found with the administration of the *B. forficata* extract may be mediated by the combined mechanisms of action of the different secondary metabolites that were detected in the samples. It could be thought that, in the procedure for obtaining the crude extract, the properties of each identified metabolite could be modified; however, there are studies indicating that the processes of obtaining and drying the extract that are similar to those used in this study in *B. forficata* do not alter the properties of metabolites such as flavonoids (e.g., quercetin and kaempferol). In addition, when the authors administered that extract at a dose of 200 mg/kg iv to Wistar rats, they observed decreases of between 46.42 and 48.17% in glucose levels after the day of administration [21]. Additionally, returning again to kaempferol, there is evidence that this metabolite decreases insulin resistance through the downregulation of IκBα and the inhibition of NF-κB pathway activation [58,59]. This supports the notion that metabolites from the dry extract of *B. forficata* also exert an influence on the expression of certain metabolic pathways that may be involved in diabetes. Furthermore, as another study points out, the dry extract of the leaves of *Bauhinia holophylla* (400 mg/kg) presented hypoglycemic activity through the inhibition of glycogen synthase kinase 3-beta and an activation in glycogenesis in mice treated with STZ [60].

Taking into account all of the previously mentioned information, we support the idea of using the *B. forficata* extract in the treatment of diseases such as diabetes in countries such as México, where a high percentage of the population makes use of herbalism. In fact, in other South American countries, the commercialization of this species in naturist preparations is already being promoted, and there are already several patents for this purpose [61]. In addition, although in several of the studies the authors used it in models of type 2 diabetes, we think it could be utilized to treat diabetes in general, as indicated by another, more recent study, in which the authors used capsules of *B. forficata* extract and found that the manner of preparing and administering the extract did not affect the therapeutic properties of the secondary metabolites [62]. In addition, after it was administered every 2 days (as it was in this work) for 3 months (herein, we administered it for 1 month and a half) to 25 volunteer patients, significant decreases in triglyceride and cholesterol levels were found [63].

4. Materials and Methods

4.1. Acquisition of the Plant Species and Processing in the Laboratory

The leaves and stems of *Bahuina forficata* Link were obtained from a legally accredited business located in the state of Nuevo León, México, and were taken to the Hormones and Behavior Laboratory of the Department of Physiology of the National School of Biological

Sciences to complete their environmental drying for 1 week. The material (both leaves and stems) was then crushed and macerated in methanol for 1 week. The macerate was subjected to reduced pressure distillation (Rotavaporator Prendo© Model 1750, Prendo, Puebla, México) to remove the methanol; the distillate was left to air dry for 1 week to obtain the dry crude extract of leaves and stems combined.

Solubility tests were performed to select the solvent to make a stock suspension of this crude extract at 50 mg/mL, and it was found that the best solvent to resuspend the crude extract for intragastric administration in mice was distilled water.

4.2. Chemicals Used in the Experiments

The chemicals 2,2-diphenyl-1-picrylhydrazyl (DPPH) and streptozocin (STZ) were purchased from Sigma-Aldrich. Giemsa dye was purchased from Hycel (México). Methanol was purchased from Golden Bell Co. (Mexico City, México).

4.3. Animals in Laboratory Settings

In this study, male Swiss albino mice (weighing 25–30 g each) of the NIH strain were used. They were obtained from the official supplier of the National School of Biological Sciences (ENCB) of the National Polytechnic Institute and housed in the animal chamber of the Department of Physiology of the ENCB, Zacatenco campus for acclimatization in communal acrylic cages (48 cm long × 22 cm wide × 20 cm high), with water and food *ad libitum* and a light-dark cycle of 12:00 (lights turning on at 08:00), as well as a room temperature of 22 ± 2 °C and under standard humidity conditions. The animals were handled and subjected to experimentation according to Mexican standards (NOM-033-ZOO-1995, NOM-062-ZOO-1999, NOM-087-ECOL-1995) and the international bioethics standards currently in force.

4.4. Qualitative Phytochemical Analysis

Samples of the crude extract of the leaves and stems of *B. forficata* were taken and subjected to the various qualitative chemical reactions described in other works [64,65] to determine secondary metabolites, mainly of a polar nature, which were identified by changes in coloration, the formation of precipitates, foaming, etc.

4.5. Spectroscopic Analysis

Fractions of the dry extract of *B. forficata* were taken and stored in vials for a series of general spectroscopic analyses. The samples were analyzed at the Center for Nanosciences and Micro and Nanotechnologies of the National Polytechnic Institute (Mexico City, México). For the analysis of high-performance liquid chromatography (HPLC), an Agilent model 1260 Infinity II device with a variable UV-Vis wavelength detector and a wavelength range of 190 to 600 nm was employed. Also, it is coupled to an Agilent mass spectrometer. Parameter conditions used were: Mobile phase, 50% Water, 50% MeOH, and 1% FA; a flow rate of 0.4–0.5 mL/min; a stop time of 25 min; a needle wash mode and standard wash injection volume of 5 µL; a column temperature of 30 °C; UV detection at 280 nm/4 nm; Ref.: OFF > 0.025 min (0.5 s response time) (10 Hz); an MS detection acquisition mode at MS1; a minimum range of 100 m/z and a maximum range of 7000 m/z; an ion polarity at positive source parameters; a gas temperature of 290 °C; a gas flow rate of 14 L/min; a nebulizer set at 20 psig; a sheath gas temperature of 400 °C; a sheath gas flow rate of 12 L/min; scan source parameters at a Vcap of 5000, V Nozzle voltage of 2000 V, fragmentor of 500 V, skimmer of 10, octopole RF peak of 750; and reference masses of 922.0098 and 1821.9523 T.

Thirty µL of sample was injected into an Agilent ZORBAX Rx-SIL, 100 × 3.0 mm, 1.8 µm column, with a flow rate of 0.4 mL/min and a mixture of 50% methanol and 50% water. A scanning spectrum with an UV-Vis Agilent 8453 spectrophotometer was obtained for the crude extracts in order to establish the absorption wavelength to be used for the HPLC variable wavelength detector, which correspond with the higher absorption peaks observed, and also to give brief information about the concentration of the compounds mixed in the crude extract. Overall, the determined concentrations of analytes ranged from 0.0530 mg/mL–0.0002 mg/mL (before dilution). In addition to the lengths of 270 and 560 nm, a wavelength of 214 nm was also utilized to verify the presence of hypsochromic shift changes due to compounds with chromophore effects.

For the Fourier transform infrared analysis (FTIR) technique, an Espertoi Lambda Series 5000 device was used.

4.6. Evaluation of In Vitro Antioxidant Activity

Four concentrations of the crude extract of *B. forficata* (50, 25, 21.5, and 6.25 mg/mL) were prepared in methanol to determine its antioxidant activity using the in vitro method of DPPH (2,2-diphenyl-1-picrylhydrazyl). A solution of 0.01 g of DPPH in 25 mL of methanol was prepared.

This method was performed on a UV-VIS spectrophotometer (Velab©; VE-5100UV, Velaquin, México city, México); quartz cells containing 1850 µL of methanol, 140 µL of DPPH free radical, and 10 µL of some of the concentrations of the crude extract diluted in methanol were prepared, and absorbance was measured at 517 nm of each solution. The absorbance value was recorded at 0 (without extract sample) and at 1, 5, 15, 20, 30, 60, and 90 min. These readings were taken in duplicate for each time, and the average value of each absorbance was substituted in Equation (1) to calculate the % of inhibition in the presence of DPPH.

$$\% \text{ DPPH inhibition} = (Absm_{t=0} - Absm_{t=n}/Absm_{t=0}) \times 100 \quad (1)$$

where: $Absm_{t=0}$ = sample absorbance at zero time (without extract). $Absm_{t=n}$ = sample absorbance at "n" time (with extract).

The percentage data were plotted for each concentration of the extract and compared against the % of inhibition in the presence of DPPH obtained for a reference solution (2% ascorbic acid).

4.7. Assessment of Genoprotective Activity

Three groups of male Swiss albino mice were formed and housed in three cages (35 cm long × 25 cm wide × 12 cm high), each containing six mice. Each group received one of the following treatments: (i) Control; administration of vehicle (mineral oil intragastrically (i.g.)) every 2 days for 1 week; taking a blood smear every 2 days for 2 weeks; (ii) Anthracene (10 mg/kg, i.g.), administration of anthracene dissolved in mineral oil, every 2 days for 1 week and with a blood smear, every 2 days for 2 weeks, and (iii) Anthracene + *B. forficata* (500 mg/kg, i.g.), administration of anthracene plus *B. forficata* extract every 2 days for 1 week and with a blood smear every 2 days for 2 weeks. All blood smears were fixed in methanol (6 min) and colored with Giemsa (40 min) to be evaluated using the micronucleus detection technique in mouse peripheral blood [43] and to be analyzed under the optical microscope (VELAB©; VE-M5, McAllen, TX, USA) with 100× magnification (immersion).

4.8. Assessment of Hypoglycemic Activity

Three groups of male Swiss albino mice were formed and housed in three cages (35 cm long × 25 cm wide × 12 cm high), each containing six mice. Each group received one of the following treatments: (i) Control mice were administered i.g. with the plant-extract dissolution vehicle every 2 days (saline, 0.9%; vol = weight/1000); each week, blood glucose was measured with a commercial device (Optium FreeStyle©, Roche, Boston, MA, USA), making a small cut in the distal part of the mouse's tail to drain one drop of blood. Additionally, the body weight of the mice was recorded (prior fasting, <12 h) for 36 days; (ii) Diabetic mice were administered with a single intraperitoneal dose (i.p.) of streptozotocin (STZ; 120 mg/kg, dissolved in citrate buffer). After 1 week of administration, blood glucose was measured with a commercial device (Optium FreeStyle©). A mouse was considered diabetic (hyperglycemic) when its blood glucose levels reached 150 mg/dL or higher. Additionally, the body weight of the mice was recorded. These animals were administered i.g. every 2 days with a vehicle and with a weekly measurement of glucose and triglycerides (prior fasting, <12 h) for 36 days; (iii) Diabetic + *B. forficata* extract (500 mg/kg, i.g.), mice administered i.g. every 2 days with the methanolic extract of *Bahuina forficata* (500 mg/kg) and with a weekly glucose measurement (prior fasting, <12 h) for 36 days.

4.9. Statistical Analysis

The data obtained in the experiments of genoprotective activity and hypoglycemic effect were analyzed with SigmaStat ver. 12.0 statistical software, utilizing repeated measures two-way ANOVA and the Student–Newman–Keuls post-hoc test to determine significant differences among the different groups. In all cases, a level of $\alpha = 0.05$ was employed as the criterion for establishing statistically significant differences.

5. Conclusions

In this work, evidence has been provided of the antioxidant, genoprotective, and hypoglycemic activity of the methanolic extract of *B. forficata* leaves and stems. We think that it could be used for both type 1 and type 2 diabetes. However, more in-depth studies on these properties still need to be conducted, and one of these would be to isolate the secondary metabolites found in the dry extract in order to administer it in the chemical model with STZ to determine whether the therapeutic effect is determined by any of the metabolites detected with the phytochemistry or whether it is due to the set of these present in the dry extract.

In summary, this study proposes the use of *B. forficata* extract as an alternative coadjunctive therapy for the treatment of diabetes, without leaving allopathic therapy to one side, which could aid in improving the quality of life of patients with this pathology and perhaps reduce the treatment cost and the severity of the side effects of several of the drugs used.

Author Contributions: Conceptualization, T.A.F.-A. and E.A.C.-B.; methodology, T.A.F.-A. and E.A.C.-B.; formal analysis, T.A.F.-A., A.M.-G., and L.A.-R.; investigation, T.A.F.-A., E.A.C.-B. and E.O.M.-S.; resources, T.A.F.-A.; data curation, T.A.F.-A., A.M.-G., and J.A.M.-P.; writing—original draft preparation, T.A.F.-A., E.A.C.-B., C.V.-V. and O.L.-M.; writing—review and editing, T.A.F.-A.; supervision, T.A.F.-A.; project administration, T.A.F.-A.; funding acquisition, T.A.F.-A. All authors have read and agreed to the published version of the manuscript.

Funding: This study was partially funded by the Research and postgraduate secretariat with research project SIP20221343 of the Escuela Nacional de Ciencias Biológicas, of Instituto Politécnico Nacional, México.

Informed Consent Statement: All authors have consented to the acknowledgement.

Data Availability Statement: Not applicable.

Acknowledgments: The authors recognize Maggie Brunner for writing and reviewing the original manuscript.

Conflicts of Interest: The authors declare no conflict of interest.

References

1. IDF Diabetes Atlas. International Diabetes Federatión. 10th Edition 2021. Available online: www.diabetesatlas.org (accessed on 20 July 2022).
2. Basto-Abreu, A.; López-Olmedo, N.; Rojas-Martínez, R.; Aguilar-Salinas, C.A.; De la Cruz-Góngora, V.; Rivera-Dommarco, J.; Shamah-Levy, T.; Romero-Martínez, M.; Barquera, S.; Villalpando, S.; et al. Prevalence of diabetes and glycemic control in Mexico: National results from 2018 and 2020. *Salud Pública Méx.* **2021**, *63*, 725–733. [CrossRef]
3. ENSANUT. Encuesta Nacional de Salud y Nutrición 2018. Presentación de Resultados (insp.mx). Available online: https://ensanut.insp.mx/encuestas/ensanut2018/doctos/informes/ensanut_2018_presentacion_resultados.pdf (accessed on 24 June 2022).

4. Lima-Martínez, M.M.; Carrera-Boadac, C.; Madera-Silva, M.D.; Maríne, W.; Contreras, M. COVID-19 y diabetes mellitus: Una relación bidireccional. *Clin. Investig. Arterioscler.* **2021**, *33*, 151–157. [CrossRef]
5. Giannouchos, T.V.; Sussman, R.A.; Mier, J.M.; Poulas, K.; Farsalinos, K. Characteristics and risk factors for COVID-19 diagnosis and adverse outcomes in Mexico: An analysis of 89,756 laboratory–confirmed COVID-19 cases. *Eur. Respir. J.* **2021**, *57*, 202144. [CrossRef]
6. Bukhman, G.; Bavuma, C.; Gishoma, C.; Gupta, N.; Kwan, G.F.; Laing, R.; Beran, D. Endemic diabetes in the world's poorest people. *Lancet Diabetes Endocrinol.* **2015**, *3*, 402–403. [CrossRef]
7. Aguilar, A.; Xolalapa, S. La herbolaria Mexicana en el tratamiento de la diabetes. *Ciencia* **2002**, *53*, 24–35.
8. Bye, R.; Linares, E. Plantas medicinales del México prehispánico. *Arqueol. Mex.* **2018**, *39*, 4–11.
9. Santos-Díaz, M.S.; Barba-de la Rosa, A.P.; Héliès-Toussaint, C.; Guéraud, F.; Nègre-Salvayr, A. *Opuntia* spp.: Characterization and benefits in chronic diseases. *Oxidative Med. Cell. Longev.* **2017**, 8634249. [CrossRef]
10. Andrade-Cetto, A.; Wiedenfeld, H. Anti-hyperglycemic effect of *Opuntia streptacantha* Lem. *J. Ethnopharmacol.* **2011**, *133*, 940–943. [CrossRef]
11. Bouhrim, M.; Elhouda-Daoudi, N.; Ouassou, H.; Benoutman, A.; Loukili, E.H.; Ziyyat, A.; Mekhfi, H.; Legssyer, A.; Aziz, M.; Bnouham, M. Phenolic content and antioxidant, antihyperlipidemic, and antidiabetogenic effects of *Opuntia dillenii* seed oil. *Sci. World J.* **2020**. [CrossRef]
12. Pingali, U.; Abid-Ali, M.; Gundagani, S.; Nutalapati, C. Evaluation of the effect of an aqueous extract of *Azadirachta indica* (Neem) leaves and twigs on Glycemic control, endothelial dysfunction and systemic inflammation in subjects with type 2 diabetes mellitus: A randomized, double-blind, placebo-controlled clinical study. *Diabetes Metab. Syndr. Obes. Targets Ther.* **2020**, *13*, 4401–4412.
13. Patil, S.M.; Shirahatti, P.S.; Ramith Ramu, R. *Azadirachta indica* A. Juss (neem) against diabetes mellitus: A critical review on its phytochemistry, pharmacology, and toxicology. *J. Pharm. Pharmacol.* **2022**, *74*, 681–710. [CrossRef]
14. Andrade-Cetto, A.; Heinrich, M. Mexican plants with hypoglycaemic effect used in the treatment of diabetes. *J. Ethnopharmacol.* **2005**, *99*, 325–348. [CrossRef]
15. Blanco, L. Pata de Vaca: Características, Hábitat, Propiedades, Ingesta. Available online: www.lifeder.com/pata-de-vaca/ (accessed on 20 June 2022).
16. Sinou, C.; Forest, F.; Bruneau, A. The genus *Bauhinia* s.l. (Leguminosae): A phylogeny based on the plastid trnLtrnF region. *Botany* **2009**, *87*, 947–960. [CrossRef]
17. Aragadvay-Yungán, R.G.; Barros-Rodríguez, M.; Ortiz, L.; Carro, M.D.; Navarro-Marcos, C.; Yasseen-Elghandour, M.M.M.M.; Mohamed-Salem, A.Z. Mitigation of ruminal methane production with enhancing the fermentation by supplementation of different tropical forage legumes. *Environ. Sci. Pollut. Res.* **2022**, *29*, 3438–3445. [CrossRef]
18. Lubkowski, J.; Durbin, S.V.; Silva, M.C.C.; Farnsworth, D.; Gildersleeve, J.C.; Oliva, M.L.V.; Wlodawe, A. Structural analysis and unique molecular recognition properties of a Bauhinia forficata lectin that inhibits cancer cell growth. *FEBS J.* **2017**, *284*, 429–450. [CrossRef]
19. Cechinel-Filho, V. Chemical composition and biological potential of plants from the genus *Bauhinia*. *Phytother. Res.* **2009**, *23*, 1347–1354. [CrossRef]
20. Cechinel-Zanchett, C.C.; de Andrade-Fonseca da Silva, R.C.M.V.; Tenfena, A.; Siebertb, D.A.; Mickeb, G.; Vitalib, L.; Cechinel-Filhoa, V.; Faloni de Andradea, S.; de Souza, P. *Bauhinia forficata* link, a Brazilian medicinal plant traditionally used to treat cardiovascular disorders, exerts endothelium-dependent and independent vasorelaxation in thoracic aorta of normotensive and hypertensive rats. *J. Ethnopharmacol.* **2019**, *243*, 112118. [CrossRef]
21. Da Cunha, A.M.; Menon, S.; Menon, R.; Couto, A.G.; Burger, C.; Biavatti, M.W. Hypoglycemic activity of dried extracts of *Bauhinia forficata* Link. *Phytomedicine* **2010**, *17*, 37–41. [CrossRef]
22. Fernandes-Salgueiro, A.C.; Folmer, V.; Pires-da Silva, M.; Loureiro-Mendez, A.S.; Pegoraro-Zemolin, A.P.; Posser, T.; Luis-Franco, J.; Luiz-Puntel, R.; Orione-Puntel, G. Effects of *Bauhinia* forficata Tea on oxidative stress and liver damage in diabetic mice. *Oxidative Med. Cell. Longev.* **2016**. [CrossRef]
23. Silva-dos-Santos, J.; Gonçalves-Cirino, J.P.; De-Oliveira-Carvalho, P.; Ortega, M.M. The Pharmacological Action of Kaempferol in Central Nervous System Diseases: A Review. *Front. Pharmacol.* **2021**, *11*, 565700. [CrossRef]
24. Szkudelski, T. The mechanism of alloxan and streptozotocin action in B cells of the rat pancreas. *Physiol. Res.* **2001**, *50*, 537–546. [PubMed]
25. Lenzen, S. The mechanisms of alloxan- and streptozotocin-induced diabetes. *Diabetologia* **2008**, *51*, 216–226. [CrossRef] [PubMed]
26. Konrad, R.J.; Mikolaenko, I.; Tolar, J.F.; Liu, K.; Kudlow, J.E. The potential mechanism of the diabetogenic action of streptozotocin: Inhibition of pancreatic β-cell O-GlcNAc-selective N-acetyl-β-D-glucosaminidase. *Biochem. J.* **2001**, *356*, 31–41. [CrossRef] [PubMed]
27. Mosic, M.; Dramicanin, A.; Ristivojevic, P.; Milojkovic-Opsenica, D. Extraction as a critical step in phytochemical Analysis. *J. AOAC Int.* **2020**, *103*, 365–372. [CrossRef] [PubMed]
28. Ajebli, M.; Khan, H.; Eddouks, M. Natural alkaloids and diabetes mellitus: A review. *Endocr. Metab. Immune Disord. Drug Targets* **2021**, *21*, 111–130. [CrossRef]
29. Chang, W.; Chen, L.; Hatch, G.M. Berberine as a therapy for type 2 diabetes and its complications: From mechanism of action to clinical studies. *Biochem. Cell Biol.* **2015**, *93*, 479–486. [CrossRef]

30. Zhang, M.; Xiao-Yan, L.; Li, J.; Zhi-Gang, X.; Chen, L. The characterization of high-fat diet and multiple low-dose streptozotocin induced type 2 diabetes rat model. *Exp. Diabetes Res.* **2008**. [CrossRef]
31. Sinan, K.I.; Zengin, G.; Zheleva-Dimitrova, D.; Etienne, O.K.; Mahomoodally, M.F.; Bouyahya, A.; Lobine, D.; Chiavaroli, A.; Ferrante, C.; Menghini, L.; et al. Qualitative phytochemical fingerprint and network pharmacology investigation of *Achyranthes aspera* Linn. extracts. *Molecules* **2020**, *25*, 1973. [CrossRef]
32. Nogueira, T.S.R.; Passos, M.S.; Pessanha-S-Nascimento, L.; Barreto-de-S-Arantes, M.; Monteiro, N.O.; Imad-da-S-Boeno, S.; De-Carvalho-Junior, A.; Azevedo, O.A.; Da-S-Terra, W.; Gonçalves-C-Vieira, M.; et al. Chemical compounds and biologic activities: A review of *Cedrela* genus. *Molecules* **2020**, *25*, 5401. [CrossRef]
33. Huang, Q.; Lu, G.; Shen, H.M.; Chung, M.C.M.; Ong, C.N. Anti-cancer properties of anthraquinones from rhubarb. *Med. Res. Rev.* **2007**, *27*, 609–630. [CrossRef]
34. Liu, Y.; Mapa, M.S.T.; Sprando, R.L. Anthraquinones inhibit cytochromes P450 enzyme activity in silico and in vitro. *J. Appl. Toxicol.* **2021**, *41*, 1438–1445. [CrossRef]
35. Li, Y.; Jiang, J.G. Health functions and structure-activity relationships of natural anthraquinones from plants. *Food Funct.* **2018**, *9*, 6063–6080. [CrossRef]
36. Ferreres, F.; Gil-Izquierdo, A.; Vinholes, J.; Silva, S.T.; Valentao, P.; Andrade, P.B. *Bauhinia forficata* Link authenticity using flavonoids profile: Relation with their biological properties. *Food Chem.* **2012**, *134*, 894–904. [CrossRef]
37. Srisawat, P.; Fukushima, E.O.; Yasumoto, S.; Robertlee, J.; Suzuki, H.; Seki, H.; Muranaka, T. Identification of oxidosqualene cyclases from the medicinal legume tree *Bauhinia forficata*: A step toward discovering preponderant a-amyrin-producing activity. *New Phytol.* **2019**, *224*, 352–366. [CrossRef]
38. De Souza, P.; Mota, L.; Boeing, T.; Somensi, L.B.; Cecconi, C.; Zanchett, C.; Campos, A.; De Medeiros, C.; Krueger, A.; Bastos, J.K.; et al. Influence of prostanoids in the diuretic and natriuretic effects of extracts and kaempferitrin from *Bauhinia forficata* Link leaves in rats. *Phytother. Res.* **2017**, *31*, 1521–1528. [CrossRef]
39. Farag, M.A.; Sakna, S.T.; El-fiky, N.M.; Shabana, M.M.; Wessjohann, L.A. Phytochemical, antioxidant and antidiabetic evaluation of eight *Bauhinia* L. species from Egypt using UHPLC–PDA–qTOF-MS and chemometrics. *Phytochemistry* **2015**, *119*, 41–50. [CrossRef]
40. Fernandes-de-Aráujo, F.; De-Paulo-Farias, D.; Neri-Numa, I.A.; Pastore, G.M. Polyphenols and their applications: An approach in food chemistry and innovation potential. *Food Chem.* **2021**, *338*, 127535. [CrossRef]
41. Rodrigues-Franco, R.; Da-Silva-Carvalho, D.; Borges-Rosa-de-Moura, F.; Benatti-Justino, A.; Guerra-Silva, H.C.; Gomes-Peixoto, L.; Salmen-Espindola, F. Antioxidant and anti-glycation capacities of some medicinal plants and their potential inhibitory against digestive enzymes related to type 2 diabetes mellitus. *J. Ethnopharmacol.* **2018**, *215*, 140–146. [CrossRef]
42. Pinafo, M.S.; Benedetti, P.R.; Gaiotte, L.B.; Costa, F.G.; Schoffen, J.P.F.; Fernandes, G.S.A.; Chuffa, L.G.A.; Seiva, F.R.F. Effects of *Bauhinia forficata* on glycaemia, lipid profile, hepatic glycogen content and oxidative stress in rats exposed to Bisphenol A. *Toxicol. Rep.* **2019**, *6*, 244–252. [CrossRef]
43. Zúñiga-González, G.; Torres-Bugarín, O.; Luna-Aguirre, J.; González-Rodríguez, A.; Zamora-Perez, A.; Gómez-Meda, B.C.; Ventura-Aguilar, A.J.; Ramos-Ibarra, M.L.; Ramos-Mora, A.; Ortíz, G.G.; et al. Spontaneous micronuclei in peripheral blood erythrocytes from 54 animal species (mammals, reptiles and birds): Part two. *Mutat. Res.* **2000**, *467*, 99–103. [CrossRef]
44. Meléndez-Gélvez, I.; Quijano-Vargas, M.J.; Quijano-Parra, A. Actividad mutagénica indicida por hidrocarburos aromáticospolicíclicos en muestras de PM$_{2.5}$ en un sector residencial de villa del rosario-norte de Santander, Colombia. *Rev. Int. Contam. Ambient.* **2016**, *32*, 435–444. [CrossRef]
45. Fenech, M.; Knasmueller, S.; Bolognesi, C.; Holland, N.; Bonassi, S.; Kirsch-Volders, M. Micronuclei as biomarkers of DNA damage, aneuploidy, inducers of chromosomal hypermutation and as sources of pro-inflammatory DNA in humans. *Mutat. Res.* **2020**, *786*, 108342. [CrossRef] [PubMed]
46. Grossi, M.R.; Berni, A.; Pepe, G.; Filippi, S.; Mosesso, P.; Shivnani, A.A.; Papeschi, C.; Natarajan, A.T.; Palitti, F. A comparative study of the anticlastogenic effects of chlorophyllin on N-methyl-N'-nitro-N-nitrosoguanidine (MNNG) or 7,12-dimethylbenz(α)anthracene (DMBA) induced micronuclei in mammalian cells in vitro and *in vivo*. *Toxicol. Lett.* **2012**, *214*, 235–242. [CrossRef] [PubMed]
47. Düsman, E.; De Almeida, I.V.; Coelho, A.C.; Balbi, T.J.; Düsman-Tonin, L.T.; Pimenta-Vicentini, V.E. Antimutagenic effect of Medicinal plants *Achillea millefolium* and *Bauhinia forficata* In Vivo. *Evid. Based Comp. Altern. Med.* **2013**. [CrossRef] [PubMed]
48. Sugunadevi, G.; Suresh, K.; Vijayaanand, M.A.; Rajalingam, K.; Sathiyapriya, J. Anti genotoxic effect of Mosinone-A on 7, 12-dimethyl benz[a] anthracene induced genotoxicity in male golden Syrian hamsters. *Pathol. Oncol. Res.* **2012**, *18*, 69–77. [CrossRef]
49. Borges-dos Santos, F.J.; Moura, D.J.; Flores-Pérez, V.; De Moura-Sperotto, A.R.; Bastos-Caramão, E.; Melo-Cavalcante, A.M.C.; Saffi, J. Genotoxic and mutagenic properties of *Bauhinia platypetala* extract, a traditional Brazilian medicinal plant. *J. Ethnopharmacol.* **2012**, *144*, 474–482. [CrossRef]
50. Ferri, F.F. Diabetes mellitus. In *Ferri's Clinical Advisor 2018*, 1st ed.; Elsevier: Alpharetta, GA, USA, 2018; 2011p.
51. Powers, A.C.; Niswender, K.D.; Evans-Molina, C. Diabetes Mellitus: Diagnosis, Classification, and Pathophysiology. In *Harrison's Principles of Internal Medicine*, 20th ed.; Jameson, J., Fauci, A.S., Kasper, D.L., Hauser, S.L., Longo, D.L., Loscalzo, J., Eds.; McGraw Hill: New York, NY, USA, 2018; Available online: https://accessmedicine.mhmedical.com/content.aspx?bookid=2129&sectionid=192288322 (accessed on 15 July 2018).

52. Hirata, Y.; Nomura, K.; Senga, Y.; Okada, Y.; Kobayashi, K.; Okamoto, S.; Minokoshi, Y.; Imamura, M.; Takeda, S.; Hosooka, T.; et al. Hyperglycemia induces skeletal muscle atrophy via a WWP1/KLF15 axis. *JCI Insight* **2019**, *4*, e124952. [CrossRef]
53. Kulkarni, Y.A.; Garud, M.S. *Bauhinia variegata* (Caesalpiniaceae) leaf extract: An effective treatment option in type I and type II diabetes. *Biomed. Pharmacother.* **2016**, *83*, 122–129.
54. Pepato, M.T.; Martins-Baviera, A.; Vendramini, R.C.; Brunetti, I.L. Evaluation of toxicity after one-months treatment with *Bauhinia forficata* decoction in streptozotocin-induced diabetic rats. *BMC Complement. Altern. Med.* **2004**, *4*, 7. [CrossRef]
55. Rodrigues-Franco, R.; Mota-Alves, V.H.; Ribeiro-Zabisky, L.F.; Benatti-Justino, A.; Machado-Martins, M.; Lopes-Saraiva, A.; Goulart, L.R.; Espindola, F.S. Antidiabetic potential of *Bauhinia forficata* Link leaves: A non-cytotoxic source of lipase and glycoside hydrolases inhibitors and molecules with antioxidant and antiglycation properties. *Biomed. Pharmacother.* **2020**, *123*. [CrossRef]
56. Sharma, D.; Tekade, R.K.; Kalia, K. Kaempferol in ameliorating diabetes-induced fibrosis and renal damage: An in vitro and in vivo study in diabetic nephropathy mice model. *Phytomedicine* **2020**, *76*, 153235. [CrossRef]
57. Trojan-Rodrigues, M.; Alves, T.L.S.; Soares, G.L.G.; Ritter, M.R. Plants used as antidiabetics in popular medicine in Rio Grande do Sul, southern Brazil. *J. Ethnopharmacol.* **2012**, *139*, 155–163. [CrossRef]
58. Luo, C.; Yang, H.; Tang, C.; Yao, G.; Kong, L.; He, H.; Zhou, Y. Kaempferol alleviates insulin resistance via hepatic IKK/NF-κB signal in type 2 diabetic rats. *Int. Immunopharmacol.* **2015**, *28*, 744–750. [CrossRef]
59. Ren, J.; Lu, Y.; Quian, Y.; Chen, B.; Wu, T.; Ji, G. Recent progress regarding kaempferol for the treatment of various diseases. *Exp. Ther. Med.* **2019**, *18*, 2759–2776. [CrossRef]
60. Saldanha, L.L.; Quintiliano-Delgado, A.; Marcourt, L.; De-Paula-Camaforte, N.A.; Ponce-Vareda, P.M.; Ebrahimi, S.N.; Vilegas, W.; Dokkedal, A.L.; Ferreira-Queiroz, E.; Wolfender, J.; et al. Hypoglycemic active principles from the leaves of *Bauhinia holophylla*: Comprehensive phytochemical characterization and in vivo activity profile. *PLoS ONE* **2021**, *16*, e0258016. [CrossRef]
61. Cardozo-De-Souza, B.V.; Dos-Reis-Moreira-Araújo, R.S.; Almeida-Silva, O.; Costa-Faustino, L.; Beserra-Gonçalves, M.F.; Lima-Dos-Santos, M.; Rocha-Souza, G.; Moura-Rocha, L.; Sousa-Cardoso, M.L.; Cunha-Nunes, L.C. *Bauhinia forficata* in the treatment of diabetes mellitus: A patent review. *Expert Opin. Ther. Pat.* **2018**, *28*, 129–138.
62. Tonelli, C.A.; Quintana-De-Oliveira, S.; Da-Silva-Vieira, A.A.; Biavatti, M.W.; Ritter, C.; Reginatto, F.H.; Machado-De-Campos, A.; Dal-Pizzol, F. Clinical efficacy of capsules containing standardized extract of *Bauhinia forficata* Link (pata-de-vaca) as adjuvant treatment in type 2 diabetes patients: A randomized, double blind clinical trial. *J. Ethnopharmacol.* **2022**, *282*, 114616. [CrossRef]
63. Córdova-Mariángel, P.; Avello-Lorca, M.; Morales-Leon, F.; Fernández-Rocca, P.; Villa-Zapata, L.; Pastene-Navarrete, E. Effects of *Bauhinia forficata* Link tea on lipid profile in diabetic patients. *J. Med. Food* **2019**, *22*, 321–323. [CrossRef]
64. Alcibar-Muñóz, M.; Alonso, S.; Berdeja-Martínez, B.; Germán-Faz, M.C.; Hernández-de-Jesús, M.L.; Razo, A.; Silva-Torres, R. Manual del curso experimental de fitoquímica para la carrera de Químico Farmaceútico Industrial. *Esc. Nac. Cienc. Biol. IPN* **2019**, *19*, 116.
65. Carbajal-Rojas, L.; Hata-Uribe, Y.; Sierra-Martínez, N.; Rueda-Niño, D. Análisis fitoquímico preliminar de hojas, tallos y semillas de Cupatá (*Strychnos schultesiana* Krunkoff). *Colomb. For.* **2009**, *12*, 161–170. [CrossRef]

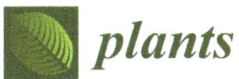

Review

The Anticancer Potential of Plant-Derived Nutraceuticals via the Modulation of Gene Expression

Maria Vrânceanu [1,†], Damiano Galimberti [2], Roxana Banc [3,*,†], Ovidiu Dragoş [4,*,†], Anamaria Cozma-Petruţ [3,†], Simona-Codruţa Hegheş [5,†], Oliviu Voştinaru [6], Magdalena Cuciureanu [7], Carmina Mariana Stroia [8], Doina Miere [3] and Lorena Filip [3,†]

1. Department of Toxicology, "Iuliu Haţieganu" University of Medicine and Pharmacy, 6 Pasteur Street, 400349 Cluj-Napoca, Romania
2. Italian Association of Anti-Ageing Physicians, Via Monte Cristallo, 1, 20159 Milan, Italy
3. Department of Bromatology, Hygiene, Nutrition, "Iuliu Haţieganu" University of Medicine and Pharmacy, 6 Pasteur Street, 400349 Cluj-Napoca, Romania
4. Department of Kinetotheraphy and Special Motricity, "1 Decembrie 1918" University of Alba Iulia, 510009 Alba Iulia, Romania
5. Department of Drug Analysis, "Iuliu Haţieganu" University of Medicine and Pharmacy, 6 Pasteur Street, 400349 Cluj-Napoca, Romania
6. Department of Pharmacology, Physiology and Physiopathology, "Iuliu Haţieganu" University of Medicine and Pharmacy, 6 Pasteur Street, 400349 Cluj-Napoca, Romania
7. Department of Pharmacology, University of Medicine and Pharmacy "Grigore T. Popa" Iasi, 16 Universităţii Street, 700115 Iași, Romania
8. Department of Pharmacy, Oradea University, 1 Universităţii Street, 410087 Oradea, Romania
* Correspondence: roxana.banc@umfcluj.ro (R.B.); ovidiu.dragos@uab.ro (O.D.); Tel.: +40-744-367-958 (R.B.); +40-733-040-917 (O.D)
† These authors contributed equally to this work.

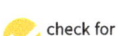

Abstract: Current studies show that approximately one-third of all cancer-related deaths are linked to diet and several cancer forms are preventable with balanced nutrition, due to dietary compounds being able to reverse epigenetic abnormalities. An appropriate diet in cancer patients can lead to changes in gene expression and enhance the efficacy of therapy. It has been demonstrated that nutraceuticals can act as powerful antioxidants at the cellular level as well as anticarcinogenic agents. This review is focused on the best studies on worldwide-available plant-derived nutraceuticals: curcumin, resveratrol, sulforaphane, indole-3-carbinol, quercetin, astaxanthin, epigallocatechin-3-gallate, and lycopene. These compounds have an enhanced effect on epigenetic changes such as histone modification via HDAC (histone deacetylase), HAT (histone acetyltransferase) inhibition, DNMT (DNA methyltransferase) inhibition, and non-coding RNA expression. All of these nutraceuticals are reported to positively modulate the epigenome, reducing cancer incidence. Furthermore, the current review addresses the issue of the low bioavailability of nutraceuticals and how to overcome the drawbacks related to their oral administration. Understanding the mechanisms by which nutraceuticals influence gene expression will allow their incorporation into an "epigenetic diet" that could be further capitalized on in the therapy of cancer.

Keywords: nutraceuticals; gene expression; epigenetic therapy; cancer

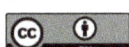

1. Introduction

Nowadays, cancer is the second leading cause of death globally, with nearly one in seven deaths being due to cancer. About one-third of deaths from cancer are determined by five main behavioral and dietary risks: high Body Mass Index (BMI), low fruit and vegetable intake, lack of physical activity, tobacco use, and alcohol consumption [1]. Several clinical and epidemiological studies support the association between nutrition and the development or progression of different malignancies [2], with prostate, colon, gastric, and breast cancer being the types of cancer most closely related to diet. There is scientific evidence that a proper diet and lifestyle can substantially reduce cancer risk. For example, adherence to the Mediterranean diet (MD) has been reported as a valuable tool against cancer, and several studies have found a significant reduction in cancer mortality in subjects following the MD. A diet designed to support cancer patients can help reduce the toxicity of radio- and chemotherapy and strengthen the immune system. In the last years, science has focused more on nutraceuticals as protective factors [3]. According to the scientific literature, nutraceuticals are a good source of molecules, able to regulate gene expression and reverse epigenetic alterations due to specific modulation mechanisms [4]. Nutraceuticals, therefore, assume the role of cellular and functional modulators, able to ensure the optimization of the physiological processes of the human body [5].

In the field of cancer research, epigenetic modifications are of particular interest, having an impact on cell proliferation, differentiation, and survival [6]. Cancer can be considered a multi-stage heterogeneous disease, driven by genetic and epigenetic anomalies. Epigenetic changes are involved in biological diversity, aging, and the pathogenesis of cancer and other diseases. All human cancers are characterized by epigenetic changes that cooperate with genetic alterations [7], allowing the uncontrollable growth of cells. The epigenetic transformations are represented by post-translational changes in nucleosomal histones, the most common being methylation, acetylation correlated with transcriptional activation, deacetylation correlated with transcriptional repression, and DNA methylation and regulation by non-coding RNAs [8,9]. The epigenetic component is influenced by exogenous and endogenous factors, including diet, lifestyle, environment, ethnicity, drug intake, exposure to toxins, xenobiotics, age, sex, exercise, and family genetic heritage. Epigenetic therapy is a new area for the development of nutraceuticals, whose low risk of toxicity can represent a valid asset in the cancer prevention strategy [10]. The great potential of this type of therapy lies in the fact that epigenetic alterations are reversible, aiming to reprogram cells to a normal state [11].

Recent advances in understanding nutrigenetics and nutrigenomic mechanisms have led to the identification of nutraceuticals and biocompounds capable of favorably influencing gene expression. A healthy diet and a balanced lifestyle combined with targeted and personalized integration can keep people healthier, favoring successful aging and preventing diseases. Nutraceuticals are able to provide the elements necessary to supply the body's defense store and to optimize the responsiveness of whole organs, intervening in DNA repair processes and counteracting the key factors correlated with whole-body aging and disease progression. Bioavailability, metabolism, and the tissue distribution of bioactive molecules derived from nutraceuticals are key factors that must be managed accurately in association with their biological effects, not only in vitro but also in vivo [12].

2. Methodology

We conducted a narrative literature review, using the academic databases Pubmed and ScienceDirect for the search and collection of literature. Major keywords, such as "nutraceuticals", "cancer", "gene expression", "microRNAs", "bioavailability", "bioactive compounds", "curcumin", "resveratrol", "sulforaphane", "indole-3-carbinol", "astaxanthin", "quercetin", "epigallocatechin-3-gallate", "lycopene", and "in vitro", "in vivo", and "clinical studies", were used individually or in combination during the literature survey. We considered original research articles written in English and based our search on their importance and relevance to the field. Due to the large number of published articles on nutraceuticals included in the study, as well as the limited number of references allowed, it was necessary to focus on the most impactful and relevant aspects, and we included published review articles where appropriate. In general, we focused on recently published articles but did not impose limits on the date of publication.

3. Nutraceuticals

The term nutraceutical combines the words nutrition and pharmaceutical and indicates those nutrient principles that are found within foods. These have beneficial health effects. Nutraceutical substances derive mainly from plants, food, and microbial sources. This term was invented in 1989 by Dr. Stephen L. De Felice, who, by combining the words "nutrition" and "pharmaceutical", came to the term "nutraceutical" to indicate a food substance that, for its functional properties, aligns precisely with the limit between food and drug [13]. In reality, we should distinguish between nutraceuticals and functional foods, where the first indicates a specific substance extracted from food, with certain medicinal qualities, while the second means a real (or added) food that directly shows beneficial properties through its introduction into a diet. Nutraceuticals are biological substances that are considered as foods, parts of foods, or dietary supplements with preventive, rebalancing, therapeutic, and protective properties. Recent studies have shown promising results for these compounds in numerous pathological complications such as cancer, diabetes, and cardiovascular or neurological disorders [14]. All these conditions are characterized by many changes, including alterations in the redox state, and most nutraceuticals have antioxidant activity with the ability to fight against this situation [15].

These natural molecules are often plant extracts titrated for a particular active ingredient. In the group of nutraceuticals, there are several substances, among which the best known are curcumin, resveratrol, astaxanthin, sulforaphane, indole-3-carbinol, quercetin, epigallocatechin-3-gallate (EGCG), lycopene, anthocyanins, ellagic acid, fisetin, capsaicin and extracts of ginger (*Zingiber officinale* Rosc.), *Ziziphus jujuba* Mill., *Uncaria tomentosa* Willd. ex Schult., *Silybum marianum* L., and *Bacopa monnieri* L., all covering various therapeutic areas and having the ability, according to the latest studies, to modulate gene expression [16–18].

For each of the plant-derived nutraceuticals selected in this study, Table 1 summarizes the plant source, their ability to modulate gene expression and regulate microRNAs, and their antitumor effect.

Table 1. Summary of the gene expression variability and antitumor activity.

Natural Source	Epigenetic Modulation	Gene Targets	Biological Effects	Micro RNAs Regulated	Cancer Types	References
			Curcumin			
Turmeric	DNMT1 DNMT3b DNMT3a HDAC1 HDAC4 HDAC7	P65, Sp1, CDK, Her2, NrF2, STAT3, BAX, p38, p53 VEGF IL6 IL23 IL1-β	Chemoprevention, cell growth inhibition, cell-cycle arrest Apoptosis, angiogenesis inhibition	miR-15a↑ miR-16↑ miR-22↑ miR-26a↑ miR-34a↑ miR-145↑ miR-146a↑ miR-200b↑ miR-200c↑ miR-203 ↑ let7↑ miR-19a,b↓ miR-21↓ miR-27a↓ miR-130a↓ miR-186↓	AML Breast Prostate Colon Lung	[19–31]

Table 1. *Cont.*

Natural Source	Epigenetic Modulation	Gene Targets	Biological Effects	Micro RNAs Regulated	Cancer Types	References
Resveratrol						
Black grapes, red wine, plum, peanuts, berries, cocoa powder, dark chocolate	DNMT HDAC	p53 p300 p16 CDK AP1 EGR1 STAT1 STAT3 SIRT1 MAPK Bcl2 hTERT MTA1	Cell growth inhibition, cell-cycle arrest Apoptosis Chemopreventive	miR34a↑ miR 663↑ miR 141↑ miR 200↑ miR17↓ miR25↓ miR92a-2↓	Colon Breast Prostate Lung	[32–39]
Sulforaphane						
Broccoli Cauliflower Cabbage Brussels sprout	DNMT1 DNMT3a DNMT3b HDCA1, 2,3,8	p21 p27 CDKN hTERT EGFR Cyclin D2 Nrf2	Chemopreventive Cell-cycle arrest Apoptosis Cell growth inhibition	miR-let-7a-e↑ miR-15a↑ miR-16↑ miR-27b↑ miR-30e↑ miR-31↑ miR-34a↑ miR-124↑ miR-200a-b-c↑ miR-219-5p↑ miR-320↑ miR-19a↓ miR-19b↓ miR-92a-2↓ miR-106a↓ miR-181a↓ miR-181b↓ miR-210-3p↓ miR-221↓ miR-495↓	Prostate Breast Lung	[40–48]
Astaxanthin						
Algae, yeast, salmon, trout, krill, shrimp, and crayfish	DNMT1 DNMT3a DNMT3b	MMP2 ZEB1 EMT EGFR XPC Rad51 NQO1 NRF2/ KEAP1	Chemopreventive Apoptosis Cell growth inhibition Cell proliferation inhibition	miR-29a-3p↑ miR-200a↑ miR-375↑ miR-478b↑ miR-221↓	Pancreatic Lung Prostate Skin	[49–55]

Table 1. *Cont.*

Natural Source	Epigenetic Modulation	Gene Targets	Biological Effects	Micro RNAs Regulated	Cancer Types	References
		Quercetin				
Onion, apple, citrus fruits, raspberries Grapes Olives Tomatoes	DNMT3a DNMT3b HDAC1 DNMT1	p53 CD1 p21 PLAU ERK1/2 KRAS BRCA1 BRCA2 IGF1 IGFBP3 JNK AR Bcl2 JAK	Cell growth inhibition Cell proliferation inhibition Chemopreventive Apoptosis Cell-cycle arrest	miR-let-7↑ miR-146a↑ miR-15a↑ miR-16↑ miR-26↑ miR-142-3p↑ miR-200b-3p↑ miR-217↑ miR-330↑ miR-27a miR-21 miR-19b miR-155 miR-148c	Breast Prostate Colon Ovarian Gastric Pancreatic Lung Leukemia	[56–66]
		EGCG				
Green tea, carob flour, apples, pistachios, prunes, peaches, avocados	DNMT1 DNMT3a DNMT3b HDCA1	GSTP1 CDX2 BMP2 TIMP3 MMP2 MMP9 IGF, IGF1, IGFBP-3 VEGF p53 Bcl2	Cell growth inhibition Cell proliferation inhibition Chemopreventive Apoptosis Cell-cycle arrest Angiogenesis decreases	miR-16↑ miR-210↑ miR-330↑ miR-21↓ miR-98-5p↓	Liver Breast Prostate Lung Bladder Gastric Colon	[67–71]
		Lycopene				
Tomatoes Apricots Guava Papaya Watermelon Pink grapefruit	DNMT3a	GSTP1 AKT2 CDK2 CDK4 p53 CCND1 CCND3	Cell growth inhibition Chemopreventive Cell-cycle arrest Apoptosis	miR-let-7f-1 ↑	Prostate cancer Breast cancer	[72–75]

↑ increases expression; ↓ decreases expression.

In this review, we have focused on the first eight of those previously mentioned as the most well-known nutraceuticals, also illustrated in Figure 1, because these are the most studied in terms of antioxidant and anticancer properties, as well as the most targeted to be used in the treatment of cancer as adjuvants in association with chemotherapeutic drugs such as gemcitabine, docetaxel, doxorubicin, and cisplatin, to enhance their efficiency or limit their toxicity. Indeed, in the international database of clinical studies (ClinicalTrials.gov), it can be observed that curcumin, resveratrol, sulforaphane, indole-3-carbinol, quercetin, EGCG, and lycopene are currently in clinical trials on various types of cancer. Several examples of such clinical studies can be seen in Table 2.

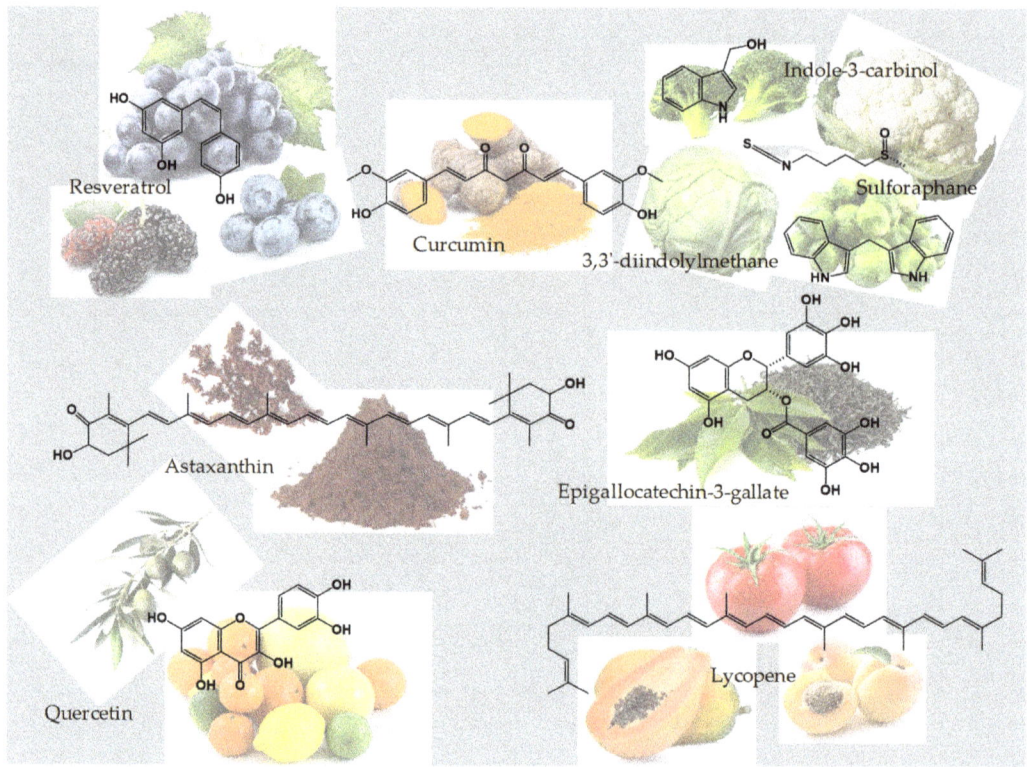

Figure 1. Main plant-derived nutraceuticals.

Table 2. List of plant-derived bioactives currently in clinical trials on various types of cancer [76].

Plant-Derived Bioactive Compound	Type of Cancer	Primary Outcome Measures	Clinical Trial Identifier
Curcumin	Breast cancer	Tumor proliferation rate	NCT03980509
Sulforaphane	Lung cancer	Prevention of lung cancer in former smokers/bronchial dysplasia index	NCT03232138
Quercetin	Squamous cell carcinoma	Prevention of squamous cell carcinoma in patients with Fanconi anemia/reduction in buccal micronuclei	NCT03476330
Epigallocatechin-3-gallate	Colorectal cancer	Change in methylation from baseline when compared to the control arm	NCT02891538
Lycopene	Metastatic colorectal cancer and skin toxicity	Skin toxicity reduction in metastatic colorectal cancer submitted to therapy with panitumumab	NCT03167268
Mixture of carotenoids, indole-3-carbinol, curcumin, EGCG, caffeine, resveratrol, lycopene, genistein, phytoestrogens	Breast and ovarian cancer syndrome	DNA damage change	NCT05306002

3.1. Curcumin

Curcuma longa L. is an herbaceous plant, perennial and rhizomatous, which belongs to the family of Zingiberaceae, as ginger (*Zingiber officinale* Rosc.) also does. The root, which is the most important component of phytotherapeutic and nutritional interest, is constituted by a cylindrical, branched, aromatic rhizome of orange-yellow color. It is used in food as a spice, especially in traditional Indian, Middle Eastern, and Thai cuisine. The plant contains more than 100 chemical compounds, but the term curcumin generally refers to 1,7-bis(4-hydroxy-3-methoxyphenyl)-1,6-heptadiene-3,5-dione, a compound known as "curcumin I". Two other best-known compounds are curcumin II (demethoxycurcumin, 1-(4-hydroxy-3-methoxyphenyl)-7-(4-hydroxyphenyl)-1,6-heptadiene-3,5-dione) and curcumin III (bisdemethoxycurcumin, 1,7-bis(4-hydroxyphenyl)-1,6-heptadiene-3,5-dione) [77]. The specific and well-known yellow curcumin color is due to "curcumin I" and the curcuminoids, bisdemethoxycurcumin and demethoxycurcumin, generally used as a natural dye in the food industry [78]. The principal essential oils of curcumin are turmerone (ar-turmerone), β-turmerone, α-turmerone, β-bisabolene, β-sesquiphellandrene, α-zingiberene, curcumol, and curcumenol [79].

Curcumin is famous for its antioxidant, anti-inflammatory, and anticancer properties and recently has been shown to act as an epigenetic modulator [25]. The role of curcumin as an epigenetic regulator includes histone modification by the regulation of histone acetyltransferase (HAT) and histone deacetylase (HDAC); DNA methylation by the inhibition of DNA methyltransferase (DNMT); microRNA modulation by the upregulation of tumor-suppressive miRNAs (miR-15a, miR-16, miR-22, miR-26a, miR-34a, miR-145, miR-146a, miR-200b, c, miR-203, and let-7) [19,20]; the downregulation of oncogenic miRNAs (miR-19a, b, miR-21, miR-27a, miR-130a, miR-186) [24]; and the activation of transcription factors, cytokines, and tumor suppressor genes [26]. DNA methylation is a great target in the treatment of acute myeloid leukemia (AML) as it is well known that the inactivation of genes due to DNA methylation has a major role in the development of AML. It has been shown that curcumin is able to downregulate DNMT1 expression in AML cell lines, in vitro and in vivo [27]. p65 and Sp1 expression, positive regulators of DNMT1, may be reduced by curcumin, which correlates with reductions in the binding of these transcription factors to the DNMT1 promoter in AML cell lines. These characteristics of curcumin make it a promising compound in the treatment of AML [28]. Due to the changes in DNA methylation, curcumin is a hypomethylating agent in breast, prostate, colon, and lung cancer.

Curcumin is able to target other, different cancer-related pathways, such as tumor suppressor genes, growth-signaling factors, transcription factors, apoptotic genes, oncoproteins, the biomarkers of inflammation, or protein kinases [29].

3.1.1. Anticancer Activity and the Suppression of Carcinogenesis

One of the main mechanisms of the anticancer effects of curcumin is due to its interference in the cell cycle and reduction in cyclin-dependent kinase (CDK) expression that controls cell-cycle progression [80]. Curcumin is able to suppress the human epidermal growth factor receptor 2, a tyrosine kinase (HER2-TK), and in this manner inhibits breast cancer cell lines [81]. By administering curcumin, there is a decrease in the activation of the PI3K (phosphoinositide 3-kinase)/AKT (AKT serine/threonine kinase) signaling pathway, resulting in an anticancer effect via the negative modulation of this cell-signaling pathway [30].

Curcumin can modulate the activity of different transcription factors, inhibiting some of them, such as nuclear factor-κB (NF-κB), activated protein-1 (AP-1), signal transducer and activator of transcription (STAT) proteins, hypoxia-inducible factor-1 (HIF-1), Notch-1, early growth response-1 (Egr-1), and β-catenin, but activating others, such as NF-E2-related factor (Nrf2) [29,31]. Transcription factors play an important role in various stages of carcinogenesis, being involved in cell proliferation, cell survival, invasion, angiogenesis, and inflammation. Most of these factors are upregulated in most cancers [31]. It has been demonstrated that curcumin inhibits STAT3 phosphorylation, which is responsible for signaling carcinogenic pathways [21]. Furthermore, curcumin is a potent inhibitor of NF-κB, and this effect is correlated with cellular apoptotic response [22]. Likewise, curcumin stimulates the expression of pro-apoptotic Bax and inhibits the activation of Mcl-1 and Bcl-2 (apoptosis regulator) antiapoptotic agents, also altering the expression of apoptotic mechanisms associated with NF-κB proteins, p38 and p53 [23].

3.1.2. Inhibition of Angiogenesis

In some tumors, curcumin inhibits angiogenesis by suppressing angiogenic cytokines, such as *IL-6*, *IL-23*, and *IL-1β* [82], and it is a direct inhibitor of angiogenesis by downregulating transcription factors, such as NF-κB, and proangiogenesis factors, such as bFGF (basic fibroblast growth factor), VEGF (vascular endothelial growth factor), and MMPs (matrix metalloproteinases), all of them linked with tumorigenesis [83].

3.1.3. Anti-Inflammatory Properties

Curcumin is a highly pleiotropic molecule, able to interact with numerous molecular targets involved in the inflammatory process, hence the strong anti-inflammatory action both in the acute phase and in the chronic phase of inflammation. Due to its strong anti-inflammatory effects, in several studies, curcumin showed the ability to prevent the development of some types of cancer by reducing the production of COX-2, lipoxygenase 2, iNOS, and related cytokines, known as mediators of the inflammatory process [84].

Furthermore, curcuminoids are able to exert antioxidant action by blocking free-circulating radicals and inhibiting the formation of new ones [85]. Curcumin can also increase the antioxidant activity, in vitro and in vivo, of the enzymes SOD, CAT, GST, and GSR, and, in this manner, curcumin directly inhibits the formation of reactive species, including superoxide radicals, nitric oxide radicals, and hydrogen peroxide. On the other hand, curcumin also increases the activity of detoxifying enzymes by reducing xenobiotics, therefore protecting against carcinogenic processes [86]. In light of these facts, research is aimed at clarifying the beneficial effects of the combination of curcumin with various antineoplastic drugs so as to improve their clinical effects and reduce their toxicity [81,87].

Although curcumin has significant medicinal properties, its poor bioavailability has limited the success of in vivo epigenetic studies, only partly bypassed by the possibility of using high dosages of the active ingredient in relation to its very low toxicity. Recently, pharmaceutical research has led to the introduction in the market of molecules with better bioavailability (phytosome technology), also opening new therapeutic horizons in terms of preventive medicine and antiaging [88].

The extremely poor bioavailability of curcumin is due to its low aqueous solubility, poor absorption, and rapid metabolism and elimination [77,89,90]. Curcumin is a hydrophobic polyphenol, practically insoluble in water between pH 1–6 [90,91]. Although some studies indicate the dissolution of curcumin in slightly basic water or aqueous buffer, there is, however, no extraordinary increase in solubility under more alkaline conditions. Moreover, curcumin becomes very susceptible to degradation, particularly around neutral pH, i.e., at a pH above 6.5 [89,92].

The low absorption rate of curcumin in the gastrointestinal tract is due to the hydrophobic nature of curcumin [77]. A series of clinical studies analyzed by Nelson et al. showed that although curcumin was administered in a high oral dose of up to 12 g/day, which was well tolerated, the absorption of the compound was negligible and curcumin could not be detected in the serum of most subjects tested [93]. Dei Cas and Ghidoni confirmed, in other two studies performed on healthy volunteers, that curcumin was detected only in the plasma of one of the subjects from the first study, and only in the plasma of two of the twenty-four subjects enrolled in the second study, respectively, and only after a high single oral dose of 10–12 g [91]. Regarding the distribution of curcumin through the body, one study shows that the compound is degraded and/or transformed before and/or after absorption, while the results of several studies suggest that curcumin is not distributed to any specific organ at appreciable levels [93]. The liver is the main organ responsible for the metabolism of curcumin, along with the intestine and intestinal microbiota. In humans, phase I metabolism consists of the reduction of the double bonds of curcumin, in enterocytes and hepatocytes, through the action of alcohol dehydrogenase, forming mostly dihydrocurcumin, tetrahydrocurcumin, hexahydrocurcumin, and octahydrocurcumin, while dihydroferulic acid and ferulic acid are minor biliary metabolites [77,90,91,93]. Curcumin and its reduced metabolites are then subjected to phase II metabolism by conjugation with glucuronic acid and sulfate at the phenolic positions [94]. Intestinal microbiota, through *Escherichia coli* and *Blautia* sp., has been shown to be responsible for an alternative metabolism of curcumin. Several studies suggest that some of the curcumin metabolites may be more active than curcumin [90,91]. After oral administration, curcumin and its metabolites are mostly excreted in the feces, the urinary excretion being extremely low [77,94].

Moreover, the clinical use of curcumin may be also limited by its photodegradation in light, being affected both the structure and properties of curcumin [95].

In order to overcome the main disadvantages related to the oral administration of curcumin, new strategies for its efficient delivery have been investigated. Among the curcumin formulation strategies used in order to enhance its absorption are lipid additions (such as turmeric oil, piperine, or turmeric oleoresin), the adsorption and dispersion of curcumin onto various matrices (such as γ-cyclodextrin or whey protein), and particle size reduction, but also modified structures of curcumin analogs and micellar and nanoparticle formulations of curcumin [94,96]. Unfortunately, some of these formulations claimed an enhanced bioavailability of curcumin only on the basis of increased solubility, without considering the solubility–permeability interplay in the gastrointestinal tract when using solubility-enabling formulations for oral lipophilic drugs [94,97]. The most important goals in the development of curcumin delivery systems are enhancing solubility, increasing bioavailability by enhancing small intestine permeation, preventing degradation in the intestinal environment, increasing content in the bloodstream, and increasing efficacy. Among the delivery systems that have shown promising results in this regard are micelles, liposomes, phospholipid complexes, nanoemulsions, microemulsions, emulsions, solid lipid nanoparticles, nanostructured lipid carriers, biopolymer nanoparticles, microgels, nanogels, etc. [94,96,98–100].

3.2. Resveratrol

Resveratrol (3,5,4′-trihydroxystilbene) is a stilbenoid, a polyphenolic phytoalexin produced by some plants in response to injury or attack by pathogens, such as fungi or bacteria. Sources of resveratrol in food include grapes (*Vitis vinifera* L.), blueberries (*Vaccinium corymbosum* L.), raspberries (*Rubus idaeus* L.), mulberries (*Morus alba* Hort. ex Loudon L.), and peanuts (*Arachis hypogaea* L.). Resveratrol presents two geometric isomers: *cis*-(Z) and *trans*-(E). The *trans* form exposed to ultraviolet radiation can undergo isomerization to the *cis form* [101]. The *cis* form is dominant in prevalence and especially in= biological activity such as cell-cycle arrest, apoptosis, differentiation, and the antiproliferation of cancer cells [102,103]. Originally, resveratrol was isolated by Takaoka in 1940, from the roots of white hellebore (*Veratrum album* L.), and in 1963, from knotweed (*Polygonum cuspidatum* Sieb. et Zucc) root. However, only in 1992 did resveratrol attract attention when its presence in wine was associated with the cardioprotective effects of this beverage. *Polygonum cuspidatum* Sieb. et Zucc. is one of the richest sources of resveratrol in nature and, for this reason, it has become a very important plant in modern herbal medicine [104,105].

3.2.1. Antioxidant and Anti-Inflammatory Activity

Resveratrol is able to exert powerful antioxidant and anti-inflammatory action. As an antioxidant, it has a superior activity to that of more known molecules, such as vitamin C and E, and is also more effective than flavonoids because it also acts upstream of the reaction, rendering copper inactive as a catalyst through its chelation [106].

In addition to the direct antioxidant effect, resveratrol also regulates the gene expression of the prooxidant and antioxidant enzymes: SOD1 and GPX1 are strengthened by resveratrol in a concentration-dependent manner. Therefore, the suppression of the expression of the prooxidant genes (via NADPH-oxidase) and the induction of antioxidant enzymes, such as SOD1 and GPX1, are important components of the antioxidant protective effect induced by resveratrol [107]. Resveratrol has been proven to be an effective scavenger of free radicals, including superoxide radical (O^{2-}), hydrogen peroxide (H_2O_2), hydroxyl radical (OH^-), nitric oxide (NO), and nitrogen dioxide (NO_2) [108,109].

However, direct scavenger activities are relatively scarce, also due to the reduced in vivo half-life of this molecule. The antioxidant properties of resveratrol in vivo, on the other hand, are due to its effect as a regulator of gene expression. Resveratrol induces the downregulation of NADPH-oxidase, with a consequent reduction in reactive oxygen species (ROS). Furthermore, by hyperstimulating tetrahydrobiopterin-GTP-cyclohydrolase, the expression of a variety of antioxidant enzymes is increased. Some of the genes regulating the effect of resveratrol are mediated by Nrf2 [110].

3.2.2. Resveratrol and Cells Apoptosis

The role of resveratrol as a modulator of cell apoptosis is fundamental. The cellular apoptosis promoted by resveratrol can be mediated by multiple mechanisms, such as the upregulation of cyclin-dependent kinase inhibitors; the activation of mitochondria and cascade of caspases, apoptosis-inducing cytokines, and related receptors; the downregulation of cell survival proteins (e.g., survivin, XIAP (X-linked inhibitor of apoptosis protein), cIAPs, cFLIP, Bcl-XL, Bcl-2); and the inhibition of cell survival kinases (e.g., MAPK, AKT/phosphoinositide 3-kinase (PI3K), PKC, EGFR kinase) and transcription survival factors (e.g., NF-κB, AP-1, HIF-1α, and signal transducer and transcription activator (STAT3)). The induction of one of these pathways by resveratrol leads to cell death [32,33].

Resveratrol regulates proteins involved in DNA and cell-cycle synthesis, such as p53 and Rb/E2F, CDK, and their inhibitors. Resveratrol influences the activity of transcription factors involved in proliferation and stress response, such as NF-κB, AP1, and EGR1. One part of these events is mediated by MAPK and tyrosine kinase, for example, SRC, and leads to the modulation of survival and apoptotic factors (e.g., members of the Bcl-2 family, inhibitors of apoptosis) as well as to the modulation of enzymes involved in carcinogenesis (e.g., cyclooxygenase (COX), nitric oxide synthase (NOS), phase I and II enzymes) [32]. Finally, resveratrol helps regulate the activity and expression of co-transcription factors such as p300 and SIRT1 [34].

A limited number of studies have demonstrated that resveratrol administration leads to the restoration of the hyper- and hypomethylated states of several oncogenic and tumor suppressor genes [111]. In HCC1806 breast cancer cells, resveratrol downregulates the DNMT1, DNMT3a, DNMT3b, and negatively regulated hTERT with the inhibition of SIRT followed by the inhibition of breast cancer cell growth [112]. In colon cancer, the administration of resveratrol increases SIRT1 expression and decreases NF-κB, with antiproliferative effects on colon cancer cell lines. In prostate cancer cells, resveratrol downregulates the metastasis-associated protein 1, MTA1, allowing the acetylation/activation of p53 [113]. Resveratrol is able to inhibit cell proliferation and metastasis by modulating genes involved in cell cycle regulation and by upregulating p53, leading to enhanced apoptosis [35]. Regarding microRNA modulation, resveratrol decreases several oncogenic microRNAs, including miR17, miR25, and miR 92a-2, and increases the expression of tumor-suppressive miR 34a and miR 663 in colon cancer [36,37]. In breast cancer, resveratrol increases the expression of miR-141 and miR-200 with the inhibition of the proliferation of cancer cells [38]. In light of these studies, resveratrol appears capable of exerting antioxidant and chemopreventive activities and could be considered an epigenetic drug.

Resveratrol also promotes the activation of sirtuins [39] (Figure 2) in synergy with melatonin. The fact that melatonin and resveratrol are present in various foods implies possible synergistic effects, suggesting combined use to promote health and longevity [114].

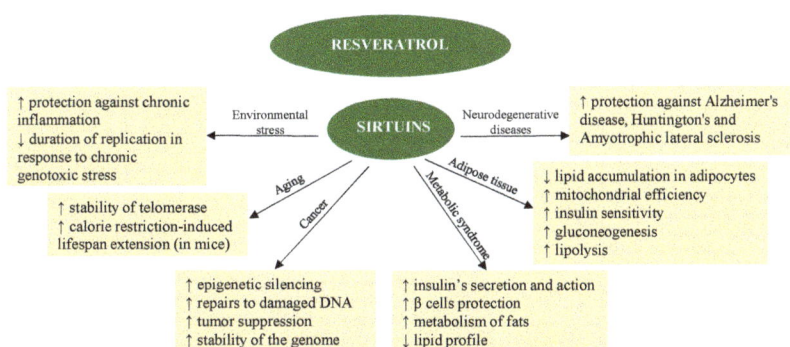

Figure 2. Resveratrol exerts different effects by activating sirtuin [4].

The mechanism of epigenetic action in the case of resveratrol also suggests its indication in the treatment of neurodegenerative diseases [115,116]. In fact, the neuroprotective and neurotrophic effects induced by resveratrol have been the subject of multiple studies, both in vitro and in vivo, and make it again a dietary epidrug in the adjuvant treatment and prevention of these diseases [116]. Resveratrol induces autophagy, directly inhibiting the mTOR pathway through interaction with the ATP-binding pocket of mTOR (it direct competes with ATP) [117]. Likewise, it induces the death of tumor cells, also thanks to the inhibition of the mTORC1 pathway [118].

It is necessary to remember that the TOR gene and the expressed mTOR protein are modulated by nutrients and regulate cell growth, motility, proliferation, survival, and protein synthesis and transcription, acting as kind of centralized modulators of various metabolic signals [118,119].

However, the reasons that limit the effectiveness of resveratrol in vivo are dosage and bioavailability. The bioavailability of resveratrol is very low because of its very fast metabolism [70]. Despite having high cellular membrane permeability and being a lipid-soluble compound, resveratrol has poor water solubility (~0.03 mg/mL) and high chemical instability that affects its bioavailability [120,121].

After ingestion, resveratrol undergoes rapid absorption [122]. At a low oral dose (25 mg), the absorption rate is high (~75%), being absorbed by various cell types, but it is not known exactly whether this rate of absorption is maintained at higher doses [123]. However, in dose-escalation studies, resveratrol showed linear pharmacokinetics, even at high doses [124]. After oral administration, resveratrol is absorbed in the intestine by passive diffusion, and once in the bloodstream, is absorbed in the liver by passive diffusion or receptor-mediated transport [120,121,125]. Then, resveratrol can undergo phase II metabolism in the liver, leading to glucuronide–resveratrol and sulfate–resveratrol derivatives, or it can be found in the blood as a free molecule, 90% in the form of complexes, being attached in a non-covalent manner to proteins, such as albumin and lipoproteins (especially LDL), and a small proportion existing in the form of a free fraction of uncomplexed resveratrol [122,126,127]. At the cell membrane level, the complexes will dissociate, following the interaction of albumin and LDL with specific receptors, leaving resveratrol free to enter the cells [121,123,127]. Of the more than 20 metabolites of resveratrol identified in humans and animals, the glucuronide and sulfate conjugates from phase II metabolism are the most abundant, with plasma levels higher than ingested resveratrol [120].

In addition to its rapid metabolism, resveratrol also undergoes rapid excretion, with 75% of the total resveratrol consumed being excreted. Two human studies showed that after the oral administration of 25 mg of resveratrol, the maximum concentration of resveratrol in circulating plasma was below 10 ng/mL, 0.5 h after the oral dose [122,127]. These results show that despite the rapid absorption of resveratrol, its plasma levels are low due to its rapid metabolism [122]. To conclude, the very low oral bioavailability of resveratrol (less than 1–2% of the dose in humans and around 40% in rats) is associated with several factors, such as poor water solubility, which affects its absorption; the high permeability of the intestinal membrane; isomerization due to light exposure; auto-oxidation; and rapid and extensive pre-systemic metabolism [125,127–130].

Although numerous in vitro studies have shown a wide variety of biological activities associated with resveratrol, these effects cannot be extrapolated in vivo. Therefore, animal studies and clinical trials have not shown similar efficacy for this molecule, as the tissue distribution of resveratrol is very low [122,126,127]. However, resveratrol has also been shown to be efficient in vivo, despite its low bioavailability. The efficacy of resveratrol in vivo may be due to the conversion of its conjugated forms to resveratrol in the liver; to the enterohepatic recirculation of its metabolites, followed by deconjugation and reabsorption; or to the activity of its metabolites [127]. Although it is not known exactly whether the efficacy of resveratrol is due to the compound itself or its metabolites, resveratrol has been shown to be more active than its metabolite, resveratrol monosulfate, in two human bladder cancer (HBC) cell lines, showing greater anti-tumor effects than resveratrol monosulfate and producing a better safety profile in vitro [124]. In contrast, evaluating the effect of resveratrol and its metabolites on the gut barrier and microbiota in a CD-1 mouse model, it was observed that its metabolite, resveratrol-3-O-sulfate, better regulates gut microbial growth and provides superior gut barrier function than resveratrol [124]. Another intensively studied resveratrol metabolite, dihydro-resveratrol, has been shown to be a more effective antioxidant than the vitamin E analog, Trolox [120,131]. In terms of piceatannol, studies show that it has similar biological effects to resveratrol, or is even stronger than its precursor [132]. It has been found in large amounts, as a resveratrol metabolite, in plasma, skin, and liver tissue after the administration of resveratrol in mouse models [120].

Resveratrol bioavailability is increased by gastric juices, so it is recommended to take it with meals [133]. In addition, the circadian rhythm and the type of meal may influence bioavailability [123,134]. Therefore, in order to increase the bioavailability of resveratrol, the best time to administer it turned out to be in the morning [134]. There are wide margins of safety and non-toxicity. Lower doses have a beneficial effect, while higher doses (2 g/day or more) can be associated with a number of side effects, such as diarrhea, nausea, abdominal pain, hypersensitivity, or frontal headache [121,123]. The best dose range, for an actual clinical benefit in vivo, is between 250 mg and 500 mg/day [135].

One of the strategies that may improve the pharmacokinetics and bioavailability of resveratrol is the synergism with other phytochemicals, such as piperine. Thus, the co-administration of resveratrol and piperine has improved the bioavailability of resveratrol by inhibiting its rapid metabolism [126,130]. The use of polydatin, a compound that is extracted from the roots of the *Polygonum cuspidatum* Sieb. et Zucc. plant and differs from resveratrol by the presence of one molecule of glucose—which makes the compound more water-soluble and, consequently, more bioavailable than resveratrol—has also been discussed [121]. It has also been considered to increase the bioavailability of orally administered resveratrol by using alternative routes of administration, such as inhalers and transdermal, buccal, and nasal–brain routes, obtaining promising results [124].

Other measures that may improve the pharmacokinetics of resveratrol, and therefore bioavailability, have focused on innovative delivery systems, such as nanoemulsions, nanosuspensions, dendrimers, liposomes and nanoliposomes, solid lipid nanoparticles, and polymeric nanoparticles [125,126,130].

3.3. Sulforaphane, Indole-3-Carbinol, and 3,3′-Diindolylmethane

The consumption of cruciferous vegetables, such as broccoli (*Brassica oleracea* var. *italica* Plenck), cabbage (*Brassica oleracea* var. *capitata* L.), brussels sprouts (*Brassica oleracea* var. *gemmifera* Zenker), cauliflower (*Brassica oleracea* var. *botrytis* L.), and kale (*Brassica oleracea* var. *viridis* DC. L.) has been associated with anticancer and antioxidant effects. Considerable evidence shows that glucosinolates (GLSs) are the main phytochemicals in cruciferous vegetables that contribute to their health effects [136]. GLSs are relatively inactive and necessitate hydrolysis by plant endogenous myrosinase (MYR) to deliver a variety of bioactive compounds, such as isothiocyanates (ITCs) and indoles. Neutral pH conditions are favorable for the formation of ITCs [137,138]. GLSs and the enzyme MYR are stored in different compartments of plant cells, requiring plant tissue to be damaged for cellular breakdown to occur and MYR to be released and act on GLSs. Therefore, the processing of cruciferous vegetables (i.e., by mastication, cutting, chopping) has an important impact on the bioavailability of GLSs and their hydrolysis products [139,140]. Furthermore, MYR tends to be denatured when cooking cruciferous vegetables, particularly in conditions of increased temperature (>80 °C) and prolonged cooking [136]. In this context, recent research has indicated steaming to be a cooking method more appropriate than boiling in increasing the bioavailability of ITCs from cruciferous vegetables [141,142]. Interesting results are also provided by a study showing that when MYR in cruciferous vegetables is denatured by heating, the supplementation of exogenous MYR can improve the conversion of GLSs to ITCs. More precisely, the study reported that the addition to cooked broccoli of an active source of MYR, in the form of powdered mustard seeds, increased over four times the bioavailability of the ITC sulforaphane (SFN) compared to the bioavailability of SFN in cooked broccoli consumed alone [143].

Nevertheless, even if MYR is inactivated by the thermal treatment of cruciferous vegetables, the ingested GLSs are able to reach the colon, where they can be metabolized by MYR-producing gut bacteria, generating hydrolysis products such as ITCs, which are absorbed or/and excreted [137,144,145]. The hydrolysis of GLSs by the human microbiota has been reported to be highly variable and diverse, a phenomenon that may be attributed to differences in microbiota composition between individuals [146].

Furthermore, the consumption of cruciferous vegetables in their raw form seems to be of interest in order to ensure a better intake of GLS hydrolysis products. Conaway et al. reported that the bioavailability of ITCs from fresh broccoli was about three times higher than that from cooked broccoli, in which MYR is inactivated [147]. Indeed, if MYR remains active in the ingested cruciferous vegetable, it will hydrolyze most GLSs in the small intestine and generate breakdown products that are absorbed at this level [137].

Concerning the assimilation by the body of the GLS hydrolysis products, absorbed ITCs are conjugated to glutathione, with the involvement of glutathione-S-transferase (GST) enzymes, and metabolized via the mercapturic acid pathway [138]. The polymorphisms of genes coding for GST may have an important effect on ITC metabolism, leading to interindividual variations in the benefits from exposure to these compounds. For instance, individuals carrying deletions in both GST M1 and GST T1 genes may show a more rapid elimination of ITCs, requiring a high intake of cruciferous vegetables in order to capitalize on their positive health effects [148]. As for the metabolism of indoles, molecules such as indole-3-carbinol (I3C) principally undergo oxidative metabolization to indole-3-carboxaldehyde and indole-3-carboxylic acid. The quantification of ITC and indole metabolites in human urine and plasma may serve as an approach to characterize the intake of bioactive compounds from cruciferous vegetables [149,150]. Indeed, it has been demonstrated that the urinary elimination of mercapturic acids after the consumption of cooked cruciferous vegetables accounts for a maximum of 20% of the ingested GLSs. If the vegetables are consumed in the raw form, the rate can reach 88% [137].

To date, the most extensively studied ITCs and indoles are SFN and I3C, respectively. SFN is the precursor of glucoraphanin, the main GLS in broccoli, accounting for about 80% of the total yield [73]. Glucobrassicin is also an important GLS in broccoli [150]. The cleavage of glucobrassicin by MYR generates predominantly I3C. In the acidic conditions at the gastric level, I3C further forms a mixture of dimers, linear and cyclic trimers, and higher oligomers, with 3,3′-diindolylmethane (DIM) being the major condensation product [149,151]. Between 20 and 40% of the ingested I3C is converted to DIM [40]. In fact, several studies have suggested that the health effects of I3C can be mainly attributed to DIM [151,152]. I3C, as well as its acid condensation products, are absorbed at the intestinal level and then distributed into several well-perfused tissues, where they exhibit their biological activities [153].

Currently, SFN, I3C, and DIM are considered promising cancer chemopreventive compounds. I3C is also recognized to have biological properties such as the inhibition of inflammation and angiogenesis, decreases in proliferation, and the promotion of tumor cell death [154].

3.3.1. Chemopreventive Activity and Epigenetic Role

There is much evidence to connect the chemopreventive properties of I3C, DIM, and SFN with epigenetic mechanisms [155]. Several studies suggest that, at least in part, the chemopreventive effects of I3C are due to the downregulation of class I HDAC isoenzymes (HDAC1, HDAC2, HDAC3, and HDAC8) by DIM. Decreased HDAC expression leads to the increased expression of the pro-apoptotic Bcl-2 (B-cell lymphoma 2)-associated X (Bax) protein, CDKNs p21, and p27 followed by the arrest of the cell cycle and increased rate of apoptosis. For this reason, HDAC inhibition may be a novel epigenetic mechanism for cancer prevention by DIM [41].

SFN may target the aberrant hypermethylation status by downregulating the expression of DNMT1 and DNMT3a in breast cancer cells [42].

Cyclin D2 is a major regulator of the cell cycle and its hypermethylation is correlated with prostate cancer progression. SFN is capable of decreasing the expression of DNMT1 and DNMT3b and epigenetically modulating cyclin D2 expression, acting as a prostate cancer chemopreventive agent [43].

I3C and DIM modulate the expression of several miRNAs and lncRNAs [82,83]. Thus, DIM increases the expression of tumor suppressor microRNAs, such as let-7a-e, miRNA-15a, miRNA-16, miR-27b, miR-30e, miR-31, miR-34a, miR-124, miR 200 a, miR 200b, miR 200c, miR-219-5p, and miR-320, and decreases the expression of oncogenic miR19a, miR19b, miR92a-2, miR 106a, miR 181a, miR 181b, miR 210-3p, miR 221, and miR 495 [40,44,45].

3.3.2. Effect of Estrogen Analog and Anticarcinogenic in Mammary Tumor Cells

I3C is capable of arresting the growth of human tumor cells in the G1 phase of the reproductive cell cycle [156]. I3C is also a potent inducer of cytochrome P450 enzymes, including CYP1A1, CYP1A2, and CYP1B1 [157,158]. These phase I metabolizing enzymes are involved in the oxidative metabolism of estrogens. I3C and DIM can alter endogenous estrogen metabolism by increasing the 2-hydroxylation reaction, resulting in an increase in the 2-OH:16-OH ratio relative to the estrogen metabolites [159]. The metabolites of these hormones can inhibit or stimulate the onset of hormone-sensitive neoplasms [160]. Several studies have demonstrated that estrone 2 (2OHE1) tends to inhibit the growth of the neoplasm, whereas estrone 16 (16OHE1) promotes tumor growth [161]. The individuals with estrone 2 prevalence are more protected than those with higher levels of estrone 16. Clinical studies have shown that the estrone 2/estrone 16 ratio is an important marker regarding the risk of breast cancer. When this ratio is lower than unity, there are severe clinical forms, while when this ratio is higher than three, the consequences are more favorable [162]. Other products resulting from estrone and estradiol conversion are 2-hydroxylated estrogens, such as 2-hydroxyestrone and 2-hydroxyestradiol, which show anticancer properties that equate them to antiestrogens, targeting several aspects of cancer cell cycle survival and regulation, including cyclin-dependent kinase activities, caspase activation, estrogen metabolism, and estrogen receptor signaling [163,164].

The positive effects of I3C and DIM are related to the fact that both are capable of modifying the estradiol hydroxylation receptor site, resulting in the diminution of 16-α-hydroxyestrone production in favor of 2-hydroxyestrone. I3C and DIM are also involved in the stimulation of liver detoxifying enzyme production, capable of neutralizing and degrading the harmful metabolites of estrogens and xenoestrogens, assimilated as environmental or food pollutants [165,166].

3.3.3. Anticancer Activity

The SFN also exhibits anticancer action by controlling the progression of tumorigenesis. In non-small cell lung cancer (NSCLC), the SFN is able to attenuate the signaling pathway of EGFR, suggesting an anticancer mechanism of action [46]. As a whole, it has shown multiple effects, including the arrest of cell growth, differentiation, and apoptosis, as recently demonstrated in the case of prostate neoplasms [47].

SFN inhibits the proliferation, in vivo, of breast cancer cells, while in normal cells the effect is insignificant. Cancer cells are characterized by the high expression of telomerase. Treatment with SFN inhibits the catalytic subunit of human telomerase reverse transcriptase (hTERT) [167]. At the same time, scientific studies have shown interference in DNA methyltransferase (DNMT) activity, in particular DNMT1 and DNMT3a, which have been reduced in breast cancer cells treated with SFN, suggesting that this compound may be able to repress hTERT through specific epigenetic pathways. Furthermore, the downregulation of hTERT expression facilitates the induction of cell apoptosis in breast cancer cells, paving the way for approaches aimed at the SFN-mediated prevention of this neoplasia and as preventive nutraceuticals [48].

3.3.4. Anti-Inflammatory Activity

Inflammation is usually associated with chronic disease and cancer. It is well known that NF-κB is a major transcription factor involved in the regulation of the expression of many pro-inflammatory genes, such as COX-2 and iNOS. I3C and DIM exert anti-inflammatory effects by the downregulation of COX-2, iNOS, CXCL5, and IL-6 expression, which may be mediated by reductions in NF-κB activation [168].

In conclusion, the GLSs present in cruciferous vegetables have beneficial effects on general health and are also potential anticancer agents, due to their antioxidant and detoxifying properties and epigenetic mechanisms, including the modification of CpG (cytosine–phosphate–guanine) methylation, which occurs predominantly in cancer-related genes, the regulation of histone modification, and changes in miRNA expression [169,170].

The daily dosage of SFN demonstrated to provide beneficial health effects is around 20–40 mg [171]. Furthermore, the recommended daily dosage for I3C ranges between 200 mg and 900 mg per day and for DIM between 25 mg and 450 mg per day, respectively. The use over time must include both urinary and blood hormone monitoring, including, in the urine, the observation of the relationship between estrone 2 and estrone 16 and, at the hematic level, of the total estrone and estradiol and total and free testosterone and androstenedione, so as to constantly adapt the therapy. A diet rich in cruciferous vegetables seems to provide SFN, I3C, and DIM in sufficient amounts for the prevention of many types of cancer, including those that are hormone-related, such as breast, ovary, uterus, and prostate neoplasms [172–174]. In contrast, to achieve therapeutic concentrations of SFN, I3C, and DIM, the intake of these compounds in the form of dietary supplements seems to be required [40,175].

The exploitation of SFN by the nutraceutical industry has faced some challenges because this ITC shows high lipophilicity, low aqueous solubility, and poor stability due to sensitivity to oxygen, heat, and alkaline conditions. However, the use of nanotechnology has allowed the increase in the aqueous solubility and bioavailability of SFN through the development of formulations such as polymeric nanoparticles, magnetic nanoparticles, micelles, liposomes, and carbon dots [175].

Likewise, the low thermal- and photostability of I3C and DIM represent important challenges for the nutraceutical application of these compounds. One approach to overcome this issue has been proposed by Luo et al. (2013), who showed that the encapsulation of I3C and DIM in zein/carboxymethyl chitosan nanoparticles can protect these bioactives against temperature- and light-induced degradation [176].

3.4. Astaxanthin

Astaxanthin (3,3′-dihydroxy-β, β′-carotene-4,4′-dione) (ASX) is a red-orange pigment, a xanthophyll carotenoid, and a member of the macro-family of carotenoids [177]. Synthesized in appropriate quantities by microalgae—*Haematococcus lacustris* (Gir.-Chantr.) Rostaf., *Chromochloris zofingiensis* (Donz) Fucikova and L. A. Lewis, *Chlorococcum sp.*, and *Phaffia rhodozyma* M.W. Mill., Yoney. and Soneda—ASX enters the food chain through crustaceans and predatory fish such as salmon, in whose meat it can easily reach 5–10 mg/kg [178].

ASX has antioxidant potential, as well as anti-inflammatory and antineoplastic activities, acting as an antioxidant and reducing oxidative stress, thereby preventing protein and lipid oxidation and DNA damage. Having antioxidant action, it helps to maintain the functionality of tissues and systems, promoting better overall homeostasis [177].

ASX affects tumor growth in different types of cancers. Several studies have demonstrated that ASX is able to resensitize gemcitabine-resistant human pancreatic cancer cells to gemcitabine [49]. ASX increases DNMT3a expression at low concentrations, but at high concentrations decreases the expression of DNMT1, 3a, and 3b and attenuates NAD(P)H Quinone Dehydrogenase 1 (NQO1) expression via the Nrf2/KEAP1 pathway, reducing cell viability in prostate and skin cancer cells [50,51]. ASX has also the ability to reduce tumor growth in prostate cancer by increasing the expression of tumor suppressor microRNAs, miR-375 and miR-478b [52]. In breast cancer, ASX negatively affects cell viability [179,180], due to apoptotic and autophagic effects that allow it to kill the cancer cells without affecting normal cells [181].

In colorectal cancer (CRC), ASX has demonstrated anti-migratory and anti-invasive activity by increasing miR-29a-3p and miR-200a expression, suppressing MMP2 and ZEB1 expression, resulting in the repression of the epithelial–mesenchymal transition (EMT) of CRC cells [53]. Regarding lung cancer, NSCLC accounts for the majority of lung cancer-related deaths [182]. There are few studies to show the effects of ASX against NSCLC or other lung cancers in vivo. In vitro, ASX is able to reduce the viability of NSCLC cells in a dose-dependent manner [183,184]. Moreover, ASX enhances apoptosis and decreases cell proliferation. ASX is able to enhance the cytotoxicity of the drugs with clinical activity in NSCLS, such as erlotinib, a selective epidermal growth factor receptor (EGFR) tyrosine kinase inhibitor. The co-administration of erlotinib and ASX has increased cytotoxicity and inhibited cell growth in NSCLC cells, associated with the downregulation of xeroderma pigmentosum complementation group C (XPC) expression [184]. The overexpression of thymidylate synthase (TS) usually causes resistance to antitumor treatment, especially pemetrexed used in advanced NSCLC forms. ASX treatment decreases TS expression, both alone and in combination with pemetrexed. Moreover, ASX administration together with mitomycin C significantly reduces Rad51 expression, which exhibits high levels in chemoresistant carcinoma [54,55].

All these in vitro findings suggest that ASX may improve the efficacy of standard treatments in lung cancer. Some studies have also suggested that ASX could be used to treat gastric cancer, based on its role in necroptotic signaling [185].

Despite its biological activities, ASX has very low bioavailability, similar to other carotenoids [55,186]. When astaxanthin is administered orally, the bioavailability varies between 10 and 50% of the given dose [187]. The very poor bioavailability of ASX is due to dissolution limitations in gastrointestinal fluids and also to the saturated capacity of incorporation into bile micelles, which limits its absorption [188,189]. Being a very lipophilic compound, it has extremely low water solubility, which prevents its dispersibility and causes a low absorption rate [55,190]. After ingestion, ASX mixes with bile acid, forming micelles in the small intestine, partially absorbed by intestinal mucosa cells, which will incorporate astaxanthin into chylomicrons [178]. After their release into the lymph within the systemic circulation, chylomicrons with ASX are digested by lipoprotein lipase, ASX is assimilated with lipoproteins and transported to tissues, and chylomicrons remnants are quickly removed by the liver and other tissues [178]. In nature, astaxanthin is predominantly found in the form of mono- and diesters, being, respectively, esterified with one or two units of fatty acids in hydroxyl groups, or in the form of carotenoproteins when conjugated with proteins [187]. Recent research shows that ASX bioavailability varies depending on its molecular structure, origin, and isomerization [187,191,192]. Therefore, in the case of natural astaxanthin in esterified form, bioavailability is improved by facilitating its incorporation into mixed micelles in the lumen, where unsaturated lipids are released by the action of bile salts and pancreatic lipases before free astaxanthin is absorbed by intestinal mucosal cells [187]. Of the esterified forms of ASX, monoesters have shown significantly higher bioavailability than astaxanthin diesters [191]. Regarding the difference in bioavailability arising from isomerization, the spatial arrangement of atoms in the case of the 3S,3′S stereoisomer has been shown to increase the bioavailability of astaxanthin compared to the 3R,3′S and 3R,3′R isomers [193,194]. While synthetic ASX is a racemic mixture of the three stereoisomers (3S,3′S; 3R,3′S; 3R,3′R), naturally occurring ASX is in the form of the isomer 3S,3′S [194]. Thus, for the most efficient 3S,3′S stereoisomer, the main primary source is the green alga *Haematococcus lacustris* (Gir.-Chantr.) Rostaf., but also other sources such as *Paracoccus carotinifaciens* Tsubokura et al. or *Salmo salar* L., while the 3R,3′S and 3R,3′R stereoisomers, respectively, have primary sources such as distilled petroleum and the yeast *Phaffia rhodozyma* M.W. Mill., Yoney. and Soneda, respectively [193,194]. In addition, due to its highly unsaturated molecular structure, ASX has reduced chemical stability during processing, storage, and digestion, being easily degraded in both acidic and alkaline environments and also under UV light, oxygen, or heat action [55,195,196]. The bioavailability of ASX has been reported to be increased in humans by its incorporation into lipid formulations of various compositions, and this may be due to the presence of conjugated bile salt and its ability to form bile salt micelles [189]. The combination of ASX with edible oils has led to both high bioavailability and stability [178,193]. Enhanced ASX absorption was demonstrated in a study with a combination of ASX and fish oil, which succeeded in promoting hypolipidemic/hypocholesterolemic effects in plasma and its increased phagocytic activity of activated neutrophils compared to ASX and fish oil separately [193,197]. Moreover, the administration of *Haematococcus lacustris* (Gir.-Chantr.) Rostaf. biomass dispersed in olive oil has shown increased bioavailability and enhanced antioxidant properties in ASX, both in rat plasma and in liver tissues [178,193]. In addition to the dietary fat content, another factor with a major influence on astaxanthin absorption is smoking. Thus, the bioavailability of astaxanthin in smokers is reduced by 40% [193].

In order to improve the water solubility, stability, and bioavailability of ASX, several delivery systems have been developed, such as complex coacervation, liposomes, emulsions and nanoemulsions, microparticles, and polymeric nanoparticles [196,198,199]. Since lipid-based nanoparticles, such as liposomes, solid-lipid nanoparticles, and niosomes have limitations, such as poor water solubility and permeability, instability, rapid metabolism, and poor oral bioavailability, polymeric nanoparticles have begun to be used to overcome these limitations. Thus, after encapsulation in polymeric nanoparticles made from biodegradable natural polymers, such as polysaccharides and proteins, water solubility, stability, and absorption in the human body were enhanced [190,199]. In terms of nanoemulsion-based delivery systems, they provide improved physical stability and increase water dispersibility and bioavailability [184].

3.5. Quercetin

Quercetin is a flavonoid belonging to the flavonols group, present in a large variety of fruits—apples (*Malus domestica* (Suckow) Borkh.), grapes (*Vitis vinifera* L.), olives (*Olea europaea* Hoffmanns. and Link L.), citrus fruits such as oranges (*Citrus sinensis* (L.) Osbeck), and raspberries (*Rubus idaeus* L.)—vegetables—tomatoes (*Solanum lycopersicum* L.), onions (*Allium cepa* L.), broccoli (*Brassica oleracea* var. *italica* Plenck), and capers (*Capparis spinosa* L.)—drinks (tea and red wine), and herbal extracts [128]. In nature, quercetin is not present in the isolated form but is the aglyconic component of some glycosides, including rutin and quercitrin. In this form it abounds, in particular, in extracts of horse chestnut (*Aesculus hippocastanum* L.), *Gingko biloba* L., marigold (*Calendula officinalis* L.), hawthorn (*Crataegus monogyna* Jacq.), chamomile (Matricaria recutita L. and *Chamaemelum nobile* L.), lovage (*Levisticum officinale* W. D. J. Koch), and St. John's wort (*Hypericum perforatum* L.) [200,201]. Quercetin is a natural anti-inflammatory, antioxidant and anti-cancer compound with many abilities, its most important functions being mentioned in Table 3.

Table 3. The most important functions of quercetin.

Quercetin's Functions	References
Ability to restore tocopherol after its transformation into tocopheryl radical.	[202]
Ability to protect the endogenous antioxidant enzymatic systems, catalase (CAT), superoxide dismutase (SOD2), glutathione peroxidase (GPX), and glutathione reductase (GR).	[203]
Ability to eliminate superoxide anion and limit nitric oxide biosynthesis during inflammatory processes.	[204]
Ability to inhibit proinflammatory pathways such as those focused on the action of 5-lipoxygenase, which would otherwise lead to the possible excessive biosynthesis of leukotriene mediators of inflammation and phospholipase A2, which generates arachidonic acid and, in turn, favors the biosynthesis of inflammatory prostaglandins.	[205]
Inhibition of multiple cellular enzymes such as tyrosine kinase (TK) including growth factor receptor EGFR, calcium-phospho-lipid-dependent protein kinase (PKC), and ornithine decarboxylase (ODC), which produces polyamines known to be involved in cell proliferation and phosphoinositide kinases PI3K and PI4P-5K, involved in the proliferative responses triggered by the mitogenic pathways of signal transduction. For these last two properties, quercetin has been extensively studied in oncology, in particular with reference to the mechanisms of cell proliferation and carcinogenesis.	[206,207]
Mimics aromatase inhibitors.	[208]
Antiplatelet and cardioprotective action that limits its use in the case of concomitant intake by the patient of anticoagulant drugs such as dicoumarols.	[209]
Neuroprotective and neurotrophic action as an adjuvant therapy in the case of neurodegenerative diseases and the prevention of the same in subjects with increased susceptibility.	[210]

Many in vitro and in vivo studies have demonstrated the anticancer effects of quercetin against breast, prostate, kidney, colorectal, ovarian, gastric, nasopharyngeal, and pancreatic cancer. The antitumor effects include the inhibition of angiogenesis proliferation, the inhibition of the cell cycle, and tumor metastasis prevention [56].

Quercetin is capable of increasing the pro-apoptotic molecules BAX, caspase-3, caspase-9, and p53 and stimulating the mitochondrial apoptosis pathway, resulting in increased proapoptotic effects [57,59]. Another important feature of quercetin is related to the arrest of the cell cycle in the G1 phase by activating p21 and decreasing D1/Cd4 and E/Cdk2 ratios [211,212]. Several studies have demonstrated that quercetin can inhibit carcinogenesis and metastasis in cancer and is capable of stabilizing p53, a key molecule in cancer therapy involved in cell death and survival regulation [60].

In gastrointestinal cancer (GC), the genes encoding for the proteins urokinase plasminogen activator (uPA) and uPA receptor (uPAR) are strongly associated with this type of cancer, being a crucial pathway for tumor invasion. Quercetin has the ability to decrease the expression of these genes, strongly associated with the suppression of cell viability, migration, and invasion. Likewise, quercetin has antimetastatic effects in GC by interfering with uPA/uPAR systems, AMPKα, NF-kβ, ERK1/2, and PKC-δ regulation [61]. In patients with CRC carrying the KRAS mutant gene, quercetin decreases cell viability and increases apoptosis by AKT pathway repression and the activation of the c-Jun N-terminal kinase (JNK) pathway in mutant KRAS cells [62].

In prostate cancer, quercetin inhibits the expression of androgen receptor (AR) and AR-mediated PSA expression at the transcriptional level with the inhibition of tumor progression. Quercetin can suppress survival protein Akt and enhance prostate cancer apoptosis in a dose-dependent manner [63].

Quercetin decreases IGF1 levels and increases IGFBP3, which is associated with an increase in proapoptotic effects and a decrease in anti-apoptotic proteins BCL2 and BCL-XL [64].

Src is a non-receptor tyrosine kinase that is deregulated in many types of cancer. Quercetin has an anti-NSCLC effect in lung cancer by inhibiting the Src-mediated Fn14/NF-κB pathway [213].

The epigenetic mechanisms associated with quercetin are the suppression of Janus kinase 2 (JAK2) with the inhibition of the proliferation, invasion, and migration of cancer cells [65]. Quercetin can also enhance apoptosis through its DNA-demethylating activity. Quercetin has an inhibiting effect on class I HDAC expression in leukemia cells due to increased proteasomal degradation [66]. Quercetin turns out to be a valid nutraceutical that can help reduce the formation of free radicals and pro-inflammatory substances, proving to be a valuable aid for human health.

Quercetin has also been shown to modulate the expression of microRNAs in different types of cancer by increasing the expression of tumor-suppressive miR-let-7, miR-15a, miR-16, miR-16, miR-22, miR-26, miR-200b-3p, miR-142-3p, miR-146a, miR-217, and miR-330 and decreasing the expression of oncogenic miR-27a, miR-155, miR-21, miR-19b, miR-148c [58].

The bioavailability of quercetin is generally poor and characterized by high interindividual variability, which could explain the conflicting results on quercetin bioactivities reported in various studies [214,215]. Pharmacokinetic studies indicate a low absorption of quercetin, with less than 1% of quercetin being absorbed in humans following oral administration [214,216]. The absorption of quercetin is related to its solubility in the vehicle used for administration [214,217]. Thus, the low solubility of quercetin in water, gastric fluids, and small intestine fluids will limit its absorption in the body [216,218]. The absorption of quercetin depends on its chemical structure. Thus, while quercetin aglycone is absorbed in both the stomach and small intestine, glycosylated forms of quercetin are not absorbed in the stomach and will be absorbed only in the small intestine, after deglycosylation, as quercetin aglycone. Quercetin biotransformation occurs by small intestinal and hepatic xenobiotic metabolism, which consists of three phases: phase I modification, phase II conjugation, and phase III elimination. Quercetin is rapidly eliminated via feces and urine. In addition to poor absorption, another factor limiting the bioavailability of quercetin is its hepatic biliary excretion, a significant proportion of absorbed quercetin being directed to biliary elimination and not to circulation [214,215].

Other factors that may affect quercetin bioavailability include the food matrix, nondigestible fiber, dietary fat, the presence of sugar moieties, and the botanical origin of quercetin. The results of a randomized crossover study, in which six women ingested the same amount of quercetin either in cereal bars or hard capsules, showed that the bioavailability of quercetin is higher when the quercetin aglycone is consumed as a whole food component [218,219]. In a study of rats, the influence of nondigestible oligosaccharides on the bioavailability of quercetin was examined. The co-administration of quercetin with short-chain fructooligosaccharides has been shown to improve the bioavailability of quercetin, as microbial degradation of the quercetin aglycone in the large intestine has been inhibited, thereby promoting the absorption of the quercetin glycoside [214,218]. Since quercetin aglycone is lipophilic, its co-ingestion along with fat has been able to increase the absorption of quercetin by incorporating it into micelles. This was observed in a study using pigs, but the improvement in the quercetin bioavailability in the case of fatty food ingestion was also demonstrated in another in vivo study in humans [214,218,219]. The bioavailability of quercetin may also be influenced by the presence or absence of the glucoside moiety, with studies in pigs showing the increased bioavailability of quercetin glycoside compared to quercetin aglycone, most likely due to the preferential absorption of quercetin glucoside, which is more water-soluble than quercetin aglycone [214]. In addition, the bioavailability of quercetin glycosides may be influenced by the type of sugar moiety [219]. Another factor on which quercetin bioavailability depends is its botanical origin. Thus, comparing the bioavailability of different forms of quercetin derivatives from onions, apples, and tea, it was observed that quercetin glycosides from onions had the highest bioavailability. The bioavailability of quercetin in humans may also be affected by health status, gut microbiota, genetic factors, and oxidative stress [218]. Various approaches have been used to improve the water solubility and bioavailability of quercetin, such as encapsulation in nanoparticles, emulsions and nanoemulsions, hydrogels, cyclodextrin complexation, size reduction (nanosuspension, nanocrystals, nanorods), co-crystallization, and amorphous solid dispersions [216,218,220].

3.6. Epigallocatechin-3-Gallate

EGCG is the most abundant catechin in tea, especially in green tea (*Camellia sinensis* L.). EGCG is a polyphenol with antioxidant and anti-inflammatory action. Besides tea, it is also found in smaller quantities in other foods, such as carob (*Ceratonia siliqua* L.) flour, apples (*Malus domestica* (Suckow) Borkh.), blackberries (*Rubus plicatus* L. Weihe and Nees), raspberries (*Rubus idaeus* L.), pistachios (*Pistacia vera* L.), prunes (*Prunus domestica* L.), peaches (*Prunus persica* (L.) Batsch), and avocados (*Persea americana* Mill.). From the tea plant, for production, the leaf bud and the two adjacent leaves are used together with their stem. Green tea is very rich in polyphenols, and among them, EGCG is the most-studied active ingredient with the highest antioxidant activity [221].

In the case of polyphenols, the antioxidant action is achieved through the oxidation of polyphenols to quinones (which, although toxic to the body, polymerize after their formation, so they are no longer absorbed) and the reduction in the relative substrates. The green tea catechins are capable of modulating epigenetic processes, reversing DNA methylation in the tumor suppressor genes, and increasing their relative transcription. They also modulate DNA methylation, mitigating the effect of DNMT1 (direct enzymatic inhibition, indirect enzymatic inhibition, reduced DNMT1 expression, and reduced translation) [67]. Another epigenetic mechanism would then be related to the redox properties of green tea catechins and their ability to inhibit histone deacetylase (HDAC) [68].

In vivo studies have also shown that the high consumption of green tea, and therefore a high intake of EGCG, has the ability, compared to placebo groups, to decrease the methylation of CDX2 and BMP-2 in gastric carcinoma, with effective epigenetic modulation [69].

EGCG, and tea polyphenols in general, are capable of mediating the epigenetic induction of metalloproteinase inhibitors (TIMP), such as TIMP-3, whose levels have a key role in suppressing the gelatinolytic activity of MMP-2 and MMP-9, involved in the metastatic process. Therefore, EGCG is considered a modulator of metalloproteinase activity, with benefits at oncological levels [70].

EGCG also has the ability to inhibit acute promyelocytic leukemia (APL) by inhibiting cell proliferation and promoting apoptosis [222]. In cell culture and animal models of prostate, breast, skin, liver, bladder, lung, and digestive tract cancer, EGCG induces the inhibition of cell proliferation and apoptosis by affecting the MAPK/ERK pathways and growth factors IGF1, IGF, and IGFBP-3. By inhibiting PI3K/AKT/p-BAD, a cell survival pathway, EGCG controls apoptosis. Moreover, EGCG is able to inhibit angiogenesis, invasion, and VEGF [69]. EGCG is an important regulator of cancer-associated microRNAs and upregulates miR-16, miR-210, and miR-330 and decreases miR-21 and miR-98-5p expression in liver, prostate, and lung cancer [71].

Despite the numerous health-promoting properties of EGCG demonstrated by in vitro and in vivo studies, its use by humans poses challenges due to poor systemic bioavailability [223]. After ingestion, EGCG requires effective intestinal absorption to further exhibit its biological activities. However, EGCG seems to be poorly absorbed by the body, reaching only a reduced concentration in the plasma and then rapidly (<8 h) becoming undetectable in the systemic circulation [224]. Overall, it has been estimated that only about 1% of the orally-consumed EGCG is absorbed into the circulatory system in order to further reach target organs [225]. For instance, research on human subjects has reported a plasma concentration of EGCG as low as 0.15 µM following the consumption of two cups of green tea [226]. Such a result may be due, at least in part, to EGCG being hydrolyzed by esterases in the saliva but also due to this compound being degraded under the alkaline pH conditions of the duodenum. In fact, the EGCG molecule undergoes autoxidation at alkaline pH, with the formation of oxidative products [227]. In addition, EGCG is extensively decomposed by intestinal microorganisms [228]. Indeed, only a minor proportion of the ingested EGCG is absorbed in the upper gastrointestinal tract. The remaining fraction of EGCG transits from the small to the large intestine, where it undergoes metabolism by local microbiota, leading to the formation of various catechin ring-fission products [229]. These latter metabolites can be excreted into urine or reabsorbed into the systemic circulation and further act as bioactives [230,231]. Anti-oxidative, anti-inflammatory, and anti-cancer effects have been reported for catechin ring-fission metabolites, suggesting that these compounds may actually contribute to some of the health benefits attributed to EGCG [224].

As concerns the intestinal absorption of EGCG, this process seems to show low efficiency, as EGCG lacks specific receptors for its absorption and is carried by passive diffusion (e.g., paracellular diffusion, transcellular diffusion) across epithelial cells. Following absorption, EGCG undergoes a phenomenon of active outflow, mediated by components of the efflux transport system (e.g., P-glycoprotein, multidrug resistance-associated proteins, breast cancer resistance proteins) that actively efflux intracellular EGCG to the extracellular intestinal space [225,232]. At the level of the small intestine and liver, EGCG is metabolized by phase II enzymes, releasing glucuronidated, sulfated, and methylated conjugates. EGCG metabolites are excreted through both bile and urine. EGCG can be further reabsorbed from the intestine through the enterohepatic recirculation process [233–235].

To capitalize on the therapeutic potential of EGCG in humans, despite its reduced bioavailability, high intakes have been suggested (e.g., the consumption of 8 to 16 cups/day of green tea) [236]. Nevertheless, using high doses of catechins may be of concern in the context of their dose-dependent toxic effects. A recent report by the European Food Safety Agency indicated a risk of liver damage following the intake of EGCG in the form of dietary supplements, at doses of 800 mg/day or above [237,238]. In order to manage these issues and improve the bioavailability of EGCG, several approaches have been identified. One approach involves the co-administration of EGCG with other bioactives. For instance, a formulation with ascorbic acid and sucrose has been demonstrated to enhance EGCG bioavailability by increasing its bioaccessibility and intestinal uptake from green tea [239]. Likewise, it has been suggested that the ingestion of EGCG on an empty stomach may improve its systemic absorption [240]. Moreover, the structural modification of EGCG by methylation, acyclization, or glycoside modification seems to allow the management of its premature degradation and reduced absorption rate [228,233]. Finally, one promising approach to protect EGCG against unfavorable gastrointestinal conditions and improve its bioavailability includes the design of nanocarriers. Examples of carriers developed for the nanodelivery of green tea catechins comprise surfactant-based nanovesicles (liposomes, phytosomes, niosomes, bilosomes), polysaccharide nanostructures, protein nanoparticles, nanoemulsions, and nanostructured lipid carriers [225,241].

3.7. Lycopene

Lycopene is a non-provitamin A carotenoid, present particularly in tomatoes (*Solanum lycopersicum* L.), but also in apricots (*Prunus armeniaca* S. X. Sun L.), guava (*Psidium guajava* L.), papaya (*Carica papaya* L.), watermelon (*Citrullus lanatus* subsp. *vulgaris* (Schrad.) Fursa), and pink grapefruit (*Citrus × paradisi* Macfad.). The level of ripeness in these fruits influences their lycopene content. For example, the content of lycopene is 50 mg/kg in ripe tomatoes, but only 5 mg/kg in unripe yellow tomatoes [242]. In addition to having a powerful antioxidant action, lycopene can improve the fluidity of the circulating blood mass and reduce the inflammatory response [243].

Carotenoids, as well as their metabolites and oxidation products, improve communication at the level of the intercellular junction gate GJC (Gap Junction Communication), which is considered one of the mechanisms of cancer prevention. GJC is deficient in many forms of cancer and the restoration of this function leads to cell proliferation reduction [244]. Several studies have demonstrated that lycopene is capable of modulating the expression of genes involved in inflammation, apoptosis, and cancer progression and, in this manner, reducing prostate cancer risk [245,246].

11. Ahuja, N.; Sharma, A.R.; Baylin, S.B. Epigenetic Therapeutics: A New Weapon in the War Against Cancer. *Annu. Rev. Med.* **2016**, *67*, 73–89. [CrossRef]
12. Sut, S.; Baldan, V.; Faggian, M.; Peron, G.; Dall'Acqua, S. Nutraceuticals, A New Challenge for Medicinal Chemistry. *Curr. Med. Chem.* **2016**, *23*, 3198–3223. [CrossRef]
13. Calvani, M.; Pasha, A.; Favre, C. Nutraceutical Boom in Cancer: Inside the Labyrinth of Reactive Oxygen Species. *Int. J. Mol. Sci.* **2020**, *21*, 1936. [CrossRef]
14. Bergamin, A.; Mantzioris, E.; Cross, G.; Deo, P.; Garg, S.; Hill, A.M. Nutraceuticals: Reviewing their Role in Chronic Disease Prevention and Management. *Pharm. Med.* **2019**, *33*, 291–309. [CrossRef]
15. Rafieian-Kopaei, M.; Baradaran, A.; Rafieian, M. Plants antioxidants: From laboratory to clinic. *J. Nephropathol.* **2013**, *2*, 152–153. [CrossRef]
16. Parsaei, P.; Karimi, M.; Asadi, S.Y.; Rafieian-kopaei, M. Bioactive components and preventive effect of green tea (*Camellia sinensis*) extract on post-laparotomy intra-abdominal adhesion in rats. *Int. J. Surg.* **2013**, *11*, 811–815. [CrossRef]
17. Santini, A.; Tenore, G.C.; Novellino, E. Nutraceuticals: A paradigm of proactive medicine. *Eur. J. Pharm. Sci.* **2017**, *96*, 53–61. [CrossRef]
18. Lachance, P.A.; Das, Y.T. Nutraceuticals. In *Comprehensive Medicinal Chemistry II*; Taylor, J.B., Triggle, D.J., Eds.; Elsevier: Oxford, UK, 2007; pp. 449–461. ISBN 9780080450445.
19. Teiten, M.H.; Dicato, M.; Diederich, M. Curcumin as a regulator of epigenetic events. *Mol. Nutr. Food Res.* **2013**, *57*, 1619–1629. [CrossRef]
20. Yang, C.H.; Yue, J.; Sims, M.; Pfeffer, L.M. The Curcumin Analog EF24 Targets NF-κB and miRNA-21, and Has Potent Anticancer Activity In Vitro and In Vivo. *PLoS ONE* **2013**, *8*, e71130. [CrossRef]
21. Qadir, M.; Naqvi, S.; Muhammad, S. Curcumin: A Polyphenol with Molecular Targets for Cancer Control. *Asian Pac. J. Cancer Prev.* **2016**, *17*, 2735–2739.
22. Vadukoot, A.K.; Mottemmal, S.; Vekaria, P.H. Curcumin as a Potential Therapeutic Agent in Certain Cancer Types. *Cureus* **2022**, *14*, e22825. [CrossRef]
23. Wang, M.; Jiang, S.; Zhou, L.; Yu, F.; Ding, H.; Li, P.; Zhou, M.; Wang, K. Potential Mechanisms of Action of Curcumin for Cancer Prevention: Focus on Cellular Signaling Pathways and miRNAs. *Int. J. Biol. Sci.* **2019**, *15*, 1200–1214. [CrossRef]
24. Zhang, J.; Zhang, T.; Ti, X.; Shi, J.; Wu, C.; Ren, X.; Yin, H. Curcumin promotes apoptosis in A549/DDP multidrug-resistant human lung adenocarcinoma cells through a miRNA signaling pathway. *Biochem. Biophys. Res. Commun.* **2010**, *399*, 1–6. [CrossRef] [PubMed]
25. Reuter, S.; Gupta, S.C.; Park, B.; Goel, A.; Aggarwal, B.B. Epigenetic changes induced by curcumin and other natural compounds. *Genes Nutr.* **2011**, *6*, 93. [CrossRef] [PubMed]
26. Hassan, F.U.; Rehman, M.S.U.; Khan, M.S.; Ali, M.A.; Javed, A.; Nawaz, A.; Yang, C. Curcumin as an alternative epigenetic modulator: Mechanism of action and potential effects. *Front. Genet.* **2019**, *10*, 514. [CrossRef]
27. Yu, J.; Peng, Y.; Wu, L.C.; Xie, Z.; Deng, Y.; Hughes, T.; He, S.; Mo, X.K.; Chiu, M.; Wang, Q.E.; et al. Curcumin Down-Regulates DNA Methyltransferase 1 and Plays an Anti-Leukemic Role in Acute Myeloid Leukemia. *PLoS ONE* **2013**, *8*, e55934. [CrossRef] [PubMed]
28. Boyanapalli, S.S.S.; Kong, A.N.T. "Curcumin, the King of Spices": Epigenetic Regulatory Mechanisms in the Prevention of Cancer, Neurological, and Inflammatory Diseases. *Curr. Pharmacol. Rep.* **2015**, *1*, 129–139. [CrossRef] [PubMed]
29. Nagoor, N.H.; Aggarwal, B. Cancer-linked targets modulated by curcumin. *Int. J. Biochem. Mol. Biol.* **2012**, *3*, 328–351.
30. Farghadani, R.; Naidu, R. Curcumin: Modulator of Key Molecular Signaling Pathways in Hormone-Independent Breast Cancer. *Cancers* **2021**, *13*, 3427. [CrossRef]
31. Zhou, H.; Beevers, C.S.; Huang, S. Targets of curcumin. *Curr. Drug Targets* **2011**, *12*, 332. [CrossRef]
32. Varoni, E.M.; Lo Faro, A.F.; Sharifi-Rad, J.; Iriti, M. Anticancer Molecular Mechanisms of Resveratrol. *Front. Nutr.* **2016**, *3*, 8. [CrossRef]
33. Issinger, O.G.; Guerra, B. Phytochemicals in cancer and their effect on the PI3K/AKT-mediated cellular signalling. *Biomed. Pharmacother.* **2021**, *139*, 111650. [CrossRef]
34. Signorelli, P.; Ghidoni, R. Resveratrol as an anticancer nutrient: Molecular basis, open questions and promises. *J. Nutr. Biochem.* **2005**, *16*, 449–466. [CrossRef]
35. Fernandes, G.F.S.; Silva, G.D.B.; Pavan, A.R.; Chiba, D.E.; Chin, C.M.; Dos Santos, J.L. Epigenetic Regulatory Mechanisms Induced by Resveratrol. *Nutrients* **2017**, *9*, 1201. [CrossRef]
36. Tili, E.; Michaille, J.J.; Alder, H.; Volinia, S.; Delmas, D.; Latruffe, N.; Croce, C.M. Resveratrol modulates the levels of microRNAs targeting genes encoding tumor-suppressors and effectors of TGFβ signaling pathway in SW480 cells. *Biochem. Pharmacol.* **2010**, *80*, 2057–2065. [CrossRef]
37. Kumazaki, M.; Noguchi, S.; Yasui, Y.; Iwasaki, J.; Shinohara, H.; Yamada, N.; Akao, Y. Anti-cancer effects of naturally occurring compounds through modulation of signal transduction and miRNA expression in human colon cancer cells. *J. Nutr. Biochem.* **2013**, *24*, 1849–1858. [CrossRef]
38. Hagiwara, K.; Kosaka, N.; Yoshioka, Y.; Takahashi, R.U.; Takeshita, F.; Ochiya, T. Stilbene derivatives promote Ago2-dependent tumour-suppressive microRNA activity. *Sci. Rep.* **2012**, *2*, 314. [CrossRef]

39. Borra, M.T.; Smith, B.C.; Denu, J.M. Mechanism of human SIRT1 activation by resveratrol. *J. Biol. Chem.* **2005**, *280*, 17187–17195. [CrossRef]
40. Williams, D.E. Indoles Derived from Glucobrassicin: Cancer Chemoprevention by Indole-3-Carbinol and 3,3′-Diindolylmethane. *Front. Nutr.* **2021**, *8*, 4334. [CrossRef]
41. Beaver, L.M.; Yu, T.W.; Sokolowski, E.I.; Williams, D.E.; Dashwood, R.H.; Ho, E. 3,3′-Diindolylmethane, but not indole-3-carbinol, inhibits histone deacetylase activity in prostate cancer cells. *Toxicol. Appl. Pharmacol.* **2012**, *263*, 345–351. [CrossRef]
42. Lubecka-Pietruszewska, K.; Kaufman-Szymczyk, A.; Stefanska, B.; Cebula-Obrzut, B.; Smolewski, P.; Fabianowska-Majewska, K. Sulforaphane Alone and in Combination with Clofarabine Epigenetically Regulates the Expression of DNA Methylation-Silenced Tumour Suppressor Genes in Human Breast Cancer Cells. *J. Nutrigenet. Nutr.* **2015**, *8*, 91–101. [CrossRef]
43. Hsu, A.; Wong, C.P.; Yu, Z.; Williams, D.E.; Dashwood, R.H.; Ho, E. Promoter de-methylation of cyclin D2 by sulforaphane in prostate cancer cells. *Clin. Epigenetics* **2011**, *3*, 3. [CrossRef]
44. Phuah, N.H.; Nagoor, N.H. Regulation of microRNAs by natural agents: New strategies in cancer therapies. *Biomed. Res. Int.* **2014**, *2014*, 804510. [CrossRef] [PubMed]
45. El-Daly, S.M.; Gamal-Eldeen, A.M.; Gouhar, S.A.; Abo-elfadl, M.T.; El-Saeed, G. Modulatory Effect of Indoles on the Expression of miRNAs Regulating G1/S Cell Cycle Phase in Breast Cancer Cells. *Appl. Biochem. Biotechnol.* **2020**, *192*, 1208–1223. [CrossRef] [PubMed]
46. Chen, C.Y.; Yu, Z.Y.; Chuang, Y.S.; Huang, R.M.; Wang, T.C.V. Sulforaphane attenuates EGFR signaling in NSCLC cells. *J. Biomed. Sci.* **2015**, *22*, 1–9. [CrossRef] [PubMed]
47. Ganai, S.A. Histone deacetylase inhibitor sulforaphane: The phytochemical with vibrant activity against prostate cancer. *Biomed. Pharmacother.* **2016**, *81*, 250–257. [CrossRef] [PubMed]
48. Meeran, S.M.; Patel, S.N.; Tollefsbol, T.O. Sulforaphane causes epigenetic repression of hTERT expression in human breast cancer cell lines. *PLoS ONE* **2010**, *5*, e11457. [CrossRef]
49. Yan, T.; Li, H.Y.; Wu, J.S.; Niu, Q.; Duan, W.H.; Han, Q.Z.; Ji, W.M.; Zhang, T.; Lv, W. Astaxanthin inhibits gemcitabine-resistant human pancreatic cancer progression through EMT inhibition and gemcitabine resensitization. *Oncol. Lett.* **2017**, *14*, 5400–5408. [CrossRef]
50. Yang, Y.; Fuentes, F.; Shu, L.; Wang, C.; Pung, D.; Li, W.; Zhang, C.; Guo, Y.; Kong, A.N. Epigenetic CpG Methylation of the Promoter and Reactivation of the Expression of GSTP1 by Astaxanthin in Human Prostate LNCaP Cells. *AAPS J.* **2017**, *19*, 421–430. [CrossRef]
51. Yang, Y.; Yang, I.; Cao, M.; Su, Z.; Wu, R.; Guo, Y.; Fang, M.; Kong, A.N. Fucoxanthin Elicits Epigenetic Modifications, Nrf2 Activation and Blocking Transformation in Mouse Skin JB6 P+ Cells. *AAPS J.* **2018**, *20*, 32. [CrossRef]
52. Ni, X.; Yu, H.; Wang, S.; Zhang, C.; Shen, S. Astaxanthin Inhibits PC-3 Xenograft Prostate Tumor Growth in Nude Mice. *Mar. Drugs* **2017**, *15*, 66. [CrossRef]
53. Kim, H.Y.; Kim, Y.M.; Hong, S. Astaxanthin suppresses the metastasis of colon cancer by inhibiting the MYC-mediated downregulation of microRNA-29a-3p and microRNA-200a. *Sci. Rep.* **2019**, *9*, 9457. [CrossRef]
54. Tomasini, P.; Barlesi, F.; Mascaux, C.; Greillier, L. Pemetrexed for advanced stage nonsquamous non-small cell lung cancer: Latest evidence about its extended use and outcomes. *Ther. Adv. Med. Oncol.* **2016**, *8*, 198–208. [CrossRef]
55. Yang, L.; Qiao, X.; Gu, J.; Li, X.; Cao, Y.; Xu, J.; Xue, C. Influence of molecular structure of astaxanthin esters on their stability and bioavailability. *Food Chem.* **2021**, *343*, 128497. [CrossRef]
56. Mirazimi, S.M.A.; Dashti, F.; Tobeiha, M.; Shahini, A.; Jafari, R.; Khoddami, M.; Sheida, A.H.; Esna Ashari, P.; Aflatoonian, A.H.; Elikaii, F.; et al. Application of Quercetin in the Treatment of Gastrointestinal Cancers. *Front. Pharmacol.* **2022**, *13*, 921. [CrossRef]
57. Zhang, Q.; Zhao, X.H.; Wang, Z.J. Cytotoxicity of flavones and flavonols to a human esophageal squamous cell carcinoma cell line (KYSE-510) by induction of G2/M arrest and apoptosis. *Toxicol. In Vitro* **2009**, *23*, 797–807. [CrossRef]
58. Kim, D.H.; Khan, H.; Ullah, H.; Hassan, S.T.S.; Šmejkal, K.; Efferth, T.; Mahomoodally, M.F.; Xu, S.; Habtemariam, S.; Filosa, R.; et al. MicroRNA targeting by quercetin in cancer treatment and chemoprotection. *Pharmacol. Res.* **2019**, *147*, 104346. [CrossRef]
59. Tan, J.; Wang, B.; Zhu, L. Regulation of survivin and Bcl-2 in HepG2 cell apoptosis induced by quercetin. *Chem. Biodivers.* **2009**, *6*, 1101–1110. [CrossRef]
60. Tanigawa, S.; Fujii, M.; Hou, D.X. Stabilization of p53 is involved in quercetin-induced cell cycle arrest and apoptosis in HepG2 cells. *Biosci. Biotechnol. Biochem.* **2008**, *72*, 797–804. [CrossRef]
61. Xi, L.; Zhang, Y.; Kong, S.; Liang, W. miR-34 inhibits growth and promotes apoptosis of osteosarcoma in nude mice through targetly regulating TGIF2 expression. *Biosci. Rep.* **2018**, *38*, 20180078. [CrossRef]
62. Yang, Y.; Wang, T.; Chen, D.; Ma, Q.; Zheng, Y.; Liao, S.; Wang, Y.; Zhang, J. Quercetin preferentially induces apoptosis in KRAS-mutant colorectal cancer cells via JNK signaling pathways. *Cell Biol. Int.* **2019**, *43*, 117–124. [CrossRef]
63. Ghafouri-Fard, S.; Shabestari, F.A.; Vaezi, S.; Abak, A.; Shoorei, H.; Karimi, A.; Taheri, M.; Basiri, A. Emerging impact of quercetin in the treatment of prostate cancer. *Biomed. Pharmacother.* **2021**, *138*, 111548. [CrossRef]
64. Vijayababu, M.R.; Arunkumar, A.; Kanagaraj, P.; Arunakaran, J. Effects of quercetin on insulin-like growth factors (IGFs) and their binding protein-3 (IGFBP-3) secretion and induction of apoptosis in human prostate cancer cells. *J. Carcinog.* **2006**, *5*, 10. [CrossRef]

65. Luo, C.L.; Liu, Y.Q.; Wang, P.; Song, C.H.; Wang, K.J.; Dai, L.P.; Zhang, J.Y.; Ye, H. The effect of quercetin nanoparticle on cervical cancer progression by inducing apoptosis, autophagy and anti-proliferation via JAK2 suppression. *Biomed. Pharmacother.* **2016**, *82*, 595–605. [CrossRef]
66. Alvarez, M.C.; Maso, V.; Torello, C.O.; Ferro, K.P.; Saad, S.T.O. The polyphenol quercetin induces cell death in leukemia by targeting epigenetic regulators of pro-apoptotic genes. *Clin. Epigenetics* **2018**, *10*, 139. [CrossRef]
67. Yiannakopoulou, E.C. Targeting DNA methylation with green tea catechins. *Pharmacology* **2015**, *95*, 111–116. [CrossRef]
68. Khan, M.A.; Hussain, A.; Sundaram, M.K.; Alalami, U.; Gunasekera, D.; Ramesh, L.; Hamza, A.; Quraishi, U. (-)-Epigallocatechin-3-gallate reverses the expression of various tumor-suppressor genes by inhibiting DNA methyltransferases and histone deacetylases in human cervical cancer cells. *Oncol. Rep.* **2015**, *33*, 1976–1984. [CrossRef]
69. Henning, S.M.; Wang, P.; Carpenter, C.L.; Heber, D. Epigenetic effects of green tea polyphenols in cancer. *Epigenomics* **2013**, *5*, 729. [CrossRef]
70. Deb, G.; Thakur, V.S.; Limaye, A.M.; Gupta, S. Epigenetic induction of tissue inhibitor of matrix metalloproteinase-3 by green tea polyphenols in breast cancer cells. *Mol. Carcinog.* **2015**, *54*, 485–499. [CrossRef] [PubMed]
71. Cadieux, Z.; Lewis, H.; Esquela-Kerscher, A. Role of Nutrition, the Epigenome, and MicroRNAs in Cancer Pathogenesis. In *MicroRNAs in Diseases and Disorders: Emerging Therapeutic Targets*; Royal Society of Chemistry: London, UK, 2019; pp. 1–35. ISBN 9781782621454.
72. Qi, W.J.; Sheng, W.S.; Peng, C.; Xiaodong, M.; Yao, T.Z. Investigating into anti-cancer potential of lycopene: Molecular targets. *Biomed. Pharmacother.* **2021**, *138*, 111546. [CrossRef] [PubMed]
73. Fu, L.-J.; Ding, Y.-B.; Wu, L.-X.; Wen, C.-J.; Qu, Q.; Zhang, X.; Zhou, H.-H. The Effects of Lycopene on the Methylation of the GSTP1 Promoter and Global Methylation in Prostatic Cancer Cell Lines PC3 and LNCaP. *Int. J. Endocrinol.* **2014**, *2014*, 1–9. [CrossRef] [PubMed]
74. Lu, Y.; Edwards, A.; Chen, Z.; Tseng, T.S.; Li, M.; Gonzalez, G.V.; Zhang, K. Insufficient Lycopene Intake Is Associated With High Risk of Prostate Cancer: A Cross-Sectional Study From the National Health and Nutrition Examination Survey (2003–2010). *Front. Public Health* **2021**, *9*, 2041. [CrossRef]
75. Li, D.; Chen, L.; Zhao, W.; Hao, J.; An, R. MicroRNA-let-7f-1 is induced by lycopene and inhibits cell proliferation and triggers apoptosis in prostate cancer. *Mol. Med. Rep.* **2016**, *13*, 2708–2714. [CrossRef]
76. Home—ClinicalTrials.gov. Available online: https://clinicaltrials.gov/ct2/home (accessed on 6 September 2022).
77. Sharifi-Rad, J.; Rayess, Y.; Rizk, A.A.; Sadaka, C.; Zgheib, R.; Zam, W.; Sestito, S.; Rapposelli, S.; Neffe-Skocińska, K.; Zielińska, D.; et al. Turmeric and Its Major Compound Curcumin on Health: Bioactive Effects and Safety Profiles for Food, Pharmaceutical, Biotechnological and Medicinal Applications. *Front. Pharmacol.* **2020**, *11*, 1021. [CrossRef]
78. Hwang, K.W.; Son, D.; Jo, H.W.; Kim, C.H.; Seong, K.C.; Moon, J.K. Levels of curcuminoid and essential oil compositions in turmerics (*Curcuma longa* L.) grown in Korea. *Appl. Biol. Chem.* **2016**, *59*, 209–215. [CrossRef]
79. Dosoky, N.; Setzer, W. Chemical Composition and Biological Activities of Essential Oils of Curcuma Species. *Nutrients* **2018**, *10*, 1196. [CrossRef]
80. Kasi, P.D.; Tamilselvam, R.; Skalicka-Woźniak, K.; Nabavi, S.F.; Daglia, M.; Bishayee, A.; Pazoki-Toroudi, H.; Nabavi, S.M. Molecular targets of curcumin for cancer therapy: An updated review. *Tumour Biol.* **2016**, *37*, 13017–13028. [CrossRef]
81. Giordano, A.; Tommonaro, G. Curcumin and Cancer. *Nutrients* **2019**, *11*, 2376. [CrossRef]
82. Mansouri, K.; Rasoulpoor, S.; Daneshkhah, A.; Abolfathi, S.; Salari, N.; Mohammadi, M.; Rasoulpoor, S.; Shabani, S. Clinical effects of curcumin in enhancing cancer therapy: A systematic review. *BMC Cancer* **2020**, *20*, 791. [CrossRef]
83. Dai, C.; Zhang, X.; Zhang, K. New Discovery of Curcumin Combination Therapy and Action Mechanism. *Evid. Based Complement. Altern. Med.* **2020**, *2020*, 4793058. [CrossRef]
84. Shanmugam, M.K.; Rane, G.; Kanchi, M.M.; Arfuso, F.; Chinnathambi, A.; Zayed, M.E.; Alharbi, S.A.; Tan, B.K.H.; Kumar, A.P.; Sethi, G. The Multifaceted Role of Curcumin in Cancer Prevention and Treatment. *Molecules* **2015**, *20*, 2728–2769. [CrossRef]
85. Abrahams, S.; Haylett, W.L.; Johnson, G.; Carr, J.A.; Bardien, S. Antioxidant effects of curcumin in models of neurodegeneration, aging, oxidative and nitrosative stress: A review. *Neuroscience* **2019**, *406*, 1–21. [CrossRef]
86. Ruan, D.; Zhu, Y.W.; Fouad, A.M.; Yan, S.J.; Chen, W.; Zhang, Y.N.; Xia, W.G.; Wang, S.; Jiang, S.Q.; Yang, L.; et al. Dietary curcumin enhances intestinal antioxidant capacity in ducklings via altering gene expression of antioxidant and key detoxification enzymes. *Poult. Sci.* **2019**, *98*, 3705–3714. [CrossRef]
87. Shaikh, S.; Shaikh, J.; Naba, Y.S.; Doke, K.; Ahmed, K.; Yusufi, M. Curcumin: Reclaiming the lost ground against cancer resistance. *Cancer Drug Resist.* **2021**, *4*, 298–320. [CrossRef]
88. Sabet, S.; Rashidinejad, A.; Melton, L.D.; McGillivray, D.J. Recent advances to improve curcumin oral bioavailability. *Trends Food Sci. Technol.* **2021**, *110*, 253–266. [CrossRef]
89. Heger, M.; van Golen, R.F.; Broekgaarden, M.; Michel, M.C. The molecular basis for the pharmacokinetics and pharmacodynamics of curcumin and its metabolites in relation to cancer. *Pharmacol. Rev.* **2013**, *66*, 222–307. [CrossRef]
90. Anand, P.; Kunnumakkara, A.B.; Newman, R.A.; Aggarwal, B.B. Bioavailability of curcumin: Problems and promises. *Mol. Pharm.* **2007**, *4*, 807–818. [CrossRef]
91. Cas, M.D.; Ghidoni, R. Dietary Curcumin: Correlation between Bioavailability and Health Potential. *Nutrients* **2019**, *11*, 2147. [CrossRef]

92. Zou, L.; Liu, W.; Liu, C.; Xiao, H.; McClements, D.J. Utilizing food matrix effects to enhance nutraceutical bioavailability: Increase of curcumin bioaccessibility using excipient emulsions. *J. Agric. Food Chem.* **2015**, *63*, 2052–2062. [CrossRef]
93. Nelson, K.M.; Dahlin, J.L.; Bisson, J.; Graham, J.; Pauli, G.F.; Walters, M.A. The Essential Medicinal Chemistry of Curcumin. *J. Med. Chem.* **2017**, *60*, 1620–1637. [CrossRef]
94. Stohs, S.J.; Chen, O.; Ray, S.D.; Ji, J.; Bucci, L.R.; Preuss, H.G. Highly Bioavailable Forms of Curcumin and Promising Avenues for Curcumin-Based Research and Application: A Review. *Molecules* **2020**, *25*, 1397. [CrossRef]
95. Paolino, D.; Vero, A.; Cosco, D.; Pecora, T.M.G.; Cianciolo, S.; Fresta, M.; Pignatello, R. Improvement of Oral Bioavailability of Curcumin upon Microencapsulation with Methacrylic Copolymers. *Front. Pharmacol.* **2016**, *7*, 485. [CrossRef]
96. Rahimi, H.R.; Nedaeinia, R.; Shamloo, A.S.; Nikdoust, S.; Oskuee, R.K. Novel delivery system for natural products: Nano-curcumin formulations. *Avicenna J. Phytomed.* **2016**, *6*, 383. [PubMed]
97. Porat, D.; Dahan, A. Active intestinal drug absorption and the solubility-permeability interplay. *Int. J. Pharm.* **2018**, *537*, 84–93. [CrossRef] [PubMed]
98. Kharat, M.; McClements, D.J. Recent advances in colloidal delivery systems for nutraceuticals: A case study—Delivery by Design of curcumin. *J. Colloid Interface Sci.* **2019**, *557*, 506–518. [CrossRef] [PubMed]
99. Hu, B.; Liu, X.; Zhang, C.; Zeng, X. Food macromolecule based nanodelivery systems for enhancing the bioavailability of polyphenols. *J. Food Drug Anal.* **2017**, *25*, 3–15. [CrossRef] [PubMed]
100. Cuomo, F.; Cofelice, M.; Venditti, F.; Ceglie, A.; Miguel, M.; Lindman, B.; Lopez, F. In-vitro digestion of curcumin loaded chitosan-coated liposomes. *Colloids Surf. B. Biointerfaces* **2018**, *168*, 29–34. [CrossRef]
101. Lamuela-Raventós, R.M.; Romero-Pérez, A.I.; Waterhouse, A.L.; de la Torre-Boronat, M.C. Direct HPLC Analysis of cis- and trans-Resveratrol and Piceid Isomers in Spanish Red Vitis vinifera Wines. *J. Agric. Food Chem.* **1995**, *43*, 281–283. [CrossRef]
102. Akinwumi, B.C.; Bordun, K.A.M.; Anderson, H.D. Biological Activities of Stilbenoids. *Int. J. Mol. Sci.* **2018**, *19*, 792. [CrossRef]
103. Anisimova, N.Y.U.; Kiselevsky, M.V.; Sosnov, A.V.; Sadovnikov, S.V.; Stankov, I.N.; Gakh, A.A. Trans-, cis-, and dihydro-resveratrol: A comparative study. *Chem. Cent. J.* **2011**, *5*, 88. [CrossRef]
104. Ducimetiere, P.; Cambien, F.; Richard, J.L.; Rakotovao, R.; Claude, J.R. Coronary heart disease in middle-aged Frenchmen. Comparisons between Paris Prospective Study, Seven Countries Study, and Pooling Project. *Lancet* **1980**, *1*, 1346–1350. [CrossRef]
105. Ferrières, J. The French paradox: Lessons for other countries. *Heart* **2004**, *90*, 107. [CrossRef]
106. Miura, T.; Muraoka, S.; Ikeda, N.; Watanabe, M.; Fujimoto, Y. Antioxidative and prooxidative action of stilbene derivatives. *Pharmacol. Toxicol.* **2000**, *86*, 203–208. [CrossRef]
107. Spanier, G.; Xu, H.; Xia, N.; Tobias, S.; Deng, S.; Wojnowski, L.; Forstermann, U.; Li, H. Resveratrol reduces endothelial oxidative stress by modulating the gene expression of superoxide dismutase 1 (SOD1), glutathione peroxidase 1 (GPx1) and NADPH oxidase subunit (NOX4). *J. Physiol. Pharmacol.* **2009**, *60*, 111–116.
108. Valko, M.; Leibfritz, D.; Moncol, J.; Cronin, M.T.D.; Mazur, M.; Telser, J. Free radicals and antioxidants in normal physiological functions and human disease. *Int. J. Biochem. Cell Biol.* **2007**, *39*, 44–84. [CrossRef]
109. Di Meo, S.; Reed, T.T.; Venditti, P.; Victor, V.M. Role of ROS and RNS Sources in Physiological and Pathological Conditions. *Oxid. Med. Cell. Longev.* **2016**, *2016*, 1245049. [CrossRef]
110. Farkhondeh, T.; Folgado, S.L.; Pourbagher-Shahri, A.M.; Ashrafizadeh, M.; Samarghandian, S. The therapeutic effect of resveratrol: Focusing on the Nrf2 signaling pathway. *Biomed. Pharmacother.* **2020**, *127*, 110234. [CrossRef]
111. Lubecka, K.; Kurzava, L.; Flower, K.; Buvala, H.; Zhang, H.; Teegarden, D.; Camarillo, I.; Suderman, M.; Kuang, S.; Andrisani, O.; et al. Stilbenoids remodel the DNA methylation patterns in breast cancer cells and inhibit oncogenic NOTCH signaling through epigenetic regulation of MAML2 transcriptional activity. *Carcinogenesis* **2016**, *37*, 656–668. [CrossRef]
112. Kala, R.; Shah, H.N.; Martin, S.L.; Tollefsbol, T.O. Epigenetic-based combinatorial resveratrol and pterostilbene alters DNA damage response by affecting SIRT1 and DNMT enzyme expression, including SIRT1-dependent γ-H2AX and telomerase regulation in triple-negative breast cancer. *BMC Cancer* **2015**, *15*, 672. [CrossRef]
113. Kai, L.; Samuel, S.K.; Levenson, A.S. Resveratrol enhances p53 acetylation and apoptosis in prostate cancer by inhibiting MTA1/NuRD complex. *Int. J. Cancer* **2010**, *126*, 1538–1548. [CrossRef]
114. Ramis, M.R.; Esteban, S.; Miralles, A.; Tan, D.X.; Reiter, R.J. Caloric restriction, resveratrol and melatonin: Role of SIRT1 and implications for aging and related-diseases. *Mech. Ageing Dev.* **2015**, *146–148*, 28–41. [CrossRef]
115. Komorowska, J.; Wątroba, M.; Szukiewicz, D. Review of beneficial effects of resveratrol in neurodegenerative diseases such as Alzheimer's disease. *Adv. Med. Sci.* **2020**, *65*, 415–423. [CrossRef]
116. Ahmed, T.; Javed, S.; Javed, S.; Tariq, A.; Šamec, D.; Tejada, S.; Nabavi, S.F.; Braidy, N.; Nabavi, S.M. Resveratrol and Alzheimer's Disease: Mechanistic Insights. *Mol. Neurobiol.* **2017**, *54*, 2622–2635. [CrossRef]
117. Park, D.; Jeong, H.; Lee, M.N.; Koh, A.; Kwon, O.; Yang, Y.R.; Noh, J.; Suh, P.G.; Park, H.; Ryu, S.H. Resveratrol induces autophagy by directly inhibiting mTOR through ATP competition. *Sci. Rep.* **2016**, *6*, 21772. [CrossRef]
118. Taniguchi, T.; Iizumi, Y.; Watanabe, M.; Masuda, M.; Morita, M.; Aono, Y.; Toriyama, S.; Oishi, M.; Goi, W.; Sakai, T. Resveratrol directly targets DDX5 resulting in suppression of the mTORC1 pathway in prostate cancer. *Cell Death Dis.* **2016**, *7*, e2211. [CrossRef]
119. Zou, Z.; Tao, T.; Li, H.; Zhu, X. MTOR signaling pathway and mTOR inhibitors in cancer: Progress and challenges. *Cell Biosci.* **2020**, *10*, 31. [CrossRef]

120. Ionescu, V.S.; Popa, A.; Alexandru, A.; Manole, E.; Neagu, M.; Pop, S. Dietary Phytoestrogens and Their Metabolites as Epigenetic Modulators with Impact on Human Health. *Antioxidants* **2021**, *10*, 1893. [CrossRef] [PubMed]
121. Quarta, A.; Gaballo, A.; Pradhan, B.; Patra, S.; Jena, M.; Ragusa, A. Beneficial Oxidative Stress-Related trans-Resveratrol Effects in the Treatment and Prevention of Breast Cancer. *Appl. Sci.* **2021**, *11*, 11041. [CrossRef]
122. Pannu, N.; Bhatnagar, A. Resveratrol: From enhanced biosynthesis and bioavailability to multitargeting chronic diseases. *Biomed. Pharmacother.* **2019**, *109*, 2237–2251. [CrossRef]
123. Vesely, O.; Baldovska, S.; Kolesarova, A. Enhancing Bioavailability of Nutraceutically Used Resveratrol and Other Stilbenoids. *Nutrients* **2021**, *13*, 3095. [CrossRef]
124. de Vries, K.; Strydom, M.; Steenkamp, V. A Brief Updated Review of Advances to Enhance Resveratrol's Bioavailability. *Molecules* **2021**, *26*, 4367. [CrossRef]
125. Santos, A.C.; Pereira, I.; Pereira-Silva, M.; Ferreira, L.; Caldas, M.; Collado-González, M.; Magalhães, M.; Figueiras, A.; Ribeiro, A.J.; Veiga, F. Nanotechnology-based formulations for resveratrol delivery: Effects on resveratrol in vivo bioavailability and bioactivity. *Colloids Surf. B. Biointerfaces* **2019**, *180*, 127–140. [CrossRef] [PubMed]
126. De Vries, K.; Strydom, M.; Steenkamp, V. Bioavailability of resveratrol: Possibilities for enhancement. *J. Herb. Med.* **2018**, *11*, 71–77. [CrossRef]
127. Gambini, J.; Inglés, M.; Olaso, G.; Lopez-Grueso, R.; Bonet-Costa, V.; Gimeno-Mallench, L.; Mas-Bargues, C.; Abdelaziz, K.M.; Gomez-Cabrera, M.C.; Vina, J.; et al. Properties of Resveratrol: In Vitro and In Vivo Studies about Metabolism, Bioavailability, and Biological Effects in Animal Models and Humans. *Oxid. Med. Cell. Longev.* **2015**, *2015*, 837042. [CrossRef]
128. Banc, R.; Loghin, F.; Miere, D.; Ranga, F.; Socaciu, C. Phenolic composition and antioxidant activity of red, rosé and white wines originating from Romanian grape cultivars. *Not. Bot. Horti Agrobot. Cluj Napoca* **2020**, *48*, 716–734. [CrossRef]
129. Amri, A.; Chaumeil, J.C.; Sfar, S.; Charrueau, C. Administration of resveratrol: What formulation solutions to bioavailability limitations? *J. Control. Release* **2012**, *158*, 182–193. [CrossRef]
130. Brotons-Canto, A.; Gonzalez-Navarro, C.J.; Gurrea, J.; González-Ferrero, C.; Irache, J.M. Zein nanoparticles improve the oral bioavailability of resveratrol in humans. *J. Drug Deliv. Sci. Technol.* **2020**, *57*, 101704. [CrossRef]
131. Zhu, Y.; Pan, W.H.; Ku, C.F.; Zhang, H.J.; Tsang, S.W. Design, synthesis and evaluation of novel dihydrostilbene derivatives as potential anti-melanogenic skin-protecting agents. *Eur. J. Med. Chem.* **2018**, *143*, 1254–1260. [CrossRef]
132. Tang, Y.L.; Chan, S.W. A review of the pharmacological effects of piceatannol on cardiovascular diseases. *Phytother. Res.* **2014**, *28*, 1581–1588. [CrossRef]
133. Neves, A.R.; Martins, S.; Segundo, M.A.; Reis, S. Nanoscale Delivery of Resveratrol towards Enhancement of Supplements and Nutraceuticals. *Nutrients* **2016**, *8*, 131. [CrossRef]
134. Almeida, L.; Vaz-da-Silva, M.; Falcão, A.; Soares, E.; Costa, R.; Loureiro, A.I.; Fernandes-Lopes, C.; Rocha, J.F.; Nunes, T.; Wright, L.; et al. Pharmacokinetic and safety profile of trans-resveratrol in a rising multiple-dose study in healthy volunteers. *Mol. Nutr. Food Res.* **2009**, *53*, S7–S15. [CrossRef]
135. Sergides, C.; Chirilă, M.; Silvestro, L.; Pitta, D.; Pittas, A. Bioavailability and safety study of resveratrol 500 mg tablets in healthy male and female volunteers. *Exp. Ther. Med.* **2016**, *11*, 164–170. [CrossRef]
136. Connolly, E.L.; Sim, M.; Travica, N.; Marx, W.; Beasy, G.; Lynch, G.S.; Bondonno, C.P.; Lewis, J.R.; Hodgson, J.M.; Blekkenhorst, L.C. Glucosinolates from Cruciferous Vegetables and Their Potential Role in Chronic Disease: Investigating the Preclinical and Clinical Evidence. *Front. Pharmacol.* **2021**, *12*, 2964. [CrossRef]
137. Barba, F.J.; Nikmaram, N.; Roohinejad, S.; Khelfa, A.; Zhu, Z.; Koubaa, M. Bioavailability of Glucosinolates and Their Breakdown Products: Impact of Processing. *Front. Nutr.* **2016**, *3*, 24. [CrossRef]
138. Iahtisham-Ul-Haq; Khan, S.; Awan, K.A.; Iqbal, M.J. Sulforaphane as a potential remedy against cancer: Comprehensive mechanistic review. *J. Food Biochem.* **2022**, *46*, e13886. [CrossRef]
139. Fahey, J.W.; Holtzclaw, W.D.; Wehage, S.L.; Wade, K.L.; Stephenson, K.K.; Talalay, P. Sulforaphane Bioavailability from Glucoraphanin-Rich Broccoli: Control by Active Endogenous Myrosinase. *PLoS ONE* **2015**, *10*, e0140963. [CrossRef] [PubMed]
140. Shekarri, Q.; Dekker, M. A physiological-based model for simulating the bioavailability and kinetics of sulforaphane from broccoli products. *Foods* **2021**, *10*, 2761. [CrossRef] [PubMed]
141. Wang, Z.; Kwan, M.L.; Pratt, R.; Roh, J.M.; Kushi, L.H.; Danforth, K.N.; Zhang, Y.; Ambrosone, C.B.; Tang, L. Effects of cooking methods on total isothiocyanate yield from cruciferous vegetables. *Food Sci. Nutr.* **2020**, *8*, 5673–5682. [CrossRef]
142. Orlando, P.; Nartea, A.; Silvestri, S.; Marcheggiani, F.; Cirilli, I.; Dludla, P.V.; Fiorini, R.; Pacetti, D.; Loizzo, M.R.; Lucci, P.; et al. Bioavailability Study of Isothiocyanates and Other Bioactive Compounds of Brassica oleracea L. var. Italica Boiled or Steamed: Functional Food or Dietary Supplement? *Antioxidants* **2022**, *11*, 209. [CrossRef]
143. Okunade, O.; Niranjan, K.; Ghawi, S.K.; Kuhnle, G.; Methven, L. Supplementation of the Diet by Exogenous Myrosinase via Mustard Seeds to Increase the Bioavailability of Sulforaphane in Healthy Human Subjects after the Consumption of Cooked Broccoli. *Mol. Nutr. Food Res.* **2018**, *62*, e1700980. [CrossRef] [PubMed]
144. Luang-In, V.; Narbad, A.; Nueno-Palop, C.; Mithen, R.; Bennett, M.; Rossiter, J.T. The metabolism of methylsulfinylalkyl- and methylthioalkyl-glucosinolates by a selection of human gut bacteria. *Mol. Nutr. Food Res.* **2014**, *58*, 875–883. [CrossRef]
145. Bouranis, J.A.; Beaver, L.M.; Ho, E. Metabolic Fate of Dietary Glucosinolates and Their Metabolites: A Role for the Microbiome. *Front. Nutr.* **2021**, *8*, 690. [CrossRef]

146. Li, F.; Hullar, M.A.J.; Beresford, S.A.A.; Lampe, J.W. Variation of glucoraphanin metabolism in vivo and ex vivo by human gut bacteria. *Br. J. Nutr.* **2011**, *106*, 408–416. [CrossRef]
147. Conaway, C.C.; Getahun, S.M.; Liebes, L.L.; Pusateri, D.J.; Topham, D.K.W.; Botero-Omary, M.; Chung, F.L. Disposition of glucosinolates and sulforaphane in humans after ingestion of steamed and fresh broccoli. *Nutr. Cancer* **2000**, *38*, 168–178. [CrossRef]
148. Aronica, L.; Ordovas, J.M.; Volkov, A.; Lamb, J.J.; Stone, P.M.; Minich, D.; Leary, M.; Class, M.; Metti, D.; Larson, I.A.; et al. Genetic Biomarkers of Metabolic Detoxification for Personalized Lifestyle Medicine. *Nutrients* **2022**, *14*, 768. [CrossRef]
149. Hauder, J.; Winkler, S.; Bub, A.; Rüfer, C.E.; Pignitter, M.; Somoza, V. LC-MS/MS quantification of sulforaphane and indole-3-carbinol metabolites in human plasma and urine after dietary intake of selenium-fortified broccoli. *J. Agric. Food Chem.* **2011**, *59*, 8047–8057. [CrossRef]
150. Sun, J.; Charron, C.S.; Novotny, J.A.; Peng, B.; Yu, L.; Chen, P. Profiling glucosinolate metabolites in human urine and plasma after broccoli consumption using non-targeted and targeted metabolomic analyses. *Food Chem.* **2020**, *309*, 125660. [CrossRef]
151. Bradlow, H.; Zeligs, M. Diindolylmethane (DIM) spontaneously forms from indole-3-carbinol (I3C) during cell culture experiments. *In Vivo* **2010**, *24*, 387–391.
152. Anderton, M.J.; Manson, M.M.; Verschoyle, R.; Gescher, A.; Steward, W.P.; Williams, M.L.; Mager, D.E. Physiological modeling of formulated and crystalline 3,3′-diindolylmethane pharmacokinetics following oral administration in mice. *Drug Metab. Dispos.* **2004**, *32*, 632–638. [CrossRef]
153. Anderton, M.J.; Manson, M.M.; Verschoyle, R.D.; Gescher, A.; Lamb, J.H.; Farmer, P.B.; Steward, W.P.; Williams, M.L. Pharmacokinetics and tissue disposition of indole-3-carbinol and its acid condensation products after oral administration to mice. *Clin. Cancer Res.* **2004**, *10*, 5233–5241. [CrossRef]
154. Acharya, A.; Das, I.; Singh, S.; Saha, T. Chemopreventive properties of indole-3-carbinol, diindolylmethane and other constituents of cardamom against carcinogenesis. *Recent Pat. Food. Nutr. Agric.* **2010**, *2*, 166–177. [CrossRef]
155. Nian, H.; Delage, B.; Ho, E.; Dashwood, R.H. Modulation of Histone Deacetylase Activity by Dietary Isothiocyanates and Allyl Sulfides: Studies with Sulforaphane and Garlic Organosulfur Compounds. *Environ. Mol. Mutagen.* **2009**, *50*, 213. [CrossRef]
156. Jump, S.M.; Kung, J.; Staub, R.; Kinseth, M.A.; Cram, E.J.; Yudina, L.N.; Preobrazhenskaya, M.N.; Bjeldanes, L.F.; Firestone, G.L. N-Alkoxy derivatization of indole-3-carbinol increases the efficacy of the G1 cell cycle arrest and of I3C-specific regulation of cell cycle gene transcription and activity in human breast cancer cells. *Biochem. Pharmacol.* **2008**, *75*, 713–724. [CrossRef]
157. Szaefer, H.; Licznerska, B.; Krajka-Kuniak, V.; Bartoszek, A.; Baer-Dubowska, W. Modulation of CYP1A1, CYP1A2 and CYP1B1 expression by cabbage juices and indoles in human breast cell lines. *Nutr. Cancer* **2012**, *64*, 879–888. [CrossRef]
158. Reed, G.A.; Arneson, D.W.; Putnam, W.C.; Smith, H.J.; Gray, J.C.; Sullivan, D.K.; Mayo, M.S.; Crowell, J.A.; Hurwitz, A. Single-dose and multiple-dose administration of indole-3-carbinol to women: Pharmacokinetics based on 3,3′-diindolylmethane. *Cancer Epidemiol. Biomark. Prev.* **2006**, *15*, 2477–2481. [CrossRef]
159. Arslan, A.A.; Koenig, K.L.; Lenner, P.; Afanasyeva, Y.; Shore, R.E.; Chen, Y.; Lundin, E.; Toniolo, P.; Hallmans, G.; Zeleniuch-Jacquotte, A. Circulating Estrogen Metabolites and Risk of Breast Cancer in Postmenopausal Women. *Cancer Epidemiol. Biomark. Prev.* **2014**, *23*, 1290. [CrossRef]
160. Zeleniuch-Jacquotte, A.; Shore, R.E.; Afanasyeva, Y.; Lukanova, A.; Sieri, S.; Koenig, K.L.; Idahl, A.; Krogh, V.; Liu, M.; Ohlson, N.; et al. Postmenopausal circulating levels of 2- and 16α-hydroxyestrone and risk of endometrial cancer. *Br. J. Cancer* **2011**, *105*, 1458–1464. [CrossRef]
161. McCann, S.E.; Wactawski-Wende, J.; Kufel, K.; Olson, J.; Ovando, B.; Kadlubar, S.N.; Davis, W.; Carter, L.; Muti, P.; Shields, P.G.; et al. Changes in 2-hydroxyestrone and 16alpha-hydroxyestrone metabolism with flaxseed consumption: Modification by COMT and CYP1B1 genotype. *Cancer Epidemiol. Biomark. Prev.* **2007**, *16*, 256–262. [CrossRef]
162. Lee, S.U.; Rhee, M.; Min, Y.K.; Kim, S.H. Involvement of peroxiredoxin IV in the 16alpha-hydroxyestrone-induced proliferation of human MCF-7 breast cancer cells. *Cell Biol. Int.* **2008**, *32*, 401–405. [CrossRef]
163. Firestone, G.L.; Sundar, S.N. Minireview: Modulation of hormone receptor signaling by dietary anticancer indoles. *Mol. Endocrinol.* **2009**, *23*, 1940–1947. [CrossRef]
164. Le, H.T.; Schaldach, C.M.; Firestone, G.L.; Bjeldanes, L.F. Plant-derived 3,3′-Diindolylmethane is a strong androgen antagonist in human prostate cancer cells. *J. Biol. Chem.* **2003**, *278*, 21136–21145. [CrossRef]
165. Bradlow, H.L.; Davis, D.L.; Lin, G.; Sepkovic, D.; Tiwari, R. Effects of pesticides on the ratio of 16 alpha/2-hydroxyestrone: A biologic marker of breast cancer risk. *Environ. Health Perspect.* **1995**, *103*, 147. [CrossRef]
166. Hodges, R.E.; Minich, D.M. Modulation of Metabolic Detoxification Pathways Using Foods and Food-Derived Components: A Scientific Review with Clinical Application. *J. Nutr. Metab.* **2015**, *2015*, 760689. [CrossRef] [PubMed]
167. Abbas, A.; Hall, J.A.; Patterson, W.L.; Ho, E.; Hsu, A.; Al-Mulla, F.; Georgel, P.T. Sulforaphane modulates telomerase activity via epigenetic regulation in prostate cancer cell lines. *Biochem. Cell Biol.* **2016**, *94*, 71–81. [CrossRef] [PubMed]
168. Kim, E.J.; Park, H.; Kim, J.; Park, J.H.Y. 3,3′-diindolylmethane suppresses 12-O-tetradecanoylphorbol-13-acetate-induced inflammation and tumor promotion in mouse skin via the downregulation of inflammatory mediators. *Mol. Carcinog.* **2010**, *49*, 672–683. [CrossRef] [PubMed]
169. Fuentes, F.; Paredes-Gonzalez, X.; Kong, A.N.T. Dietary Glucosinolates Sulforaphane, Phenethyl Isothiocyanate, Indole-3-Carbinol/3,3′-Diindolylmethane: Anti-Oxidative Stress/Inflammation, Nrf2, Epigenetics/Epigenomics and In Vivo Cancer Chemopreventive Efficacy. *Curr. Pharmacol. Rep.* **2015**, *1*, 179. [CrossRef]

170. Royston, K.J.; Tollefsbol, T.O. The Epigenetic Impact of Cruciferous Vegetables on Cancer Prevention. *Curr. Pharmacol. Rep.* **2015**, *1*, 46–51. [CrossRef]
171. Houghton, C.A. Sulforaphane: Its "Coming of Age" as a Clinically Relevant Nutraceutical in the Prevention and Treatment of Chronic Disease. *Oxid. Med. Cell. Longev.* **2019**, *2019*, 2716870. [CrossRef]
172. Thomson, C.A.; Ho, E.; Strom, M.B. Chemopreventive properties of 3,30-diindolylmethane in breast cancer: Evidence from experimental and human studies. *Nutr. Rev.* **2016**, *74*, 432–443. [CrossRef]
173. Kotsopoulos, J.; Zhang, S.; Akbari, M.; Salmena, L.; Llacuachaqui, M.; Zeligs, M.; Sun, P.; Narod, S.A. BRCA1 mRNA levels following a 4–6-week intervention with oral 3,3′-diindolylmethane. *Br. J. Cancer* **2014**, *111*, 1269. [CrossRef]
174. Fujioka, N.; Fritz, V.; Upadhyaya, P.; Kassie, F.; Hecht, S.S. Research on cruciferous vegetables, indole-3-carbinol, and cancer prevention: A tribute to Lee, W. Wattenberg. *Mol. Nutr. Food Res.* **2016**, *60*, 1228–1238. [CrossRef]
175. Wang, Q.; Bao, Y. Nanodelivery of natural isothiocyanates as a cancer therapeutic. *Free Radic. Biol. Med.* **2021**, *167*, 125–140. [CrossRef]
176. Luo, Y.; Wang, T.T.Y.; Teng, Z.; Chen, P.; Sun, J.; Wang, Q. Encapsulation of indole-3-carbinol and 3,3′-diindolylmethane in zein/carboxymethyl chitosan nanoparticles with controlled release property and improved stability. *Food Chem.* **2013**, *139*, 224–230. [CrossRef]
177. Higuera-Ciapara, I.; Félix-Valenzuela, L.; Goycoolea, F.M. Astaxanthin: A review of its chemistry and applications. *Crit. Rev. Food Sci. Nutr.* **2006**, *46*, 185–196. [CrossRef]
178. Ambati, R.R.; Moi, P.S.; Ravi, S.; Aswathanarayana, R.G. Astaxanthin: Sources, extraction, stability, biological activities and its commercial applications—A review. *Mar. Drugs* **2014**, *12*, 128–152. [CrossRef]
179. Karimian, A.; Hadi Bahadori, M.; Moghaddam, A.H.; Mir Mohammadrezaei, F.; Mohammadrezaei, F.M. Effect of Astaxanthin on cell viability in T-47D and MDA-MB-231 Breast Cancer Cell Lines. *Multidiscip. Cancer Investig.* **2017**, *124*, 151832. [CrossRef]
180. McCall, B.; McPartland, C.K.; Moore, R.; Frank-Kamenetskii, A.; Booth, B.W. Effects of Astaxanthin on the Proliferation and Migration of Breast Cancer Cells In Vitro. *Antioxidants* **2018**, *7*, 135. [CrossRef]
181. Zhang, Z.; Sun, D.; Cheng, K.W.; Chen, F. Inhibition of autophagy modulates astaxanthin and total fatty acid biosynthesis in Chlorella zofingiensis under nitrogen starvation. *Bioresour. Technol.* **2018**, *247*, 610–615. [CrossRef]
182. Jemal, A.; Bray, F.; Center, M.M.; Ferlay, J.; Ward, E.; Forman, D. Global cancer statistics. *CA. Cancer J. Clin.* **2011**, *61*, 69–90. [CrossRef]
183. Liao, K.S.; Wei, C.L.; Chen, J.C.; Zheng, H.Y.; Chen, W.C.; Wu, C.H.; Wang, T.J.; Peng, Y.S.; Chang, P.Y.; Lin, Y.W. Astaxanthin enhances pemetrexed-induced cytotoxicity by downregulation of thymidylate synthase expression in human lung cancer cells. *Regul. Toxicol. Pharmacol.* **2016**, *81*, 353–361. [CrossRef]
184. Chen, J.C.; Wu, C.H.; Peng, Y.S.; Zheng, H.Y.; Lin, Y.C.; Ma, P.F.; Yen, T.C.; Chen, T.Y.; Lin, Y.W. Astaxanthin enhances erlotinib-induced cytotoxicity by p38 MAPK mediated xeroderma pigmentosum complementation group C (XPC) down-regulation in human lung cancer cells. *Toxicol. Res.* **2018**, *7*, 1247. [CrossRef]
185. Kim, S.; Lee, H.; Lim, J.W.; Kim, H. Astaxanthin induces NADPH oxidase activation and receptor-interacting protein kinase 1-mediated necroptosis in gastric cancer AGS cells. *Mol. Med. Rep.* **2021**, *24*, 1–12. [CrossRef]
186. Honda, M.; Kageyama, H.; Hibino, T.; Osawa, Y.; Hirasawa, K.; Kuroda, I. Evaluation and improvement of storage stability of astaxanthin 3 isomers in oils and fats. *Food Chem.* **2021**, *352*, 129371. [CrossRef]
187. Martínez-Álvarez, Ó.; Calvo, M.M.; Gómez-Estaca, J. Recent Advances in Astaxanthin Micro/Nanoencapsulation to Improve Its Stability and Functionality as a Food Ingredient. *Mar. Drugs* **2020**, *18*, 406. [CrossRef]
188. Madhavi, D.; Kagan, D.; Seshadri, S. A Study on the Bioavailability of a Proprietary, Sustained-release Formulation of Astaxanthin. *Integr. Med. A Clin. J.* **2018**, *17*, 38.
189. Odeberg, J.M.; Lignell, Å.; Pettersson, A.; Höglund, P. Oral bioavailability of the antioxidant astaxanthin in humans is enhanced by incorporation of lipid based formulations. *Eur. J. Pharm. Sci.* **2003**, *19*, 299–304. [CrossRef]
190. Edelman, R.; Engelberg, S.; Fahoum, L.; Meyron-Holtz, E.G.; Livney, Y.D. Potato protein- based carriers for enhancing bioavailability of astaxanthin. *Food Hydrocoll.* **2019**, *96*, 72–80. [CrossRef]
191. Saini, R.K.; Prasad, P.; Lokesh, V.; Shang, X.; Shin, J.; Keum, Y.S.; Lee, J.H. Carotenoids: Dietary Sources, Extraction, Encapsulation, Bioavailability, and Health Benefits-A Review of Recent Advancements. *Antioxidants* **2022**, *11*, 795. [CrossRef]
192. Genç, Y.; Bardakci, H.; Yücel, Ç.; Karatoprak, G.Ş.; Akkol, E.K.; Barak, T.H.; Sobarzo-Sánchez, E. Oxidative Stress and Marine Carotenoids: Application by Using Nanoformulations. *Mar. Drugs* **2020**, *18*, 423. [CrossRef]
193. Mularczyk, M.; Michalak, I.; Marycz, K. Astaxanthin and other Nutrients from Haematococcus pluvialis-Multifunctional Applications. *Mar. Drugs* **2020**, *18*, 459. [CrossRef]
194. Snell, T.W.; Carberry, J. Astaxanthin Bioactivity Is Determined by Stereoisomer Composition and Extraction Method. *Nutrients* **2022**, *14*, 1522. [CrossRef]
195. Sorasitthiyanukarn, F.N.; Ratnatilaka Na Bhuket, P.; Muangnoi, C.; Rojsitthisak, P.; Rojsitthisak, P. Chitosan/alginate nanoparticles as a promising carrier of novel curcumin diethyl diglutarate. *Int. J. Biol. Macromol.* **2019**, *131*, 1125–1136. [CrossRef] [PubMed]
196. Yang, J.; Hua, S.; Huang, Z.; Gu, Z.; Cheng, L.; Hong, Y. Comparison of bioaccessibility of astaxanthin encapsulated in starch-based double emulsion with different structures. *Carbohydr. Polym.* **2021**, *272*, 118475. [CrossRef] [PubMed]

197. Barros, M.P.; Marin, D.P.; Bolin, A.P.; De Cássia Santos Macedo, R.; Campoio, T.R.; Fineto, C.; Guerra, B.A.; Polotow, T.G.; Vardaris, C.; Mattei, R.; et al. Combined astaxanthin and fish oil supplementation improves glutathione-based redox balance in rat plasma and neutrophils. *Chem. Biol. Interact.* **2012**, *197*, 58–67. [CrossRef] [PubMed]
198. Gomez-Estaca, J.; Comunian, T.A.; Montero, P.; Ferro-Furtado, R.; Favaro-Trindade, C.S. Encapsulation of an astaxanthin-containing lipid extract from shrimp waste by complex coacervation using a novel gelatin–cashew gum complex. *Food Hydrocoll.* **2016**, *61*, 155–162. [CrossRef]
199. Sorasitthiyanukarn, F.N.; Muangnoi, C.; Rojsitthisak, P.; Rojsitthisak, P. Chitosan-alginate nanoparticles as effective oral carriers to improve the stability, bioavailability, and cytotoxicity of curcumin diethyl disuccinate. *Carbohydr. Polym.* **2021**, *256*, 117426. [CrossRef]
200. Williamson, G.; Manach, C. Bioavailability and bioefficacy of polyphenols in humans. II. Review of 93 intervention studies. *Am. J. Clin. Nutr.* **2005**, *81*, 243S–255S. [CrossRef]
201. Toma, C.-C.; Simu, G.M.; Hanganu, D.; Olah, N.; Vata, F.M.G.; Hammami, C.; Hammami, M. Chemical composition of the Tunisian Nigella sativa. Note I. Profile on essential oil. *Farmacia* **2010**, *58*, 458–464.
202. Fabre, G.; Bayach, I.; Berka, K.; Paloncýová, M.; Starok, M.; Rossi, C.; Duroux, J.L.; Otyepka, M.; Trouillas, P. Synergism of antioxidant action of vitamins E, C and quercetin is related to formation of molecular associations in biomembranes. *Chem. Commun.* **2015**, *51*, 7713–7716. [CrossRef]
203. Li, C.; Zhang, W.J.; Choi, J.; Frei, B. Quercetin affects glutathione levels and redox ratio in human aortic endothelial cells not through oxidation but formation and cellular export of quercetin-glutathione conjugates and upregulation of glutamate-cysteine ligase. *Redox Biol.* **2016**, *9*, 220–228. [CrossRef]
204. Guo, Y.Q.; Zhao, J.; Li, Z.Z.; Tang, G.H.; Zhao, Z.M.; Yin, S. Natural nitric oxide (NO) inhibitors from Chloranthus japonicus. *Bioorg. Med. Chem. Lett.* **2016**, *26*, 3163–3166. [CrossRef]
205. Mutoh, M.; Takahashi, M.; Fukuda, K.; Matsushima-Hibiya, Y.; Mutoh, H.; Sugimura, T.; Wakabayashi, K. Suppression of cyclooxygenase-2 promoter-dependent transcriptional activity in colon cancer cells by chemopreventive agents with a resorcin-type structure. *Carcinogenesis* **2000**, *21*, 959–963. [CrossRef]
206. Kashyap, D.; Mittal, S.; Sak, K.; Singhal, P.; Tuli, H.S. Molecular mechanisms of action of quercetin in cancer: Recent advances. *Tumour Biol.* **2016**, *37*, 12927–12939. [CrossRef]
207. Khan, F.; Niaz, K.; Maqbool, F.; Hassan, F.I.; Abdollahi, M.; Nagulapalli Venkata, K.C.; Nabavi, S.M.; Bishayee, A. Molecular Targets Underlying the Anticancer Effects of Quercetin: An Update. *Nutrients* **2016**, *8*, 529. [CrossRef]
208. Park, Y.J.; Choo, W.H.; Kim, H.R.; Chung, K.H.; Oh, S.M. Inhibitory Aromatase Effects of Flavonoids from Ginkgo Biloba Extracts on Estrogen Biosynthesis. *Asian Pac. J. Cancer Prev.* **2015**, *16*, 6317–6325. [CrossRef]
209. Perez-Vizcaino, F.; Duarte, J. Flavonols and cardiovascular disease. *Mol. Aspects Med.* **2010**, *31*, 478–494. [CrossRef]
210. Spagnuolo, C.; Napolitano, M.; Tedesco, I.; Moccia, S.; Milito, A.; Luigi Russo, G. Neuroprotective Role of Natural Polyphenols. *Curr. Top. Med. Chem.* **2016**, *16*, 1943–1950. [CrossRef]
211. Gupta, K.; Panda, D. Perturbation of microtubule polymerization by quercetin through tubulin binding: A novel mechanism of its antiproliferative activity. *Biochemistry* **2002**, *41*, 13029–13038. [CrossRef]
212. Moon, S.K.; Cho, G.O.; Jung, S.Y.; Gal, S.W.; Kwon, T.K.; Lee, Y.C.; Madamanchi, N.R.; Kim, C.H. Quercetin exerts multiple inhibitory effects on vascular smooth muscle cells: Role of ERK1/2, cell-cycle regulation, and matrix metalloproteinase-9. *Biochem. Biophys. Res. Commun.* **2003**, *301*, 1069–1078. [CrossRef]
213. Dong, Y.; Yang, J.; Yang, L.; Li, P. Quercetin Inhibits the Proliferation and Metastasis of Human Non-Small Cell Lung Cancer Cell Line: The Key Role of Src-Mediated Fibroblast Growth Factor-Inducible 14 (Fn14)/ Nuclear Factor kappa B (NF-κB) pathway. *Med. Sci. Monit.* **2020**, *26*, e920537-1–e920537-11. [CrossRef]
214. Guo, Y.; Bruno, R.S. Endogenous and exogenous mediators of quercetin bioavailability. *J. Nutr. Biochem.* **2015**, *26*, 201–210. [CrossRef]
215. Guo, Y.; Mah, E.; Bruno, R.S. Quercetin bioavailability is associated with inadequate plasma vitamin C status and greater plasma endotoxin in adults. *Nutrition* **2014**, *30*, 1279–1286. [CrossRef]
216. Liu, K.; Zha, X.Q.; Shen, W.; Li, Q.M.; Pan, L.H.; Luo, J.P. The hydrogel of whey protein isolate coated by lotus root amylopectin enhance the stability and bioavailability of quercetin. *Carbohydr. Polym.* **2020**, *236*, 116009. [CrossRef]
217. Lin, J.; Teo, L.M.; Leong, L.P.; Zhou, W. In vitro bioaccessibility and bioavailability of quercetin from the quercetin-fortified bread products with reduced glycemic potential. *Food Chem.* **2019**, *286*, 629–635. [CrossRef]
218. Kandemir, K.; Tomas, M.; McClements, D.J.; Capanoglu, E. Recent advances on the improvement of quercetin bioavailability. *Trends Food Sci. Technol.* **2022**, *119*, 192–200. [CrossRef]
219. Terao, J. Factors modulating bioavailability of quercetin-related flavonoids and the consequences of their vascular function. *Biochem. Pharmacol.* **2017**, *139*, 15–23. [CrossRef]
220. Manzoor, M.F.; Hussain, A.; Sameen, A.; Sahar, A.; Khan, S.; Siddique, R.; Aadil, R.M.; Xu, B. Novel extraction, rapid assessment and bioavailability improvement of quercetin: A review. *Ultrason. Sonochem.* **2021**, *78*, 1350–4177. [CrossRef]
221. Singh, B.N.; Shankar, S.; Srivastava, R.K. Green tea catechin, epigallocatechin-3-gallate (EGCG): Mechanisms, perspectives and clinical applications. *Biochem. Pharmacol.* **2011**, *82*, 1807–1821. [CrossRef]
222. Borutinskaitė, V.; Virkšaitė, A.; Gudelytė, G.; Navakauskienė, R. Green tea polyphenol EGCG causes anti-cancerous epigenetic modulations in acute promyelocytic leukemia cells. *Leuk. Lymphoma* **2018**, *59*, 469–478. [CrossRef]

223. Sahadevan, R.; Singh, S.; Binoy, A.; Sadhukhan, S. Chemico-biological aspects of (-)-epigallocatechin-3-gallate (EGCG) to improve its stability, bioavailability and membrane permeability: Current status and future prospects. *Crit. Rev. Food Sci. Nutr.* **2022**, *62*, 1–30. [CrossRef]
224. Pervin, M.; Unno, K.; Takagaki, A.; Isemura, M.; Nakamura, Y. Function of Green Tea Catechins in the Brain: Epigallocatechin Gallate and its Metabolites. *Int. J. Mol. Sci.* **2019**, *20*, 3630. [CrossRef] [PubMed]
225. Rashidinejad, A.; Boostani, S.; Babazadeh, A.; Rehman, A.; Rezaei, A.; Akbari-Alavijeh, S.; Shaddel, R.; Jafari, S.M. Opportunities and challenges for the nanodelivery of green tea catechins in functional foods. *Food Res. Int.* **2021**, *142*, 110186. [CrossRef] [PubMed]
226. Zhang, J.; Nie, S.; Wang, S. Nanoencapsulation Enhances Epigallocatechin-3-Gallate Stability and Its Anti-atherogenic Bioactivities in Macrophages. *J. Agric. Food Chem.* **2013**, *61*, 9200–9209. [CrossRef] [PubMed]
227. Krupkova, O.; Ferguson, S.J.; Wuertz-Kozak, K. Stability of (-)-epigallocatechin gallate and its activity in liquid formulations and delivery systems. *J. Nutr. Biochem.* **2016**, *37*, 1–12. [CrossRef] [PubMed]
228. Dai, W.; Ruan, C.; Zhang, Y.; Wang, J.; Han, J.; Shao, Z.; Sun, Y.; Liang, J. Bioavailability enhancement of EGCG by structural modification and nano-delivery: A review. *J. Funct. Foods* **2020**, *65*, 103732. [CrossRef]
229. Fernández, V.A.; Toledano, L.A.; Lozano, N.P.; Tapia, E.N.; Roig, M.D.G.; Fornell, R.D.L.T.; Algar, Ó.G. Bioavailability of Epigallocatechin Gallate Administered With Different Nutritional Strategies in Healthy Volunteers. *Antioxidants* **2020**, *9*, 440. [CrossRef]
230. Rinott, E.; Meir, A.Y.; Tsaban, G.; Zelicha, H.; Kaplan, A.; Knights, D.; Tuohy, K.; Scholz, M.U.; Koren, O.; Stampfer, M.J.; et al. The effects of the Green-Mediterranean diet on cardiometabolic health are linked to gut microbiome modifications: A randomized controlled trial. *Genome Med.* **2022**, *14*, 29. [CrossRef]
231. Pira, C.; Trapani, G.; Fadda, M.; Finocchiaro, C.; Bertino, E.; Coscia, A.; Ciocan, C.; Cuciureanu, M.; Hegheş, S.C.; Vranceanu, M.; et al. Comparative Study Regarding the Adherence to the Mediterranean Diet and the Eating Habits of Two Groups-The Romanian Children and Adolescents Living in Nord-West of Romania and Their Romanian Counterparts Living in Italy. *Foods* **2021**, *10*, 2045. [CrossRef]
232. Hong, J.; Lambert, J.D.; Lee, S.H.; Sinko, P.J.; Yang, C.S. Involvement of multidrug resistance-associated proteins in regulating cellular levels of (-)-epigallocatechin-3-gallate and its methyl metabolites. *Biochem. Biophys. Res. Commun.* **2003**, *310*, 222–227. [CrossRef]
233. Mehmood, S.; Maqsood, M.; Mahtab, N.; Khan, M.I.; Sahar, A.; Zaib, S.; Gul, S. Epigallocatechin gallate: Phytochemistry, bioavailability, utilization challenges, and strategies. *J. Food Biochem.* **2022**, *46*, e14189. [CrossRef]
234. Shpigelman, A.; Israeli, G.; Livney, Y.D. Thermally-induced protein–polyphenol co-assemblies: Beta lactoglobulin-based nanocomplexes as protective nanovehicles for EGCG. *Food Hydrocoll.* **2010**, *24*, 735–743. [CrossRef]
235. Legeay, S.; Rodier, M.; Fillon, L.; Faure, S.; Clere, N. Epigallocatechin Gallate: A Review of Its Beneficial Properties to Prevent Metabolic Syndrome. *Nutrients* **2015**, *7*, 5443–5468. [CrossRef]
236. Chow, H.H.S.; Hakim, I.A.; Vining, D.R.; Crowell, J.A.; Ranger-Moore, J.; Chew, W.M.; Celaya, C.A.; Rodney, S.R.; Hara, Y.; Alberts, D.S. Effects of dosing condition on the oral bioavailability of green tea catechins after single-dose administration of polyphenon E in healthy individuals. *Clin. Cancer Res.* **2005**, *11*, 4627–4633. [CrossRef]
237. Murakami, A. Dose-dependent functionality and toxicity of green tea polyphenols in experimental rodents. *Arch. Biochem. Biophys.* **2014**, *557*, 3–10. [CrossRef]
238. Younes, M.; Aggett, P.; Aguilar, F.; Crebelli, R.; Dusemund, B.; Filipič, M.; Frutos, M.J.; Galtier, P.; Gott, D.; Gundert-Remy, U.; et al. Scientific opinion on the safety of green tea catechins I EFSA. *EFSA J.* **2018**, *16*, e05239. [CrossRef]
239. Peters, C.M.; Green, R.J.; Janle, E.M.; Ferruzzi, M.G. Formulation with ascorbic acid and sucrose modulates catechin bioavailability from green tea. *Food Res. Int.* **2010**, *43*, 95. [CrossRef]
240. Naumovski, N.; Blades, B.L.; Roach, P.D. Food Inhibits the Oral Bioavailability of the Major Green Tea Antioxidant Epigallocatechin Gallate in Humans. *Antioxidants* **2015**, *4*, 373–393. [CrossRef]
241. Wang, L.; Huang, X.; Jing, H.; Ma, C.; Wang, H. Bilosomes as effective delivery systems to improve the gastrointestinal stability and bioavailability of epigallocatechin gallate (EGCG). *Food Res. Int.* **2021**, *149*, 110631. [CrossRef]
242. Tapiero, H.; Townsend, D.M.; Tew, K.D. The role of carotenoids in the prevention of human pathologies. *Biomed. Pharmacother.* **2004**, *58*, 100–110. [CrossRef]
243. Müller, L.; Caris-Veyrat, C.; Lowe, G.; Böhm, V. Lycopene and Its Antioxidant Role in the Prevention of Cardiovascular Diseases-A Critical Review. *Crit. Rev. Food Sci. Nutr.* **2016**, *56*, 1868–1879. [CrossRef]
244. Aust, O.; Ale-Agha, N.; Zhang, L.; Wollersen, H.; Sies, H.; Stahl, W. Lycopene oxidation product enhances gap junctional communication. *Food Chem. Toxicol.* **2003**, *41*, 1399–1407. [CrossRef]
245. Ilic, D.; Misso, M. Lycopene for the prevention and treatment of benign prostatic hyperplasia and prostate cancer: A systematic review. *Maturitas* **2012**, *72*, 269–276. [CrossRef]
246. Kolberg, M.; Pedersen, S.; Bastani, N.E.; Carlsen, H.; Blomhoff, R.; Paur, I. Tomato paste alters NF-κB and cancer-related mRNA expression in prostate cancer cells, xenografts, and xenograft microenvironment. *Nutr. Cancer* **2015**, *67*, 305–315. [CrossRef]
247. Przybylska, S.; Tokarczyk, G. Lycopene in the Prevention of Cardiovascular Diseases. *Int. J. Mol. Sci.* **2022**, *23*, 1957. [CrossRef]
248. Arballo, J.; Amengual, J.; Erdman, J.W. Lycopene: A Critical Review of Digestion, Absorption, Metabolism, and Excretion. *Antioxidants* **2021**, *10*, 342. [CrossRef]

249. Boileau, T.W.M.; Boileau, A.C.; Erdman, J.W. Bioavailability of all-trans and cis-isomers of lycopene. *Exp. Biol. Med.* **2002**, *227*, 914–919. [CrossRef]
250. Moran, N.E.; Cichon, M.J.; Riedl, K.M.; Grainger, E.M.; Schwartz, S.J.; Novotny, J.A.; Erdman, J.W.; Clinton, S.K. Compartmental and noncompartmental modeling of ^{13}C-lycopene absorption, isomerization, and distribution kinetics in healthy adults. *Am. J. Clin. Nutr.* **2015**, *102*, 1436–1449. [CrossRef]
251. Wang, X.D. Lycopene metabolism and its biological significance. *Am. J. Clin. Nutr.* **2012**, *96*, 1214S–1222S. [CrossRef]
252. Vitucci, D.; Amoresano, A.; Nunziato, M.; Muoio, S.; Alfieri, A.; Oriani, G.; Scalfi, L.; Frusciante, L.; Rigano, M.M.; Pucci, P.; et al. Nutritional Controlled Preparation and Administration of Different Tomato Purées Indicate Increase of β-Carotene and Lycopene Isoforms, and of Antioxidant Potential in Human Blood Bioavailability: A Pilot Study. *Nutrients* **2021**, *13*, 1336. [CrossRef]
253. Unlu, N.Z.; Bohn, T.; Clinton, S.K.; Schwartz, S.J. Carotenoid absorption from salad and salsa by humans is enhanced by the addition of avocado or avocado oil. *J. Nutr.* **2005**, *135*, 431–436. [CrossRef]
254. Lee, A.; Thurnham, D.I.; Chopra, M. Consumption of tomato products with olive oil but not sunflower oil increases the antioxidant activity of plasma. *Free Radic. Biol. Med.* **2000**, *29*, 1051–1055. [CrossRef]
255. Amorim, A.D.G.N.; Vasconcelos, A.G.; Souza, J.; Oliveira, A.; Gullón, B.; de Souza de Almeida Leite, J.R.; Pintado, M. Bio-Availability, Anticancer Potential, and Chemical Data of Lycopene: An Overview and Technological Prospecting. *Antioxidants* **2022**, *11*, 360. [CrossRef]
256. Crowe-White, K.M.; Voruganti, V.S.; Talevi, V.; Dudenbostel, T.; Nagabooshanam, V.A.; Locher, J.L.; Ellis, A.C. Variation of Serum Lycopene in Response to 100% Watermelon Juice: An Exploratory Analysis of Genetic Variants in a Randomized Controlled Crossover Study. *Curr. Dev. Nutr.* **2020**, *4*, nzaa102. [CrossRef] [PubMed]
257. Zubair, N.; Kooperberg, C.; Liu, J.; Di, C.; Peters, U.; Neuhouser, M.L. Genetic variation predicts serum lycopene concentrations in a multiethnic population of postmenopausal women. *J. Nutr.* **2015**, *145*, 187–192. [CrossRef] [PubMed]
258. Ferrucci, L.; Perry, J.R.B.; Matteini, A.; Perola, M.; Tanaka, T.; Silander, K.; Rice, N.; Melzer, D.; Murray, A.; Cluett, C.; et al. Common variation in the β-carotene 15,15′-monooxygenase 1 gene affects circulating levels of carotenoids: A genome-wide association study. *Am. J. Hum. Genet.* **2008**, *84*, 123–133. [CrossRef] [PubMed]

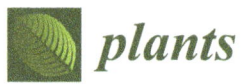

Article

The Cholesterol-Modulating Effect of the New Herbal Medicinal Recipe from Yellow Vine (*Coscinium fenestratum* (Goetgh.)), Ginger (*Zingiber officinale* Roscoe.), and Safflower (*Carthamus tinctorius* L.) on Suppressing PCSK9 Expression to Upregulate LDLR Expression in HepG2 Cells

Tassanee Ongtanasup [1,2], Nuntika Prommee [3], Onkamon Jampa [4], Thanchanok Limcharoen [1], Smith Wanmasae [5], Veeranoot Nissapatorn [2,6], Alok K. Paul [7], Maria de Lourdes Pereira [8], Polrat Wilairatana [9], Norased Nasongkla [10] and Komgrit Eawsakul [1,2,*]

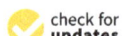

Citation: Ongtanasup, T.; Prommee, N.; Jampa, O.; Limcharoen, T.; Wanmasae, S.; Nissapatorn, V.; Paul, A.K.; Pereira, M.d.L.; Wilairatana, P.; Nasongkla, N.; et al. The Cholesterol-Modulating Effect of the New Herbal Medicinal Recipe from Yellow Vine (*Coscinium fenestratum* (Goetgh.)), Ginger (*Zingiber officinale* Roscoe.), and Safflower (*Carthamus tinctorius* L.) on Suppressing PCSK9 Expression to Upregulate LDLR Expression in HepG2 Cells. *Plants* **2022**, *11*, 1835. https://doi.org/10.3390/plants11141835

Academic Editor: José Antonio Morales-González

Received: 20 June 2022
Accepted: 9 July 2022
Published: 13 July 2022

Publisher's Note: MDPI stays neutral with regard to jurisdictional claims in published maps and institutional affiliations.

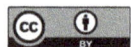

Copyright: © 2022 by the authors. Licensee MDPI, Basel, Switzerland. This article is an open access article distributed under the terms and conditions of the Creative Commons Attribution (CC BY) license (https://creativecommons.org/licenses/by/4.0/).

[1] School of Medicine, Walailak University, Nakhon Si Thammarat 80160, Thailand; tassanee.on@wu.ac.th (T.O.); thanchanok.li@wu.ac.th (T.L.)
[2] Research Excellence Center for Innovation and Health Products (RECIHP), Walailak University, Nakhon Si Thammarat 80160, Thailand; nissapat@gmail.com or veeranoot.ni@wu.ac.th
[3] Division of Applied Thai Traditional Medicine, Faculty of Public Health, Naresuan University, Phitsanulok 65000, Thailand; nuntikap@nu.ac.th
[4] Tak Community College, Nong Bua Tai 63000, Thailand; onkamon@takcc.ac.th
[5] School of Allied Health Sciences, Walailak University, Nakhon Si Thammarat 80160, Thailand; smith.wa@wu.ac.th
[6] School of Allied Health Sciences, World Union for Herbal Drug Discovery (WUHeDD), Nakhon Si Thammarat 80160, Thailand
[7] School of Pharmacy and Pharmacology, University of Tasmania, Hobart, TAS 7001, Australia; alok.paul@utas.edu.au
[8] CICECO—Aveiro Institute of Materials, Department of Medical Sciences, University of Aveiro, 3810-193 Aveiro, Portugal; mlourdespereira@ua.pt
[9] Department of Clinical Tropical Medicine, Faculty of Tropical Medicine, Mahidol University, Bangkok 10400, Thailand; polrat.wil@mahidol.ac.th
[10] Department of Biomedical Engineering, Faculty of Engineering, Mahidol University, Nakhon Pathom 73170, Thailand; norased.nas@mahidol.ac.th
* Correspondence: komgrit.ea@wu.ac.th

Abstract: PCSK9 is a promising target for developing novel cholesterol-lowering drugs. We developed a recipe that combined molecular docking, GC-MS/MS, and real-time PCR to identify potential PCSK9 inhibitors for herb ratio determination. Three herbs, *Carthamus tinctorius*, *Coscinium fenestratum*, and *Zingiber officinale*, were used in this study. This work aimed to evaluate cholesterol-lowering through a PCSK9 inhibitory mechanism of these three herbs for defining a suitable ratio. Chemical constituents were identified using GC-MS/MS. The PCSK9 inhibitory potential of the compounds was determined using molecular docking, real-time PCR, and Oil red O staining. It has been shown that most of the active compounds of *C. fenestratum* and *Z. officinale* inhibit PCSK9 when extracted with water, and *C. fenestratum* has been shown to yield tetraacetyl-d-xylonic nitrile (27.92%) and inositol, 1-deoxy-(24.89%). These compounds could inhibit PCSK9 through the binding of 6 and 5 hydrogen bonds, respectively, while the active compound in *Z. officinale* is 2-Formyl-9-[.beta.-d-ribofuranosyl] hypoxanthine (4.37%) inhibits PCSK9 by forming 8 hydrogen bonds. These results suggest that a recipe comprising three parts *C. fenestratum*, two parts *Z. officinale*, and one part *C. tinctorius* is a suitable herbal ratio for reducing lipid levels in the bloodstream through a PCSK9 inhibitory mechanism.

Keywords: cholesterol-lowering; PCSK9; *C. tinctorius*; *C. fenestratum*; *Z. officinale*; molecular docking; chemical constituents

1. Introduction

Blood cholesterol levels of total cholesterol and low-density lipoprotein (LDL) cholesterol are both major risk factors for coronary heart disease (CHD). Reduced total and LDL cholesterol levels have been shown to decrease the risk of coronary heart disease.

The most given lipid-lowering drug is statins, which potently inhibit 3-hydroxy-3-methylglutaryl-coenzyme A (HMG-CoA) reductase, the enzyme that decreases the biosynthesis of cholesterol [1–3]. This results in intracellular cholesterol depletion and subsequent upregulation of low-density lipoprotein receptors (LDLRs) expression on hepatocytes and enhanced clearance of LDL from blood circulation via the sterol regulatory element-binding protein (SREBP) pathway. Additionally, proprotein convertase subtilisin kexin type 9 (PCSK9), a member of the subtilisin-related serine protease family, has been identified as a critical regulator of low-density lipoprotein (LDL) metabolism, and inhibitors of PCSK9 are currently being investigated for their ability to lower circulating LDL via binding to its epidermal growth factor-like repeat (EGF-A) of LDLR [4–6]. Secreted PCSK9, a domain found in hepatocytes, binds to LDLR and promotes its lysosomal degradation in cells [7,8].

PCSK9 deficiency leads to a more significant number of cell surface LDLRs, and enhanced hepatic LDLR expression leads to improved plasma LDL clearance, protecting against cardiovascular disease (CVD). As a result, finding a new antihyperlipidemic drug that targets PCSK9 expression is a top priority in antihyperlipidemic research. Reducing PCSK9 transcription is a potential technique for lowering LDL. Thus, we set out to find a new recipe that inhibits PCSK9 transcription to promote plasma cholesterol-reduction effects via their effect on LDLR transcription. The new herbal recipe that induced LDLR expression may be a useful technique for treating hyperlipidemia. Complementary and alternative medicine has been utilized to control cholesterol levels and improve heart health; therefore, increasing LDLR expression from herbal drugs might be a useful antihyperlipidemic method. In addition, the use of various herbs as medicinal compounds will help to improve the effectiveness of the treatment.

Yellow vine (*Coscinium fenestratum* (Goetgh.)), commonly called 'tree turmeric', belongs to the Menispermaceae family and is a medicinally significant dioecious endangered liana [9] found in Vietnam, Singapore, Sri Lanka, and Thailand [10]. The stem and root of *C. fenestratum* are used in traditional Chinese medicine [9]. Berberine (isoquinoline alkaloids), dropalmatine, crebanine, jatrorrhizine, palmitic acid, oleic acid, and saponin have all been isolated from *C. fenestratum* [11]. These molecules possess various pharmacological effects, including anti-diabetic, anti-inflammatory, thermogenic, and antimicrobial activities [12]. Additionally, multiple studies [13–15] suggest berberine's usefulness in decreasing blood lipids. However, the usage of *C. fenestratum* for cholesterol reduction has not been explored.

Ginger (*Zingiber officinale* Roscoe), most commonly known as ginger, is a spice and flavoring ingredient used in cuisines worldwide [16]. For thousands of years, it has been used as a spice and for medicinal purposes. Its usage is attested in ancient Sanskrit and Chinese manuscripts, as well as in Arabic, Roman, and Greek medical literature [17]. *Z. officinale* is regarded as a promising medication in Ayurveda due to its efficacy as a digestive stimulant, antiasthmatic, and rubefacient [18]. It is cultivated commercially in India, China, Thailand, Australia, South Africa, and Mexico. Antioxidant activity [19–21] has been reported in vitro for *Z. officinale* aqueous and organic solvent extracts. A combination of *Z. officinale* and garlic [17] was proven to have hypoglycaemic and hypolipidemic effects in albino rats. The previous research [22] has demonstrated that ethanolic *Z. officinale* extract has considerable antihypercholesterolemic action in cholesterol-fed rabbits. It should be emphasized that *Z. officinale*'s efficacy in lowering cholesterol levels is favorable and that its usefulness should be investigated when paired with other herbs.

Safflower (*Carthamus tinctorius* L.) is an oil-producing crop that belongs to the Compositae or Asteraceae family. In Thailand, it is called Kamfoi, whereas, in China, it is called zang hong hua. *C. tinctorius* is a multifunctional crop that has been produced in Thailand

and other areas of the world for generations for a variety of purposes. It is a critical plant since it provides an alternate supply of oil. C. tinctorius research and development continue to receive little attention [23]. However, it can grow in a wide variety of environmental conditions with very high yield potential and has a variety of uses for the various plant components. However, some researchers [24,25] have reported that C. tinctorius contains linoleic acid, an unsaturated fatty acid, which is widely known and helps decrease blood cholesterol levels.

In addition, all three types of herbs—C. fenestratum, Z. officinale, and C. tinctorius—contain primary metabolite and secondary metabolite. In addition, each country has a wide range of uses as shown in Table 1.

Table 1. Primary and secondary compounds derived from plants and their therapeutic uses in different country.

Scientific Name	Primary Metabolite	Secondary Metabolite	Uses of Plants in Different Countries	Preparations/ Therapeutic Uses
Z. officinale	carbohydrate, lipids, amino acids, cinnamic acid, and vitamins [26]	oleoresin, phenolics, zingiberene, gingerols, shogaols, aromatic alcohol, and terpenoids [27]	It is distributed all over the world, such as in European countries, America, China, Japan, and India [28] with the following benefits: • reducing effect on blood lipids [29] • curing heart problems, treating stomach upset, diarrhea, headaches, and cough or nausea [30] • treating digestive problems [30] • Antibacterial agent [31] • Chemopreventive effect [32] • vomiting in motion sickness [33]	• Use both fresh and dried preparation of rhizome for medicinal use [30] • Steam distillation/supercritical CO_2 extraction for essential oil [31]
C.fenestratum	carbohy-drate, lipids, amino acids, and vitamins [34]	alkaloids, tannins, saponins, flavonoids, phenolic compounds [35]	It is distributed all over the world, such as in Sri Lanka, India, and Thailand with the following benefits: antidiabetic, diuretic, cholesterol lowering, anticancer, anti-inflammatory, antifungal, antihelmintic, antioxidant, and antimicrobial effects [36,37]	Use stem and dried preparation with solvent extractions such as • Ethanol [38] • Methanol [39] • Water [40]
C. tinctorius	formic acid, acetic acid, succinic acid, glucose, fructose, asparagine, proline, alanine, glutamine, valine, uridine, trigonelline, and choline [41]	saffloquinoside C, saffloquinoside A, anhydrosafflor yellow B, rutin, (2S)−4′,5,6,7-tetrahydroxyflavanone 6-O-β-D-glucoside, 5,7,4′-trihydroxy-6-methoxyflavone3-O-β-D-rutinoside, kaempferol-3-O-β-D-glucoside, kaempferol-3-O-rutinoside, (2S)−4′,5,7,8-tetrahydroxy-flavanone-8-O-βD-glucoside, 6-hydroxykaempferol-3,6,7-tri-O-β-D-glucoside, and kaempferol-3-O-β-D-glucosyl-(1→2)-β-D-glucoside	It is distributed all over the world, such as in India, Mexico, America, Spain, Australia, and China with the following benefits: • Promotes blood circulation and removes the stasis • relieves pain • treats headache and dizziness • protects liver and relieves jaundice [42]	• Medicinal liquor • Decoction • Pill, granule, capsule [42]

Although all three herbs have been examined for their lipid-lowering properties, none have been combined to create a lipid-lowering recipe. Therefore, in this study, new formulations from these herbs were investigated for lipid-inhibiting activity through mechanisms such as HMG-CoA, SREBP, PCSK9, and LDLR mRNA levels using molecular docking and in vitro studies. Then, the proportion of herbs in the recipe will be determined to be suitable for reducing lipid in the bloodstream.

2. Materials and Methods

2.1. Materials

2.1.1. Cell Line, Chemicals, and Computer Software

Human hepatocellular carcinoma (HepG2) was purchased from ATCC (Manassas, VA, USA). It was cultivated in Dulbecco's modified Eagle's medium (CAS No. 11965118) with 10% fetal bovine serum (CAS No. 10270), 1% PenStrep (CAS No. 15140122), and 3.7 g/L sodium bicarbonate (CAS No. 144-55-8). Filtration of the culture media was performed using a 0.22 m cellulose acetate membrane (CAS No. 11107-25-N). Cells were detached for quantification using 0.25% trypsin-EDTA (CAS No. 25200072; Gibco, Waltham, MA, USA), followed by 0.4% trypan blue staining for cultivated cell viability (CAS No. 15250061). Thiazolyl blue tetrazolium bromide (MTT, CAS No. 298-93-1) and dimethylsulfoxide (DMSO) were used to determine the viability of cells (CAS No. 67-68-5).

Oil red O was purchased from Sigma in the United States of America (CAS No. 1320-06-5) and dissolved in a stock solution by adding 100 mg oil red O to 20 mL100% isopropanol (CAS No. 67-63-0). Prior to staining, a working solution of Oil red O was made by diluting three parts stock solution with two parts DI water. This working solution was filtered using Whatman paper 42. (CAS Number 1442-110).

AutoDock 1.5.6, Python 3.8.2, MGLTools 1.5.4, Discovery Studio-2017, ArgusLab 4.0.1, ChemSketch, Avogadro, and OpenBabel were used to perform molecular docking. The research was conducted by examining the system parameters specified in the software specifications. Processor: Intel Xeon-E5-2678v3 12C/24T CPU @ 2.50 GHz–3.10 GHz, system memory: 32 GB DDR4-2133 RECC, graphics processing unit: VGA GTX 1070 TI 8G, operating system type: 64-bit, with Windows 10 as the operating system.

2.1.2. Herb Material

In August 2021, these three plants were obtained from Thailand's Vejponggosot pharmaceutical company: *C. tinctorius*, *C. fenestratum*, and *Z. officinale*. The Thai Traditional Medicine Herbarium, Department of Thai Traditional and Alternative Medicine, Bangkok, Thailand, has deposited these herbs. The voucher specimen numbers for *C. tinctorius*, *C. fenestratum*, and *Z. officinale* are TTM-c No. 1000705, TTM-c No. 1000703, and TTM-c No. 1000704, respectively.

2.2. Extraction and Isolation

Plant materials were washed and dried at 50 °C until reaching a stable weight, then ground into a powder material and prepared for extraction method.

2.2.1. Water Extraction

The powdered herb (400 g) was mixed with 1 L of warm deionized water. On a hot plate, the herb solution was heated to 100 °C for 15 min. Another 1000 mL of hot water was added to the solution because the herb absorbed the water. The final solution was boiled until only one-third of the solution remained. Prior to freeze-drying, the solution was filtered using Whatman No. 1 filter paper and stored at −20 °C. Freeze-dryer (Eyela FDU-2100, Bohemia, NY, USA) was used to lyophilize the frozen samples.

2.2.2. Ethanol Extraction

Individually, 400 g of *C. fenestratum* stem, *C. tinctorius* flower, and *Z. officinale* rhizomes were extracted with ethanol for three days using the maceration procedure. The filtrate was collected using Whatman No. 1 filter paper and evaporated using a rotary evaporator to obtain a viscous ethanolic extract (Heidolph Basic Hei-VAP ML, Schwabach, Germany). The maceration procedure was then performed twice more. Each herb's remaining ethanol was evaporated further in a vacuum drying chamber (Binder VD 23, Tuttlingen, Germany) until a stable weight was obtained.

2.3. GC-MS/MS Analysis

Scion 436 GC Bruker model performed GC-MS/MS analyses to analyze the material at a 3 mg/mL concentration. The GC-MS/MS separation of the compounds was performed with a 30-m fused silica capillary column (0.25 mm internal diameter, 0.25 µm thickness). The carrier gas was helium gas (99.999 percent) with a constant flow rate of 1 mL/min and an injection volume of 10 µL. (split ratio of 10:1). The injector was heated to 250 °C, while the ion source was heated to 280 °C. The oven temperature was kept at 110 °C for 2 min, increased to 280 °C at 5 °C/min, and then kept isothermal at 280 °C for 9-min, for a total GC run duration of 60 min. The mass analysts by ionization energy of 70 eV with 0.5 s interval scan were designed, with fragments ranging from m/z 50 to 500 Da. The intake temperature was set to 280 °C, while the source temperature was set at 250 °C. By comparing the average peak area of each component to the total areas, the relative fraction of each component was computed. MS Workstation 8 was used for handling mass spectra and chromatograms. The chemical components were identified using the NIST Version 2.0 library database of the National Institute of Standards and Technology (NIST).

2.4. Treatment of HepG2 Cells

The ATCC (Manassas, VA, USA) provided the human hepatocellular carcinoma HepG2 cell line cultured in DMEM supplemented with 10% fetal bovine serum (FBS). The cells were seeded in 96-well plates with 5×10^4 cells/mL in a normal serum medium for 24 h before being changed to DMEM without FBS overnight. For an additional 24 h, cells were treated with extracts of the *C. fenestratum*, *Z. officinale*, and *C. tinctorius*, as well as a recipe of *C. fenestratum* (3 parts), *Z. officinale* (2 parts), and *C. tinctorius* (1 part) extracted with water and ethanol at concentrations ranging from 10 to 400 µg/mL prior to cell viability testing, real-time PCR, and oil red O staining.

2.4.1. Cell Viability Analysis

An MTT assay was used to measure cell viability. Briefly, cells were treated as described above, then incubated for 4 h at 37 °C with a 1 mg/mL MTT solution [43,44]. The purple formazan crystals were dissolved in DMSO when the medium was removed. Cell viability was measured by absorbance at 550 nm of the microplate reader (Metertech M965, Taipei, Taiwan).

2.4.2. Quantitative Reverse Transcription PCR (RT-qPCR) Analysis

The total RNA mini kit (Geneaid, Taipei, Taiwan) was used to isolate total RNA from HepG2 cells. Using an iScript Mastermix (Bio-Rad, Hercules, CA, USA), a quantified 1 µg sample of total RNA was converted to cDNA. The primers for specific genes are listed in Table 2 using the Luna Master Mix. The level of mRNA expression was evaluated using a Quanti-Studio 3 (ThermoFisher, Waltham, MA, USA) according to the manufacturer's guidelines. To compare the groups, $2^{-\Delta\Delta CT}$ values were used, with GAPDH (glyceraldehyde 3-phosphate dehydrogenase) acting an endogenous control [45].

Table 2. List of real-time PCR primer sequences.

Gene	Forward Primer	Reverse Primer
GAPDH	5′-CATGAGAAGTATGACAACAGCCT-3′	5′-AGTCCTTCCACGATACCAAAGT-3′
PCSK9	5′-GCTGAGCTGCTCCAGTTTCT-3′	5′-AATGGCGTAGACACCCTCAC-3′
LDLR	5′-AGTTGGCTGCGTTAATGTGA-3′	5′-TGATGGGTTCATCTGACCAGT-3′
HMGCR	5′-TGATTGACCTTTCCAGAGCAAG-3′	5′-CTAAAATTGCCATTCCACGAGC-3′

2.4.3. Oil Red O Staining

Ice-cold PBS rinsed the fasting-induced steatosis in HepG2 cells before being fixed by ice-cold 10% formalin for 30 min. The cells were then rinsed with distilled water and stained for 30 min at room temperature with an Oil Red O working solution to generate stain lipid droplets [46]. An optical microscope was used to study and photograph the cells (Ziess AX10, Carl Zeiss, Jena, Germany). Lipid content was also determined by dissolving Oil red O in isopropanol and measuring using a microplate reader at a wavelength of 500 nm [15].

2.5. Molecular Docking

The crystal structures of PCSK9 and HMGCR with the PDB codes 6u26 [47] and 2r4f [48] were utilized. Autodock [49] was used to optimize the protein. The missing hydrogens were inserted throughout the optimization step. The final proteins were given Kollman unified atom charges and solvation parameters. Table 3 shows the grid position and size reflecting the whole protein during the docking process. Following GC-MS/MS analysis, the 3D structures of the top 5 high yielding compounds in *C. tinctorius*, *C. fenestratum*, and *Z. officinale* were chosen for docking, while positive docking controls were Alirocumab [50] and Lovastatin [51] for PCSK9 and HMGCR, respectively. All 3D structures were obtained from PubChem (https://pubchem.ncbi.nlm.nih.gov, accessed on 2 October 2021). All structures were optimized before molecular docking. Open Babel was used to add hydrogen atoms to every structure and all structures were optimized by Arguslab through semi-empirical Parametric Method 3 (PM3). Molecular docking was utilized to explore protein–ligand binding. Arguslab and Autodock were used for this docking study. In the beginning, the Arguslab engine was used for docking. The scoring function was set in default parameters. The accuracy of docking was set to regular. All docking was confirmed with Autodock3 through the Lamarckian genetic technique to ensure reliable results. The following are the optimal autodocking run parameters: number of GA runs: 50; population size: 200; and all other run parameters: default [44,52].

Table 3. The grid position and grid size of the targeted protein.

Gene	Grid Position	Grid Size
PCSK9	$34.025 \times 23.492 \times 25.638$	$110 \times 82 \times 126$
HMGCR	$73.702 \times 0.468 \times 18.849$	$122 \times 78 \times 126$

2.6. Binding Site Analysis

The structure of the compounds that resulted in lower binding energy to the targeted proteins than the standard drug was taken to visualize the binding characteristics by Discovery Studio. The ligand–protein bindings were presented as 2D and 3D. To identify the structure binding protein, the binding position was compared through CavityPlus (http://www.pkumdl.cn/cavityplus, accessed on 2 November 2021).

2.7. Statistical Analysis

The tests were carried out at least three times except molecular docking, and the results are shown as the mean ± standard deviation. SPSS 12.0 (SPSS Inc., Chicago, IL, USA) was used to perform the statistical calculations. The data were evaluated using a one-way ANOVA with Dunnet's post hoc test, with a *p*-value < 0.05 considered statistically significant.

3. Results

3.1. GC-MS/MS Analysis

The active compounds of the herbs extracted with water and ethanol were analyzed with GC-MS/MS. In this study, the five most active compounds were selected and classified into three groups: (1) the most common, which were equal to or greater than 10%; (2) the moderately common were those that were greater than 1% but less than 10%; and (3) rare compounds are substances found less than 1% of the time, which are then chosen to study binding by molecular docking. The active compounds in each herb areshown in Tables 4–6.

Table 4. Compounds identified in water-extracted C. tinctorius.

S. No.	RT	Name of the Compound	Molecular Formulae	MW	Peak Area (%)
1	6.10	D-Alanine, N-propargyloxycarbonyl-, isohexyl ester	$C_{13}H_{21}NO_4$	255	3.14
2	7.72	4H-Pyran-4-one, 2,3-dihydro-3,5-dihydroxy-6-methyl-	$C_6H_8O_4$	144	8.56
3	9.05	Acetic anhydride	$C_4H_6O_3$	102	5.72
4	9.38	Benzofuran, 2,3-dihydro-	C_8H_8O	120	23.24
5	11.14	Cyclohexasiloxane, dodecamethyl-	$C_{12}H_{36}O_6Si_6$	444	6.96
6	14.59	Sucrose	$C_{12}H_{22}O_{11}$	342	6.08
7	14.97	3,5-Dimethoxy-4-hydroxytoluene	$C_9H_{12}O_3$	168	2.46
8	15.22	3-Isopropoxy-1,1,1,7,7,7-hexamethyl-3,5,5-tris(trimethylsiloxy)tetrasiloxane	$C_{18}H_{52}O_7Si_7$	576	13.73
9	16.45	2,4-Di-tert-butylphenol	$C_{14}H_{22}O$	206	4.68
10	16.83	Methyl 4-O-acetyl-2,3,6-tri-O-ethyl-.alpha.-d-galactopyranoside	$C_{15}H_{28}O_7$	320	2.57
11	18.99	3,4-Dihydroxyphenylglycol, 4TMS derivative	$C_{20}H_{42}O_4Si_4$	458	8.94
12	22.27	3-Isopropoxy-1,1,1,7,7,7-hexamethyl-3,5,5-tris(trimethylsiloxy)tetrasiloxane-Dup1	$C_{18}H_{52}O_7Si_7$	576	4.79
13	25.21	3-Isopropoxy-1,1,1,7,7,7-hexamethyl-3,5,5-tris(trimethylsiloxy)tetrasiloxane-Dup2	$C_{18}H_{52}O_7Si_7$	576	2.71
14	27.89	Heptasiloxane, 1,1,3,3,5,5,7,7,9,9,11,11,13,13-tetradecamethyl-	$C_{18}H_{44}O_6Si_7$	504	1.79
15	29.52	Ethanol, 2,2'-(dodecylimino)bis-	$C_{16}H_{35}NO_2$	273	2.34
16	39.48	Heptacosane	$C_{27}H_{56}$	380	1.36
17	41.25	Octacosane	$C_{28}H_{58}$	394	0.92

Table 5. Compounds identified in the water-extracted C. fenestratum.

S. No.	RT	Name of the Compound	Molecular Formulae	MW	Peak Area (%)
1	6.72	Tert.-butylaminoacrylonitryl	$C_7H_{12}N_2$	124	1.67
2	7.22	N-(Trimethylsilyl)pyridin-4-amine	$C_8H_{14}N_2Si$	166	0.36
3	7.75	4H-Pyran-4-one, 2,3-dihydro-3,5-dihydroxy-6-methyl-	$C_6H_8O_4$	144	0.22
4	8.79	Catechol	$C_6H_6O_2$	110	0.9
5	9.06	Acetic anhydride	$C_4H_6O_3$	102	0.49
6	10.67	Hydroquinone	$C_6H_6O_2$	110	0.33
7	11.17	Cyclohexasiloxane, dodecamethyl-	$C_{12}H_{36}O_6Si_6$	444	0.38
8	12.67	Phenol, 2,6-dimethoxy-	$C_8H_{10}O_3$	154	1.72
9	13.92	Benzaldehyde, 3-hydroxy-4-methoxy-	$C_8H_8O_3$	152	0.24
10	15.22	3-Isopropoxy-1,1,1,7,7,7-hexamethyl-3,5,5-tris(trimethylsiloxy)tetrasiloxane	$C_{18}H_{52}O_7Si_7$	576	0.32
11	16.09	beta.-D-Glucopyranose, 1,6-anhydro-	$C_6H_{10}O_5$	162	0.78
12	16.45	2,4-Di-tert-butylphenol	$C_{14}H_{22}O$	206	0.93
13	16.6	2-Methoxy-6-methoxycarbonyl-4-pyrone	$C_8H_8O_5$	184	0.12
14	16.72	Benzoic acid, 4-hydroxy-3-methoxy-, methyl ester	$C_9H_8{10}O_4$	182	0.22

Table 5. Cont.

S. No.	RT	Name of the Compound	Molecular Formulae	MW	Peak Area (%)
15	16.83	Methyl 4-O-acetyl-2,3,6-tri-O-ethyl-.alpha.-d-galactopyranoside	$C_{15}H_{28}O_7$	320	2.1
16	16.96	2-Propanone, 1-(4-hydroxy-3-methoxyphenyl)-	$C_{10}H_{12}O_3$	180	0.7
17	17.81	Megastigmatrienone	$C_{13}H_{18}O$	190	0.31
18	18.25	Megastigmatrienone-Dup1	$C_{13}H_{18}O$	190	0.99
19	19.02	Tetraacetyl-d-xylonic nitrile	$C_{14}H_{17}NO_9$	343	27.92
20	19.31	Megastigmatrienone-Dup2	$C_{13}H_{18}O$	190	4.26
21	19.63	d-Gala-l-ido-octonic amide	$C_8H_{17}NO_8$	255	0.19
22	19.81	2,6-Dimethoxyhydroquinone	$C_8H_{10}O_4$	170	1.47
23	19.98	Benzaldehyde, 4-hydroxy-3,5-dimethoxy-	$C_9H_{10}O_4$	182	3.35
24	20.28	d-Gala-l-ido-octonic amide-Dup1	$C_8H_{17}NO_8$	255	9.75
25	20.64	Inositol, 1-deoxy-	$C_6H_{12}O_5$	164	15.58
26	20.73	Inositol, 1-deoxy–Dup1	$C_6H_{12}O_5$	164	9.31
27	21.11	3,4-Dihydrocoumarin, 4,4-dimethyl-6-hydroxy-	$C_{11}H_{12}O_3$	192	0.14
28	21.75	(E)-4-(3-Hydroxyprop-1-en-1-yl)-2-methoxyphenol	$C_{10}H_{12}O_3$	180	1.14
29	22.36	Benzoic acid, 4-hydroxy-3,5-dimethoxy-, methyl ester	$C_{10}H_{12}O_5$	212	0.24
30	26.84	trans-Sinapyl alcohol	$C_{11}H_{14}O_4$	210	1.66
31	29.52	Ethanol, 2,2'-(dodecylimino)bis-	$C_{16}H_{35}NO_2$	273	0.66
32	35.65	Hentriacontane	$C_{31}H_{64}$	436	0.39
33	37.8	Octacosane, 2-methyl-	$C_{29}H_{60}$	408	0.54
34	39.48	Heptacosane	$C_{27}H_{56}$	380	0.69
35	40.48	Octacosane, 2-methyl-Dup1	$C_{29}H_{60}$	408	0.72
36	41.25	Hentriacontane-Dup1	$C_{31}H_{64}$	436	0.66
37	41.45	Doxepin	$C_{19}H_{21}NO$	279	0.11
38	42.02	Tetratetracontane	$C_{44}H_{90}$	618	0.36
39	42.31	1,4-Methano-2H-cyclopent[d]oxepin-2,5(4H)-dione, 6-[(dimethylamino)methyl]hexahydro-8a-hydroxy-5a-methyl-9-(1-methylethyl)-, [1R-(1.alpha.,4.alpha.,5a.alpha.,6.beta.,8a.alpha.,9S*)]-	$C_{17}H_{27}NO_4$	309	0.66
40	42.66	Thieno[2,3-b]pyridine, 3-amino-2-(3,3-dimethyl-3,4-dihydroisoquinolin-1-yl)-4,6-dimethyl-	$C_{20}H_{21}N_3S$	335	5.87
41	42.84	Octacosane	$C_{28}H_{58}$	394	0.28
42	46.12	1(4H)-naphthalenone, 4-[[4-(diethylamino)phenyl]imino]-2-hydroxy-	$C_{20}H_{20}N_2O_2$	320	0.21
43	49.16	Olean-12-en-28-oic acid, 3-hydroxy-, methyl ester, (3.beta.)-	$C_{31}H_{50}O_3$	470	0.14

The water extracted from C. tinctorius contained about 17 different compounds. Benzofuran, 2,3-dihydro-, with a molecular weight of 120 and a chemical formula of C_8H_8O, had the most remarkable peak area percent of 23.24 among the seventeen compounds detected. The second most significant peak was found with 3-Isopropoxy-1,1,1,7,7,7-hexamethyl-3,5,5-tris(trimethylsiloxy)tetrasiloxane, with a molecular weight of 576 and a chemical formula of $C_{18}H_{52}O_7Si_7$, with a summative peak area percent of 21.23. The following compounds of 3,4-Dihydroxyphenylglycol, 4TMS derivative; 4H-Pyran-4-one, 2,3-dihydro-3,5-dihydroxy-6-methyl-; and Cyclohexasiloxane, dodecamethyl- had moderate peak area percent. Their respective values of peak area were 8.94, 8.56, and 6.96. $C_{20}H_{42}O_4Si_4$/458, $C_6H_8O_4$/144, and $C_{12}H_{36}O_6Si_6$/444 are their chemical formulas and molecular weights. The compounds with the lowest peak area percent are presented in Table 4 and Figure S1.

Table 6. Compounds are identified in water-extracted *Z. officinale*.

S. No	RT	Name of the Compound	Molecular Formulae	MW	Peak Area (%)
1	5.45	3(2H)-Furanone, 4-hydroxy-5-methyl-	$C_5H_6O_3$	114	0.55
2	6.13	Maltol	$C_6H_{10}O_3$	126	2.78
3	6.73	Tert.-butylaminoacrylonitryl	$C_7H_{12}N_2$	124	2.17
4	7.45	2-Propanamine, N-methyl-N-nitroso-	$C_4H_{10}N_2O$	102	0.23
5	7.75	4H-Pyran-4-one, 2,3-dihydro-3,5-dihydroxy-6-methyl-	$C_6H_8O_4$	144	2.14
6	8.76	Catechol	$C_6H_6O_2$	110	0.8
7	9.13	Decanal	$C_{10}H_{20}O$	156	1.64
8	10.65	Cyclobuta[1,2:3,4]dicyclooctene, hexadecahydro-	$C_{16}H_{28}$	220	0.44
9	11.17	Cyclohexasiloxane, dodecamethyl-	$C_{12}H_{36}O_6Si_6$	444	0.89
10	11.79	2-Methoxy-4-vinylphenol	$C_9H_{10}O_2$	150	0.48
11	14.09	10-Methyl-8-tetradecen-1-ol acetate	$C_{17}H_{32}O_2$	268	0.53
12	14.72	2-Formyl-9-[.beta.-d-ribofuranosyl]hypoxanthine	$C_{11}H_{12}N_4O_6$	296	4.37
13	14.93	Cyclopentanecarboxaldehyde	$C_6H_{10}O$	98	0.52
14	15.22	3-Isopropoxy-1,1,1,7,7,7-hexamethyl-3,5,5-tris(trimethylsiloxy)tetrasiloxane	$C_{18}H_{52}O_7Si_7$	576	0.48
15	15.83	trans-Sesquisabinene hydrate	$C_{15}H_{26}O$	222	0.40
16	15.9	Benzene, 1-(1,5-dimethyl-4-hexenyl)-4-methyl-	$C_{15}H_{22}$	202	2.8
17	16.15	Octanal, 7-hydroxy-3,7-dimethyl-	$C_{10}H_{20}O_2$	172	0.26
18	16.24	(1S,5S)-2-Methyl-5-((R)-6-methylhept-5-en-2-yl)bicyclo[3.1.0]hex-2-ene	$C_{15}H_{24}$	204	9.06
19	16.39	Alpha.-Farnesene	$C_{15}H_{24}$	204	2.1
20	16.46	Phenol, 2,5-bis(1,1-dimethylethyl)-	$C_{14}H_{22}O$	206	3.71
21	16.54	Beta.-Bisabolene	$C_{15}H_{24}$	204	2.33
22	16.81	3-Cyclohexene-1-methanol, 2-hydroxy-.alpha.,.alpha.,4-trimethyl-	$C_{10}H_8O_2$	170	1.14
23	16.95	(1S,5S)-4-Methylene-1-((R)-6-methylhept-5-en-2-yl)bicyclo[3.1.0]hexane	$C_{15}H_{24}$	204	3.77
24	17.54	2-Furanmethanol, 5-ethenyltetrahydro-.alpha.,.alpha.,5-trimethyl-, cis-	$C_{10}H_{18}O_2$	170	1.05
25	18.07	4-(1-Hydroxyallyl)-2-methoxyphenol	$C_{10}H_{12}O_3$	180	1.39
26	18.58	Ethyl N-(o-anisyl)formimidate	$C_{10}H_{13}NO_2$	179	0.49
27	18.99	Ethyl .alpha.-d-glucopyranoside	$C_8H_{16}O_6$	208	3.1
28	19.7	2-Butanone, 4-(4-hydroxy-3-methoxyphenyl)-	$C_{11}H_{14}O_3$	194	38.21
29	20.65	4-(3,4-Dimethoxyphenyl)butan-2-one	$C_{12}H_{16}O_3$	208	0.17
30	20.86	(1R,2R,4S,6S,7S,8S)-8-Isopropyl-1-methyl-3-methylenetricyclo[4.4.0.02,7]decan-4-ol	$C_{15}H_{24}O$	220	0.26
31	23.26	cis-Z-.alpha.-Bisabolene epoxide	$C_{15}H_{24}O$	220	0.49
32	23.59	2-Naphthalenemethanol, decahydro-.alpha.,.alpha.,4a-trimethyl-8-methylene-, [2R-(2.alpha.,4a.alpha.,8a.beta.)]-	$C_8H_{26}O$	222	0.47
33	24.41	trans-Z-.alpha.-Bisabolene epoxide	$C_{15}H_{24}O$	220	0.43
34	25.48	Hexadecanoic acid, methyl ester	$C_{17}H_{32}O_2$	270	0.2
35	29.52	Ethanol, 2,2′-(dodecylimino)bis-	$C_{16}H_{35}NO_2$	273	0.89
36	31	(E)-1-(4-Hydroxy-3-methoxyphenyl)dec-3-en-5-one	$C_{17}H_{24}O_3$	276	2.08
37	32.25	1-(4-Hydroxy-3-methoxyphenyl)dec-4-en-3-one	$C_{17}H_{24}O_3$	276	5.89
38	35.44	(E)-4-(2-(2-(2,6-Dimethylhepta-1,5-dien-1-yl)-6-pentyl-1,3-dioxan-4-yl)ethyl)-2-methoxyphenol	$C_{27}H_{42}O_4$	430	0.35
39	35.85	(3R,5S)-1-(4-Hydroxy-3-methoxyphenyl)decane-3,5-diyl diacetate	$C_{21}H_{42}O_4$	380	0.69
40	39.74	1-(4-Hydroxy-3-methoxyphenyl)tetradec-4-en-3-one	$C_{21}H_{32}O_3$	332	0.25

The water-extracted *C. fenestratum* contained about 43 different compounds. Tetraacetyl-d-xylonic nitrile with a molecular weight of 343 and a chemical formula of $C_{14}H_{17}NO_9$ had the most significant peak area percent of 27.92 among the forty-three compounds detected. Inositol, 1-deoxy- with a molecular weight of 164 and a chemical formula of $C_6H_{12}O_5$, had the second greatest peak, with a summative peak area of 24.89. The following compounds of d-Gala-l-ido-octonic amide, Thieno[2,3-b]pyridine,3-amino-2-(3,3-dimethyl-3,4-dihydroisoquinolin-1-yl)-4,6-dimethyl-, and Megastigmatrienone had moderate peak area percent. Their respective values of summative peak area were 9.94, 5.87, and 5.56. $C_8H_{17}NO_8/255$, $C_{20}H_{21}N_3S/335$, and $C_{13}H_{18}O/190$ are their chemical formulas and molecular weights. The compounds with the lowest peak area percent are presented in Table 5 and Figure S3.

The water-extracted *Z. officinale* contained about 42 different compounds. With a molecular weight of 194 and a chemical formula of C11H14O3, 2-Butanone, 4-(4-hydroxy-3-methoxyphenyl)- had the greatest peak area percent of 38.21 among the forty-two compounds detected. The following compounds of (1S,5S)-2-Methyl-5-((R)-6-methylhept-5-en-2-yl)bicyclo[3.1.0]hex-2-ene, 1-(4-Hydroxy-3-methoxyphenyl)dec-4-en-3-one, 2-Formyl-9-[.beta.-d-ribofuranosyl]hypoxanthine, (1S,5S)-4-Methylene-1-((R)-6-methylhept-5-en-2-yl)bicyclo[3.1.0]hexane had moderate peak area percent. Their respective values of summative peak area were 9.06, 5.89, 4.37, and 3.77. $C_{15}H_{24}/204$, $C_{17}H_{24}O_3/276$, $C_{11}H_{12}N_4O_6/296$, and $C_{15}H_{24}/204$ are their chemical formulas and molecular weights. The compounds with the lowest peak area percent are presented in Table 6 and Figure S5.

The ethanolic extracts of the three herbs are listed in Tables 7–9. The substances of the *C. fenestratum* contained mainly Inositol Inositol, 1-deoxy- at 21.46% and Megastigmatrienone, about 12.63%. *Z. officinale* contains approximately 33.27% butan-2-one, 4-(3-hydroxy-2-methoxyphenyl)- and 1-(4-Hydroxy-3-methoxyphenyl)dec-4-en. -3-one about 24.37%. Finally, *C. tinctorius* contains the main compound of 4H-Pyran-4-one, 2,3-dihydro-3,5-dihydroxy-6-methyl- approx. 12.60%.

Table 7. Compounds identified in ethanolic-extracted *C. tinctorius*.

S. No.	RT	Name of the Compound	Molecular Formulae	MW	Peak Area (%)
1	5.45	3(2H)-Furanone, 4-hydroxy-5-methyl-	$C_5H_6O_3$	114	2.82
2	5.62	Acetic anhydride	$C_4H_6O_3$	102	1.41
3	5.77	.gamma.-Dodecalactone	$C_{12}H_{22}O_2$	198	4.31
4	6.13	Maltol	$C_6H_6O_3$	126	4.2
5	6.74	Cyclopentanol	$C_5H_{10}O$	86	6.74
6	7.45	2-Propanamine, N-methyl-N-nitroso-	$C_4H_{10}N_2O$	102	2.18
7	7.75	4H-Pyran-4-one, 2,3-dihydro-3,5-dihydroxy-6-methyl-	$C_6H_8O_4$	144	7.76
8	7.87	4H-Pyran-4-one, 2,3-dihydro-3,5-dihydroxy-6-methyl–Dup1	$C_6H_8O_4$	144	4.84
9	8.37	2H-Pyran, 3,4-dihydro-	C_5H_8O	84	2.42
10	8.58	5,8,11,14-Eicosatetraenoic acid, phenylmethyl ester, (all-Z)-	$C_{27}H_{38}O_2$	394	0.69
11	8.76	Catechol	$C_6H_6O_2$	110	4.27
12	9.06	Acetamide, N-[4-(4-nitrobenzylidenamino)-3-furazanyl]-	$C_{11}H_9N_5O_4$	275	3.43
13	9.4	Benzofuran, 2,3-dihydro-	C_8H_8O	120	3.51
14	9.61	5-Hydroxymethylfurfural	$C_6H_6O_3$	126	1.33
15	10.67	Hydroquinone	$C_6H_6O_2$	110	0.82
16	10.97	2-Butanone, 4-(ethylthio)-	$C_6H_{12}OS$	132	0.97
17	11.15	Cyclohexasiloxane, dodecamethyl-	$C_{12}H_{36}O_6Si_6$	444	3.31

Table 7. Cont.

S. No.	RT	Name of the Compound	Molecular Formulae	MW	Peak Area (%)
18	11.77	2-Methyl-9-.beta.-d-ribofuranosylhypoxanthine	$C_{11}H_{14}N_4O_5$	282	2.04
19	12.66	Phenol, 2,6-dimethoxy-	$C_8H_{10}O_3$	154	0.43
20	13.31	DL-Proline, 5-oxo-, methyl ester	$C_6H_9NO_3$	143	1.76
21	13.9	4-Methyl(trimethylene)silyloxyoctane	$C_{12}H_{26}OSi$	214	1.72
22	14.16	3,7-Diacetamido-7H-s-triazolo[5,1-c]-s-triazole	$C_7H_9N_7O_2$	223	2.54
23	14.89	l-Pyrrolid-2-one, N-carboxyhydrazide	$C_5H_9N_3O_2$	143	6.13
24	14.97	Guanosine	$C_{10}H_{13}N_5O_5$	283	6.58
25	15.22	3-Isopropoxy-1,1,1,7,7,7-hexamethyl-3,5,5-tris(trimethylsiloxy)tetrasiloxane	$C_{18}H_{52}O_7Si_7$	576	1.29
26	16.45	2,4-Di-tert-butylphenol	$C_{14}H_{22}O$	206	1.41
27	18.72	d-Glycero-d-ido-heptose	$C_7H_{14}O_7$	210	1.42
28	19.44	3-Deoxy-d-mannonic acid	$C_6H_{12}O_6$	180	7.85
29	19.68	d-Glycero-d-ido-heptose-Dup1	$C_7H_{14}O_7$	210	3.94
30	19.87	2-Methyl-9-.beta.-d-ribofuranosylhypoxanthine-Dup1	$C_{11}H_{14}N_4O_5$	282	2.17
31	22.29	Heptasiloxane, 1,1,3,3,5,5,7,7,9,9,11,11,13,13-tetradecamethyl-	$C_{14}H_{44}O_6Si_7$	504	0.33
32	25.48	Hexadecanoic acid, methyl ester	$C_{17}H_{34}O_2$	270	0.76
33	29.52	Ethanol, 2,2′-(dodecylimino)bis-	$C_{16}H_{35}NO_2$	273	1.2
34	32.25	Heptacosane	$C_{27}H_{56}$	380	0.86
35	39.48	Heptacosane-Dup1	$C_{27}H_{56}$	380	1.45
36	40.34	9-Octadecenamide, (Z)-	$C_{18}H_{35}NO$	281	0.76
37	41.25	Heptacosane-Dup2	$C_{27}H_{56}$	380	0.35

Table 8. Compounds identified in the ethanolic-extracted C. fenestratum.

S. No	RT	Name of the Compound	Molecular Formulae	MW	Peak Area (%)
1	6.11	3-Acetylthymine	$C_7H_8N_2O_3$	168	0.26
2	6.72	Tert.-butylaminoacrylonitryl	$C_7H_{12}N_2$	124	1.1
3	7.22	4-Isopropylbenzenethiol, S-methyl-	$C_{10}H_{14}S$	166	0.34
4	7.75	4H-Pyran-4-one, 2,3-dihydro-3,5-dihydroxy-6-methyl-	$C_6H_8O_4$	144	0.15
5	8.78	Catechol	$C_6H_8O_2$	110	0.8
6	9.06	1-[3-(4-Bromophenyl)-2-thioureido]-1-deoxy-b-d-glucopyranose 2,3,4,6-tetraacetate	$C_{21}H_{25}BrN_2O_9S$	560	0.26
7	11.15	Cyclohexasiloxane, dodecamethyl-	$C_{12}H_{36}O_6Si_6$	444	0.09
8	11.79	2-Methoxy-4-vinylphenol	$C_9H_{10}O_2$	150	0.17
9	12.68	Phenol, 2,6-dimethoxy-	$C_9H_{10}O_3$	154	0.09
10	13.31	2-Pyrrolidinone, 5-(cyclohexylmethyl)-	$C_{11}H_{19}NO$	181	0.18
11	13.92	Benzaldehyde, 3-hydroxy-4-methoxy-	$C_8H_8O_3$	152	0.15
12	15.23	3-Isopropoxy-1,1,1,7,7,7-hexamethyl-3,5,5-tris(trimethylsiloxy)tetrasiloxane	$C_{18}H_{52}O_7Si_7$	576	0.4
13	16.11	.beta.-D-Glucopyranose, 1,6-anhydro-	$C_6H_{10}O_5$	162	0.67
14	16.46	2,4-Di-tert-butylphenol	$C_{14}H_{22}O$	206	0.37
15	16.59	2-Methoxy-6-methoxycarbonyl-4-pyrone	$C_8H_8O_5$	184	0.1

Table 8. Cont.

S. No	RT	Name of the Compound	Molecular Formulae	MW	Peak Area (%)
16	16.73	Benzoic acid, 4-hydroxy-3-methoxy-, methyl ester	$C_9H_{10}O_4$	182	0.11
17	16.84	Methyl 4-O-acetyl-2,3,6-tri-O-ethyl-.alpha.-d-galactopyranoside	$C_{15}H_{28}O_7$	320	0.19
18	16.97	2-Propanone, 1-(4-hydroxy-3-methoxyphenyl)-	$C_{10}H_{12}O_3$	180	0.26
19	17.8	Megastigmatrienone	$C_{13}H_{18}O$	190	0.19
20	18.24	Megastigmatrienone-Dup1	$C_{13}H_{18}O$	190	0.86
21	18.71	3,4,5-Trimethoxyphenol	$C_9H_{12}O_4$	184	1.91
22	19.01	Cyclopropanetetradecanoic acid, 2-octyl-, methyl ester	$C_{26}H_{50}O_2$	394	7.19
23	19.18	Tetraacetyl-d-xylonic nitrile	$C_{14}H_{17}NO_9$	343	9.47
24	19.32	Megastigmatrienone-Dup2	$C_{13}H_{18}O$	190	11.58
25	19.81	2-Oxa-3-azabicyclo[4.4.0]dec-3-ene, 5-methyl-1-trimethylsilyloxy-, N-oxide	$C_{12}H_{23}NO_3Si$	257	2
26	19.98	Benzaldehyde, 4-hydroxy-3,5-dimethoxy-	$C_9H_{10}O_4$	182	3
27	20.07	.alpha.-l-Mannose semicarbazone pentaacetate	$C_{18}H_{25}N_3O_{12}$	475	1.48
28	20.28	d-Gala-l-ido-octonic amide	$C_8H_{17}NO_8$	255	7
29	20.6	Shikimic acid	$C_7H_{10}O_5$	174	4.84
30	20.9	(E)-2,6-Dimethoxy-4-(prop-1-en-1-yl)phenol	$C_{11}H_{14}O_3$	194	8.69
31	21.13	Inositol, 1-deoxy-	$C_6H_{12}O_5$	164	6.02
32	21.46	Inositol, 1-deoxy–Dup1	$C_6H_{12}O_5$	164	15.44
33	21.75	(E)-4-(3-Hydroxyprop-1-en-1-yl)-2-methoxyphenol	$C_{10}H_{12}O_3$	180	1.26
34	22.28	3-Isopropoxy-1,1,1,7,7,7-hexamethyl-3,5,5-tris(trimethylsiloxy)tetrasiloxane-Dup1	$C_{18}H_{52}O_7Si_7$	576	0.2
35	22.37	Benzoic acid, 4-hydroxy-3,5-dimethoxy-, methyl ester	$C_{10}H_{12}O_5$	212	0.72
36	22.82	4-Hydroxy-4a,8-dimethyl-3-methylene-3,3a,4,4a,7a,8,9,9a-octahydroazuleno[6,5-b]furan-2,5-dione	$C_{15}H_{18}O_4$	262	0.12
37	25.48	Hexadecanoic acid, methyl ester	$C_{17}H_{34}O_2$	270	0.19
38	26.83	trans-Sinapyl alcohol	$C_{11}H_{14}O_4$	210	0.43
39	27.89	1,3-Dioxolo[4,5-g]isoquinolin-5(6H)-one, 7,8-dihydro-	$C_{10}H_9NO_3$	191	0.1
40	28.68	9,12-Octadecadienoic acid, methyl ester, (E,E)-	$C_{19}H_{34}O_2$	294	0.08
41	28.8	9-Octadecenoic acid (Z)-, methyl ester	$C_{19}H_{36}O_2$	296	0.15
42	29.52	Ethanol, 2,2′-(dodecylimino)bis-	$C_{16}H_{35}NO_2$	273	0.25
43	40.47	7-Isoquinolinol, 1,2,3,4-tetrahydro-1-[(3-hydroxy-4-methoxyphenyl)methyl]-6-methoxy-2-methyl-, (S)-	$C_{19}H_{23}NO_4$	329	0.09
44	41.05	Corydine	$C_{20}H_{23}NO_4$	341	0.06
45	41.45	Ethylamine, 2-((p-bromo-.alpha.-methyl-.alpha.-phenylbenzyl)oxy)-N,N-dimethyl-	$C_{18}H_{22}BrNO$	347	0.06
46	42.3	1-Undecanamine, N,N-dimethyl-	$C_{13}H_{29}N$	199	0.32
47	42.67	Thieno[2,3-b]pyridine, 3-amino-2-(3,3-dimethyl-3,4-dihydroisoquinolin-1-yl)-4,6-dimethyl-	$C_{20}H_{21}N_3S$	335	4.26
48	44.57	Berbine, 13,13a-didehydro-9,10-dimethoxy-2,3-(methylenedioxy)-	$C_{20}H_{19}NO_4$	337	1.3
49	44.69	Ergosta-5,22-dien-3-ol, acetate, (3.beta.,22E)-	$C_{30}H_{48}O_2$	440	0.28
50	45.31	Thalictricavine	$C_{21}H_{23}NO_4$	353	0.12
51	45.42	.beta.-Sitosterol	$C_{29}H_{50}O$	414	0.21
52	46.15	1(4H)-naphthalenone, 4-[[4-(diethylamino)phenyl]imino]-2-hydroxy-	$C_{20}H_{20}N_2O_2$	320	1.29
53	49.19	Olean-12-en-28-oic acid, 3-hydroxy-, methyl ester, (3.beta.)-	$C_{31}H_{50}O_3$	470	2.15
54	50.18	Urs-12-en-28-oic acid, 3-hydroxy-, methyl ester, (3.beta.)-	$C_{31}H_{50}O_3$	470	0.23
55	50.35	Urs-12-en-28-oic acid, 3-hydroxy-, methyl ester, (3.beta.)-Dup1	$C_{31}H_{50}O_3$	470	0.78

Table 9. Compounds are identified in ethanolic-extracted *Z. officinale*.

S. No.	RT	Name of the Compound	Molecular Formulae	MW	Peak Area (%)
1	9.12	Decanal	$C_{10}H_{20}O$	156	3.1
2	10.18	2,6-Octadien-1-ol, 3,7-dimethyl-, (Z)-	$C_{10}H_{18}O$	154	0.91
3	15.91	Benzene, 1-(1,5-dimethyl-4-hexenyl)-4-methyl-	$C_{15}H_{22}$	202	1.28
4	16.23	1,3-Cyclohexadiene, 5-(1,5-dimethyl-4-hexenyl)-2-methyl-, [S-(R*,S*)]-	$C_{15}H_{24}$	204	3.79
5	16.4	.alpha.-Farnesene	$C_{15}H_{24}$	204	1.19
6	16.55	.beta.-Bisabolene	$C_{15}H_{24}$	204	0.93
7	16.94	Cyclohexene, 3-(1,5-dimethyl-4-hexenyl)-6-methylene-, [S-(R*,S*)]-	$C_{15}H_{24}$	204	2.03
8	17.74	Nerolidol	$C_{15}H_{26}O$	222	0.89
9	18.07	4-(1-Hydroxyallyl)-2-methoxyphenol	$C_{10}H_{12}O_3$	180	1.35
10	19.8	Butan-2-one, 4-(3-hydroxy-2-methoxyphenyl)-	$C_{11}H_{14}O_3$	194	33.27
11	20.11	2-Naphthalenemethanol, decahydro-.alpha.,.alpha.,4a-trimethyl-8-methylene-, [2R-(2.alpha.,4a.alpha.,8a.beta.)]-	$C_{15}H_{26}O$	222	1.4
12	20.66	(1S,2R,5R)-2-Methyl-5-((R)-6-methylhept-5-en-2-yl)bicyclo[3.1.0]hexan-2-ol	$C_{15}H_{26}O$	222	0.99
13	20.87	1H-3a,7-Methanoazulen-5-ol, octahydro-3,8,8-trimethyl-6-methylene-	$C_{15}H_{24}O$	220	1.63
14	23.27	cis-Z-.alpha.-Bisabolene epoxide	$C_{15}H_{24}O$	220	1.83
15	24.43	trans-Z-.alpha.-Bisabolene epoxide	$C_{15}H_{24}O$	220	0.83
16	24.55	Acetic acid, 3-hydroxy-6-isopropenyl-4,8a-dimethyl-1,2,3,5,6,7,8,8a-octahydronaphthalen-2-yl ester	$C_{17}H_{26}O_3$	278	0.65
17	25.48	Hexadecanoic acid, methyl ester	$C_{17}H_{34}O_2$	270	0.42
18	31.02	(E)-1-(4-Hydroxy-3-methoxyphenyl)dec-3-en-5-one	$C_{17}H_{24}O_3$	276	4.96
19	31.2	3-Decanone, 1-(4-hydroxy-3-methoxyphenyl)-	$C_{17}H_{26}O_3$	278	1.5
20	32.33	1-(4-Hydroxy-3-methoxyphenyl)dec-4-en-3-one	$C_{17}H_{24}O_3$	276	24.37
21	35.48	(E)-4-(2(2-(2,6-Dimethylhepta-1,5-dien-1-yl)-6-pentyl-1,3-dioxan-4-yl)ethyl)-2-methoxyphenol	$C_{27}H_{42}O_4$	430	1.13
22	35.87	1-(4-Hydroxy-3-methoxyphenyl)dodec-4-en-3-one	$C_{19}H_{28}O_3$	304	5.23
23	38.64	(E)-1-(4-Hydroxy-3-methoxyphenyl)tetradec-3-en-5-one	$C_{21}H_{32}O_3$	332	0.74
24	39.74	1-(4-Hydroxy-3-methoxyphenyl)tetradec-4-en-3-one	$C_{21}H_{32}O_3$	332	3.24
25	40.14	1-(4-Hydroxy-3-methoxyphenyl)tetradecane-3,5-dione	$C_{21}H_{32}O_4$	348	0.35
26	42.79	(E)-4-(2(2-(2,6-Dimethylhepta-1,5-dien-1-yl)-6-pentyl-1,3-dioxan-4-yl)ethyl)-2-methoxyphenol-Dup1	$C_{27}H_{42}O_4$	430	0.61
27	45.43	.beta.-Sitosterol	$C_{29}H_{50}O$	414	1.35

3.2. Determination of Maximum Dose for HepG2

The cytotoxicity of these herbs—*C. fenestratum*, *Z. officinale*, and *C. tinctorius*—extracted with water and ethanol from concentrations of 10–400 µg/mL were investigated in HepG2 cells by MTT assays. The findings revealed that all herbs extracted with water or ethanol at concentrations less than 50 µg/mL were harmless to HepG2 cells (cell viability >80%). In Figure 1, water extraction of the *C. fenestratum*, *Z. officinale*, and *C. tinctorius* at 50 µg/mL resulted in HepG2 cell survival rates of 88.16%, 90.19%, and 97.28%, respectively. Furthermore, ethanol extraction of *C. fenestratum*, *Z. officinale*, and *C. tinctorius* at 50 µg/mL resulted in cell survival of 103.63%, 82.75%, and 102.71%, respectively. As a result, the maximum dosage of those herbs was indicated for further research at 50 µg/mL. From the experiement, it was found that *Z. officinale* extracted with ethanol had the highest toxicity. Concentration values calculated using the fitting curve showed that the maximum concentration of *Z. officinale* extracted with ethanol that made HepG2 cells non-toxicity was 54.16 ± 3.90 µg/mL. In addition, The MTT assay was used to assess the safety of this recipe. It was revealed that a 3:2:1 ratio of *C. fenestratum*, *Z. officinale*, and *C. tinctorius* could be safely used at concentrations up to 100 µg/mL in this recipe.

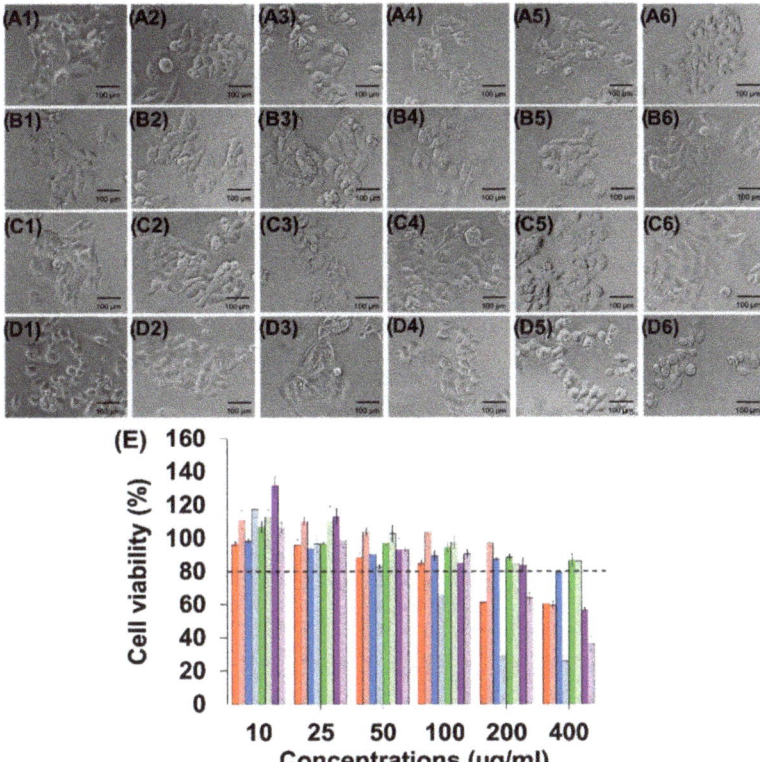

Figure 1. Cell survival and cytotoxicity testing of the HepG2 cells. (**A**) Morphology was exposed to different concentrations ((**A1**): 10 µg/mL; (**A2**): 25 µg/mL; (**A3**): 50 µg/mL; (**A4**): 100 µg/mL; (**A5**): 200 µg/mL; and (**A6**): 400 µg/mL) of *C. fenestratum* from water extraction. (**B**) Morphology was exposed to different concentrations ((**B1**): 10 µg/mL; (**B2**): 25 µg/mL; (**B3**): 50 µg/mL; (**B4**): 100 µg/mL; (**B5**): 200 µg/mL; and (**B6**): 400 µg/mL) of *Z. officinale* from water extraction. (**C**) Morphology was exposed to different concentrations ((**C1**): 10 µg/mL; (**C2**): 25 µg/mL; (**C3**): 50 µg/mL; (**C4**): 100 µg/mL; (**C5**): 200 µg/mL; and (**C6**): 400 µg/mL) of *C. tinctorius* from water extraction. (**D**) Morphology was exposed to different concentrations (**D1**): 10 µg/mL; (**D2**): 25 µg/mL; (**D3**): 50 µg/mL; (**D4**): 100 µg/mL; (**D5**): 200 µg/mL; and (**D6**): 400 µg/mL) of medicinal recipe containing *C. fenestratum*: *Z. officinale*: and *C. tinctorius* extracted with water in a ratio of 3:2:1. (**E**) MTT assay of HepG2 cells treated with different concentrations of the *C. fenestratum* (Water extract: red bar and Ethanolic: red stripes), *Z. officinale* (water extract: blue bar and ethanolic: blue stripes), *C. tinctorius* (water extract: green bar and ethanolic: green stripes), and Recipe (water extract: purple bar and ethanolic: purple stripes.

3.3. Effect of the C. fenestratum, Z. officinale, and C. tinctorius on Transcriptional Activity of HMGCR, LDLR, PCSK9, and SREBP2

The previous study [53] on the correlation between SREBP2 and PCSK9 has indicated that inhibiting transcriptional activation of the sterol regulatory element binding protein 2 (SREBP2), which regulates PCSK9, increases LDLR expression, as seen in Figure 2. It was discovered that inhibiting SREBP2 expression enhanced LDLR activation. *C. fenestratum* extracted with water and ethanol has lipid-lowering activity through upregulating hepatic LDLR. Among three herbs with two types of extraction, this study found that the most effective way to upregulate LDLR expression by up to 23.12-fold was to treat with water-extracted *C. fenestratum*, followed by water-extracted *Z. officinale*, which increased the expression of LDLR mRNA by up to 9.09-fold.

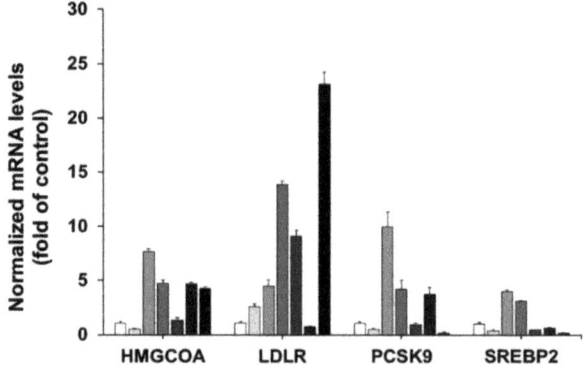

Figure 2. Effects of aqueous and ethanolic extract of *Z. officinale*, *C. tinctorius*, and *C. fenestratum* on mRNA expression levels. The bar graphs go from white (left) to black (right), indicating the control (white), the ethanolic extract of *Z. officinale* (light gray), *C. tinctorius* (medium gray), *C. fenestratum* (dark gray), the water extract of *Z. officinale* (light black), *C. tinctorius* (medium black), and *C. fenestratum* (black) respectively.

From LDLR mRNA, the number of LDLR expressions on the surface of hepatocytes is a significant factor [54]. Water-extracted *C. fenestratum* showed the most significant LDLR mRNA expression in HepG2 cells, followed by ethanol-extracted *C. fenestratum*, water-extracted *Z. officinale*, and ethanol-extracted *C. tinctorius*. The reduction of PCSK9 mRNA expression is the primary cause of LDLR mRNA expression, as seen in Figure 2. Although *Z. officinale*'s potency is less effective at inhibiting PCSK9 than the *C. fenestratum*, *Z. officinale* extract was most effective at suppressing HMGR mRNA expression, as shown in Figure 2. Therefore, the presence of *Z. officinale* in the recipe can reduce the production of lipids from the liver, resulting in lowering blood lipids. In Thai traditional medicine, in addition considering the effectiveness of treatment with main and assistance drugs, it is also essential to add an herb that makes it more appetizing by adjusting the color. Therefore, *C. tinctorius*, which gives it its reddish-orange color and is used as a lipid-lowering herb [55], is used to improve its color.

3.4. Effect of Lipid Deposition in HepG2

According to the lipid staining with Oil red O examination, the total lipid in HepG2 cells following treatment with water and ethanol extraction of the *C. fenestratum* was 0.95 and 0.77 folds; *C. tinctorius* was 0.80 and 0.86 folds; *Z. officinale* was 0.78 and 0.73 folds, and the recipe was 0.61 and 0.48 folds, respectively. We found that treating HepG2 cells for 24 h with a recipe containing *C. fenestratum*, *Z. officinale*, and *C. tinctorius* had a strong synergistic effect, causing a significant reduction in lipid deposition when compared to individual herbs. Furthermore, these herbs extracted with ethanol were discovered to play an essential role in lowering the quantity of lipid accumulated in the HepG2 cell. The low lipid accumulation in HepG2 cells was due to the suppression of lipid synthesis, which resulted in a reduction in the quantity of lipid stained in the HepG2 cells.

In this experiment, *Z. officinale* exhibited more significant inhibition of HMGCR mRNA than lovastatin (2.5 times) [56] through 0.51- and 1.34-fold increases in HMGCR mRNA expression in ethanol and water extracts, respectively, compared to the control. In addition, when comparing the HMGCR mRNA inhibition of the extracts with statins, it was found that all herbal extracts inhibited HMGCR mRNA better than all statins. The inhibition value of herbal extracts ranged from 0.52–7.69-fold. The results also compared statins such as simvastatin, pravastatin, fluvastatin, atorvastatin, and rosuvastatin, which can induce HMGCR mRNA expression by up to 15-, 12-, 11-, 9-, and 17-fold in order [56]. The HMGCR mRNA expression found that the three herbal extracts had better properties in inhibiting lipid formation than statins.

Statins have good inhibitory properties in the production of lipids from the liver. Therefore, *Z. officinale* with a mechanism of action that inhibits HMGCR mRNA expression is also effective in inhibiting lipid synthesis. As a result, the lipid accumulation in HepG2 cells was lower than in other herbs, as shown in Figure 3. However, the large amount of lipid accumulation in the HepG2 cells of *C. fenestratum* results from most of the compounds suppressing the PCSK9 expression, which results in increased LDLR expression. However, it has little effect on the expression of HMG-CoA reductase (HMGCR). This causes more lipid to be absorbed into HepG2 cells.

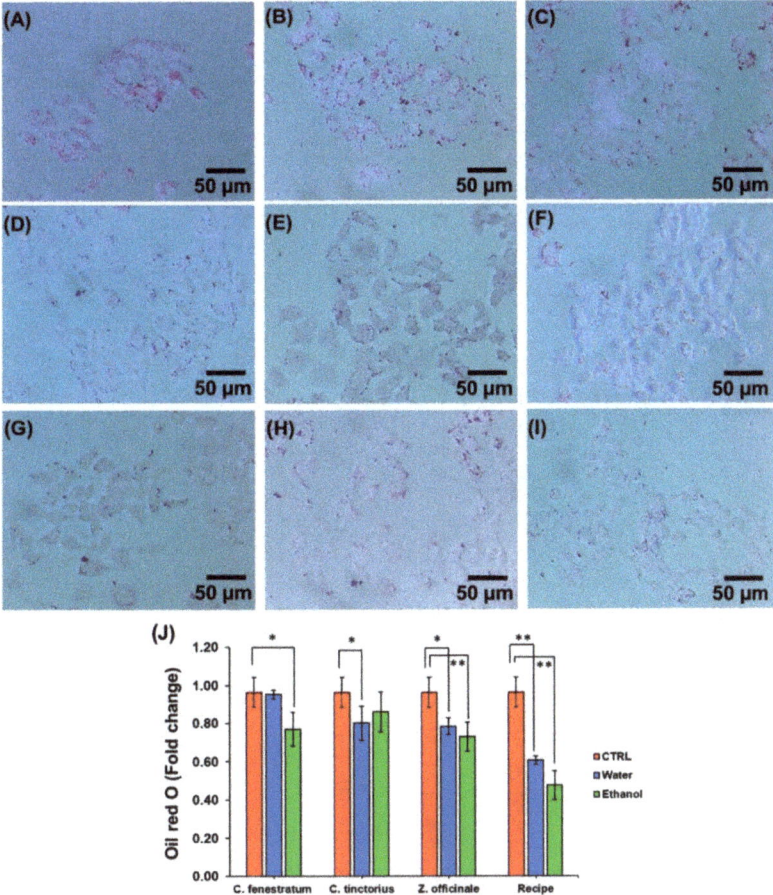

Figure 3. Effects of Oil red-O staining in HepG2 and examined using an inverted microscope. Oil red-O staining of HepG2 was incubated with water extract of (**B**) *C. fenestratum*, (**D**) *C. tinctorius*, (**F**) *Z. officinale*, and (**H**) recipe and Ethanolic extract of (**C**) *C. fenestratum*, (**E**) *C. tinctorius*, (**G**) *Z. officinale*, and (**I**) recipe compared to without treatment as (**A**) control. (**J**) Quantification of lipid accumulation by extracting oil red-O with isopropanol and measuring the OD of extract at 500 nm.

According to Thai traditional knowledge, the recipe composition is divided into three parts: the main drug, the assistance drug, and the servant drug. Therefore, the main drug was classified as the *C. fenestratum* in the highest proportion in this study. After all, it was the effect that needed to absorb lipid to the liver from the bloodstream, followed by *Z. officinale* as an assistance drug because it has properties to inhibit the production of lipid from the liver, and *C. tinctorius* as the servant drug, which helps to adjust the color of the recipe to make it more appetizing.

3.5. Molecular Docking for the Top 5 Highest Amounts of the Compound from Each Herb

Figure 4 and Table 10 show that PCSK9 has three pocket-binding sites: strong binding sites, medium binding sites, and low binding sites. Figure 4B,D shows three strong binding sites, one medium binding site, and six low binding sites. Water extraction of *C. fenestratum* including Inositol, 1-deoxy-, Tetraacetyl-d-xylonic nitrile, Megastigmatrienone, and Thieno[2,3-b]pyridine, 3-amino-2-(3,). 3-dimethyl-3,4-dihydroisoquinolin-1-yl)-4,6-dimethyl- binds to PCSK9 at a strong binding site. *Z. officinale* extract with water is 2-Formyl-9-[.beta.-d-ribofuranosyl]hypoxanthine, (1S,5S)-2-Methyl-5-((R)-6-methylhept-5-en-2-. yl)bicyclo[3.1.0]hex-2-ene, 2-Butanone, 4-(4-hydroxy-3-methoxyphenyl)-, 1-(4-Hydroxy-3-methoxyphenyl)dec-4-en-3- one, and (1S,5S)-4-Methylene-1-((R)-6-methylhept-5-en-2-yl)bicyclo[3.1.0]hexane. It was found that it was able to bind the PCSK9 region at the strong binding site. Aqueous *C. tinctorius* extract showed that Cyclohexasiloxane, dodecamethyl- binds to PCSK9 at the low binding site and 3,4-Dihydroxyphenylglycol, 4TMS derivative binds to PCSK9 at the strong binding site.

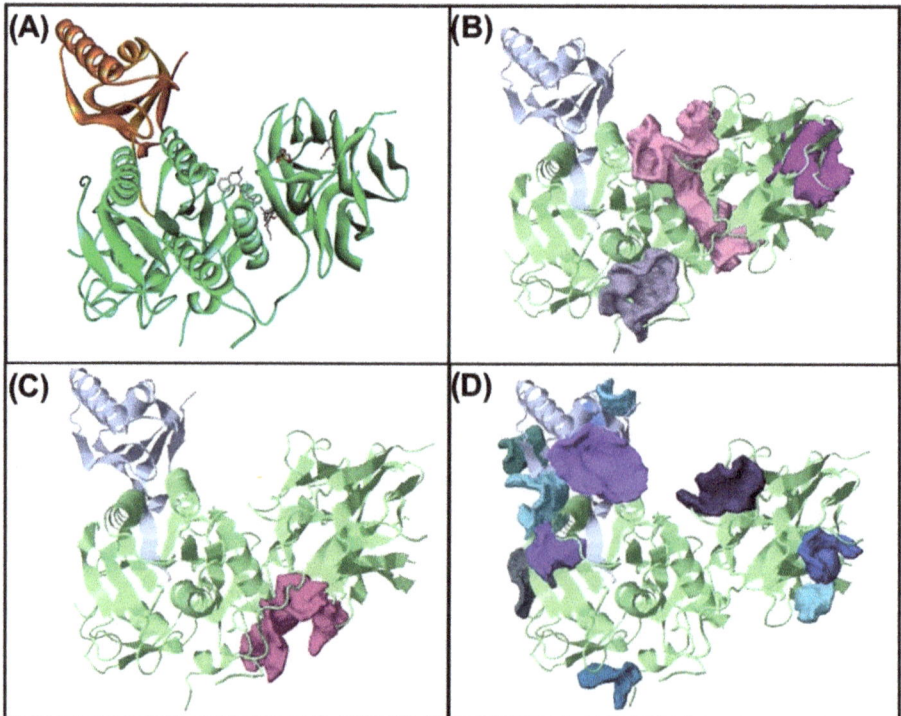

Figure 4. The pocket binding sites of the (**A**) PCSK9 protein at (**B**) high, (**C**) medium, and (**D**) low binding affinity was analyzed with CavityPlus (http://www.pkumdl.cn/cavityplus, accessed on 2 November 2021).

Table 10. The pocket binding site of PCSK9.

No.	Binding Site	Amino Acid
1	Strong No. 1	ILE:154, PRO:155, ASN:157, LEU:158, GLU:159, ARG:160, ILE:161, THR:162, PRO:163, ARG:165, TYR:166, ARG:167, ARG:237, ASP:238, ALA:239, GLY:240, VAL:241, ALA:242, LYS:243, GLY:244, GLY:394, ILE:395, ALA:397, MET:398, MET:399, LEU:400, SER:401, ALA:402, GLU:403, LEU:406, ARG:414, PHE:418, ALA:443, LEU:444, PRO:445, PRO:446, SER:447, THR:448, HIS:449, GLY:450, ALA:451
2	Strong No. 2	ALA:68:A, LYS:69:A, GLY:292, TYR:293, SER:294, ARG:295, LEU:297, ASN:298, ALA:299, ALA:300, CYS:301, GLN:302, ARG:303, LEU:304, ALA:305, ARG:306, ALA:307, GLY:308, VAL:309, THR:313, ASP:321, ALA:322, CYS:323, LEU:324, TYR:325, SER:326, PRO:327, ALA:328, SER:329, ALA:330, PRO:331, GLU:332, VAL:333, ILE:334, THR:335, GLY:356, ARG:357, CYS:358, VAL:359, ASP:360, LEU:361, THR:407, LEU:408, ALA:409, GLU:410, ARG:412, GLN:413, ILE:416, HIS:417, SER:419, ALA:420, LYS:421, ASP:422, VAL:423, ILE:424, ASN:425, GLU:426, ALA:427, PHE:429, GLU:431, ASP:432, GLN:433, ARG:434, VAL:435, LEU:436, THR:437, PRO:438, ASN:439, LEU:440, CYS:457, ARG:458, THR:459, VAL:460, TRP:461, SER:462, ALA:463, HIS:464, SER:465, GLY:466, ALA:471, THR:472, ALA:473, ILE:474, ALA:475, ARG:476, CYS:477, ALA:478, PRO:479, ASP:480, GLU:481, GLU:482, LEU:483, PHE:489, ARG:491, GLU:501, GLY:505, LYS:506, LEU:507, VAL:508, ARG:510, VAL:520, TYR:521, ALA:522, ILE:523, ARG:525, CYS:526, GLU:620, GLN:621, THR:623, VAL:624, ALA:625, CYS:626, TYR:648, ALA:649, VAL:650, ASP:651, ASN:652, THR:653, CYS:654, VAL:655, ARG:657
3	Strong No. 3	CYS:486, SER:487, SER:488, GLY:493, LYS:494, ARG:495, ARG:496, GLY:497, GLU:498, ALA:514, PHE:515, ARG:549, LEU:559, GLY:561, CYS:562, SER:563, SER:564, HIS:565, TRP:566, GLU:567, VAL:568, GLU:569, ASP:570, GLN:584, PRO:585, ASN:586, GLN:587, CYS:588, VAL:589, GLY:590, HIS:591, ARG:592, GLU:593, ALA:594, SER:595, ILE:596, HIS:597, LYS:609, VAL:610, LYS:611, GLU:612, GLY:634, CYS:635, SER:636, ALA:637, LEU:638, PRO:639, SER:642, HIS:643, VAL:644, LEU:645, GLY:646, ALA:647, TYR:648, VAL:656, ALA:671, ALA:674, VAL:675, ALA:676, ILE:677
4	Medium	GLU:159, ARG:160, ILE:161, THR:162, PRO:163, PRO:164, ARG:165, TYR:166, ASP:343, GLU:403, GLN:413, ARG:414, ILE:416, HIS:417, PHE:418, SER:419, ALA:420, LYS:421, ASP:422, VAL:423, LEU:440, VAL:441, ALA:442, ALA:443, LEU:444, PRO:445, PRO:446, SER:447, THR:448, HIS:449, GLY:450, ALA:451, GLY:452, TRP:453, GLN:454, LEU:455, PHE:456, CYS:457, ARG:458, ARG:525, LEU:606, LYS:611, ALA:625, CYS:626, GLU:627, GLU:628, GLY:629, TRP:630, THR:631, LEU:632, VAL:650, ASP:651, ASN:652, THR:653, CYS:679, ARG:680, SER:681, ARG:682

In conclusion, extracts of *C. fenestratum* and *Z. officinale* with water effectively inhibit PCSK9 at the strong binding site, resulting in the most effective inhibition of PCSK9. It was found that the extract could bind to PCSK9 in multiple pocket-binding sites, resulting in combinational inhibition efficiency [57]. After examining the active compounds in each herb via GC-MS/MS, the constituents of the active compounds were identified. The top five compounds were studied through molecular docking to determine that compounds PCSK9 and HMGCR exhibit protein-binding activities. The molecular docking binding studies showed that the effect was consistent with real-time PCR.

In Table 11, the binding between the active ingredients in the herbal aqueous extract and PCSK9 via Arguslab and Autodock showed that approximately 64.24% *C. fenestratum* including Tetraacetyl-d-xylonic nitrile, Inositol, 1-deoxy-, Thieno[2,3-b]pyridine, 3-amino-2-(3,3-dimethyl-3,4-dihydroisoquinolin-1-yl)-4, 6-dimethyl-, Megastigma-trienone binds the most to PCSK9 as it was able to bind to PCSK9 at a lower binding energy than the Alirocumab (standard drug). In Figures 5–7, the highest number of compounds found in *C. fenestratum* are 1) Tetraacetyl-d-xylonic nitrile (27.92%). It strongly binds to PCSK9, forming up to six hydrogen bonds with the amino acids HIS643, VAL644, ARG495, and TRP566. 2) Inositol, 1-deoxy- (24.89%) can bind the PCSK9 with different amino acids compared to Tetraacetyl-d-xylonic nitrile-PCSK9 binding. It can form up to five hydrogen bonds with the amino acids TRP461, ALA649, VAL435, and ASN439. Followed by the main active compounds of *Z. officinale*, including 2-Butanone, 4-(4-hydroxy-3-methoxyphenyl)-, (1S,5S)-2-Methyl-5-((R)). -6-methylhept-5-en-2-yl)bicyclo[3.1.0]hex-2-ene, 1-(4-Hydroxy-3-methoxyphenyl)dec-4-en-3-one, 2-Formyl- 9-[.beta.-d-ribofuranosyl]hypoxanthine, (1S,5S)-4-Methylene-1-((R)6-methylhept-5-en-2-yl)bicyclo[3.1.0]hexane binds to PCSK9 because the number of active compounds that can bind to PCSK9 is 61.3%, and it was found that

Z. officinale contains only 1 compound, and 2-Formyl-9-[.beta.-d-ribofuranosyl]hypoxanthine contained only 4.37% of *Z. officinale* extract to form a high 8-position hydrogen bond with the amino acids TRP461, LEU436, ASP360, ARG458, ALA649, ASP651, and THR469. The compound number of *C. fenestratum* extracts that can bind to PCSK9 is larger than the compound number of *Z. officinale* extracts, resulting in the water extract of *C. fenestratum* having a better inhibition effect than *Z. officinale*. In comparison, *C. tinctorius*'s active compounds have poor binding to PCSK9 because it contains only two compounds: 3,4-Dihydroxyphenylglycol, 4TMS derivative (8.94%), and Cyclohexasiloxane, dodecamethyl- (6.96%), which were found to total just 15.9%, resulting in poor inhibition of PCSK9. These compounds formed very few hydrogen bonds with PCSK9 binding compared to the two herbs mentioned above. Therefore, the preparation of the traditional recipe [58] suggested that the main drug with an excellent inhibitory effect in the highest proportion is *C. fenestratum* (3 parts), the assisting drug (2 parts) is *Z. officinale*, and the flavorful herb is *C. tinctorius* (1 part).

Table 11. Energy binding and phytochemical inhibition constants of herbal extracts with water at the binding sites of PCSK9 from ArgusLab and Autodock analysis and quantification of each compound through GC-MS/MS analysis.

No.	Herb	Compound Name	GC-MS/MS % Peak Area	ArgusLab Binding Energy (kcal/mol)	Autodock Binding Energy (kcal/mol)	Autodock Inhibition Constant (Ki)
1		Alirocumab (Positive control)		−7.59	−5.61	77.42 μM
2		Benzofuran, 2,3-dihydro-	23.24	−8.90	−5.43	104.25 μM
3	*C. tinctorius*	3-Isopropoxy-1,1,1,7,7,7-hexamethyl-3,5,5-tris(trimethylsiloxy)tetrasiloxane	21.23	N/B	−5.47	97.4 μM
4		3,4-Dihydroxyphenylglycol, 4TMS derivative	8.94	−8.63	−7.54	2.96 μM
5		4H-Pyran-4-one, 2,3-dihydro-3,5-dihydroxy-6-methyl-	8.56	−6.19	−6.99	7.46 μM
6		Cyclohexasiloxane, dodecamethyl-	6.96	−8.34	−7.88	1.69 μM
7		d-Gala-l-ido-octonic amide	9.94	−7.15	−6.46	18.3 μM
8		Inositol, 1-deoxy-	24.89	−8.33	−7.30	4.48 μM
9	*C. fenestratum*	Tetraacetyl-d-xylonic nitrile	27.92	−8.26	−6.76	11.05 μM
10		Thieno[2,3-b]pyridine, 3-amino-2-(3,3-dimethyl-3,4-dihydroisoquinolin-1-yl)-4,6-dimethyl-	5.87	−11.14	−10.15	36.5 nM
11		Megastigmatrienone	5.56	−10.83	−7.87	1.7 μM
12		2-Butanone, 4-(4-hydroxy-3-methoxyphenyl)-	38.21	−8.73	−7.66	2.42 μM
13		(1S,5S)-2-Methyl-5-((R)-6-methylhept-5-en-2-yl)bicyclo[3.1.0]hex-2-ene	9.06	−10.26	−7.25	4.82 μM
14	*Z. officinale*	1-(4-Hydroxy-3-methoxyphenyl)dec-4-en-3-one	5.89	−10.32	−8.35	754.12 nM
15		2-Formyl-9-[.beta.-d-ribofuranosyl]hypoxanthine	4.37	−7.62	−10.79	12.4 nM
16		(1S,5S)-4-Methylene-1-((R)-6-methylhept-5-en-2-yl)bicyclo[3.1.0]hexane	3.77	−11.26	−7.40	3.78 μM

N/B: No suitable ligand poses were discovered.

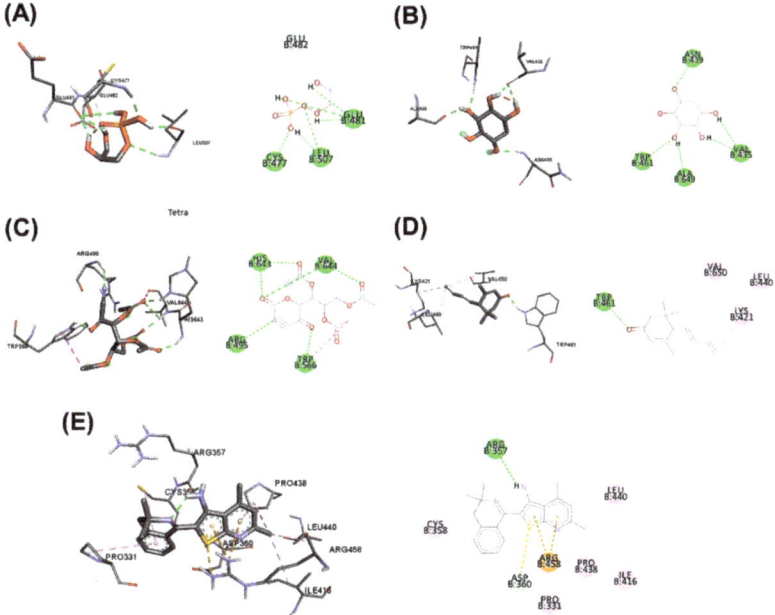

Figure 5. 3D (LHS) and 2D (RHS) Molecular docking pose visualization showing water extraction of *C. fenestratum*: (**A**) Alirocumab, (**B**) Inositol, 1-deoxy-, (**C**) Tetraacetyl-d-xylonic nitrile, (**D**) Megastigmatrienone, (**E**) Thieno[2,3-b]pyridine, 3-amino-2-(3,3-dimethyl-3,4-dihydroisoquinolin-1-yl)-4,6-dimethyl- interactions with PCSK9.

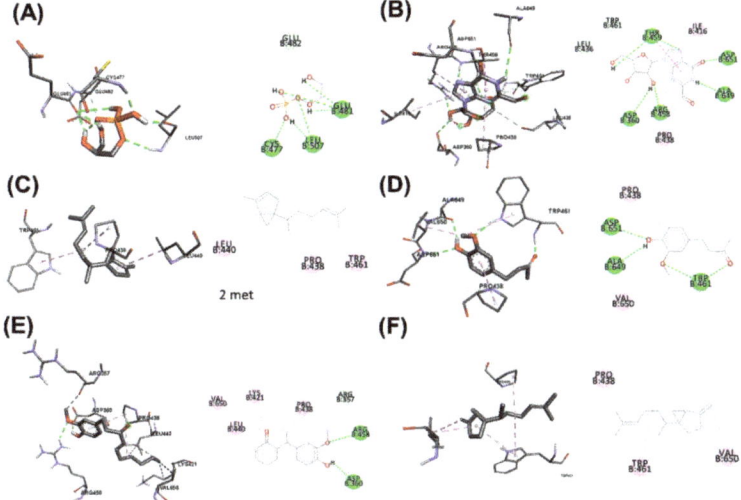

Figure 6. 3D (LHS) and 2D (RHS) Molecular docking pose visualization showing water extraction of *Z. officinale*: (**A**) Alirocumab, (**B**) 2-Formyl-9-[.beta.-d-ribofuranosyl]hypoxanthine, (**C**) (1S,5S)-2-Methyl-5-((R)-6-methylhept-5-en-2-yl)bicyclo[3.1.0]hex-2-ene, (**D**) 2-Butanone, 4-(4-hydroxy-3-methoxyphenyl)-, (**E**) 1-(4-Hydroxy-3-methoxyphenyl)dec-4-en-3-one, (**F**) (1S,5S)-4-Methylene-1-((R)-6-methylhept-5-en-2-yl)bicyclo[3.1.0]hexane interactions with PCSK9.

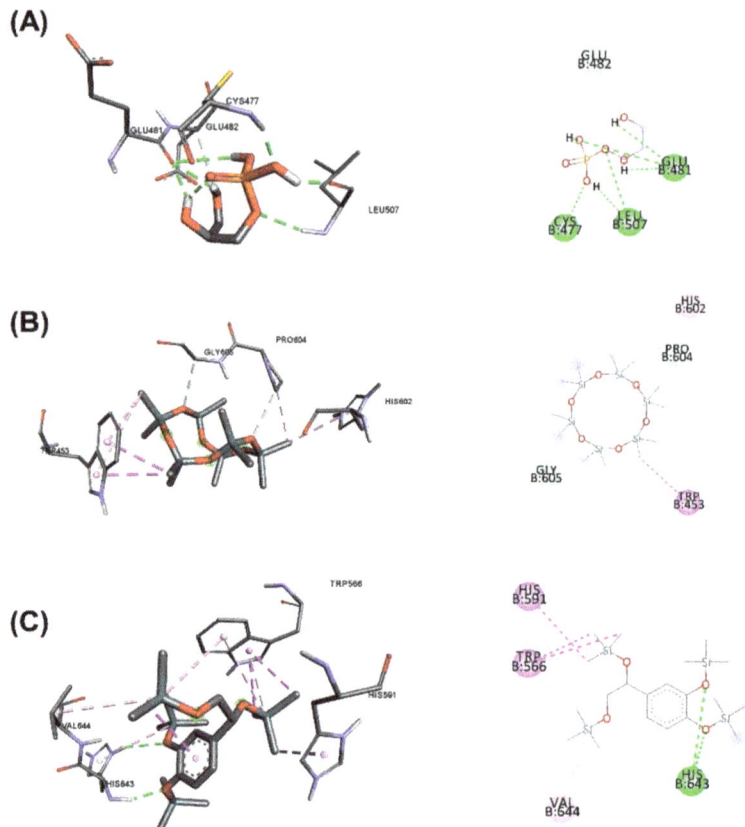

Figure 7. 3D (LHS) and 2D (RHS) Molecular docking pose visualization showing water extraction of *C. tinctorius*: (**A**) Alirocumab, (**B**) Cyclohexasiloxane, dodecamethyl-, (**C**) 3,4-Dihydroxyphenylglycol, 4TMS derivative interactions with PCSK9.

In Table 12, the binding of active compounds in herbs extracted with ethanol and PCSK9 studied via Arguslab and Autodock showed that compounds of *Z. officinale* had a 71.62% inhibitor to PCSK9 as compared to *C. fenestratum* containing a total active inhibitor of 47.04%, thus resulting in better inhibition to PCSK9 of *Z. officinale* than *C. fenestratum* when extracted with ethanol. The results are consistent with the real-time PCR results. It was concluded that the most effective inhibitor of PCSK9 was herbal extracts in water because in water extracts, it was found that the active compounds in *C. fenestratum* and *Z. officinale* extracts are 64.24% and 61.3%, respectively. By comparison, the herb extracts in ethanol provide active *C. fenestratum* and *Z. officinale* compounds at 47.04% and 71.62%, respectively. Therefore, when combining the active compounds for PCSK9 inhibition, *C. fenestratum* and *Z. officinale* suggest the best extraction in the water extract. In addition, studies on the inhibition of HMGCR through Arguslab and Autodock showed that no herbal extract was more effective at inhibiting HMGCR than lovastatin (positive control). The study in Tables 13 and 14 found that most of the compounds in *Z. officinale* had good efficacy in inhibiting HMGCR compared to extracts of *C. fenestratum* and *C. tinctorius*. The results are consistent with the effect of real-time PCR. Therefore, the mechanism of HMGCR affecting lipid formation can be best suppressed with *Z. officinale* extract and is classified as an assistance drug in this recipe.

Table 12. Energy binding and phytochemical inhibition constants of herbal extracts with ethanol at the binding sites of PCSK9 from ArgusLab and Autodock analysis and quantification of each compound through GC-MS/MS analysis.

No.	Herb	Compound Name	GC-MS/MS % Peak Area	ArgusLab Binding Energy (kcal/mol)	Autodock Binding Energy (kcal/mol)	Autodock Inhibition Constant (Ki)
1		Alirocumab (Positive control)		−7.59	−5.61	77.42 μM
2		Cyclopentanol	6.74	−8.29	−5.27	137.36 μM
3		3-Deoxy-d-mannonic acid	7.85	−7.43	−6.93	8.27 μM
4	C. tinctorius	Guanosine	6.58	−7.47	−11.31	5.16 nM
5		l-Pyrrolid-2-one, N-carboxyhydrazide	6.13	−7.27	−7.38	3.89 μM
6		4H-Pyran-4-one, 2,3-dihydro-3,5-dihydroxy-6-methyl-	12.60	−6.19	−6.99	7.46 μM
7		(E)-2,6-Dimethoxy-4-(prop-1-en-1-yl)phenol	8.69	−8.76	−7.51	3.11 μM
8		Cyclopropanetetradecanoic acid, 2-octyl-, methyl ester	7.19	−12.56	−5.14	169.81 μM
9	C. fenestratum	Megastigmatrienone	12.63	−10.83	−7.87	1.7 μM
10		Inositol, 1-deoxy-	21.46	−8.33	−7.30	4.48 μM
11		Thieno[2,3-b]pyridine, 3-amino-2-(3,3-dimethyl-3,4-dihydroisoquinolin-1-yl)-4,6-dimethyl-	4.26	−11.14	−10.15	36.5 nM
12		1,3-Cyclohexadiene, 5-)1,5-dimethyl-4-hexenyl)-2-methyl-, [S-(R*,S*)]	3.79	−10.91	−7.36	4.0 μM
13		1-(4-Hydroxy-3-methoxyphenyl)dodec-4-en-3-one	5.23	−11.29	−8.69	428.1 nM
14	Z. officinale	(E)-1-(4-Hydroxy-3-methoxyphenyl)dec-3-en-5-one	4.96	−10.40	−8.8	351.96 nM
15		Butan-2-one, 4-(3-hydroxy-2-methoxyphenyl)-	33.27	−8.25	−7.44	3.54 μM
16		1-(4-Hydroxy-3-methoxyphenyl)dec-4-en-3-one	24.37	−10.32	−8.35	754.12 nM

Table 13. Energy binding and phytochemical inhibition constants of herbal extracts with water at the binding sites of HMGR from ArgusLab and Autodock analysis and quantification of each compound through GC-MS/MS analysis.

No.	Herb	Compound Name	GC-MS/MS % Peak Area	ArgusLab Binding Energy (kcal/mol)	Autodock Binding Energy (kcal/mol)	Autodock Inhibition Constant (Ki)
1		Lovastatin (Positive control)		−9.23012	−8.55	540.36 nM
2		Benzofuran, 2,3-dihydro-	23.24	−8.19673	−5.91	46.78 μM
3		3-Isopropoxy-1,1,1,7,7,7-hexamethyl-3,5,5-tris(trimethylsiloxy)tetrasiloxane	21.23	N/B	−5.15	168.03 μM
4	C. tinctorius	3,4-Dihydroxyphenylglycol, 4TMS derivative	8.94	−7.66333	−6.60	14.6 μM
5		4H-Pyran-4-one, 2,3-dihydro-3,5-dihydroxy-6-methyl-	8.56	−6.64198	−7.22	5.07 μM
6		Cyclohexasiloxane, dodecamethyl-	6.96	−7.98578	−7.59	2.75 μM

Table 13. Cont.

No.	Herb	Compound Name	GC-MS/MS % Peak Area	ArgusLab Binding Energy (kcal/mol)	Autodock Binding Energy (kcal/mol)	Autodock Inhibition Constant (Ki)
7	C. fenestratum	d-Gala-l-ido-octonic amide	9.94	−7.64931	−5.85	51.27 μM
8		Inositol, 1-deoxy-	24.89	−8.28603	−7.34	4.15 μM
9		Tetraacetyl-d-xylonic nitrile	27.92	−7.88168	−6.49	17.48 μM
10		Thieno[2,3-b]pyridine, 3-amino-2-(3,3-dimethyl-3,4-dihydroisoquinolin-1-yl)-4,6-dimethyl-	5.87	−10.0154	−7.75	2.07 μM
11		Megastigmatrienone	5.56	−9.73578	−6.04	37.12 μM
12	Z. officinale	2-Butanone, 4-(4-hydroxy-3-methoxyphenyl)-	38.21	−9.35038	−5.90	47.54 μM
13		(1S,5S(-2-Methyl-5-((R)-6-methylhept-5-en-2-yl)bicyclo[3.1.0]hex-2-ene	9.06	−10.7714	−5.82	54.27 μM
14		1-(4-Hydroxy-3-methoxyphenyl)dec-4-en-3-one	5.89	−10.5172	−6.10	33.53 μM
15		2-Formyl-9-[.beta.-d-ribofuranosyl]hypoxanthine	4.37	−7.52531	−7.96	1.47 μM
16		(1S,5S)-4-Methylene-1-((R)-6-methylhept-5-en-2-yl)bicyclo[3.1.0]hexane	3.77	−10.1426	−5.41	108.68 μM

Table 14. Energy binding and phytochemical inhibition constants of herbal extracts with ethanol at the binding sites of HMGR from ArgusLab and Autodock analysis and quantification of each compound through GC-MS/MS analysis.

No.	Herb	Compound Name	GC-MS/MS % Peak Area	ArgusLab Binding Energy (kcal/mol)	Autodock Binding Energy (kcal/mol)	Autodock Inhibition Constant (Ki)
1		Lovastatin (Positive control)		−9.23012	−8.55	540.36 nM
2	C. tinctorius	Cyclopentanol	6.74	−8.37591	−4.72	345.87 μM
3		3-Deoxy-d-mannonic acid	7.85	−7.71546	−4.19	845.72 μM
4		Guanosine	6.58	−8.31259	−7.77	2 μM
5		l-Pyrrolid-2-one, N-carboxyhydrazide	6.13	−7.38878	−6.99	7.54 μM
6		4H-Pyran-4-one, 2,3-dihydro-3,5-dihydroxy-6-methyl-	12.60	−6.64198	−7.22	5.07 μM
7		(E)-2,6-Dimethoxy-4-(prop-1-en-1-yl)phenol	8.69	−8.90424	−6.69	12.52 μM
8		Cyclopropanetetradecanoic acid, 2-octyl-, methyl ester	7.19	−11.2679	−3.62	2.22 mM
9	C. fenestratum	Megastigmatrienone	12.63	−9.73578	−6.04	37.12 μM
10		Inositol, 1-deoxy-	21.46	−8.28603	−7.34	4.15 μM
11		Thieno[2,3-b]pyridine, 3-amino-2-(3,3-dimethyl-3,4-dihydroisoquinolin-1-yl)-4,6-dimethyl-	4.26	−10.0154	−7.75	2.07 μM

Table 14. Cont.

No.	Herb	Compound Name	GC-MS/MS % Peak Area	ArgusLab Binding Energy (kcal/mol)	Autodock Binding Energy (kcal/mol)	Autodock Inhibition Constant (Ki)
12	Z. officinale	1,3-Cyclohexadiene, 5-(1,5-dimethyl-4-hexenyl)-2-methyl-, [S-(R*,S*)]-	3.79	−10.5606	−5.80	56.41 μM
13		1-(4-Hydroxy-3-methoxyphenyl)dodec-4-en-3-one	5.23	−10.681	−5.43	104.75 μM
14		(E)-1-(4-Hydroxy-3-methoxyphenyl)dec-3-en-5-one	4.96	−10.2192	6.04	37.24 μM
15		Butan-2-one, 4-(3-hydroxy-2-methoxyphenyl)-	33.27	−8.67751	−5.68	69.13 μM
16		1-(4-Hydroxy-3-methoxyphenyl)dec-4-en-3-one	24.37	−10.5172	−6.10	33.53 μM

Tables 15 and 16 show that the ethanol extract of Z. officinale had a better binding effect on SREBP2 than the aqueous extract. Four substances of ethanol extraction of Z. officinale, consisting of (1) 1,3-Cyclohexadiene, 5-(1,5-dimethyl-4-hexenyl)-2-methyl-, [S-(R*,S*).]-, (2) 1-(4-Hydroxy-3-methoxyphenyl)dodec-4-en-3-one, (3) (E)-1-(4-Hydroxy-3-methoxyphenyl)dec-3-en-5-one, and (4) 1-(4-Hydroxy-3-methoxyphenyl)dec-4-en-3-one Z. officinale with aqueous extract were less binding to SREBP2 because there were only three active substances with energy binding less than −10 kcal/mol: (1) (1S,5S)-2-Methyl-5-((R)-6-methylhept-5-en-2-yl)bicyclo[3.1.0]hex-2-ene, (2) 1-(4- Hydroxy-3-methoxyphenyl)dec-4-en-3-one, and (3) (1S,5S)-4-Methylene-1-((R)-6-methylhept-5-en-2-yl)bicyclo[3.1.0]hexane.

Table 15. Energy binding and phytochemical inhibition constants of herbal extracts with water at the binding sites of SREBP2 from ArgusLab and Autodock analysis and quantification of each compound through GC-MS/MS analysis.

No.	Herb	Compound Name	GC MS/MS % Peak Area	ArgusLab Binding Energy (kcal/mol)	Autodock Binding Energy (kcal/mol)	Autodock Inhibition Constant (Ki)
1		Metformin (Positive control)		−5.87716	−5.56	84.25 μM
2	C. tinctorius	Benzofuran, 2,3-dihydro-	23.24	−8.62431	−5.08	189.21 μM
3		3-Isopropoxy-1,1,1,7,7,7-hexamethyl-3,5,5-tris(trimethylsiloxy)tetrasiloxane	21.23	N/B	−5.85	51.15 μM
4		3,4-Dihydroxyphenylglycol, 4TMS derivative	8.94	−7.48581	−4.38	615.35 μM
5		4H-Pyran-4-one, 2,3-dihydro-3,5-dihydroxy-6-methyl-	8.56	−6.69362	−6.49	17.62 μM
6		Cyclohexasiloxane, dodecamethyl-	6.96	−7.32463	−7.03	7.06 μM
7	C. fenestratum	d-Gala-l-ido-octonic amide	9.94	−7.16144	−5.95	43.16 μM
8		Inositol, 1-deoxy-	24.89	−7.83301	−6.89	8.83 μM
9		Tetraacetyl-d-xylonic nitrile	27.92	−7.59524	−5.13	173.8 μM
10		Thieno[2,3-b]pyridine, 3-amino-2-(3,3-dimethyl-3,4-dihydroisoquinolin-1-yl)-4,6-dimethyl-	5.87	−9.68843	−9.91	54.25 nM
11		Megastigmatrienone	5.56	−11.7348	−7.37	3.97 μM

Table 15. Cont.

No.	Herb	Compound Name	GC MS/MS	ArgusLab	Autodock	
			% Peak Area	Binding Energy (kcal/mol)	Binding Energy (kcal/mol)	Inhibition Constant (Ki)
12	Z. officinale	2-Butanone, 4-(4-hydroxy-3-methoxyphenyl)-	38.21	−8.93613	−7.39	3.82 µM
13		(1S,5S)-2-Methyl-5-((R)-6-methylhept-5-en-2-yl)bicyclo[3.1.0]hex-2-ene	9.06	−12.9835	−7.32	4.3 µM
14		1-(4-Hydroxy-3-methoxyphenyl)dec-4-en-3-one	5.89	−11.3944	−8.62	476.42 nM
15		2-Formyl-9-[.beta.-d-ribofuranosyl]hypoxanthine	4.37	−7.4906	−8.69	425.74 nM
16		(1S,5S)-4-Methylene-1-((R)-6-methylhept-5-en-2-yl)bicyclo[3.1.0]hexane	3.77	−12.7577	−7.41	3.72 µM

Table 16. Energy binding and phytochemical inhibition constants of herbal extracts with ethanol at the binding sites of SREBP2 from ArgusLab and Autodock analysis and quantification of each compound through GC-MS/MS analysis.

No.	Herb	Compound Name	GC MS/MS	ArgusLab	Autodock	
			% Peak Area	Binding Energy (kcal/mol)	Binding Energy (kcal/mol)	Inhibition Constant (Ki)
1		Metformin (Positive control)		−5.87716	−5.56	84.25 µM
2	C. tinctorius	Cyclopentanol	6.74	−7.35609	−4.51	498.19 µM
3		3-Deoxy-d-mannonic acid	7.85	−7.11679	−5.37	115.85 µM
4		Guanosine	6.58	−7.51631	−9.56	99.06 nM
5	C. fenestratum	l-Pyrrolid-2-one, N-carboxyhydrazide	6.13	−6.78964	−6.51	16.87 µM
6		4H-Pyran-4-one, 2,3-dihydro-3,5-dihydroxy-6-methyl-	12.60	−6.69362	−6.49	17.62 µM
7		(E)-2,6-Dimethoxy-4-(prop-1-en-1-yl)phenol	8.69	−9.32055	−7.45	3.49 µM
8		Cyclopropanetetradecanoic acid, 2-octyl-, methyl ester	7.19	−11.2105	−4.97	227.42 µM
9		Megastigmatrienone	12.63	−11.7348	−7.37	3.97 µM
10		Inositol, 1-deoxy-	21.46	−7.83301	−6.89	8.83 µM
11		Thieno[2,3-b]pyridine, 3-amino-2-(3,3-dimethyl-3,4-dihydroisoquinolin-1-yl)-4,6-dimethyl-	4.26	−9.68843	−9.91	54.25 nM
12	Z. officinale	1,3-Cyclohexadiene, 5-(1,5-dimethyl-4-hexenyl)-2-methyl-, [S-(R*,S*)]-	3.79	−11.7619	−7.05	6.75 µM
13		1-(4-Hydroxy-3-methoxyphenyl)dodec-4-en-3-one	5.23	−11.602	−4.88	265.67 µM
14		(E)-1-(4-Hydroxy-3-methoxyphenyl)dec-3-en-5-one	4.96	−10.7057	−6.15	30.88 µM
15		Butan-2-one, 4-(3-hydroxy-2-methoxyphenyl)-	33.27	−9.25557	−5.93	45.14 µM
16		1-(4-Hydroxy-3-methoxyphenyl)dec-4-en-3-one	24.37	−11.3944	−4.88	265.67 µM

Interestingly, the aqueous extract of *C. fenestratum* contained only one substance, megastigmatrienone. The binding of SREBP2 was lower than −10 kcal/mol, but the inhibition efficiency was higher in the ethanol extraction. This is because there are two active substances that caFn inhibit SREBP2 using energy below −10 kcal/mol: Cyclopropanetetradecanoic acid, 2-octyl-, methyl ester and Megastigmatrienone. The results are also consistent with RT-PCR regarding the expression of SREBP2.

In conclusion, the extracts with the best SREBP2 inhibition were ranked from highest to lowest efficiency. In the following order, *Z. officinale*, *C. fenestratum*, and *C. tinctorius* extracts were extracted, respectively, and it was found that the ethanol extract had a better inhibitory effect than the aqueous extract.

4. Discussion

High levels of cholesterol are a significant risk factor for atherosclerosis and cardiovascular disease. Reducing the blood lipid profile may aid in the treatment of high levels of cholesterol-related diseases and disorders, including metabolic syndrome. Statins are medications that can lower cholesterol in a blood vessel and should be taken by most individuals. However, even after taking statins, the lipids in the blood in some individuals remained high [59]. Statins merely enhance the LDLR expression. LDLR destruction stays high if PCSK9 expression is still high [7]. Even though PCSK9 inhibition is beneficial for lipid reduction, the striking benefit achieved with only statin treatments in patients with a wide range of cholesterol levels cannot be attributed to their cholesterol-lowering effect. Therefore, inhibiting PCSK9 expression is crucial for improving lipid reduction.

In this study, the lowering cholesterol activity of three plants, *C. tinctorius*, *C. fenestratum*, and *Z. officinale*, as well as the potential molecular mechanisms involved in their lowering cholesterol activity, were investigated in the human liver cell line HepG2 by using molecular docking and RT-qPCR. Furthermore, we proved that combining these plants by making three parts *C. fenestratum* (primary herb), two parts *Z. officinale* (support herb), and one part *C. tinctorius* (coloring herb) significantly reduced lipid accumulation in hepatocytes by investigating Oil red O staining.

According to these findings, water-extracted *C. fenestratum* was the most effective at downregulating PCSK9 mRNA in HepG2 cells, followed by ethanol-extracted *Z. officinale*, water-extracted ginger, and water-extracted *C. tinctorius*. PCSK9 expression was reduced, which increased LDLR expression. Water-extracted *C. fenestratum* exhibited the most significant induction of LDLR expression, followed by water-extracted *Z. officinale* and water-extracted *C. tinctorius*. Further GC-MS/MS analysis of active compounds for these herbs revealed that excellent inhibition of lipid deposition depended on the efficacy of binding to target proteins and the number of chemical compounds present in the herb. Studies have shown that the highest number of compounds found in the *C. fenestratum* are the following: (1) Tetraacetyl-d-xylonic nitrile (27.92%). It binds strongly to PCSK9, forming up to six hydrogen bonds with the amino acids HIS643, VAL644, ARG495, and TRP566. (2) Inositol, 1-deoxy- (24.89%) can bind the PCSK9 with different amino acids compared to Tetraacetyl-d-xylonic nitrile-PCSK9 binding. It can form up to five hydrogen bonds with the amino acids TRP461, ALA649, VAL435, and ASN439. *Z. officinale* contains only 1 compound, 2-Formyl-9-[.beta.-d-ribofuranosyl]hypoxanthine, which contained only 4.37% of *Z. officinale* extract to form a high 8-position hydrogen bond with the amino acids TRP461, LEU436, ASP360, ARG458, ALA649, ASP651, and THR469. Finally, *C. tinctorius*. *C. tinctorius*'s active compounds have poor binding to PCSK9 because it contains only two compounds: 3,4-Dihydroxyphenylglycol, 4TMS derivative (8.94%), and Cyclohexasiloxane, dodecamethyl-(6.96%), which were found to total just 15.9%, resulting in poor inhibition of PCSK9. These compounds formed very few hydrogen bonds with PCSK9 binding. *C. fenestratum* is the best PCSK9 inhibitor because of its high binding to the target protein and its high active compounds, followed by *Z. officinale*, which has a better PCSK9 inhibitor than the *C. fenestratum*. However, the low content of active compounds resulted in less efficacy of *Z. officinale* in inhibiting PCSK9. Finally, *C. tinctorius* was the least effective in inhibiting PCSK9 because of its fewer active compounds and poorer binding capacity than the herbs, as mentioned earlier. From the study results, an herbal recipe for reducing lipid has been designed by using the knowledge of Thai traditional medicine [58] to set the drug recipe as the main drug, which is the drug that has the highest efficiency in inhibiting lipid with the highest ratio. This recipe is three parts *C. fenestratum*. An assistance drug is a drug that will increase the efficiency of the main drug to reduce lipid with a lesser ratio. This recipe is two parts *Z. officinale*, and a colorant drug is used for adding applicability to the recipe with the lowest ratio. One part of *C. tinctorius* was added to this recipe. This recipe was tested for lipid reduction efficacy using HepG2 cells. It was found that this recipe could reduce lipid accumulation better than using the herb alone. Therefore, this is the world's first herbal recipe that helps reduce lipid through PCSK9 inhibition.

To clarify the substance structure and biological activity, the study found that the main inhibitors of PCSK9 were tetraacetyl-d-xylonic nitrile (27.92 percent) from *C. fenestratum*, and 2-Formyl-9-[.beta.-d-ribofuranosyl]hypoxanthine (4.37%) from *Z. officinale*. The study of Structure-Activity Relationship (SAR) is available through the website: http://way2drug.com/PassOnline/predict.php. The structure of a substance with a Pa value greater than 0.7 indicates that the substance can be developed as a drug for the treatment of such diseases [60]. The composition analysis of *C. fenestratum* showed that tetraacetyl-d-xylonic nitrile (CC(=O)OCC(C(C(C(=O)C#N)OC(=O)C)OC(=O) C)OC(=O)C) showed very good properties as a lipid metabolism regulator. Pa = 0.822 and *Z. officinale* containing 2-Formyl-9-[.beta.-d-ribofuranosyl] hypoxanthine (C1=NC2=C(N1C3C(C(C(O3)CO)O)O)N=C(NC2=O)C=O) has very good lipotropic properties, with Pa = 0.870. The aforementioned data clearly show that the extracts of *C. fenestratum* and *Z. officinale* have good properties in lowering lipid levels.

Although extractions involve many methods and a variety of solvents, the water and ethanol extraction methods are traditional and easy to implement. The introductions of tetraacetyl-d-xylonic nitrile and 2-Formyl-9-[.beta.-d-ribofuranosyl] hypoxanthine were assessed according to the solubility calculation with SWISSADME, tetraacetyl-d-xylonic nitrile had Log S (ESOL)[61], Log S (Ali) [62], and Log S (SILICOS-IT) [63] as -0.94, -2.22, and -0.74, respectively. The values showed that the compound had high water solubility. Formyl-9-[.beta.-d-ribofuranosyl] hypoxanthine, the values of Log S (ESOL), Log S (Ali), and Log S (SILICOS-IT) were -0.90, -1.24, and 0.20, respectively, refer to high water solubility. From the calculation of solubility, Formyl-9-[.beta.-d-ribofuranosyl] hypoxanthine has slightly better water solubility than tetraacetyl-d-xylonic nitrile. As a result, both compounds with PCSK9 inhibitory activity were better extracted with water than ethanol, consistent with the results of the GC-MS/MS study that found tetraacetyl-d-xylonic nitrile in 27.92% water extraction while extracting only 9.47% with ethanol. Moreover, 2-Formyl-9-[.beta.-d-ribofuranosyl] hypoxanthine was extracted with a 4.37% yield in water, while there are no compounds found in ethanol extraction.

5. Conclusions

In conclusion, for screening PCSK9 inhibitors from three plants, *C. tinctorius*, *C. fenestratum*, and *Z. officinale*, an efficient technique incorporating molecular docking, RT-qPCR test, in vitro cytotoxicity, and Oil red O staining assay was devised. Two chemicals had a high yield from *C. fenestratum* based on GC-MS/MS detection: tetraacetyl-d-xylonic nitrile (27.92 percent) and Inositol, 1-deoxy- (24.89 percent). These compounds could inhibit PCSK9 strongly through the binding of 6 and 5 hydrogen bonds, respectively, while the active compound in *Z. officinale* is 2-Formyl-9-[.beta.-d-ribofuranosyl] hypoxanthine (4.37%), which inhibits PCSK9 by forming 8 hydrogen bonds. According to our findings, we may utilize a formula consisting of three parts *C. fenestratum* (primary herb), two parts *Z. officinale* (assistance herb), and one part *C. tinctorius* (servant herb) to define a reasonable herbal ratio for the intervention and prevention of PCSK9-related disorders in the future. Furthermore, because of targeted screening and precise analysis, this technique is expected to be used for a broader range of applications, such as fast screening of active components from herbs, and improving herb ratios in alternative medicine.

Supplementary Materials: The following supporting information can be downloaded at: https://www.mdpi.com/article/10.3390/plants11141835/s1.

Author Contributions: T.O. and K.E. provided the concept and designed the study. T.O. and K.E. conducted the analyses and wrote the manuscript. T.O., N.P., O.J., T.L., S.W. and K.E. Participated in data analysis. N.N. and K.E. carried out experimental validation. A.K.P., M.d.L.P., P.W., V.N., N.N. and K.E. Contributed to revising and proofreading the manuscript. All authors have read and agreed to the published version of the manuscript.

Funding: This research is partially financially supported by Walailak University, Thailand (Grant no. WU-IRG-65-013) and partially supported by New Strategic Research (P2P) project, Walailak University, Thailand. Project CICECO-Aveiro Institute of Materials, UIDB/50011/2020, UIDP/50011/2020 & LA/P/0006/2020, financed by national funds through the FCT/MEC (PIDDAC).

Data Availability Statement: The datasets used and/or analyzed during the current study are available from the corresponding author Komgrit Eawsakul (komgrit.ea@wu.ac.th) on reasonable request.

Acknowledgments: We would like to thank the BioNEDD lab, Mahidol University and Center of Excellence Research for Innovation and Health Product, and the School of Medicine, Walailak University for providing laboratory facilities.

Conflicts of Interest: The authors declare that they have no conflict of interest.

References

1. Istvan, E. Statin inhibition of HMG-CoA reductase: A 3-dimensional view. *Atheroscler. Suppl.* **2003**, *4*, 3–8. [CrossRef]
2. Liu, L.; Yeh, Y.-Y. S-alk (en) yl cysteines of garlic inhibit cholesterol synthesis by deactivating HMG-CoA reductase in cultured rat hepatocytes. *J. Nutr.* **2002**, *132*, 1129–1134. [CrossRef]
3. Mahdavi, A.; Bagherniya, M.; Fakheran, O.; Reiner, Ž.; Xu, S.; Sahebkar, A. Medicinal plants and bioactive natural compounds as inhibitors of HMG-CoA reductase: A literature review. *BioFactors* **2020**, *46*, 906–926. [CrossRef] [PubMed]
4. Pearlstein, R.A.; Hu, Q.Y.; Zhou, J.; Yowe, D.; Levell, J.; Dale, B.; Kaushik, V.K.; Daniels, D.; Hanrahan, S.; Sherman, W. New hypotheses about the structure-function of proprotein convertase subtilisin/kexin type 9: Analysis of the epidermal growth factor-like repeat A docking site using WaterMap. *Proteins Struct. Funct. Bioinform.* **2010**, *78*, 2571–2586. [CrossRef] [PubMed]
5. Schroeder, C.I.; Swedberg, J.E.; Withka, J.M.; Rosengren, K.J.; Akcan, M.; Clayton, D.J.; Daly, N.L.; Cheneval, O.; Borzilleri, K.A.; Griffor, M. Design and synthesis of truncated EGF-A peptides that restore LDL-R recycling in the presence of PCSK9 in vitro. *Chem. Biol.* **2014**, *21*, 284–294. [CrossRef] [PubMed]
6. Zhang, D.-W.; Lagace, T.A.; Garuti, R.; Zhao, Z.; McDonald, M.; Horton, J.D.; Cohen, J.C.; Hobbs, H.H. Binding of proprotein convertase subtilisin/kexin type 9 to epidermal growth factor-like repeat A of low density lipoprotein receptor decreases receptor recycling and increases degradation. *J. Biol. Chem.* **2007**, *282*, 18602–18612. [CrossRef]
7. Lagace, T.A. PCSK9 and LDLR degradation: Regulatory mechanisms in circulation and in cells. *Curr. Opin. Lipidol.* **2014**, *25*, 387–393. [CrossRef]
8. Nassoury, N.; Blasiole, D.A.; Tebon Oler, A.; Benjannet, S.; Hamelin, J.; Poupon, V.; McPherson, P.S.; Attie, A.D.; Prat, A.; Seidah, N.G. The cellular trafficking of the secretory proprotein convertase PCSK9 and its dependence on the LDLR. *Traffic* **2007**, *8*, 718–732. [CrossRef]
9. Tushar, K.; George, S.; Remashree, A.; Balachandran, I. *Coscinium fenestratum* (Gaertn.) Colebr.—A review on this rare, critically endangered and highly-traded medicinal species. *J. Plant Sci.* **2008**, *3*, 133–145. [CrossRef]
10. Ved, D.; Saha, D.; Ravikumar, K.; Haridasan, K. Coscinium fenestratum. *IUCN Red List Threat. Species* **2015**, T50126585A50131325.
11. Rojsanga, P.; Gritsanapan, W.; Suntornsuk, L. Determination of berberine content in the stem extracts of Coscinium fenestratum by TLC densitometry. *Med. Princ.* **2006**, *15*, 373–378. [CrossRef] [PubMed]
12. Kashyap, S.; Kapoor, N.; Kale, R.D. Coscinium fenestratum: Callus and suspension cell culture of the endangered medicinal plant using vermicompost extract and coelomic fluid as plant tissue culture media. *Am. J. Plant Sci.* **2016**, *7*, 899. [CrossRef]
13. Dong, H.; Zhao, Y.; Zhao, L.; Lu, F. The effects of berberine on blood lipids: A systemic review and meta-analysis of randomized controlled trials. *Planta Med.* **2013**, *79*, 437–446. [CrossRef] [PubMed]
14. Wang, Y.; Tong, Q.; Shou, J.-W.; Zhao, Z.-X.; Li, X.-Y.; Zhang, X.-F.; Ma, S.-R.; He, C.-Y.; Lin, Y.; Wen, B.-Y. Gut microbiota-mediated personalized treatment of hyperlipidemia using berberine. *Theranostics* **2017**, *7*, 2443. [CrossRef] [PubMed]
15. Yang, S.-G.; Park, H.-J.; Kim, J.-W.; Jung, J.-M.; Kim, M.-J.; Jegal, H.-G.; Kim, I.-S.; Kang, M.-J.; Wee, G.; Yang, H.-Y. Mito-TEMPO improves development competence by reducing superoxide in preimplantation porcine embryos. *Sci. Rep.* **2018**, *8*, 10130. [CrossRef] [PubMed]

16. Račková, L.; Cupáková, M.; Ťažký, A.; Mičová, J.; Kolek, E.; Košťálová, D. Redox properties of ginger extracts: Perspectives of use of Zingiber officinale Rosc. as antidiabetic agent. *Interdiscip. Toxicol.* **2013**, *6*, 26. [CrossRef]
17. Bhandari, U.; Ahmed, J.; Pillai, K. An overview of Zingiber officinale (ginger); Chemistry and pharmacological profile. *Hamdard Med.* **2001**, *44*, 28–32.
18. Mascolo, N.; Jain, R.; Jain, S.; Capasso, F. Ethnopharmacologic investigation of ginger (Zingiber officinale). *J. Ethnopharmacol.* **1989**, *27*, 129–140. [CrossRef]
19. Jitoe, A.; Masuda, T.; Tengah, I.; Suprapta, D.N.; Gara, I.; Nakatani, N. Antioxidant activity of tropical ginger extracts and analysis of the contained curcuminoids. *J. Agric. Food Chem.* **1992**, *40*, 1337–1340. [CrossRef]
20. Krishnakantha, T.; Lokesh, B.R. Scavenging of superoxide anions by spice principles. *Indian J. Biochem. Biophys.* **1993**, *30*, 133–134.
21. Pulla Reddy, A.C.; Lokesh, B. Studies on spice principles as antioxidants in the inhibition of lipid peroxidation of rat liver microsomes. *Mol. Cell. Biochem.* **1992**, *111*, 117–124. [CrossRef]
22. Bhandari, U.; Pillai, K. Effect of ethanolic extract of Zingiber officinale on dyslipidaemia in diabetic rats. *J. Ethnopharmacol.* **2005**, *97*, 227–230. [CrossRef] [PubMed]
23. Gautam, S.; Bhagyawant, S.S.; Srivastava, N. Detailed study on therapeutic properties, uses and pharmacological applications of safflower (*Carthamus tinctorius* L.). *Int. J. Ayurveda Pharma Res.* **2014**, *2*, 1–4.
24. COŞGE, B.; GÜRBÜZ, B.; KIRALAN, M. Oil content and fatty acid composition of some safflower (*Carthamus tinctorius* L.) varieties sown in spring and winter. *Int. J. Nat. Eng. Sci.* **2007**, *1*, 11–15.
25. Katkade, M.; Syed, H.; Andhale, R.; Sontakke, M. Fatty acid profile and quality assessment of safflower (*Carthamus tinctorius*) oil. *J. Pharmacogn. Phytochem.* **2018**, *7*, 3581–3585.
26. Salem, M.A.; Zayed, A.; Alseekh, S.; Fernie, A.R.; Giavalisco, P. The integration of MS-based metabolomics and multivariate data analysis allows for improved quality assessment of Zingiber officinale Roscoe. *Phytochemistry* **2021**, *190*, 112843. [CrossRef]
27. Bhagyalakshmi, B.; Singh, N.S. Meristem culture and micropropagation of a variety of ginger (Zingiber officinale Rosc.) with a high yield of oleoresin. *J. Hortic. Sci.* **1988**, *63*, 321–327. [CrossRef]
28. Nair, K.P. Production, Marketing, and Economics of Ginger. In *Turmeric (Curcuma longa L.) and Ginger (Zingiber officinale Rosc.)—World's Invaluable Medicinal Spices: The Agronomy and Economy of Turmeric and Ginger*; Nair, K.P., Ed.; Springer International Publishing: Cham, Switzerland, 2019; pp. 493–518.
29. Arablou, T.; Aryaeian, N. The effect of ginger (Zingiber Officinale) as an ancient medicinal plant on improving blood lipids. *J. Herb. Med.* **2018**, *12*, 11–15. [CrossRef]
30. Sharifi-Rad, J.; Sureda, A.; Tenore, G.C.; Daglia, M.; Sharifi-Rad, M.; Valussi, M.; Tundis, R.; Sharifi-Rad, M.; Loizzo, M.R.; Ademiluyi, A.O.; et al. Biological Activities of Essential Oils: From Plant Chemoecology to Traditional Healing Systems. *Molecules* **2017**, *22*, 70. [CrossRef]
31. Wang, X.; Shen, Y.; Thakur, K.; Han, J.; Zhang, J.-G.; Hu, F.; Wei, Z.-J. Antibacterial Activity and Mechanism of Ginger Essential Oil against Escherichia coli and Staphylococcus aureus. *Molecules* **2020**, *25*, 3955. [CrossRef] [PubMed]
32. Baliga, M.S.; Haniadka, R.; Pereira, M.M.; D'Souza, J.J.; Pallaty, P.L.; Bhat, H.P.; Popuri, S. Update on the Chemopreventive Effects of Ginger and its Phytochemicals. *Crit. Rev. Food Sci. Nutr.* **2011**, *51*, 499–523. [CrossRef] [PubMed]
33. Mowrey, D.; Clayson, D. Motion Sickness, Ginger, and Psychophysics. *Lancet* **1982**, *319*, 655–657. [CrossRef]
34. Vijay, D.; Haleshi, C.; Sringeswara, A.N. Endangered Medicinal Plant *Coscinium fenestratum* (Gaertn.) Colebr A Review. *Pharmacogn. J.* **2020**, *12*, 1077–1085.
35. Goveas, S.W.; Abraham, A.; Research. Extraction and secondary metabolite analysis of *Coscinium fenestratum* (Gaertn.) Colebr: An important medicinal plant of western ghats. *Int. J. Pharm. Sci. Res.* **2014**, *5*, 3484.
36. Kothalawala, S.D.; Edward, D.; Harasgama, J.C.; Ranaweera, L.; Weerasena, O.V.D.S.J.; Niloofa, R.; Ratnasooriya, W.D.; Premakumara, G.A.S.; Handunnetti, S.M. Immunomodulatory Activity of a Traditional Sri Lankan Concoction of *Coriandrum sativum* L. and *Coscinium fenestratum* G. *Evid. Based Complement. Altern. Med.* **2020**, *2020*, 9715060. [CrossRef]
37. Reuter, J.; Huyke, C.; Casetti, F.; Theek, C.; Frank, U.; Augustin, M.; Schempp, C. Anti-inflammatory potential of a lipolotion containing coriander oil in the ultraviolet erythema test. *Der Dtsch. Dermatol. Ges.* **2008**, *6*, 847–851. [CrossRef]
38. Harisaranraj, R.; Babu, S.; Suresh, K. Antimicrobial properties of selected Indian medicinal plants against acne-inducing bacteria. *Ethnobot. Leafl.* **2010**, *14*, 84–94.
39. Suseela, V.; Poornima, K. Free radical scavenging activity of tree turmeric (*Coscinium fenestratum*). *Indian J. Nutr. Diet.* **2009**, *46*, 199–203.
40. Wongcome, T.; Panthong, A.; Jesadanont, S.; Kanjanapothi, D.; Taesotikul, T.; Lertprasertsuke, N. Hypotensive effect and toxicology of the extract from *Coscinium fenestratum* (Gaertn.) Colebr. *J. Ethnopharmacol.* **2007**, *111*, 468–475. [CrossRef]
41. Lu, J.-X.; Zhang, C.-X.; Hu, Y.; Zhang, M.-H.; Wang, Y.-N.; Qian, Y.-X.; Yang, J.; Yang, W.-Z.; Jiang, M.-M.; Guo, D.-A. Application of multiple chemical and biological approaches for quality assessment of *Carthamus tinctorius* L. (safflower) by determining both the primary and secondary metabolites. *Phytomedicine* **2019**, *58*, 152826.
42. Zhou, X.; Tang, L.; Xu, Y.; Zhou, G.; Wang, Z. Towards a better understanding of medicinal uses of *Carthamus tinctorius* L. in traditional Chinese medicine: A phytochemical and pharmacological review. *J. Ethnopharmacol.* **2014**, *151*, 27–43. [CrossRef] [PubMed]

43. Eawsakul, K.; Chinavinijkul, P.; Saeeng, R.; Chairoungdua, A.; Tuchinda, P.; Nasongkla, N. Preparation and characterizations of RSPP050-loaded polymeric micelles using poly (ethylene glycol)-b-poly (ε-caprolactone) and poly (ethylene glycol)-b-poly (D, L-lactide). *Chem. Pharm. Bull.* **2017**, *65*, 530–537. [CrossRef]
44. Nasongkla, N.; Tuchinda, P.; Munyoo, B.; Eawsakul, K. Preparation and Characterization of MUC-30-Loaded Polymeric Micelles against MCF-7 Cell Lines Using Molecular Docking Methods and In Vitro Study. *Evid. Based Complementary Altern. Med.* **2021**, *2021*, 5597681. [CrossRef] [PubMed]
45. Chen, H.-C.; Chen, P.-Y.; Wu, M.-J.; Tai, M.-H.; Yen, J.-H. Tanshinone IIA modulates low density lipoprotein uptake via down-regulation of PCSK9 gene expression in HepG2 cells. *PLoS ONE* **2016**, *11*, e0162414.
46. Leng, E.; Xiao, Y.; Mo, Z.; Li, Y.; Zhang, Y.; Deng, X.; Zhou, M.; Zhou, C.; He, Z.; He, J. Synergistic effect of phytochemicals on cholesterol metabolism and lipid accumulation in HepG2 cells. *BMC Complement. Altern. Med.* **2018**, *18*, 122. [CrossRef] [PubMed]
47. Zainab, R.; Kaleem, A.; Ponczek, M.B.; Abdullah, R.; Iqtedar, M.; Hoessli, D.C. Finding inhibitors for PCSK9 using computational methods. *PLoS ONE* **2021**, *16*, e0255523. [CrossRef]
48. Shamsara, J. CrossDocker: A tool for performing cross-docking using Autodock Vina. *SpringerPlus* **2016**, *5*, 344. [CrossRef]
49. Morris, G.M.; Goodsell, D.S.; Huey, R.; Hart, W.E.; Halliday, S.; Belew, R.; Olson, A.J. AutoDock. In *Automated Docking of Flexible Ligands to Receptor-User Guide*; The Scripps Research Institute, Molecular Graphics Laboratory, Department of Molecular Biology: La Jolla, CA, USA, 2001.
50. Roth, E.M.; Diller, P. Alirocumab for hyperlipidemia: Physiology of PCSK9 inhibition, pharmacodynamics and Phase I and II clinical trial results of a PCSK9 monoclonal antibody. *Future Cardiol.* **2014**, *10*, 183–199. [CrossRef]
51. Tobert, J.A. Lovastatin and beyond: The history of the HMG-CoA reductase inhibitors. *Nat. Rev. Drug Discov.* **2003**, *2*, 517–526. [CrossRef]
52. Eawsakul, K.; Panichayupakaranant, P.; Ongtanasup, T.; Warinhomhoun, S.; Noonong, K.; Bunluepuech, K. Computational study and in vitro alpha-glucosidase inhibitory effects of medicinal plants from a Thai folk remedy. *Heliyon* **2021**, *7*, e08078. [CrossRef]
53. Sasaki, M.; Terao, Y.; Ayaori, M.; Uto-Kondo, H.; Iizuka, M.; Yogo, M.; Hagisawa, K.; Takiguchi, S.; Yakushiji, E.; Nakaya, K. Hepatic Overexpression of Idol Increases Circulating Protein Convertase Subtilisin/Kexin Type 9 in Mice and Hamsters via Dual Mechanisms: Sterol Regulatory Element–Binding Protein 2 and Low-Density Lipoprotein Receptor–Dependent Pathways. *Arterioscler. Thromb. Vasc. Biol.* **2014**, *34*, 1171–1178. [CrossRef] [PubMed]
54. Bursill, C.; Roach, P.D.; Bottema, C.D.; Pal, S. Green tea upregulates the low-density lipoprotein receptor through the sterol-regulated element binding protein in HepG2 liver cells. *J. Agric. Food Chem.* **2001**, *49*, 5639–5645. [CrossRef] [PubMed]
55. Sakai, K.; Shimokawa, T.; Kobayashi, T.; Okuyama, H. Lipid lowering effects of high linoleate and high α-linolenate diets in rats and mice. Consequence of long-term feedings. *Chem. Pharm. Bull.* **1992**, *40*, 2129–2132. [CrossRef]
56. Jiang, S.-Y.; Li, H.; Tang, J.-J.; Wang, J.; Luo, J.; Liu, B.; Wang, J.-K.; Shi, X.-J.; Cui, H.-W.; Tang, J. Discovery of a potent HMG-CoA reductase degrader that eliminates statin-induced reductase accumulation and lowers cholesterol. *Nat. Commun.* **2018**, *9*, 5138. [CrossRef]
57. Bálint, M.; Jeszenői, N.; Horváth, I.; van der Spoel, D.; Hetényi, C. Systematic exploration of multiple drug binding sites. *J. Chemin.* **2017**, *9*, 65. [CrossRef]
58. Yuan, H.; Ma, Q.; Ye, L.; Piao, G. The Traditional Medicine and Modern Medicine from Natural Products. *Molecules* **2016**, *21*, 559. [CrossRef]
59. Mora, S.; Glynn, R.J.; Boekholdt, S.M.; Nordestgaard, B.G.; Kastelein, J.J.P.; Ridker, P.M. On-Treatment Non–High-Density Lipoprotein Cholesterol, Apolipoprotein B, Triglycerides, and Lipid Ratios in Relation to Residual Vascular Risk after Treatment with Potent Statin Therapy: JUPITER (Justification for the Use of Statins in Prevention: An Intervention Trial Evaluating Rosuvastatin). *J. Am. Coll. Cardiol.* **2012**, *59*, 1521–1528. [PubMed]
60. Ghadimi, S.; Asad-Samani, K.; Ebrahimi-Valmoozi, A.A. Synthesis, spectroscopic characterization and structure-activity relationship of some phosphoramidothioate pesticides. *J. Iran. Chem. Soc.* **2011**, *8*, 717–726. [CrossRef]
61. Delaney, J.S. ESOL: Estimating Aqueous Solubility Directly from Molecular Structure. *J. Chem. Inf. Comput. Sci.* **2004**, *44*, 1000–1005. [CrossRef]
62. Ali, J.; Camilleri, P.; Brown, M.B.; Hutt, A.J.; Kirton, S.B. Revisiting the General Solubility Equation: In Silico Prediction of Aqueous Solubility Incorporating the Effect of Topographical Polar Surface Area. *J. Chem. Inf. Modeling* **2012**, *52*, 420–428. [CrossRef]
63. Daina, A.; Michielin, O.; Zoete, V. SwissADME: A free web tool to evaluate pharmacokinetics, drug-likeness and medicinal chemistry friendliness of small molecules. *Sci. Rep.* **2017**, *7*, 42717. [CrossRef] [PubMed]

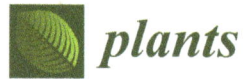 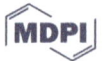

Article

Anti-Biofilm and Associated Anti-Virulence Activities of Selected Phytochemical Compounds against *Klebsiella pneumoniae*

Idowu J. Adeosun, Itumeleng T. Baloyi and Sekelwa Cosa *

Department of Biochemistry, Genetics and Microbiology, Division of Microbiology, University of Pretoria, Private Bag X20, Hatfield, Pretoria 0028, South Africa; u21747050@tuks.co.za (I.J.A.); u18372882@tuks.co.za (I.T.B.)
* Correspondence: sekelwa.cosa@up.ac.za

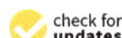

Citation: Adeosun, I.J.; Baloyi, I.T.; Cosa, S. Anti-Biofilm and Associated Anti-Virulence Activities of Selected Phytochemical Compounds against *Klebsiella pneumoniae*. *Plants* 2022, 11, 1429. https://doi.org/10.3390/plants11111429

Academic Editor: Veronique Seidel

Received: 3 May 2022
Accepted: 24 May 2022
Published: 27 May 2022
Corrected: 8 March 2023

Publisher's Note: MDPI stays neutral with regard to jurisdictional claims in published maps and institutional affiliations.

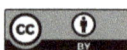

Copyright: © 2022 by the authors. Licensee MDPI, Basel, Switzerland. This article is an open access article distributed under the terms and conditions of the Creative Commons Attribution (CC BY) license (https:// creativecommons.org/licenses/by/ 4.0/).

Abstract: The ability of *Klebsiella pneumoniae* to form biofilm renders the pathogen recalcitrant to various antibiotics. The difficulty in managing *K. pneumoniae* related chronic infections is due to its biofilm-forming ability and associated virulence factors, necessitating the development of efficient strategies to control virulence factors. This study aimed at evaluating the inhibitory potential of selected phytochemical compounds on biofilm-associated virulence factors in *K. pneumoniae*, as well as authenticating their antibiofilm activity. Five phytochemical compounds (alpha-terpinene, camphene, fisetin, glycitein and phytol) were evaluated for their antibacterial and anti-biofilm-associated virulence factors such as exopolysaccharides, curli fibers, and hypermucoviscosity against carbapenem-resistant and extended-spectrum beta-lactamase-positive *K. pneumoniae* strains. The antibiofilm potential of these compounds was evaluated at initial cell attachment, microcolony formation and mature biofilm formation, then validated by in situ visualization using scanning electron microscopy (SEM). Exopolysaccharide surface topography was characterized using atomic force microscopy (AFM). The antibacterial activity of the compounds confirmed fisetin as the best anti-carbapenem-resistant *K. pneumoniae*, demonstrating a minimum inhibitory concentration (MIC) value of 0.0625 mg/mL. Phytol, glycitein and α-terpinene showed MIC values of 0.125 mg/mL for both strains. The assessment of the compounds for anti-virulence activity (exopolysaccharide reduction) revealed an up to 65.91% reduction in phytol and camphene. Atomic force microscopy detected marked differences between the topographies of untreated and treated (camphene and phytol) exopolysaccharides. Curli expression was inhibited at both 0.5 and 1.0 mg/mL by phytol, glycitein, fisetin and quercetin. The hypermucoviscosity was reduced by phytol, glycitein, and fisetin to the shortest mucoid string (1 mm) at 1 mg/mL. Phytol showed the highest antiadhesion activity against carbapenem-resistant and extended-spectrum beta-lactamase-positive *K. pneumoniae* (54.71% and 50.05%), respectively. Scanning electron microscopy correlated the in vitro findings, with phytol significantly altering the biofilm architecture. Phytol has antibiofilm and antivirulence potential against the highly virulent *K. pneumoniae* strains, revealing it as a potential lead compound for the management of *K. pneumoniae*-associated infections.

Keywords: antibacterial; exopolysaccharides; hypermucoviscosity; *Klebsiella pneumoniae*; phytochemical compounds

1. Introduction

Biofilms are typical forms of bacterial communities that grow on living and non-living solid surfaces, which are often immersed in a self-producing matrix [1,2]. Biofilm-associated cells can attach irreversibly to several surfaces and have become a critical worldwide health concern because of their ability to withstand antibiotics, human defense mechanisms, and other external stimuli, contributing to persistent chronic infections [3]. The adsorption of molecules to surfaces, bacterial adherence to the surface, the release of extracellular polymeric substances (EPS), microcolony formation, and biofilm maturation are all stages involved in biofilm formation [4] which have been reported in several bacteria communities.

Klebsiella pneumoniae, a Gram-negative bacterium belonging to the family *Enterobacteriaceae*, has been reported to form biofilms that often adhere to surfaces such as lungs, livers, and central venous catheters which are implicated in prominent nosocomial and community-acquired infections [5]. These infections include pneumonia, urinary tract infections (UTIs), bloodstream infections, necrotizing fasciitis, pyogenic liver abscess, endophthalmitis, and meningitis, among others, subsequently affecting the morbidity and mortality rate, particularly in critically ill and immunocompromised patients [6]. The interest in studying *K. pneumoniae* ATCC BAA-1705 was contingent on its ability to produce carbapenemases (KPC), which is a prevalent mechanism of resistance generated by *Klebsiella pneumoniae*, resulting in increased therapeutic dilemma and a global health threat linked to high rates of mortality [7]. Carbapenem-resistant *K. pneumoniae* is often characterized by its capacity to spread rapidly, having extensive antibiotic resistance phenotypes, yet only a few treatment options exist [7]. Furthermore, *K. pneumoniae* ATCC 700603 was also studied because it produces extended-spectrum beta-lactamases (ESBL). According to [8], the global spread of *K. pneumoniae* producing extended-spectrum lactamase (ESBL-Kp) is a serious issue; hence, the World Health Organization (WHO) categorized it alongside other ESBL-producing *Enterobacteriaceae* as a priority pathogen listed for the research and development of new antibiotics. Several antimicrobial treatments are critical in lowering the global burden imposed by this pathogen, but nonetheless, the evolution of antibiotic-resistant *K. pneumoniae* strains has become a serious public health concern [9]. *K. pneumoniae* can elude the effects of antimicrobial treatment due to the acquisition of resistance genes and the production of biofilms facilitated by EPS, making them exceedingly difficult to manage or control [10].

Antibiotic-resistant *K. pneumoniae*, which often forms biofilms, is associated with high virulence due to the nature of biofilm populations [4]. Biofilm associated virulence factors such as exopolysaccharide production, hypermucoviscosity, and the formation of curli and fimbriae also enhance the pathogenicity of this organism [11]. Bacteria protected by biofilm exopolysaccharides are up to 1000 times more resistant to antibiotics than planktonic cells [2], posing substantial therapeutic challenges and complicating treatment options.

Hypervirulent strains of *K. pneumoniae*, especially hypermucoviscous strains, also have capsule polysaccharides (CPS) for survival and immune evasion during infection, which allows them to consistently escape neutrophil-mediated intracellular killing and form abscesses at various sites, including the liver [12]. Fimbriae, another major virulence component that contributes to biofilm development in *K. pneumoniae*, consists of MrkA (capable of initiating biofilm formation) and MrkD subunits which control the binding capability and confer adhesive properties [11]. Furthermore, curli known as thin aggregative fimbriae connects directly to the substratum, which produces interbacterial bundles, allowing a cohesive and stable attachment of cells in biofilm, thereby playing an important role in biofilm development [13].

Since biofilm formation has been reported to increase virulence in *K. pneumoniae*, posing a remarkable therapeutic challenge and having developed resistance to almost all classes of conventional antibiotics [14], the development of alternative treatment options which target biofilms and related virulence factors in this pathogen is paramount.

This, therefore, necessitates the exploration of promising alternatives, which includes the search for naturally occurring compounds of plant origin capable of disrupting biofilms and their associated virulence activities. Historically, biologically active phytochemical compounds have been a valuable source of natural products, which are prominent in the prevention and treatment of diseases, helping to maintain human health [15]. The phytochemical compounds considered in this study were selected based on good docking scores and improved binding energy when bound to the SdiA protein (a transcriptional regulator which has been linked to cell division and the expression of virulence factors) in *K. pneumoniae*, as well as their drug-likeness properties which were observed during the virtual screening carried out prior to this study. The research of phytochemicals for antibacterial action, particularly against multidrug-resistant Gram-negative bacteria, has received a lot of attention in the last ten years, especially as these organisms are posing a global health challenge as well as significant economic concerns due to the rising healthcare costs [16]. This study therefore assessed the antibacterial activity and the effect of phytochemical compounds (alpha-terpinene, camphene, fisetin, glycitein and phytol) in disrupting biofilm at different stages, as well as biofilm-related virulence factors for the development of new therapeutic strategies in place of the existing conventional antibiotics.

2. Results

2.1. In Vitro Antibacterial Validation of Selected Compounds on K. pneumoniae Strains

The antibacterial activities of five phytochemical compounds (alpha-terpinene, camphene, fisetin, glycitein and phytol) against *K. pneumoniae* strains showed minimum inhibitory concentration (MIC) values ranging from 0.0625 mg/mL to 0.250 mg/mL (Table 1). The best MIC value was shown by fisetin (0.0625 mg/mL) for *K. pneumoniae* (ATCC BAA-1705). Phytol, glycitein and alpha-terpinene showed MIC values of 0.125 mg/mL for both strains; however, camphene revealed a higher MIC value of 0.250 mg/mL. The positive controls, quercetin, a known quorum-sensing inhibitor, and ciprofloxacin, revealed significant MIC values of 0.0625 mg/mL and 0.0025 mg/mL, respectively, against both strains of *K. pneumoniae*, (Table 1). The negative control showed no inhibitory activity against both strains of *K. pneumoniae*.

Table 1. MIC values of selected phytochemical compounds on *K. pneumoniae* strains.

Compounds	*K. pneumoniae* Strains and MIC (mg/mL) Values	
	K. pneumoniae (ATCC BAA-1705)	*K. pneumoniae* (ATCC 700603)
Alpha-terpinene	0.125	0.125
Camphene	0.250	0.250
Fisetin	0.0625	0.125
Glycitein	0.125	0.125
Phytol	0.125	0.125
Controls		
Ciprofloxacin	0.0025	0.0025
Quercetin	0.0625	0.0625

The MIC values are presented as the mean values of triplicates.

2.2. Inhibition of K. pneumoniae Exopolysaccharides

The quantity of EPS observed following the phenol-sulfuric acid method depicted a decrease at respective MIC values in both test pathogens. Good linearity was indicated by the correlation coefficient (R), which yielded a value of 0.971. The quantification of EPS was determined following the regression equation obtained from the standard curve Y = 0.348X − 0.074, where Y represents the absorbance obtained from the unknown samples. Figure 1 presents the EPS quantification and percentage inhibition of *K. pneumoniae* EPS by the compounds. Out of all the compounds active against the EPS production in *K. pneumoniae* ATCC 700603, the highest percentage of EPS inhibition was shown by phytol and camphene (65.91%) (Figure 1A), both having the lowest EPS yield (OD value = 1.91) (Table S1). This percentage can be compared with the result obtained for the positive control ciprofloxacin (68.45%) with a low OD value of 1.05, although the quercetin (QSI control) showed a low percentage reduction of EPS (23.21%) with an OD value of 2.68.

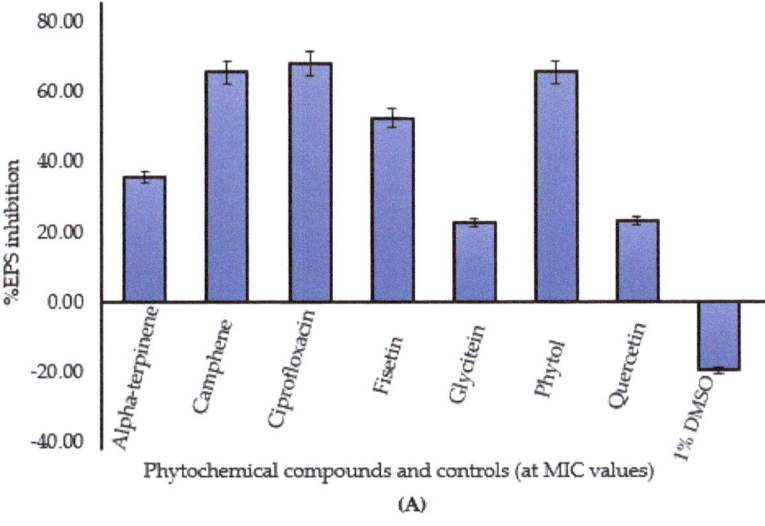

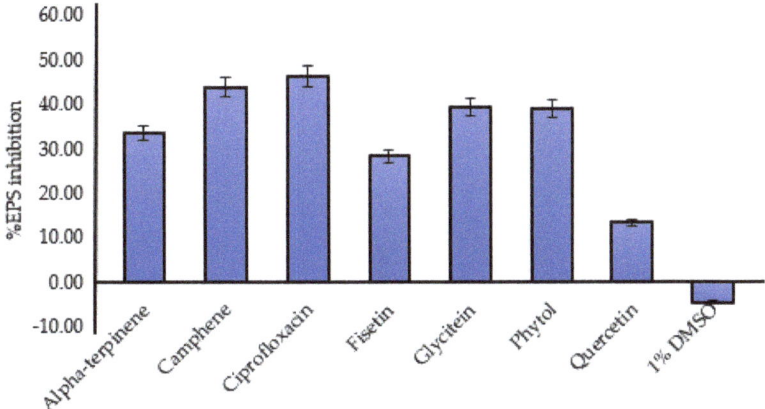

Figure 1. Quantification and percentage inhibition of exopolysaccharide present in *K. pneumoniae* ATCC 700603 (**A**) and *K. pneumoniae* ATCC BAA-1705 (**B**) treated with phytochemical compounds.

Furthermore, of all the active compounds against EPS production in *K. pneumoniae* ATCC BAA-1705, camphene showed the highest percentage inhibition and/or anti-slime activity (43.80%), having the lowest EPS yield (OD value = 2.22), similar to the results observed for ciprofloxacin (EPS inhibition at 46.26% and EPS yield at 2.01 OD value) (Figure 1B). Conversely, the untreated EPS showed enhanced production for both strains of *K. pneumoniae*.

2.3. Microscopic Surface Topography Characterization of K. pneumoniae exopolysaccharides Using Atomic Force Microscopy

The planar (2D) and cubic (3D) views of the surface topography of studied *K. pneumoniae* exopolysaccharides (EPS) are shown in Figure 2. AFM detected marked differences between the topographies of untreated and treated (camphene and phytol) EPS, selected due to the significant reduction in EPS. The AFM analysis revealed the irregularity and surface roughness of the EPS produced by untreated *K. pneumoniae* ATCC BAA-1705 and ATCC 700603 strains, mainly composed of unevenly distributed lumps which were clearly visible as cloudy areas around the cells (Figure 2(A1,F1)). Microscopically, the exopolysaccharides of both test strains exhibited a compact and tubular structure. Topologically, the EPS revealed a consistent polymer with a maximum height of the irregular lumps at 1.4 μm and 1.1 μm for untreated *K. pneumoniae* ATCC BAA-1705 and ATCC 700603, respectively, as shown in the 2D images (Figure 2(A1,F1)), while the average roughness (Ra) was recorded at 183 nm and 141 nm for *K. pneumoniae* ATCC BAA-1705 and ATCC 700603, respectively. The roughness parameters were obtained using the nanoscope analysis (v 8.15) software. The surface roughness is shown in the 3D images (Figure 2(A2,F2)).

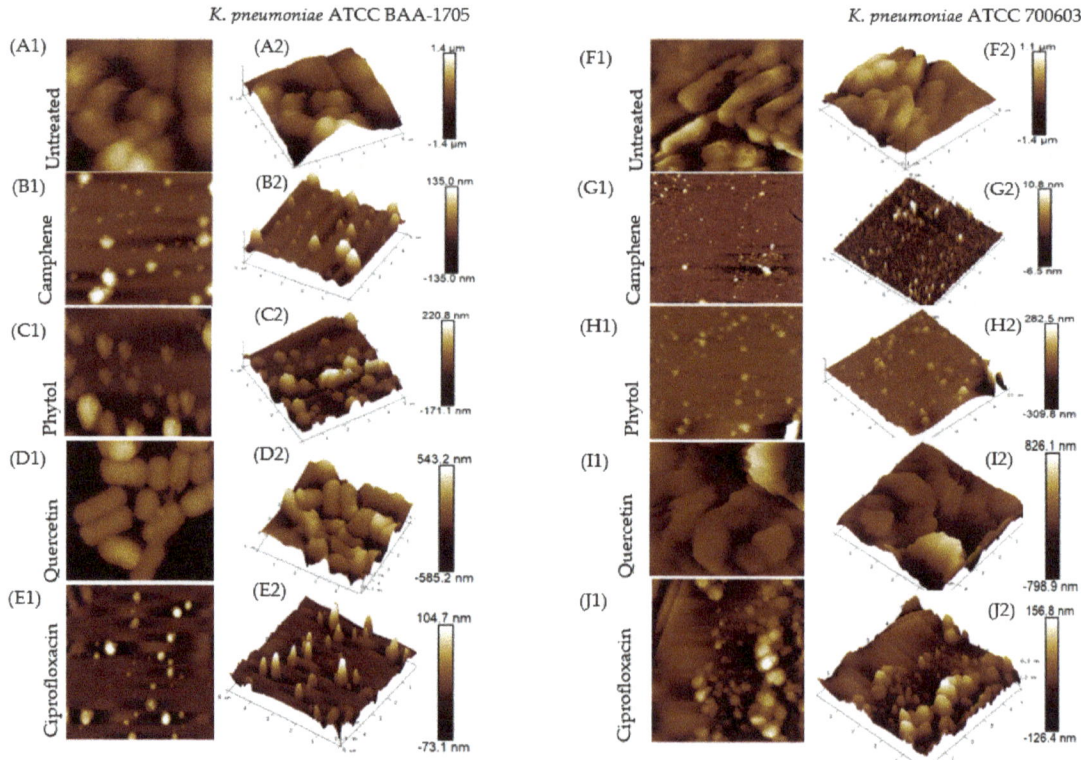

Figure 2. AFM images showing two-dimensional (2D) and three-dimensional (3D) surface topography of EPS produced by untreated and treated *K. pneumoniae* (ATCC BAA-1705 and ATCC 700603) strains at a scan size of 5.00 μm (5000 nm). 2D images of untreated and treated *K. pneumoniae* EPS are shown in (**A1–J1**). Corresponding 3D images are shown in (**A2–J2**).

The EPS treated with camphene and phytol at the MIC value revealed visible differences in height and surface roughness in comparison with the untreated EPS. The camphene-treated EPS showed maximum lump heights of 135 nm and 10.8 nm for *K. pneumoniae*, ATCC BAA-1705 and ATCC 700603, respectively (Figure 2(B1,G1)). A significantly reduced surface roughness is shown in the 3D images (Figure 2(B2,G2)). The average roughness (Ra) was recorded at 15.6 nm for *K. pneumoniae* ATCC BAA-1705 and 1.25 nm for *K. pneumoniae* ATCC 700603.

On the other hand, EPS treated with phytol had a maximum height of 220.8 nm and 282.5 nm for *K. pneumoniae* ATCC BAA-1705 and ATCC 700603, respectively

(Figure 2(C1,H1)). The average roughness (Ra) for phytol-treated EPS was 34.8 nm for *K. pneumoniae* ATCC BAA-1705 and 25.0 nm for *K. pneumoniae* ATCC 700603. Figure 2(C2,H2) revealed a reduction in surface roughness when compared with the untreated EPS.

The EPS treated with the positive controls (quercetin and ciprofloxacin) also revealed a significant reduction in the surface roughness and height, although ciprofloxacin showed improved results with a maximum lump height at 104.7 nm and average roughness at 8.80 nm for *K. pneumoniae* ATCC BAA-1705 (Figure 2(E1,E2)). Morever, ciprofloxacin-treated *K. pneumoniae* ATCC 700603 had a maximum height of 156.8 nm and average roughness of 27.6 nm (Figure 2(J1,J2)).

2.4. Curli Expression Reduction in K. pneumoniae Strains by Phytochemical Compounds

The impact of the test compounds on the occurrence of curli fibers in both strains of *K. pneumoniae* is shown in Table 2. The results show that all compounds tested at 0.125 mg/mL and 0.250 mg/mL did not inhibit curli expression in the *K. pneumoniae* strains. However, phytol, glycitein, fisetin and quercetin (positive control) at concentrations of 0.5 and 1.0 mg/mL reduced the curli expression of both strains. In addition, ciprofloxacin showed a reduction in curli expression for both strains at varying concentrations (0.125 to 1.0 mg/mL) (Table 2). On the contrary, no inhibition was shown by camphene and alpha-terpinene at all concentrations. No changes were observed in bacterial colonies (which appeared red in the presence of these compounds), similarly to the negative control.

Table 2. Effect of compounds on curli fiber synthesis in *Klebsiella pneumoniae* strains.

Compounds	Concentration (mg/mL) (A)					Concentration (mg/mL) (B)				
	Control	0.125	0.250	0.5	1.0	Control	0.125	0.250	0.5	1.0
Alpha-terpinene	+	+	+	+	+	+	+	+	+	+
Camphene	+	+	+	+	+	+	+	+	+	+
Fisetin	+	+	+	-	-	+	+	+	-	-
Glycitein	+	+	+	-	-	+	+	+	-	-
Phytol	+	+	+	-	-	+	+	+	-	-
Controls										
Ciprofloxacin	+	-	-	-	-	+	-	-	-	-
Quercetin	+	+	+	-	-	+	+	+	-	-
Untreated	+	+	+	+	+	+	+	+	+	+

Key: + (Present), - (Absent), A = ATCC BAA-1705, B = ATCC 700603.

Figure 3 shows the representative images where no inhibition of curli expression was observed for the negative control (Figure 3a) versus observed inhibition for the phytol compound (Figure 3b).

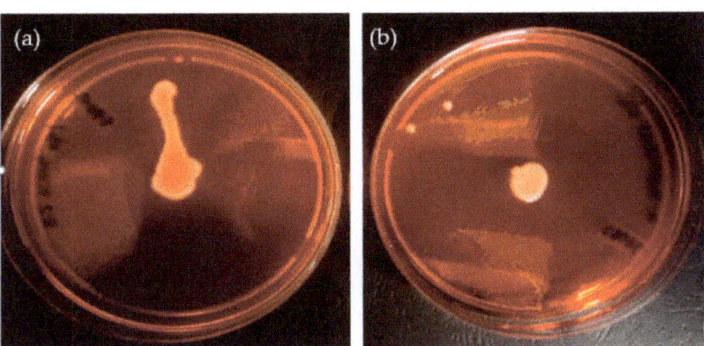

Figure 3. Representative images of curli expression in *K. pneumoniae*. (a) Negative control (untreated), showing curli-producing *K. pneumoniae*, which binds Congo red dye. (b) Inhibition of curli expression in *K. pneumoniae* subjected to phytol, as indicated by the appearance of white colonies on the brain–heart infusion agar plates supplemented with Congo red dye.

2.5. K. pneumoniae Hypermucoviscosity Reduction Using the String Test

The effect of the test compounds on hypermucoviscosity is shown in Figure 4. The string test showed that an increase in compound concentration led to a gradual decrease in the viscosity of the test strains.

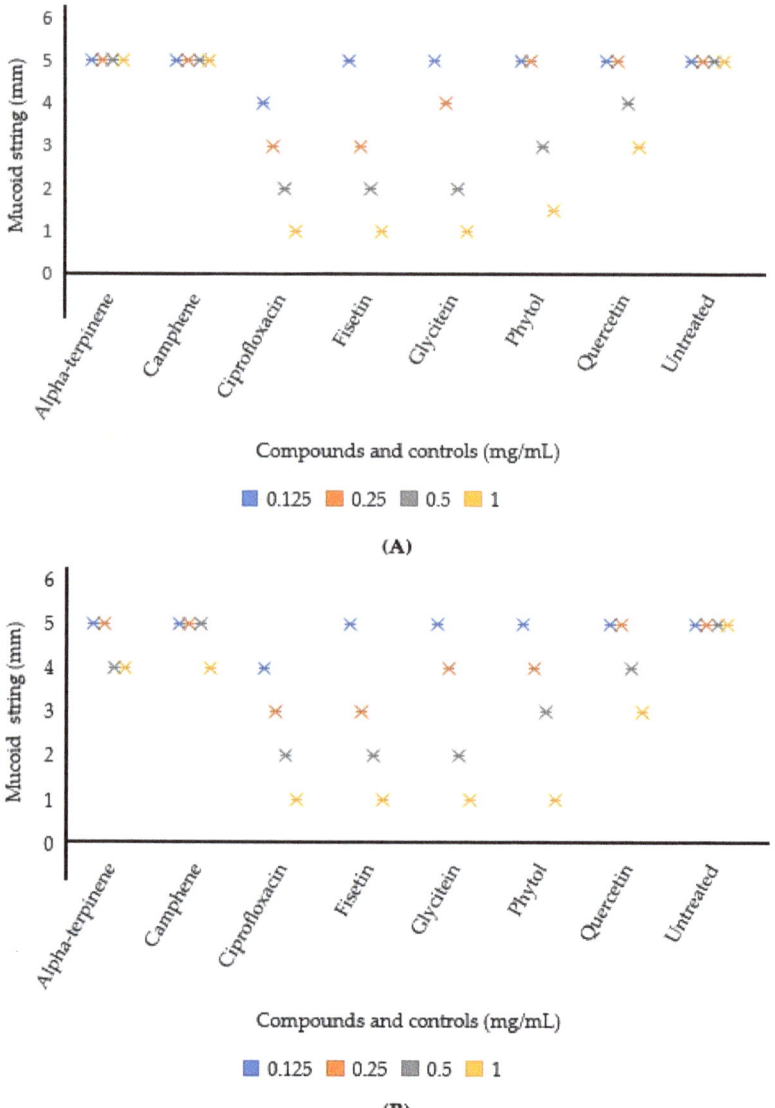

Figure 4. Effect of compounds on the inhibition of *K. pneumoniae* hypermucoviscosity. (**A**) For *K. pneumoniae* ATCC BAA-1705 (**B**) For *K. pneumoniae* ATCC 700603.

For *K. pneumoniae* ATCC BAA-1705 (Figure 4A), glycitein and fisetin revealed the potent hypermucoviscosity inhibitory activity, both showing the shortest mucoid string (1 mm) at 1.0 mg/mL (represented by the yellow *), followed by phytol (1.5 mm at 1.0 mg/mL), while no inhibitory activity was observed for camphene and alpha-terpinolene for all the concentrations tested, as seen in the negative control. Furthermore, none of the compounds showed a reduction in the hypermucoviscosity phenotype at the lowest concentration (0.125 mg/mL) tested.

Similarly, for *K. pneumoniae* ATCC 700603 (Figure 4B), glycitein, fisetin and phytol revealed potent hypermucoviscosity inhibitory activity, showing the shortest mucoid string (1 mm) at 1.0 mg/mL. However, at 0.5 mg/mL, the prominent viscosity reduction activity was shown by glycitein and fisetin, both having a mucoid string length of 2 mm. In addition, fisetin showed a potent result at the lowest concentration of 0.25 mg/mL in terms of mucoid string length reduction (3 mm), compared with the other compounds. For *K. pneumoniae* ATCC BAA-1705, no reduction in the hypermucoviscosity phenotype was shown by all the compounds at the lowest concentration tested (0.125 mg/mL), similarly to the negative control. In contrast, the positive controls (quercetin and ciprofloxacin) revealed a good reduction, with ciprofloxacin showing the highest reduction in the mucoid string length at varying concentrations for both strains (Figure 4A,B).

2.6. Inhibition of Biofilm Formation

2.6.1. Effect of Phytochemical Compounds on Initial Cell Attachment

The results of the anti-adhesion (initial attachment) assay against *K. pneumoniae* ATCC BAA-1705 and *K. pneumoniae* ATCC 700603 treated with test compounds are shown in Table 3. The results show that phytol had the highest inhibition of initial cell attachment for both strains tested, with 54.71% and 50.05%, respectively, followed by glycitein, which showed inhibition at 48.35% and 44.34%, respectively for both strains (Table 3). The least anti-adhesion activity was shown by camphene at 22.27% for *K. pneumoniae* ATCC BAA-1705 and 18.53% for *K. pneumoniae* ATCC 700603. Quercetin and ciprofloxacin revealed an initial cell attachment inhibition at 42.57% and 69.25% for *K. pneumoniae* ATCC BAA-1705, while for *K. pneumoniae* ATCC 700603, 40.66% and 62.45% were observed for quercetin and ciprofloxacin, respectively. No inhibition was revealed by the negative control (Table 3). A statistically significant difference was observed between phytol and the other compounds tested (ANOVA GLM, F = 14.14, DF = 5, R^2 = 0.049, $p < 0.05$). Phytol showed potent activity since it revealed >50% inhibition, while glycitein, camphene, fisetin and alpha-terpinene showed weak activity, having percentage inhibition values between 0 and 49%.

Table 3. Effect of phytochemical compounds on initial cell attachment (anti-adhesion) and biofilm development of *K. pneumoniae* strains.

Compounds	Percentage (%) Inhibition of Initial Cell Attachment		Percentage (%) Inhibition of Biofilm Development	
	K. pneumoniae (ATCC BAA-1705)	*K. pneumoniae* (ATCC 700603)	*K. pneumoniae* (ATCC BAA-1705)	*K. pneumoniae* (ATCC 700603)
Alpha-terpinene	33.71 ± 0.01 [a,b]	37.05 ± 0.00 [a,b]	17.23 ± 0.04 [b,c]	19.04 ± 0.03 [a,b]
Camphene	22.27 ± 0.08 [a]	18.53 ± 0.01 [a]	14.58 ± 0.04 [a]	11.08 ± 0.02 [a]
Fisetin	39.81 ± 0.01 [a,b]	32.59 ± 0.04 [a]	25.79 ± 0.00 [a,b]	29.93 ± 0.02 [a,b]
Glycitein	48.35 ± 0.02 [b,c]	44.34 ± 0.02 [c]	39.61 ± 0.01 [d]	32.77 ± 0.04 [b]
Phytol	54.71 ± 0.01 [c]	50.05 ± 0.00 [c]	43.81 ± 0.01 [e]	40.02 ± 0.01 [b]
Controls				
Ciprofloxacin	69.25 ± 0.03 [d]	62.45 ± 0.04 [d]	56.42 ± 0.03 [f]	51.77 ± 0.03 [c]
Quercetin	42.57 ± 0.03 [b,c]	40.66 ± 0.01 [b,c]	35.15 ± 0.01 [c,d]	31.81 ± 0.02 [a,b]
1% DMSO	−3.72 ± 0.04 [a]	−9.76 ± 0.01 [a]	−5.06 ± 0.03 [a]	−8.24 ± 0.02 [a]

Mean values of triplicate independent experiments ± SD. Comparison of percentage inhibition at MIC value for each treatment against *K. pneumoniae*. Different letters ([a-f]) indicate a significant difference at $p < 0.05$ between the different treatments (per column) at the same MIC value.

2.6.2. Effect of Phytochemical Compounds on Preformed Biofilm Inhibition: Biomass Measurement

The inhibition of biofilm microcolonies formed by the test strains upon treatment with the phytochemical compounds was assessed, and the results are shown in Table 3.

The percentage inhibition of preformed biofilm by the compounds was observed to be slightly less compared with the initial cell attachment, with the highest biofilm reduction of 43.81% shown by phytol for *K. pneumoniae* ATCC BAA-1705. Glycitein also revealed 39.61% inhibition for *K. pneumoniae* ATCC BAA-1705 and 32.77% inhibition for *K. pneumoniae* ATCC 700603, which is slightly higher than the results obtained for quercetin, showing 35.15% and 31.81% inhibition for *K. pneumoniae* ATCC BAA-1705 and *K. pneumoniae* ATCC 700603, respectively. However, the highest percentage inhibition was observed for ciprofloxacin at 56.42% and 51.77% for *K. pneumoniae* ATCC BAA-1705 and *K. pneumoniae* ATCC 700603, respectively (Table 3). The negative control did not reveal any inhibitory effect on the biofilm development, except for a slightly enhanced biofilm formation.

2.6.3. Disruption of Mature Biofilm by Phytochemical Compounds

Mature biofilms formed by *K. pneumoniae* strains determined under dynamic and static conditions are shown in Table 4. The highest disruption of mature biofilms under dynamic conditions was shown by phytol at 24.94% and 25.88% for *K. pneumoniae* (ATCC BAA-1705) and *K. pneumoniae* (ATCC 700603), respectively. The least inhibition was shown by camphene at 5.24% for *K. pneumoniae* (ATCC BAA-1705) and 2.06% for *K. pneumoniae* (ATCC 700603).

Table 4. Disruption of mature *K. pneumoniae* biofilms formed by various compounds under dynamic and static conditions.

Compounds	Percentage (%) Inhibition of Mature Biofilm Formed under Dynamic Condition (with Shaking)		Percentage (%) Inhibition of Mature Biofilm Formed under Static Condition (without Shaking)	
	K. pneumoniae (ATCC BAA-1705)	*K. pneumoniae* (ATCC 700603)	*K. pneumoniae* (ATCC BAA-1705)	*K. pneumoniae* (ATCC 700603)
Alpha-terpinene	18.55 ± 0.02 [b]	17.22 ± 0.13 [b]	15.18 ± 0.05 [b]	12.15 ± 0.03 [c,d]
Camphene	5.24 ± 0.01 [a,b]	2.06 ± 0.05 [b]	4.56 ± 0.01 [a,b]	4.08 ± 0.05 [b,d]
Fisetin	14.83 ± 0.02 [a,b]	12.33 ± 0.02 [b]	−8.52 ± 0.01 [a,b]	−32.43 ± 0.02 [a,b]
Glycitein	8.89 ± 0.01 [a,b]	−5.71 ± 0.01 [b]	6.89 ± 0.01 [a,b]	−12.53 ± 0.01 [b,c]
Phytol	24.94 ± 0.04 [b]	25.88 ± 0.00 [b]	20.32 ± 0.02 [b]	18.07 ± 0.01 [d]
Controls				
Ciprofloxacin	44.73 ± 0.04 [c]	51.88 ± 0.00 [c]	42.24 ± 0.02 [b]	39.15 ± 0.01 [e]
Quercetin	−27.08 ± 0.01 [a]	−44.55 ± 0.01 [a]	−35.46 ± 0.02 [a]	−52.25 ± 0.02 [a]
1% DMSO	−39.01 ± 0.01 [a]	−58.35 ± 0.01 [a]	−45.67 ± 0.02 [a]	−68.25 ± 0.02 [a]

Mean values are of triplicate independent experiments ± SD. Comparison of percentage inhibition at MIC value for each treatment against *K. pneumoniae*. Different letters ([a]–[e]) indicate a significant difference at $p < 0.05$ between the different treatments (per column) at the same MIC value.

Under static conditions, phytol again revealed higher inhibitory activity (20.32% and 18.07% for both strains), followed by alpha-terpinene (Table 4), with statistical differences found between the compounds (ANOVA GLM, F = 25.84, DF = 5, R2 = 0.0139, $p < 0.05$). The least inhibitory activity for this group was also shown by camphene at 4.56% for *K. pneumoniae* (ATCC BAA-1705) and 4.08% for *K. pneumoniae* (ATCC 700603). Moreover, fisetin and quercetin showed no inhibitory activity on mature biofilms formed by both strains under static conditions.

Overall, less inhibitory activity was shown by the compounds on mature biofilms under static conditions compared with dynamic conditions. This was also observed for the positive control of ciprofloxacin (Table 4).

2.7. In Situ Visualisation of Biofilms Using Scanning Electron Microscopy

To further investigate the detailed effects of the *K. pneumoniae* biofilms formed after treatment with the best active or potent compounds (phytol and glycitein) on antibiofilm assay results, a scanning electron microscope analysis was carried out. Figure 5 shows the SEM micrographs of the biofilms formed by the two *K. pneumoniae* strains upon exposure to phytol and glycitein (0.1 mg/mL), the positive controls (quercetin; 0.1 mg/mL and ciprofloxacin; 0.001 mg/mL), and the untreated biofilms.

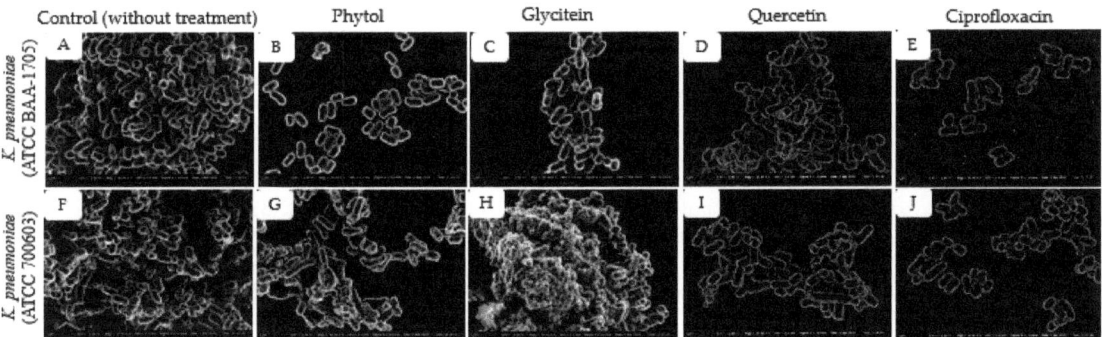

Figure 5. SEM micrographs showing the biofilm inhibitory activity of phytol and glycitein against *K. pneumoniae* ATCC BAA-1705 and ATCC 700603 at ×20,000 magnification. (**A**) *K. pneumoniae* ATCC BAA-1705 (without treatment). (**B**) *K. pneumoniae* ATCC BAA-1705 (treated with phytol). (**C**) *K. pneumoniae* ATCC BAA-1705 (treated with glycitein). (**D**) *K. pneumoniae* ATCC BAA-1705 (treated with quercetin). (**E**) *K. pneumoniae* ATCC BAA-1705 (treated with ciprofloxacin). (**F**) *K. pneumoniae* ATCC 700603 (without treatment). (**G**) *K. pneumoniae* ATCC 700603 (treated with phytol). (**H**) *K. pneumoniae* ATCC 700603 (treated with glycitein). (**I**) *K. pneumoniae* ATCC 700603 (treated with quercetin). (**J**) *K. pneumoniae* ATCC 700603 (treated with ciprofloxacin).

Phytol revealed potent antibiofilm activity for *K. pneumoniae* (ATCC BAA-1705) and *K. pneumoniae* (ATCC 700603), as evidenced in Figure 5B,G, where fewer clumps of attached microcolonies were observed, revealing a notable lessening in the quantity of biofilms with some of the cells being distances apart. A similar observation was recorded for ciprofloxacin, showing very few clumps of scattered cells (Figure 5E,J).

In comparison, the untreated biofilms formed by the two strains of *K. pneumoniae* revealed a compact arrangement of interconnected *K. pneumoniae* cells, thereby presenting continuous clumps and large aggregates of cells (Figure 5A,F). However, biofilms treated with glycitein only revealed a slight distance amongst the cells of *K. pneumoniae* (ATCC BAA-1705) (Figure 5C) while the treatment was shown to shrink and disrupt cells of *K. pneumoniae* (ATCC 700603) with extruding materials and cell debris (Figure 5H). Quercetin was less effective compared with phytol and glycitein (Figure 5D,I); moreover, it showed lesser clumps of cells than the untreated biofilms.

3. Discussion

Plants have been known for their antibacterial effects against microbial pathogens since ancient times due to their secondary metabolites [17,18]. Phytochemicals have vast advantages over synthetic compounds, including green status and unique modes of action, which could aid in the fight against antibiotic resistance. Hence, phytochemicals are emphasized as a valuable source of novel bioactive compounds that is both sustainable and abundant [18]. Furthermore, they have been identified as a promising source of quorum-sensing inhibitors, disrupting bacterial cell-to-cell communication, which enables pathogenicity and for bacteria to withstand antimicrobial substances through biofilm formation and other virulence factors [19]. These phytochemicals often have a wide range of chemical variety, structural complexity, and biological activity [19], making them promising tools for the management of illnesses, especially biofilm-related infections in an era where the supply of effective antibiotics is no longer guaranteed [20]. New sources of antimicrobials and tactics for effective biofilm inhibition and/or eradication are unquestionably necessary. Therefore, the discovery of phytochemicals targeting distinct stages of biofilm formation, such as adhesion, motility and EPS generation, including other biofilm-related virulence factors, is imperative [16]. As such, this study explored the effects of phytochemical compounds at different stages of biofilm formation and associated virulence factors in *K. pneumoniae* ATCC BAA-1705 and *K. pneumoniae* ATCC 700603.

The five studied compounds (alpha-terpinene, camphene, fisetin, glycitein and phytol) were first validated for their antibacterial effect on the growth of *K. pneumoniae* ATCC BAA-1705 and *K. pneumoniae* ATCC 700603 strains. The findings reveal MIC values ranging from 0.0625 to 0.25 mg/mL (Table 1). Of the five compounds, fisetin showed anMIC value of 0.0625 for *K. pneumoniae* (ATCC BAA-1705), as well as quercetin and ciprofloxacin (the positive controls), which indicated significant activity. This suggests that fisetin and quercetin are potential antibacterial agents against the studied pathogen. Their potent activity can be attributed to the mode of action of flavonoids, which includes the interaction of phytochemical compounds with bacterial proteins and cell wall structures [21]. This is congruent with the suggestions of Gibbons [22] and Mamabolo [23], where the antimicrobial activity of a phytochemical compound or single entity compound is defined as significant when the MIC value is ≤ 0.064 mg/mL or ≤ 0.01 mg/mL, respectively.

Other tested compounds revealed MIC values greater than 0.1 mg/mL; hence, they are regarded as compounds with low antibacterial activity. According to Mbaveng et al. [24], the MIC activity of a compound is considered low when it is greater than 100 µg/mL or 0.1mg/mL. The low MIC values obtained may be due to the protective outer membrane present in *K. pneumoniae*, being a Gram-negative bacterium [25]. In addition, they can also be attributed to the ability of *K. pneumoniae* to actively efflux the compounds from the cell, forming a capsule that shields the cell from being penetrated by the compounds or changing its phytocompound target. The low MIC values, however, do not completely rule out the bioactive potentials of these compounds as they possess a broad range of biological activities. Cosa et al. [26] and Vasavi et al. [27] reported that in some cases, compounds of natural origin may yield poor MIC values, but they are able to interfere with the quorum-sensing signaling mechanism and inhibit virulence at sub-MIC concentrations. Hence, the compounds were further assessed for their biofilm-associated anti-virulence activities.

Because biofilms are supported by a matrix of polymeric compounds known as extracellular polymeric substances (EPS), often composed of exopolysaccharides that are secreted into the environment [28], we assessed this as one of the contributing virulence factors. *Klebsiella pneumoniae*'s exopolysaccharides generally contain rare sugars such as L-fucose, L-rhamnose, or uronic acids [29,30]. Based on our findings, the exopolysaccharide reduction assay revealed that both phytol and camphene showed the highest percentage inhibition of EPS (65.91%) for *K. pneumoniae* ATCC 700603, while camphene revealed the greatest reduction in exopolysaccharide production (43.80%) in *K. pneumoniae* ATCC BAA-1705 (Figure 1).

Similar findings were reported by Srinivasan et al. [31], where phytol significantly inhibited the EPS production in *Serratia marcescens* to the level of 32% and 39% at 5 and 10 µg/mL concentrations, respectively, while no significant level of EPS inhibition was shown by the control. The bioactive potential of camphene observed in this study is congruent with the submission of Hachlafi et al. [32], where camphene inhibited pathogenicity in a wide range of pathogenic bacteria, such as *Klebsiella pneumoniae*, *Staphylococcus aureus* and *Escherichia coli*. Based on our findings, the reduction in EPS in *K. pneumoniae* by the active phytochemical compounds suggests their potential to disrupt biofilm-associated virulence factors. This is because EPS production is a key factor which forms the framework in microbial biofilms.

The validation of reduced exopolysaccharides in *K. pneumoniae* was performed using atomic force microscopy (AFM), a powerful technique for imaging the surfaces of microbial cells [33]. It has been reported as a vital tool in characterizing the topographic features of microbial exopolysaccharides [34]. Dufrene [35] also confirmed that AFM imaging allows the observation of cell wall components directly on live cells, such as polysaccharides, peptidoglycan, teichoic acids, among others, and has aided in elucidating their roles in cellular processes such as adhesion. When AFM imaging was employed in our study to analyze the surface topology of treated and untreated *K. pneumoniae* exopolysaccharides, the untreated strains resulted in the formation of a clear detectable EPS network composed of unevenly distributed and compact lumps (Figure 2(A1,F1)). The lumps may be formed due to the intra- and intermolecular aggregation of polysaccharide macromolecules [36]. This high conformational rigidity of EPS might function as a polymeric scaffold used by bacteria to build biofilms [37]. The surface topography of EPS treated with phytol and camphene on the other hand revealed scarce EPS polymers which were generally thinner and often showed irregular shapes, similar to the positive control (ciprofloxacin) (Figure 2(B1,C1,G1,H1)). These compounds showed a significant reduction in the height and surface roughness of *K. pneumoniae* EPS. This validates the results obtained from the phenol sulfuric acid method of EPS biomass measurement.

Curli, a type of fimbriae composed of proteins called curlins and functional amyloid surface fiber, is another prominent virulence factor in *K. pneumoniae* known to be involved in cell attachment to surfaces, as well as cell aggregation, which allows the formation of biofilms [38]. Curli are effective inducers of the host inflammatory response and often mediate host cell adhesion and invasion [39]. Our results clearly demonstrate that phytochemicals such as phytol, glycitein, fisetin and quercetin (0.5 and 1.0 mg/mL) efficiently inhibited the formation of curli in the *K. pneumoniae* strains (Table 2). According to a study by Gupta et al. [40], cranberry, which contains diverse bioactive phytochemical compounds, inhibited the expression of curli in *Escherichia coli* and resulted in a loss of epithelial cell colonization. This suggests that certain phytochemical compounds can bind to curli, and fimbriae as observed in our study, thereby preventing them from attaching to host tissue. According to Kikuchi et al. [13], studies have shown that curli and other cell surface structures play a significant role in the development of biofilm in *E. coli*, an *Enterobacteriaceae* similar to *K. pneumoniae*. Understanding and inhibiting biofilm-forming structures such as curli are crucial for the development of therapeutics that can reduce biofilm formation and host colonization [41].

Furthermore, virulence in *K. pneumoniae* can also be attributed to efficient iron uptake, poor sedimentation and the copious synthesis of a capsule, which confers a hypermucoviscous phenotype [42,43]. The effect of the studied phytochemical compounds on the hypermucoviscosity of *K. pneumoniae* was examined using the string test. The results reveal glycitein and fisetin as the compounds showing the best inhibition at 1.0 mg/mL for both strains, alongside phytol for *K. pneumoniae* ATCC 700603 (Figure 4). The viscosity-lowering effect of the compounds, as seen in this study, is proportional to their concentrations, as none of the compounds examined at the lowest concentration (0.125 mg/mL) showed any reduction in the hypermucoviscosity phenotype. A similar observation was also recorded in the study of Jabuk [44], where viscosity inhibition was observed in a dose-dependent manner. Lin et al. [45] reported a decrease in *K. pneumoniae* mucoviscosity, and capsular polysaccharide production by *Fructus mume* in a dose-dependent manner, thereby reducing the resistance of *K. pneumoniae* to serum killing.

K. pneumoniae can produce a thick extracellular matrix that promotes bacterial adhesion to living or non-living surfaces, preventing antibiotic penetration and lowering the effects of treatments [46]. Again, the host defenses may be improved if any stage in the formation of biofilm's structure is interrupted, resulting in better treatment outcomes. Hence, this study examined the effect of phytochemical compounds on initial cell attachment, preformed biofilm, and mature biofilm formation.

The results of the initial cell attachment inhibition reveal that phytol showed good activity on both strains of *K. pneumoniae* tested following the criteria stated by Famuyide et al. [47], having >50% inhibition (Table 3). Reports on the anti-adhesion activity of the studied compounds on *K. pneumoniae* are limited; however, Ramanathan et al. [48] reported a good anti-biofilm activity of phytol, showing up to 60% biofilm inhibition in another notorious biofilm former, *Acinetobacter baumannii*, at concentrations ranging from 5 to

640 µg/mL. Congruent to our findings, Srinivisan et al. [31] also reported a decrease in the level of metabolically active cells involved in biofilm formation in phytol treatment compared with their respective controls. This corroborates the submission of Ramanathan et al. [48], that phytol is a potential anti-biofilm agent, as it can inhibit or halt the formation of biofilms, making them more receptive to treatments. On the other hand, glycitein, camphene, fisetin, alpha-terpinene and quercetin showed weak anti-adhesion activity, having percentage inhibition values <49%. The weak activity observed might be attributed to the interference of the hydrogen bonds, electrostatic forces, and van der Waals forces of interaction within the biofilm, which often mediates the initial attachment of the sessile group of cells to solid surfaces [21].

Furthermore, our results reveal a reduced inhibition of the microcolony formation stage by the compounds (Table 3). This suggests that biofilms can be better inhibited during the initial cell attachment stage than when they begin to develop. A similar trend was observed for the inhibition of mature biofilm, where the biofilms had accumulated biomass. These findings are in tandem with results obtained in a study carried out by Mombeshora et al. [5], where the compound tested did not have any disruptive effect on mature (72 h) biofilms of *P. aeruginosa*, a Gram-negative bacterium like *K. pneumoniae*. This can also be attributed to the opinion of Kelmanson et al. [49], who noted that more resistance to external agents is often shown once biofilms have been fully established; therefore, the disruption of mature biofilms tends to require higher doses of disrupting agents than those needed to destroy planktonic cells. Additionally, difficulty in the disruption of mature biofilms might result from the slow or incomplete penetration of the treatments to the established biofilm population or an altered biochemical microenvironment within the biofilm [50]. Other studies by Baloyi et al. [51] and Sarkar et al. [52] have also shown that eradicating biofilms is challenging, as various biofilm-forming microorganisms have demonstrated resilience.

The effect of the phytochemical compounds on the inhibition of mature *K. pneumoniae* biofilm was assessed under both static and dynamic conditions. The results revealed that *K. pneumoniae* biofilms formed under static (non-shaking) conditions had lower inhibition percentages compared with the mature biofilm formed under dynamic conditions (Table 4). This could be because more mature biofilms were formed without shaking compared with the biofilms formed while shaking; hence, the treatment showed higher inhibitory activity on less mature biofilms formed while shaking. This result corroborates the findings of [53], where a decrease was observed in the biofilm biomass attached to substratum surfaces under dynamic conditions compared with the static condition. The difference in mature biofilms generated with and without shaking can be attributed to shear force, which is one of the most decisive factors in the formation of biofilms in hydrodynamic conditions [53]. Due to shear forces, bacteria that settled but could not adhere securely to the substratum surface might have been resuspended in the bulk liquid, resulting in relatively low levels of adherent biomass under dynamic conditions. Bacterial adhesion, which contributes to mature biofilm formation, is often inhibited when there is an increase in shear stress [54].

An additional remarkable mechanism in biofilm formation is the distinctive biofilm architecture [48]. SEM micrographs of the structurally complex matrix architecture and the bacteria in that matrix were used to visually validate the inhibitory effect of phytol and glycitein against biofilms formed by the two *K. pneumoniae* strains. Exceptionally, phytol treatment led to a huge collapse in the extracellular matrix architecture of *K. pneumoniae* (ATCC BAA-1705) biofilms, resulting in individual cells and loose microcolonies adhered to the coverslip (Figure 5B). The images correlated well with the quantitative results of the crystal violet staining assay, which indicated that phytol possessed good antibiofilm activity against *K. pneumoniae*. Furthermore, glycitein influenced the integrity of the *K. pneumoniae* (ATCC 700603) cell wall (Figure 5F), making the cells incapable of maintaining their typical morphology in the presence of the treatment. Damaged cell walls and cellular leakages resulting from phytochemical compound treatment can eventually cause the death of microbial cells [55].

The inhibition of the biofilm-forming ability and associated virulence factors in *K. pneumoniae* by selected phytochemical compounds could be an effective approach in controlling pathogenicity in this pathogen.

4. Materials and Methods

4.1. Chemicals, Media and Compounds Used in Assays

Chemicals used in the study, including dimethyl sulfoxide (DMSO), iodonitrotetrazolium (INT), hexamethyldisilazane (HMDS), Congo red and crystal violet were purchased from Sigma-Aldrich (Johannesburg, South Africa). Luria Bertani agar (LBA), Luria Bertani broth (LBB), brain–heart infusion agar (BHIA), blood agar (BA) and Muller–Hinton broth (MHB) were purchased from Lasec (Johannesburg, South Africa). Compounds and positive controls used in the study, including phytol (lot no: 0001452396), glycitein (lot no: MFCD00016679), camphene (lot no: MKCL4074), fisetin (lot no: 82542), alpha-terpinene (lot no: BCCD2529), quercetin (lot no: LRAB7760) and ciprofloxacin (lot no: 098M4006V), were purchased from Sigma-Aldrich (Johannesburg, South Africa).

4.2. Bacterial Strains and Growth Conditions

American Type Culture Collection strains of *K. pneumoniae* (ATCC BAA-1705 and ATCC 700603) were obtained from the NextGen Health unit at the Council for Scientific and Industrial Research (CSIR), South Africa. The bacterial strains were kept as glycerol stocks at -80 °C until required for use. The two strains of *K. pneumoniae* used in this study were prepared in Mueller–Hinton (MH) medium during MIC assay and incubated at 37 °C to obtain active bacterial cultures. One or two colonies were often transferred to sterile distilled water to obtain an absorbance ($OD_{600\ nm}$) of 0.1. The cell suspension was adjusted to achieve a 0.5 McFarland standard equivalent.

Ethics approval for the use of the *K. pneumoniae* strains was sought and obtained from the University of Pretoria, Faculty of Natural and Agricultural Sciences Ethics Committee (reference number: NAS157/2021).

4.3. Antibacterial Activity of Phytochemical Compounds against K. pneumoniae Strains

The MIC of the phytochemical compounds was determined following the broth dilution method as described by Alves et al. [56], with slight modifications. Stock concentrations (1 mg/mL) of the compounds were prepared and 100 µL of MH broth was transferred into each well of a 96-well microtiter plate. A 100 µL aliquot of each phytochemical compound (in triplicate) was transferred into the first row of microtiter plates. Serial dilutions were performed in the direction from A to H, resulting in decreasing concentrations over the range of 0.25–0.0019 mg/mL. Subsequently, 100 µL of the standardized bacterial strains ($OD_{600\ nm}$ = 0.08–0.1) was transferred into each well. Each plate was prepared with a set of positive and negative controls. Quercetin and ciprofloxacin were used as the positive controls at a concentration of 1 mg/mL and 0.01 mg/mL, respectively, while 100 µL of 1% DMSO was used as the negative control. Following incubation at 37 °C for 24 h, 40 µL of a 0.20 mg/mL solution of p-iodonitrotetrazolium violet (INT) was added to each well and incubated at 37 °C for 30 min. The MIC value for each phytochemical compound was visually assessed and recorded. The MIC was recorded as the minimum concentration of the compounds at which there was no visible growth of the test strain. The antibacterial assay was carried out in triplicate.

4.4. Inhibition of Biofilm-Associated Virulence Factor—Exopolysaccharide Assay

Reduction in EPS was carried out according to the method described by Gopu and Shetty [57]. A sterile LB broth with and without the active compound(s) was inoculated with 1% *Klebsiella pneumoniae* and incubated at 37 °C. Biofilms that adhered to the walls of the test tubes were harvested to obtain crude EPS. Briefly, late log phase cells were removed by centrifugation at $5000 \times g$ for 30 min at 2 °C. The filtered supernatant was added to three volumes of chilled ethanol and incubated overnight at 2 °C to precipitate the dislodged

EPS. Precipitated EPS was collected by centrifugation at 8000×g for 30 min then dissolved in 1 mL of deionized water and stored at −40 °C until further use. EPS was quantified by mixing 1 mL of EPS solution with an equal volume of 5% phenol and 5 mL of concentrated sulfuric acid to develop a red color. Glucose with a concentration range between 0.25 and 1 mg/mL was used as a standard to determine the R^2 value in the calibration and for the quantification of crude EPS. The intensity of the color developed was measured using a microplate reader (Biotek, United States of America) at 490 nm.

4.5. Assessment of Exopolysaccharide Inhibition Using Atomic Force Microscopy

The effect of the best two compounds (phytol and camphene) shown to reveal noteworthy exopolysaccharide inhibition in *K. pneumoniae* strains was monitored using atomic force microscopy following the method described by Santana et al. [58]. Two *K. pneumoniae* strains (ATCC BAA-1705 and ATCC 700603) were grown overnight in LB media, centrifuged (2000× g, room temperature, 15 min), washed three times in phosphate buffer (5 mM, pH 6.5), and approximately 10^8 CFU ml-1 were resuspended into tubes containing the same buffer. The phytochemical compounds were diluted to 1 mg/mL and 100 μL of compounds were added to 3 mL of the cell suspensions. The samples were incubated for 4 h at 37 °C. Cell suspensions without the addition of the compounds were used as controls.

After incubation, samples of 1 mL were collected from each treatment, centrifuged (6000×g, at room temperature for 15 min) and a smear of cells was prepared in a glass slide (191 cm). The slides were air dried and viewed using the atomic force microscope at the Microscopy Unit, University of Pretoria, South Africa.

Samples were observed in a contact imaging mode using a Veeco atomic force microscope (Dimension icon with Scan Asyst) and silicon tip on nitride lever (cantilever 0.55–0.75 μm). A nominal constant of 32 Nm-1 and resonance frequency of ≈300 kHz was used with a scan rate of 0.100 Hz and scan size of 5.00 μm. Imaging analysis was performed using the Nanoscope analysis Scan Asyst software (Nanoscope version 8.15).

4.6. Inhibition of Curli Expression

The effect of five test compounds on curli expression was assessed according to the method described by Jabuk [44] with slight modifications. The bacterial suspension was prepared by inoculating 100 μL of standardized *K. pneumoniae* strains and 100 μL of the compounds in 3 mL of LB broth. The suspension was incubated at 37 °C for 24 h. After incubation, 3 μL of the bacterial suspension was inoculated onto plates containing brain–heart infusion (BHI) agar supplemented with Congo red (CRI) dye and sucrose. Curli-producing *K. pneumoniae* bound to Congo red dye and formed red colonies, whereas curli-negative bacteria formed white colonies, which indicated a loss of curli fimbriae. Control cultures contained no compounds.

4.7. Reduction in Hypermucoviscosity Using the String Test

A variation of the string test was used to determine the effect of the studied compounds on the hypermucoviscousity (HMV) phenotype of *K. pneumoniae* strains according to the method described by Wiskur et al. [59] and Jabuk [44]. K. pneumoniae strains were inoculated on BHI plates containing the five phytochemical compounds with varying concentrations (0.125–1.0 mg/mL) and incubated overnight at 37 °C. A standard bacteriological loop was used to vertically stretch a mucoviscous string from a single colony. Each strain was defined as mucoid or regarded as a hypermucoviscous (HMV+) phenotype when string-like growth or a mucoid string of >5 mm was observed, respectively. The control culture contained no compounds.

4.8. Effect of Phytochemical Compounds on Biofilm Formation—Initial Cell Attachment, Preformed Biofilm and Mature Biofilm

Anti-adhesion (initial cell attachment), preformed biofilm (biomass measurement) and mature biofilms were assessed for inhibition by the phytochemical compounds, following the method described by Baloyi et al. [51] and Blando et al. [60], with slight modifications.

Five phytochemical compounds (alpha-terpinene, camphene, fisetin, glycitein and phytol) were tested against *K. pneumoniae* strains (ATCC BAA-1705 and ATCC 700603) for initial cell attachment, preformed and mature biofilm inhibition. For the initial cell attachment inhibition assay, 100 µL of standardized bacterial suspension (OD$_{600\,nm}$ = 0.1), 100 µL of MH broth and 100 µL of the compound were added to the wells. The positive controls (quercetin 0.1 mg/mL and ciprofloxacin, 0.001 mg/mL) and negative control (1% DMSO) were also added into the wells, which were then incubated at 37 °C for 24 h.

For preformed and mature biofilm assays, 100 µL of standardized bacterial suspension and 100 µL of MH broth were added to the wells and incubated at 37 °C for 8 h for preformed biofilm, while for mature biofilm, wells were incubated at 37 °C with and without shaking for 24 h. Following incubation, 100 µL of the compounds was transferred to individual wells and incubated for another 24 h. The modified crystal violet (CV) assay was used to analyze initial cell attachment, biofilm biomass, and mature biofilms. To eliminate planktonic cells and medium, the 96-well plates containing developed biofilm were rinsed with sterile distilled water. Afterwards, the plates were dried in the oven for 45 min at 60 °C. After drying, the remaining biofilm was stained for 15 min in the dark with a 1% CV solution (Sigma-Aldrich, Johannesburg, South Africa). To eliminate any unabsorbed stain, the wells were washed with sterile distilled water. Destaining the wells with 125 µL of 95% ethanol allowed for the semiquantitative measurement of biofilm formation. Approximately 100 µL of the destaining solution was transferred to a new plate and the absorbance (OD$_{585\,nm}$) was read using a multi-mode microplate reader (SpectraMax® paradigm). The % inhibition of test compounds was calculated from the untreated broth culture. The formula below was used in calculating the percentage of inhibition:

$$\text{Biofilm reduction (\%)} = (\text{Control}_{585nm} - \text{Test}_{585nm}) / (\text{Control}_{585nm}) \times 100$$

Results were interpreted following the criterion described by Famuyide et al. [47]. Values between 0 and 100% were interpreted as inhibitory activity; however, it was further broken down as follows: $\geq$ 50% was interpreted as good activity, and values between 0 and 49% were interpreted as weak activity, while negative values indicated a growth increase rather than the inhibition of biofilm.

4.9. In Situ Visualization of Biofilms Using Scanning Electron Microscopy

Subinhibitory biofilm inhibitory concentrations of the two most active compounds (phytol and glycitein) were fixed and visualized in a field emission gun scanning electron microscope to observe the cell density and morphology of biofilms following the method described by Wijesundara and Rupasinghe [61] with slight modifications. Biofilms were fixed (while still in a microtiter plate) over a minimum of 2 h in 0.1 M sodium cacodylate buffer (pH 7.2) containing 2% glutaraldehyde immediately after being rinsed in PBS. The biofilms were further rinsed three times with phosphate washing buffer 3 times for 15 min each. Then, the samples were dehydrated through an ethanol gradient series (35%, 50%, 75%, 90% and 100%). All the steps in the gradient involved 15 min exposure times, with the final 100% ethanol treatment being repeated three times. Drying of samples was achieved through an ethanol gradient series (25:75, 50:50, 75:25 and 100:0) for 15 min at each concentration. The 100:0 dilution step was repeated three times. A 50:50 mixture of hexamethyldisilazane (HMDS) and 100% ethanol was added and allowed to stay for 1 h with the samples covered. The HMDS–ethanol mixture was removed and fresh HMDS was added. Plates were air-dried under the fume hood for 2 h. Finally, fixed biofilms were mounted on aluminum stubs. Then, sputters were coated with gold–palladium (15 nm) and visualized using a Zeiss crossbeam 540 scanning electron microscope with operational conditions of an acceleration voltage of 10 kV, emission current of 14–16 µA, working distance of 10–12 mm and analysis lens mode.

4.10. Statistical Analysis

All results were presented as mean ± standard deviations for each sample and treatment. Data were generated in independent experimental repeats with each sample in triplicates. The ANOVA generalized linear model (Proc GLM) was used to analyze the means of inhibitory activities of the compounds and controls. All statistical analyses were carried out using the Statistical Analysis System (SAS) program version 9.4 from Stats Inc., 100 SAS Campus Drive, Cary, NC, USA, with $p < 0.05$ values considered statistically significant.

5. Conclusions

In this study, a better knowledge of the efficacy of selected phytochemical compounds was acquired by investigating antivirulence and antibiofilm activities. AFM proved to be a useful tool for visualizing the effect of compounds on EPS production in order to corroborate the in vitro findings. Amongst the phytochemical compounds evaluated in this study, phytol proved to be the most potent antivirulence antibiofilm agent, inhibiting initial cell attachment as well as exopolysaccharide production, curli expression and hypermucoviscosity. Consequently, this intriguing compound can be employed as a model in the search for new medications or as an alternative in regulating the pathogenicity of *K. pneumoniae*.

Supplementary Materials: The following supporting information can be downloaded at https://www.mdpi.com/article/10.3390/plants11111429/s1, Table S1: Exopolysaccharide reduction in *K. pneumoniae* (ATCC 700603 and ATCC BAA-1705) by studied phytochemical compounds

Author Contributions: Conceptualization, S.C.; methodology, I.J.A.; formal analysis, I.J.A.; investigation, I.J.A.; resources, S.C.; data curation, I.J.A. and I.T.B.; writing—original draft preparation, I.J.A.; writing—review and editing, I.J.A., I.T.B. and S.C.; supervision, S.C. All authors have read and agreed to the published version of the manuscript.

Funding: This study was mostly funded by the South African Medical Research Council—Self-Initiated Research (SAMRC-SIR) and partly by the South African National Research Foundation (NRF) Thuthuka Grant (grant no. 113244).

Institutional Review Board Statement: Ethics approval was granted by the University of Pretoria, Faculty of Natural and Agricultural Sciences Ethics Committee (reference number: NAS157/2021).

Informed Consent Statement: Not applicable.

Data Availability Statement: Not applicable.

Acknowledgments: The authors acknowledge the NextGen Health Unit at the Council for Scientific and Industrial Research (CSIR), South Africa, for supplying the hypervirulent *K. pneumoniae* strains. We also acknowledge the Microscopy Unit of the University of Pretoria for assisting while carrying out the microscopy analysis in this study.

Conflicts of Interest: The authors declare no conflict of interest.

References

1. Cameel, I.; Elshafie, H.S.; Caputo, L.; Sakr, S.H.; De Feo, V. *Bacillus mojavensis*: Biofilm Formation and Biochemical Investigation of Its Bioactive Metabolites. *J. Biol. Res.* **2019**, *92*, 39–45. [CrossRef]
2. Sánchez, E.; Rivas Morales, C.; Castillo, S.; Leos-Rivas, C.; García-Becerra, L.; Ortiz Martínez, D.M. Antibacterial and antibiofilm activity of methanolic plant extracts against nosocomial microorganisms. *Evid.-Based Complement. Altern. Med.* **2016**, *2016*, 1572697. [CrossRef]
3. De la Fuente-Núñez, C.; Reffuveille, F.; Fernández, L.; Hancock, R.E.W. Bacterial biofilm development as a multicellular adaptation: Antibiotic resistance and new therapeutic strategies. *Curr. Opin. Microbiol.* **2013**, *16*, 580–589. [CrossRef]

4. Divakar, S.; Lama, M.; Asad, U.K. Antibiotics versus Biofilm: An emerging battleground in microbial communities | enhanced reader. *Antimicrob. Resist. Infect. Control* **2019**, *8*, 76.
5. Mombeshora, M.; Chi, G.F.; Mukanganyama, S. Antibiofilm activity of extract and a compound isolated from *Triumfetta welwitschii* against *Pseudomonas aeruginosa*. *Biochem. Res. Int.* **2021**, *2021*, 9946183. [CrossRef]
6. Martin, R.M.; Bachman, M.A. Colonization, infection, and the accessory genome of *Klebsiella pneumoniae*. *Front. Cell. Infect. Microbiol.* **2018**, *8*, 4. [CrossRef]
7. Yao, B.; Xiao, X.; Wang, F.; Zhou, L.; Zhang, X.; Zhang, J. Clinical and molecular characteristics of multi-clone carbapenem-resistant hypervirulent (Hypermucoviscous) *Klebsiella pneumoniae* isolates in a tertiary hospital in Beijing, China. *Int. J. Infect. Dis.* **2015**, *37*, 107–112. [CrossRef]
8. Fils, P.E.L.; Cholley, P.; Gbaguidi-Haore, H.; Hocquet, D.; Sauget, M.; Bertrand, X. ESBL-Producing *Klebsiella pneumoniae* in a University Hospital: Molecular features, diffusion of epidemic clones and Evaluation of cross-transmission. *PLoS ONE* **2021**, *16*, e0247875. [CrossRef]
9. Adeosun, I.J.; Oladipo, E.K.; Ajibade, O.A.; Olotu, T.M.; Oladipo, A.A.; Awoyelu, E.H.; Alli, O.A.T.; Oyawoye, O.M. Antibiotic susceptibility of *Klebsiella pneumoniae* isolated from selected Tertiary Hospitals in Osun State, Nigeria. *Iraqi J. Sci.* **2019**, *60*, 1423–1429. [CrossRef]
10. De Paula Ramos, L.; Da Rocha Santos, C.E.; Camargo Reis Mello, D.; Nishiama Theodoro, L.; De Oliveira, F.E.; Back Brito, G.N.; Campos Junqueira, J.; Cardoso Jorge, A.O.; Dias De Oliveira, L. *Klebsiella pneumoniae* planktonic and biofilm reduction by different plant extracts: In vitro Study. *Sci. World J.* **2016**, *2016*, 3521413. [CrossRef]
11. Chung, P.Y. The emerging problems of *Klebsiella pneumoniae* infections: Carbapenem resistance and biofilm formation. *FEMS Microbiol. Lett.* **2016**, *363*, fnw219. [CrossRef]
12. Li, B.; Zhao, Y.; Liu, C.; Chen, Z.; Zhou, D. Molecular pathogenesis of *Klebsiella pneumoniae*. *Future Microbiol.* **2014**, *9*, 1071–1081. [CrossRef]
13. Kikuchi, T.; Mizunoe, Y.; Takade, A.; Naito, S.; Yoshida, S.I. Curli fibers are required for development of biofilm architecture in *Escherichia coli* K-12 and enhance bacterial adherence to human uroepithelial cells. *Microbiol. Immunol.* **2005**, *49*, 875–884. [CrossRef]
14. Boucher, H.W.; Talbot, G.H.; Bradley, J.S.; Edwards, J.E.; Gilbert, D.; Rice, L.B.; Scheld, M.; Spellberg, B.; Bartlett, J. Bad bugs, no drugs: No ESKAPE! An update from the Infectious Diseases Society of America. *Clin. Infect. Dis.* **2009**, *48*, 1–12. [CrossRef]
15. Karuppiah, P.; Mustaffa, M. Antibacterial and antioxidant activities of *Musa* Sp. leaf extracts against multidrug resistant clinical pathogens causing nosocomial infection. *Asian Pac. J. Trop. Biomed.* **2013**, *3*, 737–742. [CrossRef]
16. Barbieri, R.; Coppo, E.; Marchese, A.; Daglia, M.; Sobarzo-Sánchez, E.; Nabavi, S.F.; Nabavi, S.M. Phytochemicals for human disease: An update on plant-derived compounds antibacterial activity. *Microbiol. Res.* **2017**, *196*, 44–68. [CrossRef]
17. Elshafie, H.S.; Sakr, S.; Bufo, S.A.; Camele, I. An attempt of biocontrol the Tomato-Wilt disease caused by *Verticillium dahliae* using *Burkholderia gladioli* Pv. *Agaricicola* and its bioactive secondary metabolites. *Int. J. Plant Biol.* **2017**, *8*, 57–60. [CrossRef]
18. Borges, A.; Abreu, A.C.; Ferreira, C.; Saavedra, M.J.; Simões, L.C.; Simões, M. Antibacterial activity and mode of action of selected glucosinolate hydrolysis products against bacterial pathogens. *J. Food Sci. Technol.* **2015**, *52*, 4737–4748. [CrossRef]
19. Borges, A.; Abreu, A.C.; Dias, C.; Saavedra, M.J.; Borges, F.; Simões, M. New perspectives on the use of phytochemicals as an emergent strategy to control bacterial infections including biofilms. *Molecules* **2016**, *21*, 877. [CrossRef]
20. Monte, J.; Abreu, A.C.; Borges, A.; Simões, L.C.; Simões, M. Antimicrobial activity of selected phytochemicals against *Escherichia coli* and *Staphylococcus aureus* and their biofilms. *Pathogens* **2014**, *3*, 473–498. [CrossRef]
21. Lahiri, D.; Dash, S.; Dutta, R.; Nag, M. Elucidating the effect of anti-biofilm activity of bioactive compounds extracted from plants. *J. Biosci.* **2019**, *44*, 52. [CrossRef]
22. Gibbons, S. Anti-Staphylococcal plant natural products. *Nat. Prod. Rep.* **2004**, *21*, 263–277. [CrossRef]
23. Mamabolo, M.P.; Muganza, F.M.; Tabize Olivier, M.; Olaokun, O.O.; Nemutavhanani, L.D. Evaluation of Antigonorrhea activity and cytotoxicity of *Helichrysum caespititium* (DC) harv. whole plant extracts. *Biol. Med.* **2018**, *10*, 1–4. [CrossRef]
24. Mbaveng, A.T.; Sandjo, L.P.; Tankeo, S.B.; Ndifor, A.R.; Pantaleon, A.; Nagdjui, B.T.; Kuete, V. Antibacterial activity of nineteen selected natural products against multi-drug resistant gram-negative phenotypes. *Springerplus* **2015**, *4*, 823. [CrossRef]
25. Cosa, S.; Rakoma, J.R.; Yusuf, A.A.; Tshikalange, T.E. *Calpurnia aurea* (Aiton) benth extracts reduce Quorum sensing controlled virulence factors in *Pseudomonas aeruginosa*. *Molecules* **2020**, *25*, 2283. [CrossRef]
26. Cosa, S.; Chaudhary, S.K.; Chen, W.; Combrinck, S.; Viljoen, A. Exploring common culinary herbs and spices as potential anti-quorum sensing agents. *Nutrients* **2019**, *11*, 739. [CrossRef]
27. Vasavi, H.S.; Arun, A.B.; Rekha, P.D. Anti-quorum sensing activity of flavonoid-rich fraction from *Centella Asiatica* L. against *Pseudomonas aeruginosa* PAO1. *J. Microbiol. Immunol. Infect.* **2016**, *49*, 8–15. [CrossRef]
28. Rabin, N.; Zheng, Y.; Opoku-Temeng, C.; Du, Y.; Bonsu, E.; Sintim, H.O. Biofilm formation mechanisms and targets for developing antibiofilm agents. *Future Med. Chem.* **2015**, *7*, 493–512. [CrossRef]
29. Kumar, A.S.; Mody, K.; Jha, B. Bacterial *Exopolysaccharides*—A perception. *J. Basic Microbiol.* **2007**, *47*, 103–117. [CrossRef]
30. Patro, L.P.P.; Rathinavelan, T. Targeting the sugary armor of *Klebsiella* species. *Front. Cell. Infect. Microbiol.* **2019**, *9*, 367. [CrossRef]
31. Srinivasan, R.; Mohankumar, R.; Kannappan, A.; Raja, V.K.; Archunan, G.; Pandian, S.K.; Ruckmani, K.; Ravi, A.V. Exploring the anti-quorum sensing and antibiofilm efficacy of phytol against *Serratia marcescens* associated acute pyelonephritis infection in Wistar rats. *Front. Cell. Infect. Microbiol.* **2017**, *7*, 498. [CrossRef]

32. Hachlafi, N.E.L.; Aanniz, T.; Menyiy, N.; El Baaboua, A.; El Omari, N.; El Balahbib, A.; Shariati, M.A.; Zengin, G.; Fikri-Benbrahim, K.; Bouyahya, A. In vitro and in vivo biological investigations of camphene and its mechanism insights: A review. *Food Rev. Int.* **2021**, 1–28. [CrossRef]
33. Huang, Q.; Wu, H.; Cai, P.; Fein, J.B.; Chen, W. Atomic force microscopy measurements of bacterial adhesion and biofilm formation onto clay-sized particles. *Sci. Rep.* **2015**, *5*, 16857. [CrossRef]
34. Zhao, D.; Jiang, J.; Du, R.; Guo, S.; Ping, W.; Ling, H.; Ge, J. Purification and characterization of an *Exopolysaccharide* from *Leuconostoc Lactis* L2. *Int. J. Biol. Macromol.* **2019**, *139*, 1224–1231. [CrossRef]
35. Dufrêne, Y.F. Atomic force microscopy in microbiology: New structural and functional insights into the microbial cell surface. *MBio* **2014**, *5*, e01363-14. [CrossRef]
36. Banerjee, A.; Das, D.; Rudra, S.G.; Mazumder, K.; Andler, R.; Bandopadhyay, R. Characterization of *Exopolysaccharide* produced by *Pseudomonas* Sp. PFAB4 for Synthesis of EPS-coated AgNPs with antimicrobial properties. *J. Polym. Environ.* **2020**, *28*, 242–256. [CrossRef]
37. Foschiatti, M.; Cescutti, P.; Tossi, A.; Rizzo, R. Inhibition of cathelicidin activity by bacterial *Exopolysaccharides*. *Mol. Microbiol.* **2009**, *72*, 1137–1146. [CrossRef]
38. Anes, J.; Hurley, D.; Martins, M.; Fanning, S. Exploring the genome and phenotype of multi-drug resistant *Klebsiella pneumoniae* of clinical origin. *Front. Microbiol.* **2017**, *8*, 1913. [CrossRef]
39. Chaudhary, M.; Payasi, A. Role of EDTA and CSE1034 in curli formation and biofilm eradication of *Klebsiella pneumoniae*: A comparison with other drugs. *J. Antibiot.* **2012**, *65*, 631–633. [CrossRef]
40. Gupta, A.; Dwivedi, M.; Mahdi, A.A.; Gowda, G.A.N.; Khetrapal, C.L.; Bhandari, M. Inhibition of adherence of multi-drug resistant *E. coli* by *Proanthocyanidin*. *Urol. Res.* **2012**, *40*, 143–150. [CrossRef]
41. Barnhart, M.M.; Chapman, M.R. Plaque assay for detecting lysogeny. *Annu. Rev. Microbiol.* **2010**, *60*, 131–147. [CrossRef]
42. Sánchez-López, J.; García-Caballero, A.; Navarro-San Francisco, C.; Quereda, C.; Ruiz-Garbajosa, P.; Navas, E.; Dronda, F.; Morosini, M.I.; Cantón, R.; Diez-Aguilar, M. Hypermucoviscous *Klebsiella pneumoniae*: A challenge in community acquired infection. *IDCases* **2019**, *17*, e00547. [CrossRef]
43. Mikei, L.A.; Starki, A.J.; Forsyth, V.S.; Vornhagen, J.; Smith, S.N.; Bachman, M.A.; Mobley, H.L.T. A systematic analysis of Hypermucoviscosity and capsule reveals distinct and overlapping genes that impact *Klebsiella pneumoniae* fitness. *PloS Pathog.* **2021**, *17*, e1009376. [CrossRef]
44. Jabuk, S.I.A. In vitro and in vivo effect of three aqueous plant extract on pathogenicity of *Klebsiella pneumoniae* isolated from patient with urinary tract infection. *World J. Pharm. Res.* **2016**, *3*, 160–179.
45. Lin, T.H.; Huang, S.H.; Wu, C.C.; Liu, H.H.; Jinn, T.R.; Chen, Y.; Lin, C.T. Inhibition of *Klebsiella pneumoniae* growth and capsular *Polysaccharide* biosynthesis by Fructus Mume. *Evid.-Based Complement. Altern. Med.* **2013**, *2013*, 621701. [CrossRef]
46. Nirwati, H.; Sinanjung, K.; Fahrunissa, F.; Wijaya, F.; Napitupulu, S.; Hati, V.P.; Hakim, M.S.; Meliala, A.; Aman, A.T.; Nuryastuti, T. Biofilm formation and antibiotic resistance of *Klebsiella pneumoniae* isolated from clinical samples in a tertiary Care Hospital, Klaten, Indonesia. *BMC Proc.* **2019**, *13*, 20. [CrossRef]
47. Famuyide, I.M.; Aro, A.O.; Fasina, F.O.; Eloff, J.N.; McGaw, L.J. Antibacterial and antibiofilm activity of Acetone leaf extracts of nine under-investigated South African *Eugenia* and *Syzygium* (*Myrtaceae*) species and their selectivity indices. *BMC Complement. Altern. Med.* **2019**, *19*, 141. [CrossRef]
48. Ramanathan, S.; Arunachalam, K.; Chandran, S.; Selvaraj, R.; Shunmugiah, K.P.; Arumugam, V.R. Biofilm inhibitory efficiency of Phytol in combination with Cefotaxime against nosocomial pathogen *Acinetobacter baumannii*. *J. Appl. Microbiol.* **2018**, *125*, 56–71. [CrossRef]
49. Kelmanson, J.E.; Jager, A.K.; Van Staden, J. Zulu medicinal plants with antibacterial activity. *J. Ethnopharmacol.* **2000**, *69*, 241–246. [CrossRef]
50. Lebeaux, D.; Ghigo, J.-M.; Beloin, C. Biofilm-related infections: Bridging the gap between clinical management and fundamental aspects of Recalcitrance toward antibiotics. *Microbiol. Mol. Biol. Rev.* **2014**, *78*, 510–543. [CrossRef]
51. Baloyi, I.T.; Adeosun, I.J.; Yusuf, A.A.; Cosa, S. In silico and in vitro screening of antipathogenic properties of *Melianthus comosus* (Vahl) against *Pseudomonas aeruginosa*. *Antibiotics* **2021**, *10*, 679. [CrossRef] [PubMed]
52. Sarkar, R.; Chaudhary, S.K.; Sharma, A.; Yadav, K.K.; Nema, N.K.; Sekhoacha, M.; Karmakar, S.; Braga, F.C.; Matsabisa, M.G.; Mukherjee, P.K.; et al. Anti-biofilm activity of Marula—A study with the Standardized bark extract. *J. Ethnopharmacol.* **2014**, *154*, 170–175. [CrossRef] [PubMed]
53. Wang, J.; Liu, Q.; Dong, D.; Hu, H.; Wu, B.; Ren, H. In-Situ monitoring of the unstable bacterial adhesion process during Wastewater Biofilm formation: A comprehensive study. *Environ. Int.* **2020**, *140*, 105722. [CrossRef] [PubMed]
54. Moreira, J.M.R.; Gomes, L.C.; Araújo, J.D.P.; Miranda, J.M.; Simões, M.; Melo, L.F.; Mergulhão, F.J. The effect of glucose concentration and shaking conditions on *Escherichia coli* biofilm formation in Microtiter plates. *Chem. Eng. Sci.* **2013**, *94*, 192–199. [CrossRef]
55. Wijesinghe, G.K.; Feiria, S.B.; Maia, F.C.; Oliveira, T.R.; Joia, F.; Barbosa, J.P.; Boni, G.C.; Höfling, J.F. In-vitro antibacterial and antibiofilm activity of *Cinnamomum Verum* leaf oil against *Pseudomonas aeruginosa*, *Staphylococcus aureus* and *Klebsiella pneumoniae*. *An. Acad. Bras. Cienc.* **2021**, *93*, 1–11. [CrossRef] [PubMed]
56. Alves, M.J.; Ferreira, I.C.F.R.; Froufe, H.J.C.; Abreu, R.M.V.; Martins, A.; Pintado, M. Antimicrobial activity of phenolic compounds identified in Wild Mushrooms, SAR Analysis and docking studies. *J. Appl. Microbiol.* **2013**, *115*, 346–357. [CrossRef]

57. Gopu, V.; Shetty, P.H. Cyanidin inhibits quorum Signalling pathway of a food borne opportunistic pathogen. *J. Food Sci. Technol.* **2016**, *53*, 968–976. [CrossRef]
58. Santana, H.F.; Barbosa, A.A.T.; Ferreira, S.O.; Mantovani, H.C. Bactericidal activity of ethanolic extracts of propolis against *Staphylococcus aureus* isolated from mastitic cows. *World J. Microbiol. Biotechnol.* **2012**, *28*, 485–491. [CrossRef]
59. Wiskur, B.J.; Hunt, J.J.; Callegan, M.C. Hypermucoviscosity as a Virulence factor in experimental *Klebsiella pneumoniae* endophthalmitis. *Investig. Ophthalmol. Vis. Sci.* **2008**, *49*, 4931–4938. [CrossRef]
60. Blando, F.; Russo, R.; Negro, C.; De Bellis, L.; Frassinetti, S. Antimicrobial and antibiofilm activity against *Staphylococcus aureus* of *Opuntia ficus-Indica* (L.) Mill. cladode polyphenolic extracts. *Antioxidants* **2019**, *8*, 117. [CrossRef]
61. Wijesundara, N.M.; Rupasinghe, H.P.V. Essential Oils from *Origanum vulgare* and *Salvia Officinalis* Exhibit antibacterial and anti-biofilm activities against *Streptococcus pyogenes*. *Microb. Pathog.* **2018**, *117*, 118–127. [CrossRef] [PubMed]

MDPI
St. Alban-Anlage 66
4052 Basel
Switzerland
www.mdpi.com

Plants Editorial Office
E-mail: plants@mdpi.com
www.mdpi.com/journal/plants

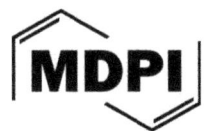

Disclaimer/Publisher's Note: The statements, opinions and data contained in all publications are solely those of the individual author(s) and contributor(s) and not of MDPI and/or the editor(s). MDPI and/or the editor(s) disclaim responsibility for any injury to people or property resulting from any ideas, methods, instructions or products referred to in the content.

www.ingramcontent.com/pod-product-compliance
Lightning Source LLC
LaVergne TN
LVHW070455100526
838202LV00014B/1729